Female Genitourinary and Pelvic Floor Reconstruction

Francisco E. Martins •
Henriette Veiby Holm •
Jaspreet S. Sandhu •
Kurt A McCammon
Editors

Female Genitourinary and Pelvic Floor Reconstruction

Volume 2

With 422 Figures and 78 Tables

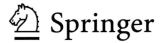

Editors
Francisco E. Martins
University of Lisbon
Lisbon, Portugal

Henriette Veiby Holm
University of Oslo
Oslo, Norway

Jaspreet S. Sandhu
Memorial Sloan Kettering Cancer Center
New York, NY, USA

Kurt A McCammon
Eastern Virginia Medical School
Norfolk, VA, USA

ISBN 978-3-031-19597-6   ISBN 978-3-031-19598-3 (eBook)
https://doi.org/10.1007/978-3-031-19598-3

© Springer Nature Switzerland AG 2023

This work is subject to copyright. All rights are solely and exclusively licensed by the Publisher, whether the whole or part of the material is concerned, specifically the rights of translation, reprinting, reuse of illustrations, recitation, broadcasting, reproduction on microfilms or in any other physical way, and transmission or information storage and retrieval, electronic adaptation, computer software, or by similar or dissimilar methodology now known or hereafter developed.
The use of general descriptive names, registered names, trademarks, service marks, etc. in this publication does not imply, even in the absence of a specific statement, that such names are exempt from the relevant protective laws and regulations and therefore free for general use.
The publisher, the authors, and the editors are safe to assume that the advice and information in this book are believed to be true and accurate at the date of publication. Neither the publisher nor the authors or the editors give a warranty, expressed or implied, with respect to the material contained herein or for any errors or omissions that may have been made. The publisher remains neutral with regard to jurisdictional claims in published maps and institutional affiliations.

This Springer imprint is published by the registered company Springer Nature Switzerland AG.
The registered company address is: Gewerbestrasse 11, 6330 Cham, Switzerland

Paper in this product is recyclable.

First, I would like to thank my co-editors for their outstanding and tireless contribution, and support with this book. I would also like to express my appreciation and gratitude to my several surgical mentors, my countless good colleagues, and my dedicated fellows and residents who have taught, supported, and encouraged my vocation in the field of male and female urologic reconstruction. To all the patients that I had the privilege to treat, care for, learn from, and who teach me daily the meaning of dignity in the face of adversity, my sincere thanks. To the ones I will always love, most especially my recently departed wife and colleague Natasha and our children Filipe, Daniela, and Tomás for the unswerving inspiration, strength, love, unconditional support, and sacrifice they shared with me for the long hours dedicated to this project and life in general. This book is my humble dedication to them. I certainly would never have made it without them.

Francisco E. Martins

Foreword

It was with pleasure that I accepted the invitation from Professor Martins to write a Foreword for this most impressive textbook, which covers virtually all aspects of lower urinary, genital, and pelvic floor abnormalities in women and their relevant anatomy, physiology, pathophysiology, and management. The co-editors are all experts with sub-specialization in various areas of such as pathology and dysfunction and have chosen their individual chapter authors with great care. The chapter authors are all experts in their own right with a history of referenced experience in the areas of their particular contributions. The book covers all the major subjects described in its title and, in addition, various subjects such as the history, basic science, epidemiology, and diagnostic evaluation in this field. Besides topics strictly related to genitourinary and pelvic floor reconstruction, readers will find within the 65 chapter, the topics of lower urinary tract storage and emptying disorders, fecal incontinence, and defecatory dysfunction. Genitourinary and pelvic trauma, congenital defects, and genital-affirming surgery are covered as well. The book should find a place in the libraries of urologists, urogynecologists, pelvic surgeons, and trauma surgeons and should stand the test of time quite well.

Emeritus Founders Professor Alan J. Wein, MD, PhD (hon), FACS
Chief of Urology and Program Director
Department of Surgery
Perelman School of Medicine at the
University of Pennsylvania
Philadelphia, Pennsylvania

Foreword

Gender medicine is quite a young discipline and historically evolved from the International Women's Movement in the 1960s and 1970s. In 2001, the American Institute of Medicine published its report "Exploring the biological contributions to human health: does sex matter?" [1], representing a starting point of gender-specific medicine, which since then steadily evolved to the present date. Against this background, embracing female genitourinary and pelvic floor reconstruction in one book is a perfect contribution to personalized medicine for females. I would like to thank and congratulate the editors Francisco Martins, Henriette V. Holm, Jaspreet Sandhu, and Kurt McCammon for their commitment to further improve health care in women by this book.

Including 65 chapters the book covers the history, anatomy, physiology, and all areas of specific problems. It starts with the historical milestones in genitourinary and pelvic floor reconstruction and gives an insight on the embryology and development of congenital anomalies in females. Pelvic floor disorders and incontinence are increasing with age. Taking the demographic changes in industrial countries into consideration, a significant rise can be expected with a major socioeconomic impact and burden to the healthcare systems. Thus, there is an urgent need for established standards with respect to diagnostics, treatments, and follow-up. Consequently, a large part of the book focusses on the evaluation and management (conservative and surgical) of the underlying disorders and diseases. For reconstruction, minimal invasive techniques are addressed as well as open surgical procedures. In addition, there is a focus on possible and common complications and their management. Besides common diseases and disorders, rare conditions such as urethral strictures or diverticula are also addressed. Solutions are offered for challenging conditions as for trauma, bladder pain syndrome, or severe irradiation damage. In principle, all types of urinary diversion can be used in females but some, such as neobladders, might have a different functional outcome compared to males – a topic also addressed in the book. Gender-assigning surgery has become an increasing part of genitourinary reconstructions in males as well as females, another actual and important subject covered. Moreover, a chapter on stem cells and tissue engineering provides a careful look into potential future treatment. Even though the same principles for reconstruction of the genitourinary tract are used in males and females, there are significant differences in the surgical approach and steps. In this book, the surgical techniques for reconstruction are described in detail by well-known and experienced surgeons. The editors succeeded in bringing together experts from all over the world as authors, thus guaranteeing a sophisticated and global perspective.

It always needs someone to take the initiative for such a contribution, which means a tremendous amount of work in addition to our daily routine and patient care. I would like to thank my colleague and dear friend Francisco Martins for taking this step. It undermines his dedication to the field of reconstructive urology and his active role in the international community of reconstructive urologists.

I highly recommend this book to everyone interested in reconstructive urology.

Professor of Urology Margit Fisch, M.D., FEAPU, FEBU
Past President ESGURS
Past President GURS
Past President DGU

References

1. Wizemann TM, Mary-Lou P, Hrsg. Exploring the biological contributions to human health: Does sex matter? Washington: National Academies Press; 2001.

Preface

This book on female genitourinary and pelvic floor reconstruction is the end-result of the work of an international panel of renowned experts in the field, who kindly lent their time, efforts, and patience to make this project a on historical perspectives, innovations, challenges, and controversies in the field of female genitourinary and pelvic floor disorders.

As the human population lives longer and general health has improved, the prevalence of these genitourinary and pelvic floor problems has also been on the rise. The term female pelvic medicine has been adopted recently to incorporate a broad array of inter-related clinical conditions that range from lower urinary tract dysfunctions and disorders, pelvic organ prolapses and anatomical anomalies, urinary voiding dysfunctions, defecatory dysfunction, sexual dysfunction, to several chronic pelvic pain problems. It has been reported and estimated that more than half of the adult females will suffer from one or more of these problems for some period in their lifetimes and about 11% will undergo surgical treatment for genitourinary and pelvic floor problems by 80 years of age. Financial costs and global healthcare burden associated with genitourinary and pelvic floor disorders result in huge adverse psychosocial impact, which ultimately reflects on quality of life. Both the increase and demand for healthcare services related to these problems will, at least, double the growth rate of the world population over the next 40 years.

Research in genitourinary and pelvic floor disorders is based on and supported by a few principles. The first principle is to increase knowledge on pathophysiology of the specific disorders, a principle that is transversal to other medical specialties. Clinical research to enhance patient outcomes is another important principle. A third principle, critical and unique to reconstructive surgery, deals with advances in wound healing, an essential component for the success of any reconstructive surgery as well as the optimization of overall clinical management.

International interest in genitourinary and pelvic floor disorders of the female patient has promoted awareness of the high prevalence of these health problems in an increasingly ageing population. A widespread need for education and training in the field of genitourinary and pelvic floor disorders and reconstructive surgery is critical as demands are on the rise and both quantity and quality of life have become an increasingly relevant issue.

This book includes 65 chapters divided into 10 sections. Section 1 includes chapters 1 through 6 and features a historical perspective of the field, dating millennia back in time, as well as its basic science and epidemiology. Section 2 includes chapters 7 through 11 and features clinical diagnosis and essential diagnostic tools needed for the various disorders included. Section 3 includes chapters 12 through 27 and features disorders of bladder storage and emptying. Section 4 includes chapters 28 through 38 and features pelvic organ prolapse disorders. Section 5 groups chapters 39 through 49 and describes urethral reconstruction associated with fistulae, diverticula, and urethral strictures. Section 6 includes chapters 50 and 51 that deal with ureteral injuries and their surgical reconstruction. Section 7 includes chapters 52 through 54 and discusses chronic pelvic pain, irritative voiding disorders, and female sexual dysfunction. Section 8 comprises chapters 55 and 56 and discusses fecal incontinence and defecatory prolapse and dysfunction. Section 9 covers chapters 57 through 59 and deals with the use of bowel in genitourinary and pelvic reconstruction. Section 10 includes chapters 60 and 61 that cover genitourinary and pelvic trauma inflicted iatrogenically, by obstetric trauma and by genital mutilation, an unfortunate procedure still perpetrated in some parts of the globe in the twenty-first century. Finally, section 11 includes chapters 62 through 65 that discuss topics related to vaginoplaty, neovagina construction due to congenital anomalies and trauma, and gender-affirming surgery. All authors in this book are hand-picked experts that have detailed the best approaches and thoughts on these challenging disorders and their respective reconstructions. We could not feel more grateful and proud. We hope that this book will be a valuable resource and an important reference text to help improve scientific knowledge and standards of clinical practice of all involved with genitourinary and pelvic floor reconstruction to take better care of their patients.

Lisbon, Portugal	Francisco E. Martins
Oslo, Norway	Henriette Veiby Holm
New York, USA	Jaspreet S. Sandhu
Norfolk, USA	Kurt A McCammon
October 2023	Editors

Acknowledgments

The editors would like to thank all contributors of this book for their hard efforts, precious time, inexhaustible patience, and kind help devoted to this challenging project and for making it a reality. We would also like to thank the Springer editorial staff, especially Monika Conji, for the tremendous volume of administrative collaboration, support, and exemplary work, including an enormous, tireless, overzealous, and prompt assistance with this project. All these generous attributes facilitated this project immensely.

Finally, a word of appreciation and enormous gratitude to all our family members and friends for their patience, understanding, and encouragement.

Francisco E. Martins
Henriette Veiby Holm
Jaspreet S. Sandhu
Kurt A McCammon

Contents

Volume 1

Part I History, Basic Science, and Epidemiology 1

1 **Historical Milestones in Female Genitourinary and Pelvic Floor Reconstruction** 3
Francisco E. Martins, Natalia Martins, and Liliya Tryfonyuk

2 **Embryology and Development of Congenital Anomalies of the Pelvis and Female Organs** 29
Vishen Naidoo, Ejikeme Mbajiorgu, and Ahmed Adam

3 **Neuroanatomy and Neurophysiology** 49
John T. Stoffel

4 **Pathophysiology of Female Micturition Disorders** 71
Alex Gomelsky, Ann C. Stolzle, and William P. Armstrong

5 **The Epidemiology and Socioeconomic Impact of Female GU and Pelvic Floor Disorders** 85
Gabriela Gonzalez and Jennifer T. Anger

6 **Measurement of Urinary Symptoms, Health-Related Quality of Life, and Outcomes of Treatment of Genitourinary and Pelvic Floor Disorders** 97
Ly Hoang Roberts, Annah Vollstedt, Priya Padmanabhan, and Larry T. Sirls

Part II Diagnostic Evaluation 111

7 **Clinical Evaluation of the Female Lower Urinary Tract and Pelvic Floor** 113
Stephanie Gleicher and Natasha Ginzburg

8 **Ultrasound Imaging of the Female Lower Urinary Tract and Pelvic Floor** 125
Lewis Chan, Vincent Tse, and Tom Jarvis

xv

9	**Electrophysiologic Evaluation of the Pelvic Floor** Simon Podnar and David B. Vodušek	139
10	**Urodynamic Evaluation: Traditional, Video, and Ambulatory Approaches** Miguel Miranda and Ricardo Pereira e Silva	157
11	**Endoscopic Evaluation** Francisco E. Martins, Natalia Martins, Liliya Tryfonyuk, and José Bernal Riquelme	179

Part III Bladder Storage and Emptying Disorders **195**

12	**Idiopathic Urinary Retention in the Female** Abdulghani Khogeer, Lysanne Campeau, and Mélanie Aubé-Peterkin	197
13	**Overview of Diagnosis and Pharmacological Treatment of Overactive and Underactive Bladder Disorders** S. Saad, N. Osman, O. A. Alsulaiman, and C. R. Chapple	207
14	**Behavioral Modification and Conservative Management of Overactive Bladder and Underactive Bladder Disorders** Alain P. Bourcier and Jean A. Juras	221
15	**Bladder Dysfunction and Pelvic Pain: The Role of Sacral, Tibial, and Pudendal Neuromodulation** Ly Hoang Roberts, Annah Vollstedt, Jason Gilleran, and Kenneth M. Peters	255
16	**Voiding Dysfunction After Female Pelvic Surgery** Shirin Razdan and Angelo E. Gousse	275
17	**Bladder Augmentation and Urinary Diversion** Henriette Veiby Holm	301
18	**Pathophysiology and Diagnostic Evaluation of Stress Urinary Incontinence: Overview** Helal Syed and Matthias Hofer	323
19	**Pudendal Nerve Entrapment Syndrome: Clinical Aspects and Laparoscopic Management** Renaud Bollens, Fabienne Absil, and Fouad Aoun	333
20	**Retropubic Suspension Operations for Stress Urinary Incontinence** Jennifer A. Locke, Sarah Neu, and Sender Herschorn	361
21	**Sling Operations for Stress Urinary Incontinence and Their Historical Evolution: Autologous, Cadaveric, and Synthetic Slings** Felicity Reeves and Tamsin Greenwell	371

22	**Complications of Stress-Urinary Incontinence Surgery**	395
	Bilal Chughtai, Christina Sze, and Stephanie Sansone	
23	**Artificial Urinary Sphincter for Female Stress Urinary Incontinence**	407
	Amélie Bazinet, Emmanuel Chartier-Kastler, and Stéphanie Gazdovich	
24	**Urethral Bulking Agents**	437
	Quentin Alimi, Béatrice Bouchard, and Jacques Corcos	
25	**Laparoscopic Burch**	449
	Tamara Grisales and Kathryn Goldrath	
26	**Management of Urinary Incontinence in the Female Neurologic Patient**	457
	Oluwarotimi S. Nettey, Katherine E. Fero, and Ja-Hong Kim	
27	**Stem Cell and Tissue Engineering in Female Urinary Incontinence**	487
	Elisabeth M. Sebesta and Melissa R. Kaufman	

Part IV Pelvic Organ Prolapse **505**

28	**Etiology, Diagnosis, and Management of Pelvic Organ Prolapse: Overview**	507
	Connie N. Wang and Doreen E. Chung	
29	**Transvaginal Repair of Cystocele**	519
	Rita Jen, Atieh Novin, and David Ginsberg	
30	**Laparoscopic Paravaginal Repair**	533
	Nikolaos Thanatsis, Matthew L. Izett-Kay, and Arvind Vashisht	
31	**Minimally Invasive Approaches in the Treatment of Pelvic Organ Prolapse: Laparoscopic and Robotic**	551
	Justina Tam, Dena E. Moskowitz, Katherine A. Amin, and Una J. Lee	
32	**Complications of the Use of Synthetic Mesh Materials in Stress Urinary Incontinence and Pelvic Organ Prolapse**	569
	Michelle E. Van Kuiken and Anne M. Suskind	
33	**Vaginal Vault Prolapse: Options for Transvaginal Surgical Repair**	593
	Michele Torosis and Victor Nitti	
34	**Role of Vaginal Hysterectomy in the Treatment of Vaginal Middle Compartment Prolapse**	607
	Luiz Gustavo Oliveira Brito, Cassio Luis Zanettini Riccetto, and Paulo Cesar Rodrigues Palma	

35	**Minimally Invasive Sacrocolpopexy** .... 617 Priyanka Kancherla and Natasha Ginzburg
36	**Open Abdominal Sacrocolpopexy** .... 631 Frederico Ferronha, Jose Bernal Riquelme, and Francisco E. Martins
37	**Management of Vaginal Posterior Compartment Prolapse: Is There Ever a Case for Graft/Mesh?** .... 643 Olivia H. Chang and Suzette E. Sutherland
38	**Vaginal Surgery Complications** .... 657 Jamaal C. Jackson and Sarah A. Adelstein

Volume 2

Part V Urethral Reconstruction: Fistulae, Diverticula, and Strictures 675

39	**Overview, Epidemiology, and Etiopathogenetic Differences in Urogenital Fistulae in the Resourced and Resource-Limited Worlds** .... 677 Heléna Gresty, Madina Ndoye, and Tamsin Greenwell
40	**Urethrovaginal Fistula Repair** .... 693 Christopher Gonzales-Alabastro, Bailey Goyette, and Stephanie J. Kielb
41	**Reconstruction of the Absent or Severely Damaged Urethra** .... 707 Elisabeth M. Sebesta, W. Stuart Reynolds, and Roger R. Dmochowski
42	**Vesicovaginal Fistula Repair: Minimally Invasive Approach** .... 731 Caroline A. Brandon and Benjamin M. Brucker
43	**Vesicovaginal Fistula Repair: Vaginal Approach** .... 761 Annah Vollstedt, Ly Hoang Roberts, and Larry T. Sirls
44	**Vesicovaginal Fistula Repair: Abdominal Approach** ...... 785 F. Reeves and A. Lawrence
45	**Rectovaginal Fistula** .... 805 Christine A. Burke, Jennifer E. Park, and Tamara Grisales
46	**Ureterovaginal Fistula Repair** .... 821 Kelsey E. Gallo, Michael W. Witthaus, and Jill C. Buckley
47	**Female Urethral Reconstruction** .... 829 Ignacio Alvarez de Toledo

Contents

48 Surgical Reconstruction of Pelvic Fracture Urethral Injuries in Females 841
Pankaj M. Joshi, Sanjay B. Kulkarni, Bobby Viswaroop, and Ganesh Gopalakrishnan

49 Surgical Repair of Urethral Diverticula 857
S. Saad, N. Osman, O. A. Alsulaiman, and C. R. Chapple

Part VI Ureteral Reconstruction 869

50 Surgical Reconstruction of Ureteral Defects: Strictures, External Trauma, Iatrogenic, and Radiation Induced 871
Gillian Stearns and Jaspreet S. Sandhu

51 Techniques of Ureteral Reimplantation 885
Andrew Lai, Rabun Jones, Grace Chen, and Diana Bowen

Part VII Pelvic Pain, Irritative Voiding Disorders, and Female Sexual Dysfunction 907

52 Pathophysiology and Clinical Evaluation of Chronic Pelvic Pain 909
Elise J. B. De and Jan Alberto Paredes Mogica

53 Bladder Pain Syndrome: Interstitial Cystitis 931
Francisco Cruz, Rui Pinto, and Pedro Abreu Mendes

54 Female Sexual Dysfunction 959
Francisco E. Martins, Farzana Cassim, Oleksandr Yatsina, and Jan Adlam

Part VIII Fecal Incontinence and Defecatory Dysfunction 995

55 Pathophysiology, Diagnosis, and Treatment of Defecatory Dysfunction 997
Amythis Soltani, Domnique Malacarne Pape, and Cara L. Grimes

56 Management of Fecal Incontinence, Constipation, and Rectal Prolapse 1013
Johannes Kurt Schultz and Tom Øresland

Part IX Use of Bowel in Genitourinary and Pelvic Reconstruction and Other Complex Scenarios 1031

57 Indications and Use of Bowel in Female Lower Urinary Tract Reconstruction: Overview 1033
Warren Lo and Jun Jiet Ng

58 **Options for Surgical Reconstruction of the Heavily Irradiated Pelvis** 1063
Jas Singh, Margaret S. Roubaud, Thomas G. Smith III, and O. Lenaine Westney

59 **Use and Complications of Neobladder and Continent Urinary Diversion in Female Pelvic Cancer** 1099
Bastian Amend, Kathrin Meisterhofer, Jens Bedke, and Arnulf Stenzl

Part X Genitourinary and Pelvic Trauma: Iatrogenic and Violent Causes (War and Civil Causes) 1127

60 **Surgical Reconstruction of the Urinary Tract Following Obstetric and Pelvic Iatrogenic Trauma** 1129
Farzana Cassim, Jan Adlam, and Madina Ndoye

61 **Female Genital Mutilation/Cutting** 1163
Madina Ndoye, Serigne Gueye, Lamine Niang, Farzana Cassim, and Jan Adlam

Part XI Vaginoplasty and Neovagina Construction in Congenital Defects, Trauma, and Gender Affirming Surgery 1183

62 **(Neo) Vaginoplasty in Female Pelvic Congenital Anomalies** 1185
Manuel Belmonte Chico Goerne, David Bouhadana, Mohamed El-Sherbiny, and Mélanie Aubé-Peterkin

63 **Genital Reconstruction in Male-to-Female Gender Affirmation Surgery** 1209
Marta R. Bizic, Marko T. Bencic, and Mirosav L. Djordjevic

64 **Complications of Gender-Affirmation Surgery** 1227
Silke Riechardt

65 **Functional and Aesthetic Surgery of Female Genitalia** 1235
S. Pusica, B. Stojanovic, and Mirosav L. Djordjevic

Index 1253

About the Editors

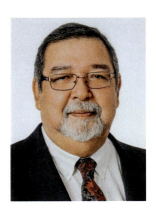

Francisco E. Martins is a Consultant Urologist with specialization on male and female genitourinary reconstruction, focusing on the complications of the treatments of pelvic malignancies, minimally invasive treatment options for penile and urethral cancers, and andrology. He obtained his Medical Degree from the Faculty of Medicine, University of Lisbon, in 1983. He was conferred the title Specialist in Urology by the Portuguese Medical Association, College of Urology, in 1993. He did temporary Urology residency training at the Brigham and Women's Hospital, Harvard University in Boston (International Exchange Urology Residency Program, September–December 1991), and a research and clinical fellowship at the University of Southern California in Los Angeles (1993–1994). His areas of major clinical and research interest are in Genito-urethral and Pelvic Trauma Reconstruction, Vesicovaginal and Rectovaginal Fistula, Female Pelvic Medicine, Erectile Dysfunction, Urinary Diversion, and Penile and Urethral Cancer. He has been Consultant Urological Surgeon at Santa Maria University Hospital (2008–present).

In May 2017, he was elected to the GURS Board of Directors (Genitourinary Reconstructive Surgeons). In October 2017, September 2018, and March 2021, he was awarded Honorary Membership of the Hungarian Urological Association (HUA), the South African Urological Association (SAUA), and the Philippine Society of Genitourinary Reconstructive Society, respectively. In May 2019, he was elected President of the GURS (Society of Genito-Urinary Reconstructive Surgeons). He is a member of several national and international societies and associations, including the Portuguese Urological Association, European Association of Urology (EAU), American Urological Association, Société Internationale d'Urologie (SIU), Canadian Urological Association (CUA), Hungarian Urological Society (HUA), and Society of Urodynamics and Functional Urology (SUFU).

He is a member of the first EAU Guidelines Panel for Urethral Strictures and a peer reviewer for several journals, including *Actas Urológicas Españolas*, *Advances in Urology*, *Biomed Research International*, *British Journal of Medicine and Medical Research*, *European Urology*, *International Urology and Nephrology*, *Journal of Men's Health*, *Journal of Surgery*, *World Journal of Urology and Journal of Urology*, and *Urology Video Journal*. He has presented and lectured at numerous national and international meetings, conferences, and congresses and has published and co-authored over 80 articles in peer-reviewed journals and 7 book chapters and has edited 4 books on erectile dysfunction, penile cancer, and male, as well as female, genitourethral reconstruction. He has also published four special issues for *Advances in Urology*, *Biomed Research International*, *Translational Andrology and Urology*, and *Journal of Clinical Medicine*.

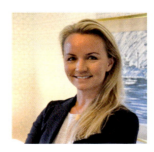

Henriette Veiby Holm is a consultant urological surgeon with specialization on female and male genitourinary reconstruction. She has a special focus on the complications of the treatments of pelvic lower urinary tract disorders, both benign and malignant, and other pelvic disorders. Female and male urethral surgery, urological implants, and andrological surgery are among her specialities. She also specializes in neurogenic dysfunction of the lower urinary tract and offers minor and major reconstructive urological surgery.

Holm obtained her medical degree from the Faculty of Medicine, Semmelweis University in Budapest, in 2004 and her Ph.D. from the Faculty of Medicine, University of Oslo, in 2015. She was conferred the title Specialist in Urology by the Norwegian Medical Association in 2020. She currently works as consultant urological surgeon at the Section of Reconstructive Urology and Neurourology, Department of Urology, Oslo University Hospital Rikshospitalet, Norway. She is member of several national and international societies and associations, including the Norwegian Urological Association, Nordic Urological Association, European Association of Urology (EAU), Société Internationale d'Urologie (SIU), and Society of Genito-Urinary Reconstructive Surgeons (GURS).

Holm is chair of the Nordic Urological Association Collaboration Group on Lower Urinary Tract Disorders and is a member of the editorial board of the *Scandinavian Journal of Urology*. She is a peer reviewer for several international journals including the *British Journal of Urology International*, *Journal of Urology*, *Neurourology and Urodynamics*, and *Scandinavian Journal of Urology*. She is a member of the Nordic Implanter Advisory Board and a former member of the Nordic Advisory Board on Botulinumtoxin in Urology.

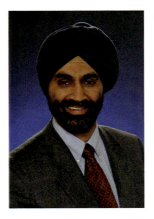

Jaspreet S. Sandhu is an Attending Urologist within the Department of Surgery (Urology Service) at Memorial Sloan Kettering Cancer Center. His primary interest is to understand, predict, prevent, and treat voiding dysfunction caused by cancer or its treatments, with a focus on the treatment of male and female incontinence and urinary tract/pelvic reconstruction. In addition, Dr. Sandhu has a strong interest in the surgical treatment of benign prostatic hyperplasia and voiding dysfunction caused by advanced cancers. He has been active, serving on committee and as faculty for annual meetings, in the American Urological Association; the Society of Urodynamics, Female Pelvic Medicine, and Urogenital Reconstruction; the Society of Genitourinary Reconstructive Surgeons; and the Society for International Urology. Dr. Sandhu has authored over 200 peer-reviewed manuscripts, review articles, and book chapters.

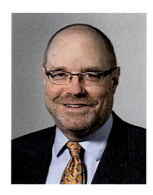

Kurt A McCammon is the Devine Chair in Genitourinary Reconstructive Surgery and Chairman and Professor of the Department of Urology at Eastern Virginia Medical School. He is the Program Director of the Urology Residency Program and also the Program Director of the Adult and Pediatric Genitourinary Reconstructive Surgery Fellowship Program at Eastern Virginia Medical School. He received his medical degree from the Medical College of Ohio and then went on to do his urology residency at Eastern Virginia Medical School (EVMS) followed by a 2 year fellowship in genitourinary reconstructive surgery also at EVMS. He received the Distinguished Alumnus Award from the University of Toledo in October 2011.

Dr. McCammon is past president of the Society of Genitourinary Surgeons and is the Chair of the Board of IVUmed. He is a member of the American Urological Association (AUA) and currently is the Mid-Atlantic representative to the AUA. He is also a member of the American College of Surgeons, the IVUmed, and Société Internationale d'Urologie. He is Diplomate of the American Board of Urology.

Dr. McCammon lectures both nationally and internationally on the topics of male and female reconstruction and has also authored numerous chapters and publications on pelvic reconstruction. His clinical interests include female urology, pelvic reconstruction, urethral reconstruction, and male incontinence.

Contributors

Fabienne Absil Gynaecology, Epicura Hospital, Ath, Belgium

Ahmed Adam Division of Urology, University of the Witwatersrand, Johannesburg, South Africa

Sarah A. Adelstein Rush University Medical Center, Chicago, IL, USA

Jan Adlam Department of Obstetrics and Gynaecoogy, Stellenbosch University/Tygerberg Hospital, Cape Town, South Africa

Quentin Alimi Department of Urology, McGill University, Jewish General Hospital, Montreal, QC, Canada

O. A. Alsulaiman Department of Urology, Sheffield Teaching Hospitals NHS Foundation Trust, Sheffield, UK

Ignacio Alvarez de Toledo Buenos Aires British Hospital, University of Buenos Aires, Buenos Aires, Argentina

Bastian Amend Department of Urology, University Hospital of Tuebingen, Eberhard Karls University, Tuebingen, Germany

Katherine A. Amin Department of Urology, University of Miami Miller School of Medicine, Miami, FL, USA

Jennifer T. Anger Department of Urology, University of California, San Diego School of Medicine, La Jolla, CA, USA

Fouad Aoun Urology, Hôtel Dieu de France, Université Saint Joseph, Beyrouth, Lebanon

William P. Armstrong LSU Health Shreveport School of Medicine, Shreveport, LA, USA

Mélanie Aubé-Peterkin Department of Surgery/Urology, McGill University Health Center and Lachine Hospital, Montreal, QC, Canada

Amélie Bazinet Department of Urology, Maisonneuve-Rosemont Hospital, University of Montreal, QC, Canada

Jens Bedke Department of Urology, University Hospital of Tuebingen, Eberhard Karls University, Tuebingen, Germany

Manuel Belmonte Chico Goerne Sexual Medicine and Genitourinary Reconstructive Surgery, McGill University Health Center, Montreal, QC, Canada

Marko T. Bencic Department of Urology, Faculty of Medicine, University of Belgrade, Belgrade, Serbia

Belgrade Center for Urogenital Reconstructive Surgery, Belgrade, Serbia

Marta R. Bizic Department of Urology, Faculty of Medicine, University of Belgrade, Belgrade, Serbia

Belgrade Center for Urogenital Reconstructive Surgery, Belgrade, Serbia

Renaud Bollens Urology, Centre Hospitalier de Wallonie Picarde, Tournai, Belgium

Urology Department, Catholic University of North of France, Lille, France

Béatrice Bouchard Department of Urology, McGill University, Jewish General Hospital, Montreal, QC, Canada

David Bouhadana McGill University, Montreal, QC, Canada

Alain P. Bourcier Centre d'Imagerie Médicale Cardinet, International Committee of Postpartum Management, Paris, France

Diana Bowen Department of Urology, Northwestern University Feinberg School of Medicine, Chicago, IL, USA

Caroline A. Brandon New York University School of Medicine, New York, NY, USA

Luiz Gustavo Oliveira Brito Division of Gynecological Surgery, Department of Obstetrics and Gynecology, Faculty of Medical Sciences, State University of Campinas – UNICAMP, Campinas, Brazil

Benjamin M. Brucker New York University School of Medicine, New York, NY, USA

Jill C. Buckley UC San Diego Health, San Diego, CA, USA

Christine A. Burke University of California Los Angeles, Los Angeles, CA, USA

Lysanne Campeau Department of Urology, Jewish General Hospital, Montreal, QC, Canada

Farzana Cassim Division of Urology, Stellenbosch University/Tygerberg Hospital, Cape Town, South Africa

Lewis Chan Department of Urology, Concord Repatriation General Hospital and University of Sydney, Sydney, NSW, Australia

Olivia H. Chang Division of Female Urology, Voiding Dysfunction and Pelvic Reconstructive Surgery, Department of Urology, University of California Irvine, Irvine, CA, USA

C. R. Chapple Department of Urology, Sheffield Teaching Hospitals NHS Foundation Trust, Sheffield, UK

Emmanuel Chartier-Kastler Department of Urology, Sorbonne Université, Academic Hospital Pitié-Salpêtrière, Paris, France

Grace Chen Department of Urology, University of Illinois at Chicago, Chicago, IL, USA

Bilal Chughtai Department of Urology, Weill Cornell Medicine/New York Presbyterian, New York, NY, USA

Department of Obstetrics and Gynecology, Weill Cornell Medicine/New York Presbyterian, New York, NY, USA

Doreen E. Chung Department of Urology, Columbia University Irving Medical Center, New York, NY, USA

Jacques Corcos Department of Urology, McGill University, Jewish General Hospital, Montreal, QC, Canada

Francisco Cruz Department of Urology, Faculty of Medicine of University of Porto, Hospital São João, I3S Institute for Investigation and Innovation in Health, Porto, Portugal

Elise J. B. De Massachusetts General Hospital, Boston, MA, USA

Mirosav L. Djordjevic Belgrade Center for Urogenital Reconstructive Surgery, Belgrade, Serbia

Roger R. Dmochowski Department of Urology, Vanderbilt University Medical Center, Nashville, TN, USA

Mohamed El-Sherbiny Department of Surgery and Pediatric surgery, McGill University Health Center and Montreal Children's Hospital, Montreal, QC, Canada

Katherine E. Fero Department of Urology, David Geffen School of Medicine at UCLA, Los Angeles, CA, USA

Frederico Ferronha Centro Hospitalar e Universitário Lisboa Central, Lisbon, Portugal

Kelsey E. Gallo UC San Diego Health, San Diego, CA, USA

Stéphanie Gazdovich Department of Urology, Maisonneuve-Rosemont Hospital, University of Montreal, QC, Canada

Jason Gilleran William Beaumont School of Medicine, Beaumont Hospital, Oakland University, Royal Oak, MI, USA

David Ginsberg USC Institute of Urology, Los Angeles, CA, USA

Natasha Ginzburg Department of Urology, SUNY Upstate Medical University, Syracuse, NY, USA

Stephanie Gleicher Department of Urology, Vanderbilt University Medical Center, Nashville, TN, USA

Kathryn Goldrath University of California Los Angeles, Los Angeles, CA, USA

Alex Gomelsky Department of Urology, LSU Health Shreveport, Shreveport, LA, USA

Christopher Gonzales-Alabastro Department of Urology, Northwestern University Feinberg School of Medicine, Chicago, IL, USA

Gabriela Gonzalez Department of Urology, University of California, Davis School of Medicine, Sacramento, CA, USA

Ganesh Gopalakrishnan Vedanayagam Hospital, Coimbatore, India

Angelo E. Gousse Department of Urology, Larkin Hospital Palm Springs Teaching Hospital, Miami, FL, USA

Bailey Goyette Division of Urology, Department of Surgery, University of MIssouri, Columbia, USA

Tamsin Greenwell University College London Hospitals, London, UK

Heléna Gresty University College London Hospitals, London, UK

Cara L. Grimes Departments of Obstetrics and Gynecology and Urology, New York Medical College, Valhalla, NY, USA

Tamara Grisales University of California Los Angeles, Los Angeles, CA, USA

Serigne Gueye Cheikh Anta Diop University/Hospital General Idrissa Poueye, Dakar, Senegal

Sender Herschorn Sunnybrook Health Sciences Centre, Toronto, ON, Canada

Ly Hoang Roberts William Beaumont School of Medicine, Beaumont Hospital, Oakland University, Royal Oak, MI, USA

Matthias Hofer Urology San Antonio, San Antonio, TX, USA

Henriette Veiby Holm Section of reconstructive urology and neurourology, Department of Urology, Oslo University Hospital Rikshospitalet, Oslo, Norway

Matthew L. Izett-Kay Department of Urogynaecology, The John Radcliffe Hospital, Oxford University Hospitals, Oxford, UK

Nuffield Department of Women's and Reproductive Health, Women's Centre, Oxford University, Oxford, UK

Jamaal C. Jackson Rush University Medical Center, Chicago, IL, USA

Tom Jarvis Department of Urology, Prince of Wales Hospital and University of NSW, Randwick, NSW, Australia

Rita Jen USC Institute of Urology, Los Angeles, CA, USA

Rabun Jones Department of Urology, University of Illinois at Chicago, Chicago, IL, USA

Pankaj M. Joshi UROKUL, Pune, India

Jean A. Juras Centre d'Imagerie Médicale Cardinet, Paris, France

Priyanka Kancherla Department of Urology, SUNY Upstate Medical University, Syracuse, NY, USA

Melissa R. Kaufman Department of Urology, Vanderbilt University Medical Center, Nashville, TN, USA

Abdulghani Khogeer Department of Surgery, Faculty of Medicine, Rabigh, King Abdulaziz University, Jeddah, Saudi Arabia

Stephanie J. Kielb Department of Urology, Northwestern University Feinberg School of Medicine, Chicago, IL, USA

Ja-Hong Kim Division of Pelvic Medicine and Reconstructive Surgery, David Geffen School of Medicine at UCLA, Los Angeles, CA, USA

Department of Urology, David Geffen School of Medicine at UCLA, Los Angeles, CA, USA

Michelle E. Van Kuiken Department of Urology, University of California, San Francisco, CA, USA

Sanjay B. Kulkarni UROKUL, Pune, India

Andrew Lai Department of Urology, University of Illinois at Chicago, Chicago, IL, USA

A. Lawrence Counties Manukau and Auckland Hospital, Auckland, New Zealand

Una J. Lee Section of Urology and Renal Transplantation, Virginia Mason Franciscan Health, Seattle, WA, USA

Warren Lo Urology, Hospital Kuala Lumpur, Kuala Lumpur, Malaysia

Jennifer A. Locke Sunnybrook Health Sciences Centre, Toronto, ON, Canada

Francisco E. Martins Department of Urology, Reconstructive Urology Unit, School of Medicine, Hospital Santa Maria, CHULN, University of Lisbon, Lisbon, Portugal

Natalia Martins Urology Division, Armed Forces Hospital, Lisbon, Portugal

Ejikeme Mbajiorgu School of Anatomical Sciences, University of the Witwatersrand, Johannesburg, South Africa

Kathrin Meisterhofer Department of Urology, University Hospital of Tuebingen; Eberhard Karls University, Tuebingen, Germany

Pedro Abreu Mendes Department of Urology, Faculty of Medicine of University of Porto, Hospital São João, I3S Institute for Investigation and Innovation in Health, Porto, Portugal

Miguel Miranda Urology Department, Centro Hospitalar Universitário Lisboa Norte, Lisbon, Lisboa, Portugal

Dena E. Moskowitz Department of Urology, University of California Irvine, Irvine, CA, USA

Vishen Naidoo Division of Urology, University of the Witwatersrand, Johannesburg, South Africa

Madina Ndoye Department of Urology, Cheikh Anta Diop University/Hospital General Idrissa Poueye, Dakar, Senegal

Oluwarotimi S. Nettey Scott Department of Urology, Baylor College of Medicine, Houston, Texas, USA

Sarah Neu Sunnybrook Health Sciences Centre, Toronto, ON, Canada

Jun Jiet Ng Urogynecology, Hospital Kuala Lumpur, Kuala Lumpur, Malaysia

Lamine Niang Cheikh Anta Diop University/Hospital General Idrissa Poueye, Dakar, Senegal

Victor Nitti Division of Female Pelvic Medicine and Reconstructive Surgery, Departments of Urology and Obstetrics and Gynecology, David Geffen School of Medicine at UCLA, Los Angeles, CA, USA

Atieh Novin USC Institute of Urology, Los Angeles, CA, USA

Tom Øresland Faculty of Medicine University of Oslo, Oslo, Norway

N. Osman Department of Urology, Sheffield Teaching Hospitals NHS Foundation Trust, Sheffield, UK

Priya Padmanabhan Oakland University William Beaumont School of Medicine, Beaumont Hospital, Royal Oak, MI, USA

Paulo Cesar Rodrigues Palma Department of Surgery, Faculty of Medical Sciences, State University of Campinas – UNICAMP, Campinas, Brazil

Domnique Malacarne Pape Departments of Obstetrics and Gynecology and Urology, New York Medical College, Valhalla, NY, USA

Jan Alberto Paredes Mogica Anahuac University, Mexico City, Mexico

Jennifer E. Park University of California Los Angeles, Los Angeles, CA, USA

Ricardo Pereira e Silva Urology, Faculdade de Medicina, Universidade de Lisboa; Centro Hospitalar Universitário Lisboa Norte, Lisbon, Portugal

Kenneth M. Peters William Beaumont School of Medicine, Beaumont Hospital, Oakland University, Royal Oak, MI, USA

Rui Pinto Department of Urology, Faculty of Medicine of University of Porto, Hospital São João, I3S Institute for Investigation and Innovation in Health, Porto, Portugal

Simon Podnar Division of Neurology, University Medical Centre Ljubljana, Ljubljana, Slovenia

S. Pusica Belgrade Center for Urogenital Reconstructive Surgery, Belgrade, Serbia

Shirin Razdan Department of Urology, Icahn School of Medicine at Mount Sinai Hospital, New York, NY, USA

F. Reeves Department of Urology, The Royal Melbourne Hospital, Melbourne, Australia

Felicity Reeves Addenbrookes Hospital, Cambridge, UK

W. Stuart Reynolds Department of Urology, Vanderbilt University Medical Center, Nashville, TN, USA

Cassio Luis Zanettini Riccetto Division of Female Urology, Department of Surgery, Faculty of Medical Sciences, State University of Campinas – UNICAMP, Campinas, Brazil

Silke Riechardt Department of Urology, University Hospital Hamburg-Eppendorf, Hamburg, Germany

Jose Bernal Riquelme Urology Division, Hospital Sotero Del Rio, Santiago, Chile

Margaret S. Roubaud Department of Plastic Surgery, Division of Surgery, The University of Texas MD Anderson Cancer Center, Houston, TX, USA

S. Saad Department of Urology, Sheffield Teaching Hospitals NHS Foundation Trust, Sheffield, UK

Jaspreet S. Sandhu Memorial Sloan Kettering Cancer Center, New York, NY, USA

Stephanie Sansone Department of Urology, Weill Cornell Medicine/New York Presbyterian, New York, NY, USA

Department of Obstetrics and Gynecology, Weill Cornell Medicine/New York Presbyterian, New York, NY, USA

Johannes Kurt Schultz Department of GI Surgery, Akershus University Hospital, Lørenskog, Norway

Elisabeth M. Sebesta Department of Urology, Vanderbilt University Medical Center, Nashville, TN, USA

Jas Singh Department of Urology, Division of Surgery, The University of Texas MD Anderson Cancer Center, Houston, TX, USA

Larry T. Sirls Oakland University William Beaumont School of Medicine, Beaumont Hospital, Royal Oak, MI, USA

Thomas G. Smith III Department of Urology, Division of Surgery, The University of Texas MD Anderson Cancer Center, Houston, TX, USA

Amythis Soltani Department of Obstetrics and Gynecology, Westchester Medical Center, Valhalla, NY, USA

Gillian Stearns Carolinas Medical Center, Charlotte, NC, USA

Arnulf Stenzl Department of Urology, University Hospital of Tuebingen; Eberhard Karls University, Tuebingen, Germany

John T. Stoffel University of Michigan, Ann Arbor, MI, USA

B. Stojanovic Belgrade Center for Urogenital Reconstructive Surgery, Belgrade, Serbia

School of Medicine, University of Belgrade, Belgrade, Serbia

Ann C. Stolzle LSU Health Shreveport School of Medicine, Shreveport, LA, USA

Anne M. Suskind Department of Urology, University of California, San Francisco, CA, USA

Suzette E. Sutherland UW Medicine Pelvic Health Center, Department of Urology, University of Washington School of Medicine, Seattle, WA, USA

Helal Syed Division of Urology, Department of Surgery, Children's Hospital Los Angeles | University of Southern California Keck School of Medicine, Los Angeles, CA, USA

Christina Sze Department of Urology, Weill Cornell Medicine/New York Presbyterian, New York, NY, USA

Justina Tam Section of Urology and Renal Transplantation, Virginia Mason Franciscan Health, Seattle, WA, USA

Urogynecology, Stony Brook Medicine, Stony Brook, NY, USA

Nikolaos Thanatsis Urogynaecology and Pelvic Floor Unit, University College London Hospital, London, UK

Michele Torosis Division of Female Pelvic Medicine and Reconstructive Surgery, Departments of Urology and Obstetrics and Gynecology, David Geffen School of Medicine at UCLA, Los Angeles, CA, USA

Liliya Tryfonyuk Urology Division, Rivne Regional Hospital, Rivne, Ukraine

Vincent Tse Department of Urology, Concord Repatriation General Hospital and University of Sydney, Sydney, NSW, Australia

Arvind Vashisht Urogynaecology and Pelvic Floor Unit, University College London Hospital, London, UK

Bobby Viswaroop Vedanayagam Hospital, Coimbatore, India

David B. Vodušek Institute of Clinical Neurophysiology, Division of Neurology, University Medical Centre Ljubljana, Ljubljana, Slovenia

Annah Vollstedt Department of Urology, University of Iowa Hospitals and Clinics, Iowa City, IA, USA

Connie N. Wang Department of Urology, Columbia University Irving Medical Center, New York, NY, USA

O. Lenaine Westney Department of Urology, Division of Surgery, The University of Texas MD Anderson Cancer Center, Houston, TX, USA

Michael W. Witthaus UC San Diego Health, San Diego, CA, USA

Oleksandr Yatsina Department of Urological Surgery, National Cancer Institute, Kyiv, Ukraine

Part V

Urethral Reconstruction: Fistulae, Diverticula, and Strictures

Overview, Epidemiology, and Etiopathogenetic Differences in Urogenital Fistulae in the Resourced and Resource-Limited Worlds

39

Heléna Gresty, Madina Ndoye, and Tamsin Greenwell

Contents

Introduction	678
Anatomical Overview and Classification of Urogenital Fistulae	678
Etiology and Epidemiology of Fistulae in the Resourced and Resource-Limited World	679
Consequences of Urogenital Fistulae in Resource-Limited Countries	681
Presenting Symptoms of Urogenital Fistulae	682
Diagnosis of Urogenital Fistulae	682
Treatment of Urogenital Fistulae	684
Outcomes of Urogenital Fistula Repair	686
Conclusion	688
References	689

Abstract

Urogenital fistulae are abnormal communications between the female genital tract and lower urinary tract, or bowel. The incidence and etiology of urogenital fistulae vary geographically and remain a serious, debilitating global healthcare problem for women worldwide where it is associated with poverty. It predominantly results from childbirth complications in low-resourced countries, especially in Africa and Asia, and iatrogenic injury in well-resourced countries. Currently, the published evidence is of relatively low quality, mainly consisting of retrospective case series. A few systematic reviews conducted over the last three decades reported that 95.2% of fistulae in developing countries were a consequence of obstetric complications, and according to the WHO, there are around 2 million women suffering from untreated urogenital fistulae worldwide with an estimated 50,000 to 100,000 new cases adding to the cohort each year, mostly in Sub-Saharan Africa. The recent estimates of the

H. Gresty · T. Greenwell (✉)
University College London Hospitals, London, UK

M. Ndoye
Department of Urology, Cheikh Anta Diop University/Hospital General Idrissa Poueye, Dakar, Senegal

global prevalence of untreated obstetric fistula vary from 654,000 to 3,500,000, especially involving countries such as Uganda, Malawi, Nigeria, Benin, Sierra Leone, and Ethiopia. Further, it is an indicator of maternal mortality and morbidity.

In this chapter, we evaluated the available evidence for etiology, intervention, and outcomes of urogenital fistulae in both low- and well-resourced worlds and highlight their inherent differences.

Keywords

Vesicovaginal fistula · Urogenital fistula · Childbirth trauma · Obstetric fistula · Obstetric trauma · Complex urogenital fistula

Introduction

Urogenital fistulae affect millions of people worldwide and have different etiologies in the well-resourced and relatively resource-limited world. In this chapter we review the classification, causes, presentation, diagnosis prevention, and treatment of urogenital fistulae with reference not only to the medical management but also the social and cultural factors that contribute to this condition.

Anatomical Overview and Classification of Urogenital Fistulae

A urogenital fistula is an abnormal connection between the urinary tract (bladder, ureter, or urethra) and the genital tract (uterus or vagina). They usually, but not always, result in continuous leakage of urine through the vagina. Vesicovaginal fistulae (VVF) are the most common, at least three times more frequently seen than ureterovaginal (UrVF), with urethrovaginal (UVF) and utero-vesical (UtVF) being rare (Fig. 1).

There are several classification systems for urogenital fistulae but currently no singularly accepted system has gained universal use. The most widely used classification systems for VVF are the Goh classification and the Waldjik classifications (Tables 1 and 2).

The ideal classification system would not only describe the fistula but also accurately predict the approach needed for repair and the outcomes of repair. Indeed, while the prognosis in terms of

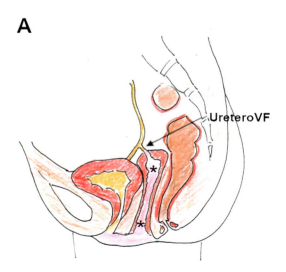
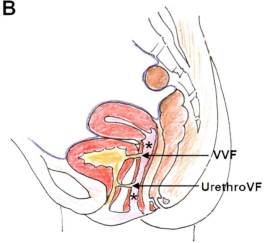

Fig. 1 Schematic representation of urogenital fistulae. (**a**) ureterovaginal fistula (**b**) vesicovaginal fistula (VVF) and urethrovaginal fistula (UVF). Note absent uterus in (**a**). Vagina indicated by asterisk (*), urine in yellow, stools in brown. (Tonolini, M. Elucidating vaginal fistulas on CT and MRI. *Insights Imaging* 10, 123 (2019). https://doi.org/10.1186/s13244-019-0812-9. Copyright © 2019, Springer Nature)

Table 1 The Goh genitourinary fistula classification [1]

Type – distance from meatus	Type 1 – distal edge of fistula >3.5 cm from external urinary meatus	Type 2 – distal edge of fistula 2.5–3.5 cm from external urinary meatus	Type 3 – distal edge of fistula 1.5–2.5 cm from external urinary meatus	Type 4 – distal edge of fistula <1.5 cm from external urinary meatus
Size – largest diameter	a) <1.5 cm	b) 1.5–3 cm	c) >3 cm	
Additional considerations	i) Mild or no fibrosis and/or vaginal length > 6 m, normal capacity	ii) Moderate or severe fibrosis and/or reduced vaginal length and/or capacity	iii) Special consideration, e.g., post-radiation, ureteric involvement, circumferential previous repair	

Table 2 The Waaldijk genitourinary fistula classification. Type II fistulae can be subclassified into type A/B and a/b as shown [2]

Involvement of closure mechanism	I – not involving urethral closure mechanism	II – involving urethral closure mechanism	III – involving ureter and exceptions
Urethral involvement	A) Without (sub)total urethral involvement	B) With (sub)total urethral involvement	
Circumferential defect	a) Without circumferential defect	b) With circumferential defect	

anatomical closure and continence restoration worsens with grade in both classification systems, they are not useful in all settings [3, 4]. In the well-resourced (previously termed "developed") world, most VVF are type 1 and neither the Goh nor Waldjik system appears to have practical relevance to predict outcomes [4]. In resource-limited countries (previously termed "developing") the critical factors for outcomes of VVF repair include the size, position, and proximity to the urethral closure mechanism and/or ureters as well as the degree of vaginal scarring [5]. The Goh classification appears superior to the Waldjik in comparative studies to predict closure rate [6, 7]. However, all systems rely on subjective application and accuracy depends on individual interpretation and surgical experience.

Etiology and Epidemiology of Fistulae in the Resourced and Resource-Limited World

Urogenital fistulae are a major health issue in resource-limited countries. Women in these geographical regions are more likely to develop and suffer from a urogenital fistula but also have less access to support and treatment.

Most fistulae occur in sub-Saharan Africa or South Asia where health systems are poorly resourced [8]. Fistulae are thought to have the highest prevalence in regions of high maternal mortality (Fig. 2) [8]. The World Health Organization estimates that between 50,000 and 100,000 women worldwide develop obstetric fistula each year [9]. This estimate is based on scantily reported data and the true burden is likely to be higher. It is estimated that there are one million women living with VVF in Nigeria alone [10] and that 1/1000 deliveries in Nigeria and Kenya are complicated by obstetric fistula [10–12]. As many women live for decades with this condition without access to surgical repair, it is estimated around 3.5 million women suffer with this condition [13].

In resource-limited countries, urogenital fistulae usually result from a prolonged, obstructed labor. This contrasts to well-resourced countries as shown in Table 3. Prolonged labor causes a sustained pressure necrosis from the anterior vaginal wall onto the bladder. This may be averted by delivery with a skilled birth attendant, particularly in a well-resourced healthcare setting where

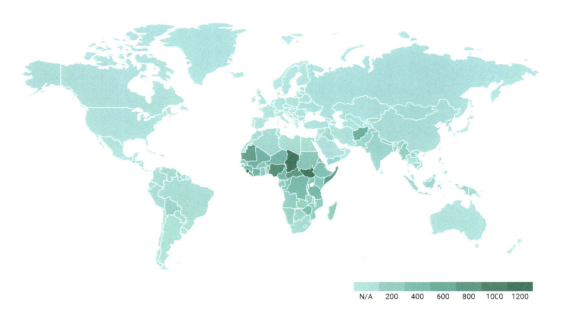

Fig. 2 Maternal mortality ratio, (maternal deaths per 100,000 live births) [14]. (Requested permission from WHO ref. ID 388774)

Table 3 Etiology of fistulae in resourced and resource-limited world. Table uses data presented in Hillary et al. [20]

Etiology	Low-resource settings	High-resource settings
Obstetric causes	95.2%	3.5%
Prolonged, obstructed labor	44.9%	0.1%
Surgical causes	4.4%	83.2%
Abdominal hysterectomy	1.2%	46.2%
Radical hysterectomy	0%	4.2%
Vaginal hysterectomy	0.4%	1.9%
Other pelvic surgery	1.6%	12.7%
Radiotherapy	0.2%	13%

Caesarian section is available [12, 15, 16]. In resource-limited countries, women are more likely to deliver outside of a healthcare setting and are out of reach of timely intervention [12]. The three main factors leading to delay are subdivided into, firstly a delay in the community to seek care, secondly a delay in transportation to a care facility, and thirdly a delay in the receipt of adequate care at a healthcare facility [17, 18]. In Ghana, studies have shown that less than a quarter of the poorest women deliver with a skilled birth attendant, compared to over 95% of the richest women [19]. The reasons for this trend include poor access to health facilities and some sociocultural factors that discourage use of health facilities for delivery.

Another factor that may contribute to the high rate of urogenital fistulae in resource-limited countries includes childbearing at young age [12]. A 2018 UNICEF publication looking at West and Central Africa reported a prevalence of child marriage (defined as being aged under 18) of 41%, with a 14% of girls under 15 being married [21]. These women may not have completed pelvic growth, particularly if they suffer with calcium and vitamin D malnutrition [19].

This may contribute to cephalo-pelvic disproportion.

These women are more likely to have a poor education, live in poverty, and live in rural areas, compounding the risk of complicated labor [21].

Harmful cultural practices such as female genital mutilation (FGM) may contribute to the development of fistulae [4, 22]. FGM is categorized as shown in Fig. 3. Type 3, involving the cutting and narrowing of the vaginal opening has been found to be more associated with fistula development [17, 23].

Type 1: This is the partial or total removal of the clitoral glans (the external and visible part of the clitoris, which is a sensitive part of the female genitals), and/or the prepuce/clitoral hood (the fold of skin surrounding the clitoral glans)

Type 2: This is the partial or total removal of the clitoral glans and the labia minora (the inner folds of the vulva), with or without removal of the labia majora (the outer folds of skin of the vulva)

Type 3: Also known as infibulation, this is the narrowing of the vaginal opening through the creation of a covering seal. The seal is formed by cutting and repositioning the labia minora, or labia majora, sometimes through stitching, with or without removal of the clitoral prepuce/clitoral hood and glans

Type 4: This includes all other harmful procedures to the female genitalia for nonmedical purposes, e.g., pricking, piercing, incising, scraping, and cauterizing the genital area

In contrast, urogenital fistulae in resourced countries are rare. In 2013, 371 new diagnoses of genitourinary fistulae were coded in Hospital Episode Statistics (HES data is a database of all admissions, Accident and Emergency attendances, and outpatient contacts in England and Wales [26].

Most urogenital fistulae in the well-resourced world are associated with surgical intervention for gynecological dysfunction or pelvic cancer. A systematic review of 2055 urogenital fistulae in well-resourced healthcare settings identified that 83.2% resulted from surgical intervention. Hysterectomy was by far the most common causative procedure, accounting for 75% of surgical causes [20]. A UK study has estimated a 0.12% incidence of VVF following hysterectomy, with the highest rate following radical hysterectomy and the lowest following vaginal hysterectomy [27]. Radiotherapy accounts for around 13% of cases recorded [20]. Presentation post radiotherapy is often delayed for up to 15–20 years and results from ongoing tissue ischemia, endothelial cell damage, endarteritis, and fibrosis. Other predisposing patient factors contributing to VVF formation include diabetes, small vessel disease previous uterine surgery, and endometriosis [4, 28, 29].

Consequences of Urogenital Fistulae in Resource-Limited Countries

The consequences of developing an obstetric fistula in a resource-limited country include not only urinary and/or fecal incontinence but also fetal

Fig. 3 The World Health Organization classification of female genital mutilation [24, 25]

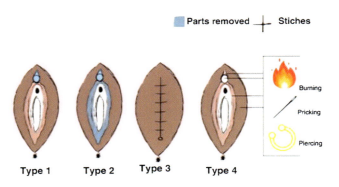

death, lower limb and pelvic girdle injuries alongside significant psychological, social, and financial adverse effects [30–32]. Evidence shows that approximately 90% of women who develop obstetric genitourinary fistulae deliver a stillborn baby [33]. Women may be marginalized or even become outcasts in the community [11, 34]. They may be considered unclean because they are soiled, malodorous and continually wet. Research has shown high rates of relationship breakdown and divorce as well as abstinence of sexual intercourse among women with fistulae [8].

Presenting Symptoms of Urogenital Fistulae

Many women in poorly resourced regions may live with a fistula for several years before presenting to a healthcare facility and up to 80% of women with fistula may never seek treatment [8, 35, 36]. When they do present, vesicovaginal fistulae classically leads to insenate urinary leakage though the vagina. Urinary incontinence can range from continuous (large and low fistulae) to intermittent and postural (small and high fistulae). In large volume leak, the woman may no longer void; instead emptying the bladder through the fistula. VVF may present alongside dyspareunia, pelvic pain, hematuria, recurrent UTIs, and vaginal narrowing as well as other sites of fistulation.

Urethrovaginal fistulae (UVF) usually present alongside a VVF in resource-limited countries and will result in continuous leakage through the vagina if sited proximal to the sphincter complex. A ureterovaginal fistula (UrVF) causes insenate leakage through the vagina but may also be associated with loin pain from an obstructed or infected renal unit. A utero-vesical (UtVF) fistula usually presents after Caesarian section where there has been simultaneous injury to the bladder and uterus. Youssef's syndrome describes a triad of cyclical hematuria, amenorrhea, and urinary continence (so long as the cervix is competent) due to a UtVF [37].

Urogenital fistulae presenting in the resource-limited world may be part of the "obstructed labour injury complex." This cluster of conditions includes the fistulous tract between the urogenital organs but also other sequalae of pressure necrosis from obstructed labor. The urogenital fistula may not present immediately at delivery, instead taking some time for the tract to form as necrotic tissues sloughs off. Other components in the complex include rectovaginal fistulae, renal damage as a result of ureteric stricture, and genital tract injury to the vagina, cervix or uterus, nerve plexus injury including foot drop, levator muscle injury, and bony pelvic injury. Further secondary sequalae include dermatitis reactions, mental health and social problems, lower limb contractures, malnourishment, and infertility.

Diagnosis of Urogenital Fistulae

Vesicovaginal fistulae are easy to identify on examination with a Sims speculum as shown in Figs. 4, 5, 6 and 7. Conversely, small "pin hole" fistulae may not be detectable on examination. Urethrovaginal, ureterovaginal, and rectovaginal fistulae may also be detected on examination. Both the fistula defect and urine pooling in the vagina may be evident. Note should be made of the size and position of the fistula and whether the urethra/bladder neck is involved.

Additional diagnostic tests may also aid in diagnosis and characterization of the fistula. The "three swab test" involves placement of three white swabs into the vagina followed by

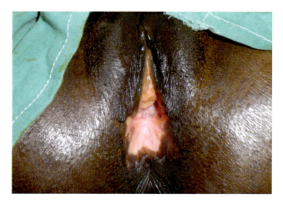

Fig. 4 Obstetric VVF on examination – perineal loss

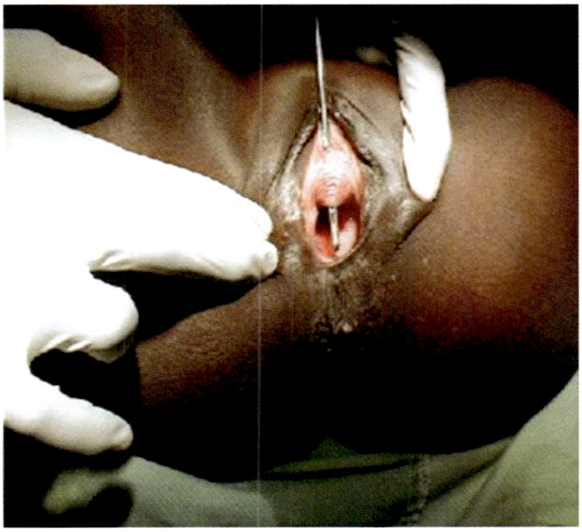

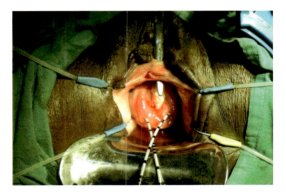

Fig. 5 Obstetric VVF on examination – urethrovesicovaginal fistula

Fig. 6 Obstetric VVF – Involving urethra and bladder neck. Stents in the ureteric orifices

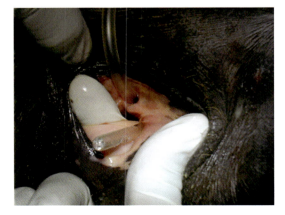

Fig. 7 Rectovaginal fistula

instillation of methylene blue dye into the bladder through a catheter as shown in Fig. 8. A wet but uncolored high swab suggests a UrVF (ureterovaginal fistula) but blue dye *may* be seen if there is reflux up the ureter. A blue high or middle swab suggests a VVF (although note a false positive with refluxing ureter to a ureterovaginal fistula as described). A blue lowest swab suggests either a UVF (urethrovaginal fistula) or leakage of dye from the urethral meatus into the vagina (vaginal reflux).

Simultaneous cystoscopy with vaginal examination remains the gold standard for diagnosis and characterization of urogenital fistulae. This can be combined with ureteric retrograde fluoroscopic studies or proctoscopy if necessary. Associated infection, inflammation, and tissue friability should be recorded and would prompt delay of repair to allow these to be treated first. Vaginal length, width, scarring, and mobility are also important to assess and determine the route of repair (Fig. 9).

In equivocal or complex cases additional imaging may aid diagnosis and also help to characterize the fistula and associated pathology. In practical terms, cross-sectional imaging is almost universally adopted in the well-resourced world. Fluoroscopic cystogram studies, Computed Tomography (CT), as well as Magnetic Resonance Imaging (MRI) may reveal fistulae (examples in Figs. 10 and 11). Contrast can be instilled intravenously as a CT-Urogram or instilled retrograde directly to the bladder (cystogram) or to the uterus (hysterogram). Dynamic voiding fluoroscopy may improve detection of a UVF. CT-Urogram has the advantage of opacification of the upper urinary tract and ureters to look for UrVF or ureteric stricture. A UrVF rarely occurs in isolation and are associated with VVF in 10–25% cases [29, 39–41]. Similarly, a UrVF should be suspected and excluded in all cases of VVF [29].

It is also important, where resources allow, to exclude other causes of urinary incontinence such as stress, urgency, mixed, and overflow incontinence. Rarely patients with long-standing refractory urinary incontinence have been found to have VVF as the cause of their problems.

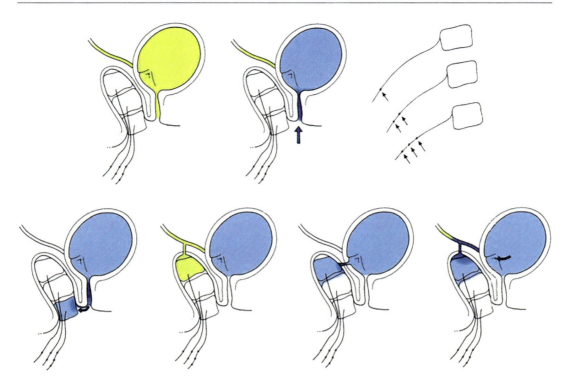

Fig. 8 The three-swab test. Tying knots in the strings attached to the swabs helps with subsequent interpretation of the results. Note the false positive with a urethrovaginal fistula associated with vesico-ureteric reflux. (Reprinted with permission from Chapple [38])

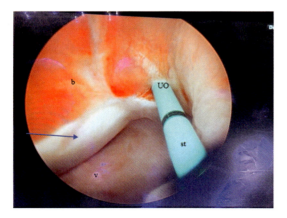

Fig. 9 Cystoscopy image showing a VVF (arrowed). The ureteric orifice (stented) is on the margin of the fistula. This was repaired vaginally. *B* bladder, *st* stent, *UO* ureteric orifice, *v* vagina. (Picture personal picture from Ms. T J Greenwell & Ms. H Gresty with patient permission)

Treatment of Urogenital Fistulae

Spontaneous closure of VVF may occur in some women (7–8% in some series) with the use of an indwelling catheter to drain the bladder [42–44]. This initial trial is especially important in resource-limited settings [28]. Factors that may favor spontaneous healing with a catheter include a short time to develop the fistula and small size of the fistula. However, if healing has not occurred within 6 weeks of the injury, then surgical repair is likely required. In selected cases, repair may be offered within 2–3 weeks of the precipitating injury. Most definitive surgery occurs 3–6 months after the injury to allow inflammation and infection to settle [4, 42, 45]. In poorly resourced countries malnourishment,

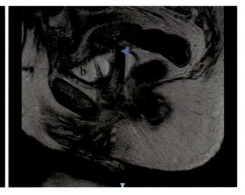

Fig. 10 (**a**) CT-Urogram and (**b**) T2-weighted MRI imaging both showing catheterized bladder (**b**), VVF (marked with arrow) and urine pooling in vagina. (Picture personal picture from Ms. T J Greenwell & Ms. H Gresty)

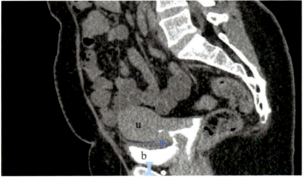
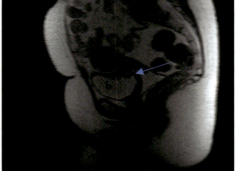

Fig. 11 CTU (left) and T2-weighted MRI (right) demonstrating a utero-vesical fistula (marked with arrow). *b* bladder, *u* uterus. At abdominal repair, there was a 2 cm fistula at the inferior anterior uterus at the junction of the cervix to the posterior bladder. (Picture personal picture from Ms. T J Greenwell and Ms. H Gresty)

helminthic infections, schistosomiasis, lymphogranuloma, tuberculosis, bladder stones, and other infections may require urgent attention before repair.

The three key principles in fistula repair include (a) wide dissection around the fistula to ensure removal of devascularized tissue and adequate exposure (b) a tension-free closure that is watertight and ideally has a tissue interposition graft, and (c) placement of a urinary drainage system postoperatively to allow healing. Choice of tissue for interposition ranges from a labial Martius fat pad, paravaginal fascia, or omental tissue. Excision of the tract is not usually advised or needed (Fig. 12).

The majority of VVFs are amenable to repair vaginally with very few requiring an abdominal approach. Those with an associated UrVF, an obstructed ureter requiring reimplant, colonic pathology or colovaginal/colovesical fistula will require an abdominal approach. Selected distal UrVF can be managed with a ureteric reconstruction via the vagina [46] but otherwise a ureteric reimplant + − Boari bladder flap may be warranted. Unfortunately, in practice, choice of route is mainly based on surgeon experience and preference. This is not the best management for women – as the morbidity acutely and in the long term from vaginal fistula repair is far less than for abdominal fistula repair [28, 47]. It is universally accepted that the most likely successful closure of a fistula is the first attempt [28]. If local surgeons are unable to perform vaginal fistula repair women are best referred to surgeons who can do

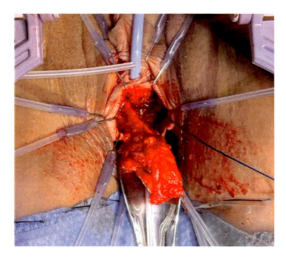

Fig. 12 Example of a Martius fat interposition fat pad harvested from the right labia. (Personal picture of Ms. T J Greenwell and Ms. H Gresty with patient permission)

so, and only if there is no alternative should they have abdominal repair for a VVF without the absolute indications cited above. In poorly resourced settings, hubs of excellence have been established to offer surgical expertise [48]. Similar pooling of expertise is seen in resourced settings with surgeons with Urogenital Reconstructive experience (Fig. 13).

Some complex urogenital fistulae will require a transabdominal approach, which can be performed open but minimally invasive routes such as laparoscopic and robotic have also been employed and are likely to develop in the future where appropriate [49]. The classical descriptions of abdominal VVF repair involve access through cystostomy through dome and anterior bladder wall and then mobilization of the bladder from the vaginal wall before watertight closure with interposition grafting [50]. Fistulae can be repaired with an extraperitoneal dissection along the back wall of the bladder alone minimizing bladder trauma and allowing easy access of omental interposition through a small peritoneal window.

A trial of conservative measures with urethral catheterization will not treat a UVF. Distal fistulae below the level of the sphincter may be asymptomatic or cause minimal symptoms and may not require intervention. Symptomatic distal UVF may be managed through a meatotomy but with a warning to women regarding the risk of an altered direction of their urinary stream. Surgical repair of more complex UVF can be challenging but follow the same principles as a vaginal VVF repair. Reconstruction using rotational vaginal, buccal mucosal, vesical flaps, or even ilium may be needed if there is significant urethral loss [51–53]. In fistulae secondary to foreign bodies such as continence mesh, removal of the foreign material is needed as seen in Fig. 14.

Utero-vesical fistulae, UtVF, may close spontaneously in around 5%, particularly the fistula is small and if hormonal manipulation is used to prevent menstruation [27, 54, 55]. However, surgical repair is often required. Different approaches to repair have been proposed. If access is amenable, vaginal repair may be possible [27]. Alternatively, an open, laparoscopic, or robotic repair using omentum as an interposition is employed [27]. Hysterectomy at the time of intra-abdominal UtVF repair is not always necessary, and uterine preservation is generally preferred if possible.

A minority of women will have an "irreparable" fistula and either fail multiple attempts at repair or have catastrophic injuries or radiotherapy damage that are not salvageable with reconstruction. These women are few in number, with a case series in Nigeria, for example, showing only 0.6% of their patients needed a urinary diversion to manage their fistula [56]. Diversion should be a last resort for women and reconstruction the preferred option if at all possible.

Outcomes of Urogenital Fistula Repair

Primary closure is achieved in up to 96% of cases of VVF via the vaginal route [4, 40, 42]. A systematic review of the literature in 2016 suggested an overall median closure rate in well-resourced countries of 94.6% (range, 75.8–98.6%) and comparable success rates from resource-limited countries of a median closure rate of 87.0% (range 58.0–100) [20]. Large, complex, or obstetric fistulae and those associated with radiotherapy have lower success rates [40, 46]. Although there are no randomized controlled trials to compare outcomes

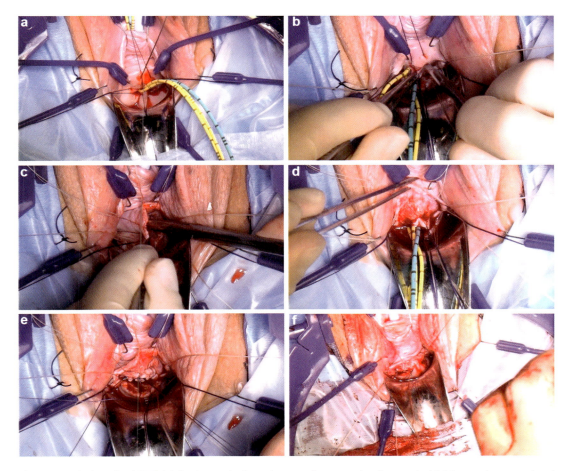

Fig. 13 Vaginal repair of VVF. (**a**) fistula margins brought forward with nylon sutures and lumen of fistula catheterized. Ureters are stented. (**b**) Fistula is circumscribed, and (**c**) mobilized free of the vaginal wall to allow a tension free repair. (**d**) Monocryl sutures placed on vaginal margin. (**e**) Bladder is closed. (**f**) Vaginal skin is closed. (Personal picture of Ms. T J Greenwell with patient permission)

of vaginal and abdominal repair, series have consistently reported lower primary closure rates for abdominal repair [22, 40]. A recently published systematic review of VVF repair cites a success rate for a vaginal closure of 91% versus 84% for abdominal repairs [57]. The author's experience is that vaginal closure of VVF is possible in approaching 90% of VVF cases in their institution with equal or higher primary closure rates to abdominal closure.

Closure rates for simple UVF after one surgery are 90% and up to 99% after a second or more operations [58–60]. For complex UVF, anatomical closure rates vary between 25% and 80% depending on etiology of the UVF and the complexity of the reconstruction required [61–63].

Continence following urogenital fistula repair is dependent on the nature of the fistula and the mode of repair. A urogenital fistula involving the bladder neck or urethral sphincter complex causing sphincteric incompetence unsurprisingly result in relatively high rates of urinary incontinence following repair – up to 50% in some series [62]. However, a systematic review of stress incontinence following VVF repair reported an average estimated rate of 6.5% in well-resourced countries and 10% in low-resourced countries [20]. In obstetric fistulae a bulbocavernosus

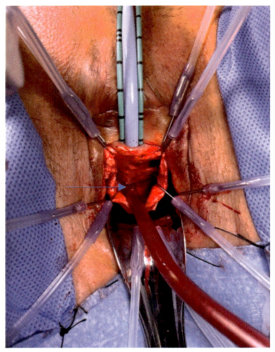 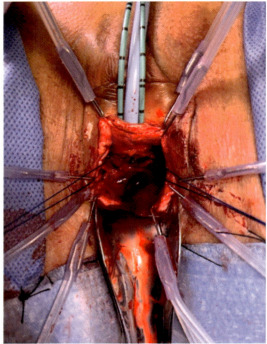

Fig. 14 Vaginal approach to a synthetic urethral mesh, which had extruded into the urethra causing a UVF. Blue urethral catheter and green ureteric catheters seen. Arrow marks the position of the tape. (Operative picture personal picture from Ms. T J Greenwell and Ms. H Gresty with patient's permission)

muscle flap has been employed with reasonable success to manage continence [64]. Continence procedures such as slings (autologous or mesh) and colposuspension may be required to treat persistent stress incontinence. Alternative causes of incontinence such as overactive bladder may need different modes of therapy such as medications, intravesical botox™, or sacral neuromodulation.

Women suffering the effects of urogenital fistulae suffer wide-reaching and sometimes devastating effects on their wider health and well-being. Women may need contraceptive advice, suffer with infertility, or need care regarding planning of future pregnancies. Holistic care to support the psychosocial needs is relevant in the well-resourced and resource-limited world. Additional needs in some areas include that around education and a return to a meaningful role in relationships and society. The United Nations pledged in 2016 an aim to "end obstetric fistula" within a generation by 2030 [48] but there remains a vital need to increase access to and strengthen the capacity of health facilities to provide high quality services for repair and care of women living with fistulae if this is to be met.

Conclusion

Urogenital fistulae affect over 3.5 million women worldwide. In poorly resourced countries they are primarily related to preventable negligence of obstetric care and can have a devastating impact on women's health and psychosocial well-being. In the well-resourced world, urogenital fistulae can still cause serious adverse effects and are usually iatrogenic. Successful repair of urogenital fistulae can lead to a dramatic improvement in women's quality of life. Moving forward, the prevention and treatment of urogenital fistulae require national, regional, and international efforts to improve access to decent, affordable medical care with additional expertise in fistula repair.

References

1. Goh JT. A new classification for female genital tract fistula. Aust N Z J Obstet Gynaecol. 2004;44:502–4. https://doi.org/10.1111/j.1479-828X.2004.00315.x.
2. Waaldijk K. Surgical classification of obstetric fistulas. Int J Gynaecol Obstet. 1995;49:161–3. https://doi.org/10.1016/0020-7292(95)02350-l.
3. Goh JT, Browning A, Berhan B, Chang A. Predicting the risk of failure of closure of obstetric fistula and residual urinary incontinence using a classification system. Int Urogynecol J Pelvic Floor Dysfunct. 2008;19:1659–62. https://doi.org/10.1007/s00192-008-0693-9.
4. Beardmore-Gray A, Pakzad M, Hamid R, Ockrim J, Greenwell T. Does the Goh classification predict the outcome of vesico-vaginal fistula repair in the developed world? Int Urogynecol J. 2017;28:937–40. https://doi.org/10.1007/s00192-016-3186-2.
5. Nsambi J, Mukuku O, Kakudji P, Kakoma JB. [Model predicting failure in surgical repair of obstetric vesicovaginal fistula]. Pan Afr Med J. 2019;34:91. https://doi.org/10.11604/pamj.2019.34.91.20547.
6. Bernard L, Giles A, Fabiano S, Giles S, Hudgins S, Olson A, Shrime MG, Feldman S, Riviello R. Predictors of obstetric fistula repair outcomes in Lubango, Angola. J Obstet Gynaecol Can. 2019;41:1726–33. https://doi.org/10.1016/j.jogc.2019.01.025.
7. Capes T, Stanford EJ, Romanzi L, Foma Y, Moshier E. Comparison of two classification systems for vesicovaginal fistula. Int Urogynecol J. 2012;23:1679–85. https://doi.org/10.1007/s00192-012-1671-9.
8. Adler AJ, Ronsmans C, Calvert C, Filippi V. Estimating the prevalence of obstetric fistula: a systematic review and meta-analysis. BMC Pregnancy Childbirth. 2013;13:246. https://doi.org/10.1186/1471-2393-13-246.
9. Tunçalp Ö, Tripathi V, Landry E, Stanton CK, Ahmed S. Measuring the incidence and prevalence of obstetric fistula: approaches, needs and recommendations. Bull World Health Organ. 2015;93:60–2. https://doi.org/10.2471/blt.14.141473.
10. Cowgill, K.D.; Bishop, J.; Norgaard, A.K.; Rubens, C.E.; Gravett, M.G. Obstetric fistula in low-resource countries: an under-valued and under-studied problem–systematic review of its incidence, prevalence, and association with stillbirth. BMC Pregnancy Childbirth 2015, 15, 193, doi:https://doi.org/10.1186/s12884-015-0592-2.
11. Ijaiya MA, Rahman AG, Aboyeji AP, Olatinwo AW, Esuga SA, Ogah OK, Raji HO, Adebara IO, Akintobi AO, Adeniran AS, et al. Vesicovaginal fistula: a review of nigerian experience. West Afr J Med. 2010;29:293–8. https://doi.org/10.4314/wajm.v29i5.68247.
12. Muleta M. Obstetric fistula in developing countries: a review article. J Obstet Gynaecol Can. 2006;28:962–6. https://doi.org/10.1016/s1701-2163(16)32305-2.
13. Bello OO, Morhason-Bello IO, Ojengbede OA. Nigeria, a high burden state of obstetric fistula: a contextual analysis of key drivers. Pan Afr Med J. 2020;36:22. https://doi.org/10.11604/pamj.2020.36.22.22204.
14. WHO, UNICEF, UNFPA, World Bank Group and the United Nations Population Division. Trends in maternal mortality 2000 to 2017: estimates. Geneva: World Health Organization; 2019.
15. Hilton, P.; Cromwell, D.A. The risk of vesicovaginal and urethrovaginal fistula after hysterectomy performed in the English National Health Service–a retrospective cohort study examining patterns of care between 2000 and 2008. BJOG 2012, 119, 1447-1454, doi:https://doi.org/10.1111/j.1471-0528.2012.03474.x.
16. Donnay F, Weil L. Obstetric fistula: the international response. Lancet. 2004;363:71–2. https://doi.org/10.1016/s0140-6736(03)15177-x.
17. Swain D, Parida SP, Jena SK, Das M, Das H. Obstetric fistula: a challenge to public health. Indian J Public Health. 2019;63:73–8. https://doi.org/10.4103/ijph.IJPH_2_18.
18. Thaddeus S, Maine D. Too far to walk: maternal mortality in context. Soc Sci Med. 1994;38:1091–110. https://doi.org/10.1016/0277-9536(94)90226-7.
19. Afulani PA. Rural/urban and socioeconomic differentials in quality of antenatal care in Ghana. PLoS One. 2015;10:e0117996. https://doi.org/10.1371/journal.pone.0117996.
20. Hillary CJ, Osman NI, Hilton P, Chapple CR. The aetiology, treatment, and outcome of urogenital fistulae managed in well- and low-resourced countries: a systematic review. Eur Urol. 2016;70:478–92. https://doi.org/10.1016/j.eururo.2016.02.015.
21. Unicef. Child marriage in West and Central Africa. 2018.
22. Beardmore-Gray A, Pakzad M, Hamid R, Ockrim JL, Greenwell T. 905 Factors associated with success or failure in VVF repair. Eur Urol Suppl. 2016;15:e905. https://doi.org/10.1016/S1569-9056(16)60907-7.
23. Matanda DJ, Sripad P, Ndwiga C. Is there a relationship between female genital mutilation/cutting and fistula? A statistical analysis using cross-sectional data from Demographic and Health Surveys in 10 sub-Saharan Africa countries. BMJ Open. 2019;9:e025355. https://doi.org/10.1136/bmjopen-2018-025355.
24. WHO. WHO guidelines on the management of health complications from female genital mutilation. Geneva: World Health Organisation; 2016.
25. Jones LL, Albert J. Identifying and responding to female genital mutilation: reflections from a UK research–practice partnership. Springer eBook. Springer Nature. 2021.
26. Department of Health, UK. Hospital Episode Statistics (HES). http://www.hesonline.nhs.uk

27. Hadzi-Djokic JB, Pejcic TP, Colovic VC. Vesico-uterine fistula: report of 14 cases. BJU Int. 2007;100: 1361–3. https://doi.org/10.1111/j.1464-410X.2007.07067.x.
28. Beardmore-Gray A, Greenwell T. Vesico-vaginal fistulae in the resource-limited setting: current status and the challenges that lie ahead, all you need to know for those practicing in a well-resourced setting. J Clin Urol. 2018;11:316–24. https://doi.org/10.1177/2051415818764593.
29. Greenwell TJ, O.J. Surgical management of urinary tract-vaginal fistulae in the developed world. BJUI Knowledge. 2019;
30. Arrowsmith S, Hamlin EC, Wall LL. Obstructed labor injury complex: obstetric fistula formation and the multifaceted morbidity of maternal birth trauma in the developing world. Obstet Gynecol Surv. 1996;51: 568–74. https://doi.org/10.1097/00006254-199609000-00024.
31. Bashah DT, Worku AG, Mengistu MY. Consequences of obstetric fistula in sub Sahara African countries, from patients' perspective: a systematic review of qualitative studies. BMC Womens Health. 2018;18:106. https://doi.org/10.1186/s12905-018-0605-1.
32. Ngongo CJ, Raassen T, Lombard L, van Roosmalen J, Weyers S, Temmerman M. Delivery mode for prolonged, obstructed labour resulting in obstetric fistula: a retrospective review of 4396 women in East and Central Africa. BJOG. 2020;127:702–7. https://doi.org/10.1111/1471-0528.16047.
33. Ahmed S, Anastasi E, Laski L. Double burden of tragedy: stillbirth and obstetric fistula. Lancet Glob Health. 2016;4:e80–2. https://doi.org/10.1016/s2214-109x(15)00290-9.
34. Muleta M, Hamlin EC, Fantahun M, Kennedy RC, Tafesse B. Health and social problems encountered by treated and untreated obstetric fistula patients in rural Ethiopia. J Obstet Gynaecol Can. 2008;30: 44–50. https://doi.org/10.1016/s1701-2163(16)32712-8.
35. Miller S, Lester F, Webster M, Cowan B. Obstetric fistula: a preventable tragedy. J Midwifery Womens Health. 2005;50:286–94. https://doi.org/10.1016/j.jmwh.2005.03.009.
36. Wall LL, Wilkinson J, Arrowsmith SD, Ojengbede O, Mabeya H. A code of ethics for the fistula surgeon. Int J Gynaecol Obstet. 2008;101:84–7. https://doi.org/10.1016/j.ijgo.2007.10.005.
37. Youssef AF. Menouria following lower segment cesarean section; a syndrome. Am J Obstet Gynecol. 1957;73:759–67. https://doi.org/10.1016/0002-9378(57)90384-8.
38. Chapple CR. Urethral Diverticula, Urethro-Vaginal Fistulae, Vesico-Vaginal Fistulae. EAU Updat Ser. 2003;1:178–85. https://doi.org/10.1016/S1570-9124(03)00040-0.
39. Benchekroun A, Lachkar A, Soumana A, Farih MH, Belahnech Z, Marzouk M, Faik M. [Uretero-vaginal fistulas. 45 cases]. Ann Urol (Paris). 1998; 32:295–9.
40. Goodwin WE, Scardino PT. Vesicovaginal and ureterovaginal fistulas: a summary of 25 years of experience. J Urol. 1980;123:370–4. https://doi.org/10.1016/s0022-5347(17)55941-8.
41. Selzman AA, Spirnak JP, Kursh ED. The changing management of ureterovaginal fistulas. J Urol. 1995;153:626–8. https://doi.org/10.1097/00005392-199503000-00020.
42. Hilton P. Urogenital fistula in the UK: a personal case series managed over 25 years. BJU Int. 2012;110: 102–10. https://doi.org/10.1111/j.1464-410X.2011.10630.x.
43. Mohr S, Brandner S, Mueller MD, Dreher EF, Kuhn A. Sexual function after vaginal and abdominal fistula repair. Am J Obstet Gynecol. 2014;211(74):e71–6. https://doi.org/10.1016/j.ajog.2014.02.011.
44. Tayler-Smith K, Zachariah R, Manzi M, van den Boogaard W, Vandeborne A, Bishinga A, De Plecker E, Lambert V, Christiaens B, Sinabajije G, et al. Obstetric fistula in Burundi: a comprehensive approach to managing women with this neglected disease. BMC Pregnancy Childbirth. 2013;13:164. https://doi.org/10.1186/1471-2393-13-164.
45. Ockrim JL, Greenwell TJ, Foley CL, Wood DN, Shah PJ. A tertiary experience of vesico-vaginal and urethro-vaginal fistula repair: factors predicting success. BJU Int. 2009;103:1122–6. https://doi.org/10.1111/j.1464-410X.2008.08237.x.
46. Toia, B.; Ockrim, J.J.; Greenwell, T.J. Ureteric reimplantation via vaginal route: a new surgical technique. J Surg Case Rep 2019, 2019, rjz235, doi:https://doi.org/10.1093/jscr/rjz235.
47. Singh O, Gupta SS, Mathur RK. Urogenital fistulas in women: 5-year experience at a single center. Urol J. 2010;7:35–9.
48. United Nations General Assembly: Report of the Secretary General: intensifying efforts to end obstetric fistula. 2016.
49. Miklos JR, Moore RD, Chinthakanan O. Laparoscopic and robotic-assisted vesicovaginal fistula repair: a systematic review of the literature. J Minim Invasive Gynecol. 2015;22:727–36. https://doi.org/10.1016/j.jmig.2015.03.001.
50. O'Conor VJ Jr. Review of experience with vesicovaginal fistula repair. J Urol. 1980;123:367–9. https://doi.org/10.1016/s0022-5347(17)55939-x.
51. Elkins TE, Ghosh TS, Tagoe GA, Stocker R. Transvaginal mobilization and utilization of the anterior bladder wall to repair vesicovaginal fistulas involving the urethra. Obstet Gynecol. 1992;79:455–60. https://doi.org/10.1097/00006250-199203000-00026.
52. Kannaiyan L, Sen S. Urethral substitution with ileum in traumatic bladder neck-vagina fistula. J Indian Assoc Pediatr Surg. 2009;14:76–7. https://doi.org/10.4103/0971-9261.55159.
53. Wang Y, Hadley HR. The use of rotated vascularized pedicle flaps for complex transvaginal procedures. J Urol. 1993;149:590–2. https://doi.org/10.1016/s0022-5347(17)36157-8.

54. Jóźwik M, Jóźwik M. Spontaneous closure of vesicouterine fistula. Account for effective hormonal treatment. Urol Int. 1999;62:183–7. https://doi.org/10.1159/000030388.
55. Novi JM, Rose M, Shaunik A, Ramchandani P, Morgan MA. Conservative management of vesicouterine fistula after uterine rupture. Int Urogynecol J Pelvic Floor Dysfunct. 2004;15:434–5. https://doi.org/10.1007/s00192-004-1165-5.
56. Wall LL, Karshima JA, Kirschner C, Arrowsmith SD. The obstetric vesicovaginal fistula: characteristics of 899 patients from Jos, Nigeria. Am J Obstet Gynecol. 2004;190:1011–9. https://doi.org/10.1016/j.ajog.2004.02.007.
57. El-Azab AS, Abolella HA, Farouk M. Update on vesicovaginal fistula: a systematic review. Arab J Urol. 2019;17:61–8. https://doi.org/10.1080/2090598x.2019.1590033.
58. Blaivas JG, Mekel G. Management of urinary fistulas due to midurethral sling surgery. J Urol. 2014;192:1137–42. https://doi.org/10.1016/j.juro.2014.04.009.
59. Gerber GS, Schoenberg HW. Female urinary tract fistulas. J Urol. 1993;149:229–36. https://doi.org/10.1016/s0022-5347(17)36045-7.
60. Rangnekar NP, Imdad Ali N, Kaul SA, Pathak HR. Role of the martius procedure in the management of urinary-vaginal fistulas. J Am Coll Surg. 2000;191:259–63. https://doi.org/10.1016/s1072-7515(00)00351-3.
61. Neu S, Locke J, Goldenberg M, Herschorn S. Urethrovaginal fistula repair with or without concurrent fascial sling placement: a retrospective review. Can Urol Assoc J. 2021;15:E276–e280. https://doi.org/10.5489/cuaj.6786.
62. Pushkar DY, Dyakov VV, Kosko JW, Kasyan GR. Management of urethrovaginal fistulas. Eur Urol. 2006;50:1000–5. https://doi.org/10.1016/j.eururo.2006.08.002.
63. Roenneburg ML, Wheeless CR Jr. Traumatic absence of the proximal urethra. Am J Obstet Gynecol. 2005;193:2169–72. https://doi.org/10.1016/j.ajog.2005.08.053.
64. Browning A. Prevention of residual urinary incontinence following successful repair of obstetric vesicovaginal fistula using a fibro-muscular sling. BJOG. 2004;111:357–61. https://doi.org/10.1111/j.1471-0528.2004.00080.x.

Urethrovaginal Fistula Repair

Christopher Gonzales-Alabastro, Bailey Goyette, and Stephanie J. Kielb

Contents

Introduction	694
Epidemiology	694
Anatomy of the Female Urethra	695
Risk Factors	695
Etiology/Pathogenesis	696
Obstetric	696
Radiation Therapy	697
Inflammatory	697
Traumatic (Non-obstetric)	697
Postsurgical (Iatrogenic)	697
Prevention	697
Clinical Presentation	698
Diagnosis	698
Treatment and Outcomes	700
Primary Closure with Vaginal Flap	700
Rectus Abdominis Muscle Flap	702
Gracilis Muscle Flap	702
Conclusion	703
Cross-References	704
References	704

C. Gonzales-Alabastro · S. J. Kielb (✉)
Department of Urology, Northwestern University Feinberg School of Medicine, Chicago, IL, USA

B. Goyette
Division of Urology, Department of Surgery, University of MIssouri, Columbia, USA

Abstract

Urethrovaginal fistulas are abnormal communications between the female urethra and vagina. For the reconstructive surgeon, there are many challenging aspects to the diagnosis and management of urethrovaginal fistulas. This is due in large part to the unique and

© Springer Nature Switzerland AG 2023
F. E. Martins et al. (eds.), *Female Genitourinary and Pelvic Floor Reconstruction*,
https://doi.org/10.1007/978-3-031-19598-3_41

complex anatomy often present, the surgical expertise required in the operating room, and the risk of postoperative morbidity or recurrence. Fortunately, urethrovaginal fistulas are rare in practice and most commonly the result of iatrogenic injuries in the developed world. In contrast, most urethrovaginal fistulas result from obstructed labor in the developing world. Surgical repair is the mainstay of definitive treatment for urethrovaginal fistulas. General principles of other urogenital fistula repair also apply to urethrovaginal fistulas including identification of adequately vascularized tissue, tension-free suture lines, and initial diversion of urine. Compared to those of vesicovaginal fistulas, options for urethrovaginal fistula repair may be more limited given the urethra's tenuous blood supply, limited mobility, and delicate interposing tissue planes. Techniques of repair vary depending on the complexity of the fistula and are usually performed with primary excision and closure of a vaginal flap. Interpositional flaps and grafts are reserved for more advanced disease. Postoperative complications include stress urinary incontinence (SUI), obstructed voiding secondary to stricture, and fistula recurrence.

Keywords

Urethrovaginal fistula · Women's health · Obstructed labor

Introduction

Urogenital fistulas are aberrant connections between the female genital tract and the urethra, bladder, or ureters. Urethrovaginal fistulas more specifically are abnormal communications between the female urethra and vagina and must be distinguished conceptually from vesicovaginal fistulas (VVF). For the reconstructive urologist, there are many challenging aspects to the diagnosis and management of urethrovaginal fistulas. Diagnosis is challenging because urethrovaginal fistulas can present in a multitude of ways including urinary incontinence, urinary drainage per vaginum, intermittent positional wetness, recurrent urinary tract infections (UTIs), perineal skin irritation, vaginal fungal infections, or asymptomatic and incidentally found lesions [1]. Definitive repair is also challenging given the unique and complex anatomy often present, the surgical expertise required in the operating room, and the risk of postoperative morbidity or recurrence. Definitive surgical management most commonly includes direct primary anatomical closure, interpositional tissue flaps or grafts, and urethral reconstruction. Postoperative complications include stress urinary incontinence (SUI), obstructed voiding secondary to stricture, and fistula recurrence.

Fortunately, urethrovaginal fistulas are rare in practice as the urethra in females is an anatomically well-protected structure. In adults, particularly in the developed world, urethrovaginal fistulas are most commonly the result of iatrogenic injuries. The use of synthetic mesh slings in the repair of stress urinary incontinence is a well-described culprit as the synthetic mesh will gradually wear down the native tissue, particularly if the mesh is under tension. Other iatrogenic causes of urethrovaginal fistulas include following urethral diverticulum repair, anterior colporrhaphy, and obstetric forceps rotations. In contrast to the developed world, most urethrovaginal fistulas result from obstructed labor in the developing world.

Epidemiology

It is estimated that there are currently 3.5 million women currently living with urogenital fistulas worldwide with 50,000–130,000 new cases annually, although the true prevalence and incidence remain unknown [2]. Urogenital fistulas demonstrate varied geographic distribution with the highest prevalence in sub-Saharan Africa and South Asia. Obtaining quality data on the incidence and prevalence of urogenital fistulas is difficult given the poor quality of data collection methods in developing countries, relative rarity of urogenital fistulas, and the tendency of affected women to conceal their condition [3]. Even less is known of the epidemiology of specific urogenital fistulas such as urethrovaginal fistulas. It is important to distinguish the etiology of urogenital fistulas in developing countries compared to developed countries. The vast majority of urogenital fistulas in developing countries is caused by obstructed labor, termed obstetric fistulas. In developed countries, the majority of urogenital fistulas are caused by iatrogenic injuries during gynecologic or urologic surgery.

In the United States, where iatrogenic causes predominate, the incidence of urethrovaginal fistula after urethral diverticulectomy ranges from 0.9% to 5% [4]. A study out of the United Kingdom demonstrated a 0.13% incidence of urogenital fistula following all types of hysterectomy [5].

Anatomy of the Female Urethra

The female urethra connects the bladder to the vulva and terminates at the external urethral meatus in the vulvar vestibule directly above the vaginal introitus. The female urethra passes through the perineal membrane in the retropubic space. It averages approximately 2–3 cm in length and 6 mm in diameter. The female urethra can be divided into four distinct layers histologically that include mucosa, submucosa, internal urethral sphincter, and external urethral sphincter. The internal sphincter is composed of smooth muscle, and the external sphincter is composed of striated skeletal muscle. The smooth muscle is innervated by the autonomic nerves of the pelvic plexus, and the striated skeletal muscle is innervated by branches of the pudendal nerve [6]. Importantly, the submucosal layer is highly vascular. The blood supply of the female urethra (Fig. 1) comes from extensions of the pudendal vessels and the vesical vessels [7]. The tenuousness of the blood supply of the female urethra contributes to both the pathogenesis of urethrovaginal fistulas as well as the difficulty of surgical repair.

Risk Factors

Risk factors for urethrovaginal fistulas should be conceptually divided into risk factors for obstetric fistulas and risk factors for iatrogenic urethrovaginal fistulas. Obstetric fistulas are caused by direct pressure of the trapped fetus over a wide area of the pelvis for a prolonged period of time, leading to tissue ischemia [8]. The prolonged tissue ischemia leads to significant scarring, fibrosis, and widespread

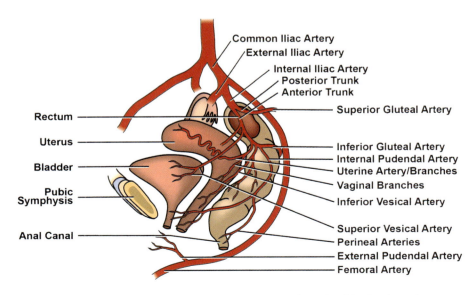

Fig. 1 The anatomy of the female pelvis, with an emphasis on the blood supply of the female urethra

destruction of the vagina resulting in vesicovaginal and urethrovaginal fistulas [8].

Iatrogenic urethrovaginal fistulas are a known complication of mid-urethral synthetic mesh sling placement, urethral diverticulectomy, urethrolysis procedures, anterior colporrhaphy, and obstetric forceps rotations. Many of the urinary tract injuries which result in urogenital fistulas are not recognized intraoperatively. Intraoperative risk factors for vesicovaginal fistula at the time of hysterectomy include uterus weight of greater than 250 g, longer operative times (longer than 5 h), and simultaneous ureteral injury [9]. At this time, intraoperative risk factors for urethrovaginal fistulas specifically have not been studied, and further research is indicated.

Other risk factors for urethrovaginal fistulas include non-obstetric trauma and pelvic radiation and systemic chemotherapy. Pelvic radiation in the form of external beam radiotherapy as well as brachytherapy also represents risk factors for urethrovaginal fistulas.

Etiology/Pathogenesis

Obstetric

Obstetric causes, particularly obstructed labor, have been shown to cause urethrovaginal fistulas. Every year between 50,000 and 100,000 women are impacted by obstetric fistulas worldwide [10]. Obstructed labor is not only a cause of urogenital fistulas, but it is also a major cause of maternal mortality and accounts for up to 6% of all maternal deaths [10] as both conditions are heavily influenced by the availability of emergency obstetric care. These vulnerable women often times suffer constant incontinence, shame, social segregation, and a multitude of other health issues [10]. It is estimated that at least two million women live with untreated urogenital fistulas, primarily in sub-Saharan Africa and South Asia [10]. It is important to know that obstetric fistulas are preventable. They can be prevented by delaying the age of first pregnancy, stopping harmful traditional practices (genital cutting or vaginal "salt packing"), and increasing access to timely obstetric care [10].

Obstructed labor leads to significant direct pressure of the obstructed fetus causing tissue ischemia to large portions of the pelvis [8]. Cephalopelvic disproportion results in the fetal head being unable to advance through the birth canal. This process can occur despite strong uterine contractions. Obstructed labor is not unique to developing countries as all pregnant women are at risk. The problem arises when treatment for obstructed labor is delayed or not diagnosed. The prolonged tissue ischemia that develops as a result of obstructed labor leads to significant scarring, fibrosis, and widespread destruction of the vaginal wall resulting in urethrovaginal fistulas [8]. The mechanism of injury is a form of pressure necrosis that occurs in the maternal soft tissues between the bony plates of the fetal head and maternal pelvic bones. The widespread devascularized tissue in the pelvis also tends to complicate future surgical interventions. Typically, the fistula will become evident within the first 2 weeks following delivery.

There are a multitude of factors that lead to delays in diagnosis, inadequate treatment, and ultimately the formation of urethrovaginal and other urogenital fistulas in developing countries. Common factors include limited or complete lack of access to emergency obstetric services; structural and economic barriers to travel; the low social, economic, and political status of women resulting in poor maternal health services; delivery at home with care by untrained birth attendants; lack of or poor quality of secondary and tertiary healthcare services; and low quality healthcare in general [11]. Other less common causes of urogenital fistulas in developing countries include genital cutting and vaginal "salt packing" [12, 13]. Genital cutting is practiced in many countries as a rite of passage to womanhood [13–15]. The low social status of women in these countries is typified by harmful practices like these. Vaginal "salt packing" is also a traditional practice that has become far less common in recent years. The mineral salts are falsely believed to aid in postpartum healing. These mineral salts are able to cause fistulas by chemical burning.

Radiation Therapy

Radiation therapy for cancers in the pelvis has been shown to cause a progressive small vessel endarteritis that impairs the vascular supply to tissues within the radiation field [16]. This can slow or prevent the healing process that occurs after surgical procedures and ultimately lead to urethrovaginal fistulas. Unfortunately, not very much can be done to mitigate this risk other than using good surgical technique, which includes limited handling of tissue and sharp dissection. Tissue devascularization can lead to a "frozen pelvis," which makes surgical dissection very difficult. Other etiologies of a frozen pelvis include cancer and endometriosis. Given the pathogenesis of radiation-induced urethrovaginal fistulas, one surgical group has pioneered using a vascular rectus abdominis flap without closure of the fistulous tracts [17].

Inflammatory

On the opposite end of the spectrum from radiation therapy, inflammation can lead to hypervascularized and friable tissue. This also leads to poor surgical healing and is a setup for postoperative fistula formation if exceptional care isn't taken to preserve the tissue. Localized inflammation in or near the pelvis is the most likely culprit, usually from pelvic inflammatory disease (PID), inflammatory bowel disease (IBD), or diverticulitis.

Traumatic (Non-obstetric)

Urethral injuries due to pelvic fractures are more common in males than females [18]. This is primarily due to anatomical differences that include greater mobility, relatively protected location, and shorter length of the female urethra. Female urethrovaginal fistulas are a rare occurrence in the setting of pelvic trauma [19]. If the urethral injury secondary to pelvic fractures is not acutely repaired, a urethrovaginal fistula may develop.

Postsurgical (Iatrogenic)

While urethrovaginal fistulas are still rare, they are increasing in incidence in industrialized countries due to the use of synthetic mesh slings for the treatment of stress urinary incontinence in women [20]. There are multiple ways that synthetic mesh slings can lead to the development of urethrovaginal fistulas. They can erode into the urethra when under too much tension, become infected, or be placed in the wrong plane (e.g., deep into the pubocervical fascia). Urethrovaginal fistulas can also occur following urethral diverticulectomy. This most likely occurs due to failure to obtain a tension-free closure of the urethral defect following excision of the diverticulum. Scarring can occur between the urethra and cervix following caesarean section or placement of cerclage sutures. This can also lead to the development of urethrovaginal fistulas. Other less common causes include urethrolysis procedures, prolapse repair, mesh removal, anterior colporrhaphy, vaginal hysterectomy, and pressure necrosis from indwelling catheters.

Prevention

Obstetric fistulas are preventable with proper diagnosis and prompt treatment of obstructed labor. Delays in diagnosis, delays in deciding to seek emergency obstetric care, and a lack of quality healthcare infrastructure all contribute to the development of obstetric fistulas. Specific preventive measures that can be initiated to prevent obstetric fistulas include operative vaginal delivery or cesarean section to treat obstructed labor and routine use of indwelling urinary catheters in cases of protracted labor. They can also be prevented by delaying the age of first pregnancy and stopping the harmful traditional practices mentioned above [7]. Postsurgical or iatrogenic urethrovaginal fistulas can only be prevented by utilizing proper surgical technique. Prompt diagnosis and repair of any surgical injuries are critical to preventing the subsequent development of urethrovaginal fistulas.

Clinical Presentation

Most urogenital fistulas present with urinary drainage per vaginum immediately following direct trauma to the lower urinary tract [8]. An exception to this is for fistulas resulting from cesarean delivery, hysterectomy, and radiation. Fistulas from cesarean delivery or hysterectomy typically present 7–30 days out from surgery, while fistula tracts following radiation therapy tend to develops weeks or months from the last radiation treatment [8].

Urethrovaginal fistulas in general can present on a spectrum from a tiny pinpoint vaginal lesion manifested by vaginal voiding to extensive urethral damage with florid urinary incontinence [1]. These patients can also present with intermittent positional wetness, recurrent urinary tract infections (UTI), perineal skin irritation, vaginal fungal infections, or asymptomatic and incidentally found lesions [1].

The specific location of the fistula tract correlates with the patient's presenting symptoms. Proximal or middle urethrovaginal fistulas typically present with either constant urinary incontinence from the vagina or intermittent positional wetness. In contrast, fistulas in the distal third of the urethra, which are beyond the external urethral sphincter, typically present with vaginal urinary leakage only during or after voiding [1]. Often times these patients are continent and only minimally symptomatic [1]. There is also evidence that urethrovaginal fistulas due to synthetic tape erosion may present with urethritis and pelvic pain as compared to the symptomatology mentioned above [21].

Approximately 90% of urogenital fistulas associated with iatrogenic causes are symptomatic within 7–30 days postoperatively [1]. In contrast, approximately 75% of obstetric fistulas present within the first 24 h following delivery [1]. Similar to iatrogenic causes, radiation-induced urethrovaginal fistulas tend to present later. They can manifest anywhere from 30 days to several years after the last radiation therapy session [22].

Diagnosis

A thorough medical and surgical history is critical to making the diagnosis of urethrovaginal fistula. It is also important to have a high index of suspicion as the diagnosis of urogenital fistulas is notoriously challenging. Important characteristics of a thorough history in this setting include symptom onset and duration as well as a thorough pelvic health history. A pelvic health history should include questions related to a history of trauma, obstructed labor, cancer, and any cancer treatments such as radiation or chemotherapy. Specific questions should be asked to ascertain symptom characteristics such as smell, color, consistency, and leakage volume. This is an important step in the history as it is necessary to exclude hematuria, vaginal bleeding, or discharge. Cervical discharge is typically a watery discharge, whereas vaginal discharge has a thicker consistency. It is also possible to have endometrial or fallopian tube discharge as well as drainage postoperatively from a seroma. Determining whether the leakage of urine is continuous, intermittent, or positional is also important as intermittent positional wetness is a sign of proximal or middle urethrovaginal fistulas, for example. A primary goal of the history is to rule out other causes of urinary incontinence.

The physical exam should involve a thorough genitourinary exam using a speculum as some urethrovaginal fistulas may be diagnosed on visual inspection. For the best results, perform a split speculum exam where only the lower blade of the speculum is utilized. This allows improved visualization of the anterior vaginal wall. Recently formed fistulas tend to be seen as small, red areas of granulation tissue. At this stage they typically lack a visible opening, although occasionally a visual opening is seen. A dye test can be done in the office or under anesthesia. The bladder is filled with methylene blue via a urinary catheter while examining with the lower bladder of a speculum. Advancing the catheter to move the inflated balloon off the bladder neck can aid in diagnosis of fistulas originating from the proximal urethra/bladder neck area. It is important to not compress the anterior vaginal wall with the speculum for best visualization. In the case of more mature fistulas, sometimes it can be difficult to visualize the vaginal orifice. It is possible that multiple fistulas or multiple structures are present or involved. If this test is negative, then it is appropriate to perform the phenazopyridine tampon test which is used to diagnosis ureteral vaginal fistulas. If the urethral fistula is proximal to the external sphincter, you will be able to see the blue dye. Post-hysterectomy vesicovaginal fistulas are typically located either at the vaginal cuff or in the upper third of the vagina. Occasionally urine leakage is seen during the exam itself, for example, in patients with vesicovaginal fistulas. There can also be pooling of urine seen at the end of the exam or just the odor of urine present. The blue dye test is standard for evaluating VVF. This test should be performed in all cases to assess for the location of the leakage. The blue dye test does not need to be performed under anesthesia, but anesthesia can be utilized in select, difficult cases.

The differential diagnosis for a patient presenting with symptoms of a urethrovaginal fistula includes other causes or urinary incontinence. It is helpful conceptually to break down the etiologies of urinary incontinence into four broad categories that include stress incontinence, urgency incontinence, mixed incontinence, and overflow incontinence. Stress urinary incontinence (SUI) is involuntary urinary leakage with increases in intra-abdominal pressure. This occurs in the absence of a bladder contraction. SUI is the most common type of incontinence in younger women with the highest incidence in patients 45–49 years of age [23]. The mechanisms underlying SUI include urethral hypermobility and intrinsic sphincter deficiency. Urgency urinary incontinence (UUI) is involuntary urinary leakage accompanied by the sudden urge to void. UUI follows under the umbrella of overactive bladder, which can occur in patients with and without incontinence. UUI is understood to result from detrusor muscle overactivity and is more common in older women and in those with other medical comorbidities. Spinal cord injuries and other neurologic conditions are known causes of overactive bladder and UUI. Mixed urinary incontinence occurs in women who present with symptoms of both stress and urgency incontinence. Overflow urinary incontinence is urinary leakage in the setting of incomplete bladder emptying. Of the types of urinary incontinence, overflow incontinence is the most likely to be constant. It is for this reason that overflow incontinence is the most likely of the types of urinary incontinence to be confused for a urethrovaginal fistula. Concomitant symptoms include urinary hesitancy, urinary frequency, weak or intermittent urinary stream, and nocturia. The mechanisms underlying overflow incontinence include detrusor underactivity and bladder outlet obstruction.

Other items on the differential diagnosis for a patient presenting with urinary leakage include urinary tract infections (UTIs), genitourinary syndrome of menopause, vaginal atrophy, urethral diverticula, ectopic ureters, neurologic disorders, cognitive impairment, functional incontinence, medications, constipation, alcohol and caffeine intake, and cancer. The differential diagnosis for urinary leakage is extensive, and the initial evaluation always includes a urinalysis in addition to a history and physical exam.

Adjunct tests including the tampon dye test can help identify upper and lower urinary tract fistulas to the vagina but are not specific to urethrovaginal fistula. Dye testing is useful in finding small fistulas. The dye (methylene blue, indigo carmine, or sterile infant formula) is mixed with sterile saline and instilled into the bladder using a bladder catheter [24]. The steps of the procedure include compressing the urethra with a gauze sponge to prevent accidental egress of dye from the urethra. After that, the bladder is filled incrementally with 60 mL aliquots of the sterile dye fluid. Next, the author (S.J.K.) favors utilizing a speculum with a built-in light source to directly assess for leakage (demonstrated by visualizing egress of blue dye from the vagina) as this allows localization of the fistula orifice and quality and mobility of the surrounding tissues for surgical planning.

Alternatively, a tampon can be placed in the vagina and then removed to check for any dye stains. Large cotton swabs can be used if a tampon is not readily available. Blue staining indicates a vesicovaginal or urethrovaginal fistula. In the case that no leakage of dye is seen, the patient is then asked to perform the Valsalva maneuver or cough. In addition, the foley catheter should be adjusted if no leakage is seen, as the balloon could be obstructing a fistula at the bladder neck level. It is important to perform this troubleshooting measure while observing the anterior vaginal wall and to remember that more than one fistula can be present.

Direct visualization of a urethrovaginal fistula may also be achieved through cystourethroscopy. Cystourethroscopy is useful in assessing the number of intravesical or intraurethral fistula orifices and their proximity to the ureteral orifices. It can also be used to assess for residual injury or any residual surgical materials.

With regard to radiographic diagnostic testing, a voiding cystourethrogram may be diagnostic of urethrovaginal fistula though detection rate is not known. The role of cross-sectional imaging in diagnosis remains to be further evaluated. Although infrequently done, magnetic resonance imaging (MRI) or double-balloon urethral catheter under fluoroscopic guidance can be utilized for the diagnosis and assessment of complex urethral fistulas. In a study of women with obstetric vesicouterine fistulas, it was shown that pelvic MRI is more sensitive than both computed tomography (CT) and intravenous pyelogram (IVP) [25]. As MRI technology has become increasingly advanced, soft tissue visualization has gotten to be of acceptable quality for diagnosis.

Treatment and Outcomes

Surgical repair remains the mainstay for the definitive treatment for urethrovaginal fistulas. A subset of patients with fistula disease distal to the external sphincter experience only abnormal stream during urination without incontinence at rest. They may decide to pursue observation without further intervention if they are not bothered by their symptoms. Similar to other urological fistula disease, successful repairs are best achieved during the initial surgical correction [26]. There is no clear consensus for the timing of repair from identification of the fistula. Waaldijk et al. has reported high success rates in immediate management of obstetric urogenital fistulas [27]. However, certain groups have advocated for delayed repair of about 2–3 months if fistula is discovered a few days after inciting injury [22, 26, 28]. Surgical optimization determining timing of repair include other factors including, but not limited to, presence of active urinary tract infections and history of radiation. Appropriate treatment of urinary and local soft tissue infections should precede fistula repair to allow for appropriate healing [29]. A delayed repair is considered for radiation-associated injuries. General principles of any fistula repair also apply to urethrovaginal fistulas including identification of adequately vascularized tissue, tension-free suture lines, and initial diversion of urine. Compared to those of vesicovaginal fistulas, options of urethrovaginal fistula repair can be sparse given the urethra's blood supply, limited mobility, and delicate interposing tissue planes. Techniques of repair vary depending on the complexity of the fistula and are usually conducted with primary excision and closure of a vaginal flap or with the use of interposition flaps for more advanced disease.

Primary Closure with Vaginal Flap

Simple fistulas can be managed with excision and primary closure using a vaginal flap. A thorough pelvic exam as well as cystourethroscopy should be performed to identify the exact location of both openings of the fistula. A urethral foley catheter should subsequently be placed and the balloon inflated. The vaginal flap should then be created with an inverted U incision along the center of the anterior vaginal wall extending just proximal to the fistula tract (Fig. 2a). Vaginal epithelia should be undermined and dissected to allow for adequate mobilization. The fistula tract should then be dissected circumferentially toward the level of the healthy urethral tissue. Fistula closure in two perpendicular layers has been described, which

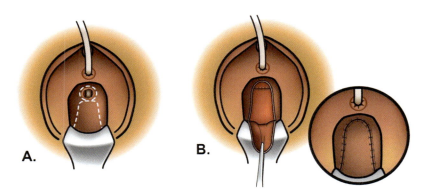

Fig. 2 (**a**) Vaginal flap incision with inverted U and circumscribing incision of urethrovaginal fistula. (**b**) Vaginal flap advancement over the repaired fistula

can incorporate closing the urethral layer transversely followed by the periurethral layer in a vertical fashion. Care should be taken to ensure that tissue tension is minimized with adequate mobilization and dissection prior to this. Finally, the vaginal U flap should be placed over the two-layered fistula repair and closed (Fig. 2b). Pushkar et al. reported a single-center experience of 71 patients with a urethrovaginal fistula repair success rate of 90.14% after primary repair using a vaginal advancement flap alone and 98.5% success after a second revision operation [22].

Martius Flap

When tissues are insufficient for a primary closure, a Martius flap, a pedicled interposition fat pad flap, can be utilized for further reinforcement and has been advocated for use as an initial approach for repair [29]. The adipose tissue of the labia majora is harvested in this approach. Interposition of the flap is performed immediately before the closure of the vaginal flap in the previously discussed procedure. Laterality of the harvest site depends on the shortest distance required to cover the fistula repair to decrease tension and ensure optimal vascularization of the flap. To harvest the flap, an incision along the groove between the labia minora and labia majora should be made. The pedicled fat pad of the labia majora should be identified and dissected with care to preserve the blood supply (Fig. 3a). The deep branch of the external pudendal artery supplies a more anterior flap favorable for the location of urethrovaginal fistulas; it also received a branch inferiorly from the internal pudendal and a branch from the obturator artery. Once dissected, this can then be tunneled under the vaginal wall to the repaired fistula site and sutured to the periurethral tissue while minimizing tension (Fig. 3b). The vaginal U flap should then be closed in the same aforementioned fashion along with the paralabial incision. A drain may be left at the discretion of the surgeon postoperatively depending on the extent of their dissection. Regarding outcomes of Martius flaps, groups have demonstrated more durable results when comparing urethrovaginal fistula repair with Martius flap versus primary closure alone [30].

Reconstruction for Recurrent or Complex Fistulas with Myofascial Flaps

Despite the high rates of successful primary vaginal flap closure and Martius flap interposition repairs, recurrent fistula disease and larger complex urogenital fistulas may require more extensive intervention. Limited options exist for reconstruction of recalcitrant urethrovaginal fistula disease after initial repair. Pedicled muscle flaps are often utilized by plastic surgeons in extensive reconstruction. These techniques have also been described within urological space in pelvic floor reconstruction [31]. In similar fashion, myofascial flaps can provide support for recurrent and complex urethrovaginal fistula

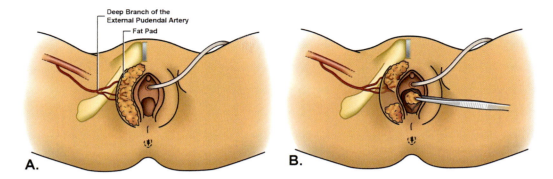

Fig. 3 (**a**) Martius flap from the labia majora fat pad one branch blood supply. (**b**) Martius flap tunneled through the vaginal wall to cover the fistula repair

which include the rectus abdominis and gracilis muscles. Since presentation of urethrovaginal fistula requiring adjunct myofascial flap reconstruction is rare, there is a paucity of published studies describing repairs in large numbers.

Rectus Abdominis Muscle Flap

Utilization of a rectus abdominis muscle flap has been described by Bruce et al. in six women with recurrent urethrovaginal fistula disease after failure of a previous Martius flap repair [32]. Similar to the Martius flap approach, interposition of the rectus abdominis flap is performed after the inverted U vaginal flap dissection is performed, circumscribing the fistula. Each rectus abdominis muscle is supplied by the superior epigastric artery superiorly and the deep inferior epigastric artery from the external iliac inferiorly. The flap is harvested by transecting one of the rectus abdominis muscles at the first tendinous intersection and tubularizing it while maintaining the inferior epigastric artery for the pedicle's supply (Fig. 4a). This is then passed through the endopelvic fascia inferiorly into to the introitus to cover the urethral repair (Fig. 4b). The distal portion can be fixed on the contralateral side on the obturator fascia, arcus tendinous, or Cooper's ligament. The vaginal U flap is then closed over the repair along with the abdominal incision. Bruce et al. reported successful repair without fistula recurrence in all six patients after a mean follow-up of 23 months [32].

Gracilis Muscle Flap

The proximity of a gracilis muscle and its vascular pedicle within the region of urogenital fistulas makes it another reasonable option for interposition in urethrovaginal fistula repair. Use of gracilis muscle in vesicovaginal fistulas and larger urethrovesicovaginal fistulas has been described in the literature [28]. As in the aforementioned repairs, the interposition takes place after dissection of the anterior vaginal wall circumscribing the fistulous tract and initial repair of the urethral defect. The gracilis muscle derives its vascular pedicle from medial circumflex branches originating from the deep femoral artery. Harvest of the flap is started by dividing the tendinous portion of the muscle just superior to the medial condyle followed by careful dissection proximally while preserving its vascular supply (Fig. 5a). The pedicled flap should then be mobilized to the introitus through a sublabial tunnel and deep to the vaginal epithelium covering the urethral repair (Fig. 5b). Described by Patil et al., the flap can be fixed to the lateral vaginal fascia and the connective tissue overlying the periosteum of the ischiopubic ramus [28]. The vaginal U flap is then closed over the repair along with the medial thigh incision.

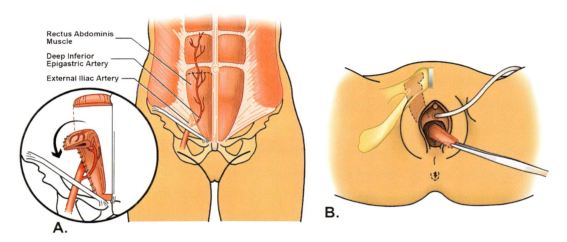

Fig. 4 (**a**) Rectus abdominis muscle flap, transected at the first tendinous intersection, and its blood supply. (**b**) Rectus abdominis muscle flap tunneled through the endopelvic fascia to cover the fistula repair

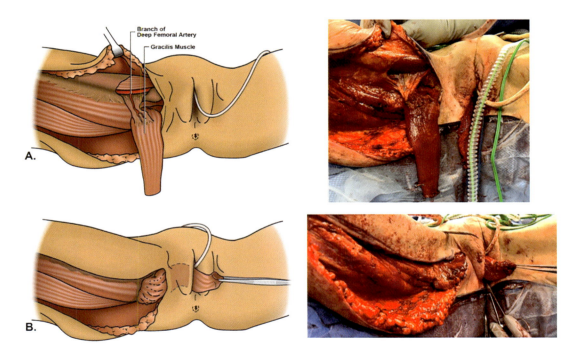

Fig. 5 (**a**) Gracilis muscle flap with its blood supply including intraoperative photograph. (**b**) Gracilis muscle flap tunneled through the sublabial tunnel to cover the fistula repair including intraoperative photograph

Conclusion

For the reconstructive surgeon, there are numerous challenging aspects to the diagnosis and management of urethrovaginal fistulas. These fistulas are increasingly rare in practice as more women have access to emergency obstetric care and the quality of our healthcare infrastructure continues to improve. The etiology of urethrovaginal fistulas differs between developed and developing countries. In the developed world, urethrovaginal fistulas most commonly result from iatrogenic injuries and from obstructed labor in the developing world. Surgical repair is the mainstay of definitive treatment for urethrovaginal fistulas. General principles of other urogenital fistula repair also apply to urethrovaginal fistulas. Techniques of repair vary depending on the complexity of the fistula and are usually performed with primary excision and closure of a vaginal flap. Interpositional flaps and grafts are reserved for more advanced disease. Specific flaps and grafts used for the repair of urethrovaginal fistulas include the Martius flap, myofascial flap, rectus abdominis muscle flap, and gracilis muscle flap. Postoperative complications include stress urinary incontinence (SUI), obstructed voiding secondary to stricture, and fistula recurrence.

Cross-References

- Reconstruction of the Absent or Severely Damaged Urethra
- Rectovaginal Fistula
- Ureterovaginal Fistula Repair
- Vesicovaginal Fistula Repair: Abdominal Approach
- Vesicovaginal Fistula Repair: Minimally Invasive Approach
- Vesicovaginal Fistula Repair: Vaginal Approach

References

1. Pushkar DY, Sumerova NM, Kasyan GR. Management of urethrovaginal fistulae. Curr Opin Urol. 2008;18:389–94.
2. Wall LL. Obstetric vesicovaginal fistula as an international public-health problem. Lancet Lond Engl. 2006;368:1201–9.
3. Tunçalp Ö, Tripathi V, Landry E, Stanton CK, Ahmed S. Measuring the incidence and prevalence of obstetric fistula: approaches, needs and recommendations. Bull World Health Organ. 2015;93:60–2.
4. Mackinnon M, Pratt JH, Pool TL. Diverticulum of the female urethra. Surg Clin North Am. 1959;39:953–62.
5. Hilton P, Cromwell DA. The risk of vesicovaginal and urethrovaginal fistula after hysterectomy performed in the English National Health Service – a retrospective cohort study examining patterns of care between 2000 and 2008. BJOG Int J Obstet Gynaecol. 2012;119:1447–54.
6. Colleselli K, Stenzl A, Eder R, Strasser H, Poisel S, Bartsch G. The female urethral sphincter: a morphological and topographical study. J Urol. 1998;160:49–54.
7. Rahn DD, Bleich AT, Wai CY, Roshanravan SM, Wieslander CK, Schaffer JI, Corton MM. Anatomic relationships of the distal third of the pelvic ureter, trigone, and urethra in unembalmed female cadavers. Am J Obstet Gynecol. 2007;197:668.e1–4.
8. Wong MJ, Wong K, Rezvan A, Tate A, Bhatia NN, Yazdany T. Urogenital fistula. Female Pelvic Med Reconstr Surg. 2012;18:71–8. quiz 78
9. Duong TH, Taylor DP, Meeks GR. A multicenter study of vesicovaginal fistula following incidental cystotomy during benign hysterectomies. Int Urogynecology J. 2011;22:975–9.
10. World Health Organization Obstetric fistula. https://www.who.int/news-room/facts-in-pictures/detail/10-facts-on-obstetric-fistula. Accessed 16 Aug 2021.
11. Cichowitz C, Watt MH, Mchome B, Masenga GG. Delays contributing to the development and repair of obstetric fistula in northern Tanzania. Int Urogynecol J. 2018;29:397–405.
12. Fahmy K. Cervical and vaginal atresia due to packing the vagina with salt after labor. Am J Obstet Gynecol. 1962;84:1466–9.
13. Tahzib F. Vesicovaginal fistula in Nigerian children. Lancet Lond Engl. 1985;2:1291–3.
14. Browning A, Allsworth JE, Wall LL. The relationship between female genital cutting and obstetric fistulae. Obstet Gynecol. 2010;115:578–83.
15. Ouedraogo I, McConley R, Payne C, Heller A, Wall LL. Gurya cutting and female genital fistulas in Niger: ten cases. Int Urogynecol J. 2018;29:363–8.
16. Kinsella TJ, Bloomer WD. Tolerance of the intestine to radiation therapy. Surg Gynecol Obstet. 1980;151:273–84.
17. Sværdborg M, Birke-Sørensen H, Bek KM, Nielsen JB. A modified surgical technique for treatment of radiation-induced vesicovaginal fistulas. Urology. 2012;79:950–3.
18. Aggarwal A, Pandey S, Singh V, Sinha RJ. Post-traumatic bony impingement into vagina: a rare cause of urethrovaginal fistula. BMJ Case Rep. 2018;2018:bcr2018226004.
19. Jiang D, Chen Z, He L, Lin H, Jin L, Xu M, Xu G, Fang X, Geng H. Repair of urethrovaginal fistula secondary to pelvic fracture with a labia minora skin flap in young girls. Urology. 2017;103:227–9.
20. Blaivas JG, Purohit RS. Post-traumatic female urethral reconstruction. Curr Urol Rep. 2008;9:397–404.
21. Siegel AL. Urethral necrosis and proximal urethrovaginal fistula resulting from tension-free vaginal tape. Int Urogynecol J Pelvic Floor Dysfunct. 2006;17:661–4.
22. Pushkar DY, Dyakov VV, Kosko JW, Kasyan GR. Management of urethrovaginal fistulas. Eur Urol. 2006;50:1000–5.

23. Minassian VA, Bazi T, Stewart WF. Clinical epidemiological insights into urinary incontinence. Int Urogynecol J. 2017;28:687–96.
24. Moir JC. Personal experiences in the treatment of vesicovaginal fistulas. Am J Obstet Gynecol. 1956;71: 476–91.
25. Abou-El-Ghar ME, El-Assmy AM, Refaie HF, El-Diasty TA. Radiological diagnosis of vesicouterine fistula: role of magnetic resonance imaging. J Magn Reson Imaging JMRI. 2012;36:438–42.
26. Mellano EM, Tarnay CM. Management of genitourinary fistula. Curr Opin Obstet Gynecol. 2014;26:415–23.
27. Waaldijk K. The immediate management of fresh obstetric fistulas. Am J Obstet Gynecol. 2004;191:795–9.
28. Patil U, Waterhouse K, Laungani G. Management of 18 difficult vesicovaginal and urethrovaginal fistulas with modified Ingelman-Sundberg and Martius operations. J Urol. 1980;123:653–6.
29. Webster GD, Sihelnik SA, Stone AR. Urethrovaginal fistula: a review of the surgical management. J Urol. 1984;132:460–2.
30. Rangnekar NP, Imdad Ali N, Kaul SA, Pathak HR. Role of the martius procedure in the management of urinary-vaginal fistulas. J Am Coll Surg. 2000;191: 259–63.
31. Tobin GR. Pelvic, vaginal, and perineal reconstruction in radical pelvic surgery. Surg Oncol Clin. 1994;3:397–413.
32. Bruce RG, El-Galley RE, Galloway NT. Use of rectus abdominis muscle flap for the treatment of complex and refractory urethrovaginal fistulas. J Urol. 2000;163:1212–5.

Reconstruction of the Absent or Severely Damaged Urethra

Elisabeth M. Sebesta, W. Stuart Reynolds, and Roger R. Dmochowski

Contents

Introduction	708
Anatomy and Function of the Female Urethra	708
Mechanisms of Severe Female Urethral Injury	709
Iatrogenic	709
Trauma	710
Preoperative Evaluation	711
Diagnosis	711
Timing of Reconstructive Surgery	712
Surgical Management	713
Techniques for Urethral Reconstruction	713
Bladder Neck Closure or Urinary Diversion	722
Repair after Eroded Synthetic Sling	725
Autologous Fascial Pubovaginal Sling for Associated Stress Urinary Incontinence	725
Conclusions	726
Cross-References	726
References	726

Abstract

Female urethral injury is a rare condition, and reconstruction of the female urethra after severe damage or urethral loss can be a technically challenging task often involving complex reconstructive techniques. Appropriate diagnosis requires knowledge of the anatomy and function of the female urethra and high clinical suspicion. Diagnostic evaluation should be careful and thoughtful, with the purpose of also aiding in surgical planning. Goals for reconstructive surgery in such patients are to achieve urethral continence and establish means for passage of urine from the bladder in a manner that improves the individual patient's quality of life. With careful evaluation and surgical planning, it is often that these goals can be accomplished in a single surgical procedure. In this chapter we discuss the normal anatomy and function of the female

E. M. Sebesta · W. S. Reynolds · R. R. Dmochowski (✉)
Department of Urology, Vanderbilt University Medical Center, Nashville, TN, USA
e-mail: roger.dmochowski@vumc.org

urethra, mechanisms of severe urethral injury or urethral loss in women, and a review of the surgical management options including local tissue flaps, bladder flaps, and bladder neck closure or urinary diversion.

Keywords

Urethral reconstruction · Urethral injury · Female urethra · Vaginal flap urethroplasty · Labial pedicle graft · Tissue interposition flaps · Bladder neck closure · Urinary diversion

Introduction

Female urethral injury is a rare condition, and reconstruction of the female urethra after severe damage or urethral loss can be a technically challenging task often involving complex reconstructive techniques. Appropriate diagnosis requires knowledge of the anatomy and function of the female urethra and high clinical suspicion. Diagnostic evaluation should be careful and thoughtful, with the purpose of also aiding in surgical planning. Goals for reconstructive surgery in such patients are to achieve urethral continence and establish means for passage of urine from the bladder in a manner that improves the individual patient's quality of life. With careful evaluation and surgical planning, it is often that these goals can be accomplished in a single surgical procedure. In this chapter, we discuss the normal anatomy and function of the female urethra, mechanisms of severe urethral injury or urethral loss in women, and a review of the surgical management options including local tissue flaps, bladder flaps, and bladder neck closure or urinary diversion.

Anatomy and Function of the Female Urethra

The female urethra is a short and thin musculofascial tube, about 2–4 cm in length. The urethra extends from the bladder neck to the urethral meatus in the vaginal vestibule, and it is responsible for drainage of urine from the bladder in addition to urinary continence.

There are two fascial attachments of the urethra which provide important anatomic support – the pubourethral and urethropelvic ligaments. The pubourethral ligaments are located between the urethra and the pubic symphysis. This point of attachment often serves as the anatomic division between proximal and distal urethra. The urethropelvic ligament is a sheet of connective tissue which suspends the urethra from the pelvic sidewall and pelvic fascia or arcus tendineus. The urethropelvic ligament is composed of two layers of pelvic fascia that are fused – the endopelvic fascia (on the abdominal side) and the periurethral fascia (on the vaginal side). These structures work to provide a hammock-like support of the urethra.

The urethra is composed of multiple tissue layers and different cell types. The inner layer consists of the mucosal epithelium while the outer layer is muscular. The inner mucosal layer consists of multiple folds, which acts as a fairly effective seal and therefore aids in urinary continence. Under the mucosa lies a thick and richly vascular elastic tissue like the corpus spongiosum. The urethral lumen itself is lined by a urothelial layer proximally which is continuous with the bladder urothelium and changes gradually to nonkeratinized stratified squamous cells distally.

The outermost layer of the urethra is a sphincter of striated muscle which spans much of the urethra length, but is most prominent in the mid-urethra. Proximally, the sphincter muscles are circular and circumferential. Distally, however, the muscle is horseshoe shaped and only spanning the ventral surface. This horseshoe-shaped muscle connects to the anterior vaginal wall as the urethrovaginal sphincter and extends along the inferior pubic ramus as the compressor urethrae. The female urethra is key in storage of urine in the bladder and maintenance of continence. The urethral sphincter is composed of slow-twitch muscle fibers, which are able to maintain the constant muscular tone needed for continence. It has been demonstrated that the amount of striated muscle declines with age which is associated with a decline in innervation [1, 2].

The smooth muscle of the urethra is continuous with that of the trigone and consists of an inner longitudinal layer and an outer circular layer. These layers are present only in the upper or proximal urethral and lie just inside the striated muscle sphincter. It is thought that these layers may aid in continence and voiding – with the circular layers constricting the urethral lumen, while the longitudinal layer may shorten the urethra and bladder neck during voiding [3].

The area where the proximal urethra passes through the musculature at the base of the bladder is referred to as the bladder or vesical neck. It contains the urethral lumen, and the detrusor musculature surrounds the internal urinary meatus. It is both part of the bladder and the urethra, and also a unique entity on its own. There is sympathetic innervation to the bladder neck that when damaged, results in the bladder neck to be open at rest [4].

The blood supply of the urethra is dual. Proximally, the blood supply is that of the bladder. Distally, the urethra is supplied by the terminal branches of the inferior vesical artery through the vaginal artery running along the superior-lateral vagina [5]. The female urethra is innervated by the pudendal nerve – S2 through S4. Afferents are through the pelvic splanchnic nerves.

Understanding of the normal anatomy and function of the female urethra is key in order to understand complex surgical reconstructive procedures. Additionally, recreating the normal anatomy and layers of the urethra surgically may help avoid secondary surgical complications after extensive reconstructions.

Mechanisms of Severe Female Urethral Injury

Significant damage to the female urethra which requires complex reconstruction is often attributable to either iatrogenic injury or pelvic or obstetric trauma. In industrialized nations, causes of urethral injury tend to be postsurgical iatrogenic injuries. In developing nations, however, the most common cause tends to be obstetric trauma due to prolonged obstructed labor.

Iatrogenic

Iatrogenic postsurgical urethral injury is the most common cause of significant urethral loss in developed countries. Anterior vaginal or urethral surgery may result in urethral injury, or fistula formation with urethral erosion. Less commonly, urethral erosions from prolonged indwelling urethral catheters may also obliterate the urethral tissue. Finally, radiation from pelvic malignancies is a significant source of urethral loss as well [6].

In a review of 98 cases of significant female urethral damage, previous vaginal or urethral surgery was the cause in 88% of patient [7]. The surgeries that result in urethral loss include transvaginal bladder neck suspensions, urethral diverticulectomy, anterior colporrhaphy, Kelly plication, vaginal hysterectomy, and other pelvic surgery [8]. The result is essentially a urethrovaginal fistula which presents as urinary incontinence [9, 10].

Additionally, insertion of a synthetic suburethral sling for the management of stress urinary incontinence (SUI) may contribute to urethral injury. At the time of placement, intraoperative urethral injury occurs in 0.2–2.5% of cases [11]. If at the time of synthetic sling placement, a urethral injury is noted during either vaginal dissection or trocar passage, it is recommended that the surgeon abandon placement of mesh, as the risk of urethral extrusion of the mesh is dramatically increased [12]. Additionally, after a successful sling placement, late erosion of mesh into the urethral lumen may result in significant urethral loss. The incidence of urethral mesh extrusion after synthetic mid-urethral sling (MUS) is less than 1% the large retrospective or randomized controlled trials; however, when it occurs, it may result in loss of significant urethral tissue [13]. Factors that may contribute to urethral extrusion are tissues with compromised blood supply (e.g., from pelvic radiation or overaggressive dissection resulting in urethral devascularization), sling over-tensioning, unnoticed iatrogenic urethral injury at time of sling placement, or traumatic urethral catheterizations postoperatively [14]. In some cases, urethral extrusion may occur many years after sling surgery. The complications of urethral sling placement are discussed in detail elsewhere in this book.

Finally, long-term urethral catheterization can result in urethral erosions that can cause dramatic urethral tissue loss and necessitate complex urethral reconstructive surgery. In one series of 13 women with spinal cord injuries whose urologic management consisted of indwelling urethral catheters, after a mean follow-up of 7 years, urethral erosions were present in 6 of the women (46%) [15]. In one retrospective review of 64 patients who underwent transvaginal or transabdominal bladder neck closure, 90% of the patients in this cohort were neurogenic patients with long-term indwelling catheters resulting in severe urethral erosions [16]. The underlying mechanism of this phenomenon is thought to be primarily due to pressure necrosis, as the indwelling catheter may result in pressure on the urethra over time [17].

Trauma

Traumatic urethral injury may result from either obstetric trauma or pelvic fracture. Obstetric trauma is secondary to obstructed labor resulting in prolonged fetal head compression of the urethra and surrounding structures against the pelvic bone. This causes decreased perfusion and pressure necrosis of the tissues with subsequent urethrovaginal fistula formation [18]. This type of injury has been described as a broad field injury to the pelvis which results in a combination of vascular and neurologic injury to multiple pelvic structures [19]. Obstetric trauma is relatively rare in developed countries, as modern obstetrical care has virtually eliminated this type of injury. However, in developing nations, this type of obstetric genitourinary injury is estimated to occur in up to 4 women per 1000 vaginal deliveries [20]. The majority of the time obstructed labor results in bladder necrosis and vesicovaginal fistulas; however, in a prospective case series of 180 women with genitourinary fistula after obstructed labor in Niger, Africa, 17% of fistulas also involved the proximal urethra, which is understandably the most vulnerable part of the urethra to this type of injury [21]. In this series, the fistulas were quite large, with the majority being 1.5–3 cm in size. Additionally, over half of the patients (56%) had complete circumferential destruction of the proximal urethra. The remainder of patients had a partial urethral injury resulting in loss of the ventral and lateral parts of the proximal urethra. Those with complete urethral injury had a blind-ending urethra with inability to catheterize the bladder per urethra, with the communication between the bladder and the anterior vaginal wall as the means of urine passage.

Injury to the urethra due to pelvic fracture is much less common in women than in men, ranging from 0% to 6% in contemporary series versus 10% in male patients [7, 22]. In an analysis of the National Trauma Data Bank from 2001 to 2005, of 31,380 patients with pelvic fractures, overall genitourinary injury was more commonly sustained in men as compared to women (66% vs. 34% respectively) [23]. However, while the incidence of bladder injury with pelvic fracture in men and women was observed to be about the same (3.41% in men vs. 3.37% in women), the risk of urethral injury was much higher in men, albeit still lower than other series (1.54% in men vs. 0.15% in women). This difference in urethral injury rate between men and women is thought to be due to several different anatomic reasons. The vagina and female urethra are more flexible and are inherently quite elastic [24]. Additionally, the female urethra is shorter in length and relatively protected [7]. It is also hypothesized that pelvic fractures in female patients are less severe and more frequently stable than in male patients [24].

A few series have examined urethral injuries after pelvic fractures in women. Most of the available literature has been in female children under the age of 17, rather than adult women [25]. Female children are thought to be perhaps more vulnerable to urethral injuries due to greater compressibility of the pelvic bones, or adult women are possibly more likely to die from associated injuries if severe enough to sustain urethral trauma, and therefore urethral injuries in adult women may go underdiagnosed [26–28]. Traumatic female urethral injuries are historically categorized as either complete (transverse) injuries which are complete transection or disruption of the urethra or partial (longitudinal) which are lacerations in the urethra [24]. Some series have noted that the majority of injuries are longitudinal lacerations [27]. In one case series of six women with urethral injuries, this type of urethral laceration was overlooked initially, as the patients were still able to be catheterized. Other series, however, have reported complete urethral disruptions or avulsions are more common and are often associated with concomitant vaginal or rectal injuries [25, 29]. These injuries are less likely to be overlooked, as they are associated with inability to pass a catheter per urethra and therefore prompt further examination. A contemporary systematic review of the literature regarding female urethral injuries associated with pelvic fractures identified 158 female patients with urethral trauma [24]. Of these, 63% were in children under the age of 17 and 37% in adult women. Of the patients in this review, 53% were managed acutely, with either catheter realignment or anastomotic repair; however, the remainder went on to require delayed repair. The surgical management specifically of urethral injury from pelvic fractures will be discussed at length in another chapter.

Preoperative Evaluation

As severe female urethral injuries and urethral loss are quite rare, it is paramount for clinicians to maintain a high index of suspicion to appropriately diagnose these patients at the time of initial encounter. The diagnostic evaluation relies largely on physical examination as well as cystoscopy; however, other adjuncts including imaging or urodynamic studies may be of use as well.

Diagnosis

The first step in diagnosing a significant urethral injury or urethral loss in a female patient is to be acutely aware of the previously discussed mechanisms of injury in the patient's history. The most common presenting complaint is urinary incontinence in the setting of vaginal or urethral surgery, pelvic fracture, long-term catheterization, obstetric injury, or pelvic radiation [8]. Occasionally, however, the patients will simply present with overactive bladder or other voiding symptoms. In patients who have undergone a sling placement, patients may have quite varied presenting symptoms, including dysuria, urethral or vaginal pain, recurrent urinary tract infections, persistent gross or microscopic hematuria, vaginal bleeding or discharge, urinary retention, urgency or urge urinary incontinence (UUI), or persistent SUI [8, 14].

If a patient's history sparks suspicion for a significant urethral injury, the first step in diagnosis is a thorough physical examination. This should include a thorough pelvic examination, preferably a complete exam with use of a vaginal speculum in the lithotomy position. However, many urethral defects are visible upon immediate inspection of the anterior vaginal wall [7]. In the case of urethral injury after pelvic fracture, 21% are diagnosed in the acute setting at the time of attempted urethral catheterization with physical exam alone [24]. In the setting of delayed diagnosis of urethral loss due to an iatrogenic injury or obstetric injury resulting in urethrovaginal fistula, it is important for the physician to examine for leakage of urine on pelvic examination with a comfortably full bladder. Additionally, palpation of the anterior vaginal wall for possible foreign body or mesh should be performed. Although the urethral injury may be clearly evident on pelvic exam, some urethral injuries may be more insidious and require further evaluation.

Endoscopic evaluation with cystourethroscopy is almost universally recommended in the diagnosis of urethral injuries and is usually quite revealing. This can be performed in the office with flexible cystoscopy or in the operating room with rigid cystoscopy along with an exam under anesthesia. Cystourethroscopy allows for direct visualization of mucosal defects or foreign body and is recommended for full characterization of the location and extent of the injury. Additionally, it allows for the clinician to evaluate the remainder of viable urethra for reconstructive surgical planning and to evaluate the sphincteric function [8]. If there is concern for a fistula that is difficult to visualize, methylene blue can be instilled in the bladder during cystoscopy to aid in diagnosis [30]. In the case of urethral erosions due to long-term catheterization, cystoscopy should also be completed to evaluate for bladder malignancy prior to planning of reconstructive surgery. Difficult cystoscopy may indicate a urethral stricture, or blind-ending urethra in the setting of a prior severe urethral avulsion injury or urethral mesh erosion resulting in obstruction or disruption of the urethra in the setting of prior urethral sling procedure.

The majority of urethral injuries are diagnosed on some combination of history, physical examination, and cystourethroscopy, and therefore the benefit or necessity of further testing including radiographic is unclear. However, in the case of equivocal office examination, further imaging may be of some benefit. Traditionally, this has involved voiding cystourethrogram (VCUG) with or without retrograde urethrogram (RUG) in order to document the presence of urethral fistula with contrast extravasation or urethral stricture. Endovaginal magnetic resonance imaging (MRI) may also be used in the diagnosis of urethral defects due to its superior soft tissue imaging capabilities. Pelvic MRI is also useful in the setting of concern for urethral tumors or other pelvic malignancies or urethral diverticulum [31]. Additionally, if there is concern regarding malignancy, cytology and/or tissue biopsy should also be considered as part of the diagnostic workup prior to reconstructive surgery [7]. In the setting of extensive urethrovaginal fistulas also involving the bladder neck and/or trigone, it is important to also evaluate the upper tracts and ureters, usually with retrograde pyelography or computed tomography (CT) scans with delayed-phase contrast for their involvement in the fistula.

Urodynamic testing prior to surgical intervention may provide important adjunct information. It is important to remember that neither a urethrovaginal fistula nor a destroyed urethral distally alone causes urinary incontinence. Damage must also occur more proximally or at the bladder neck. If the patient is completely asymptomatic but has distal loss of the urethra discovered incidentally, there may be no reason to offer this patient surgical intervention. Therefore, evaluating the patient's incontinence preoperatively with urodynamics may be important for patient counseling, in addition to determining the need for possible concomitant anti-incontinence procedure. Videourodynamics may also provide information regarding bladder compliance, vesicoureteral reflux, detrusor instability, outlet obstruction, and presence of a fistula which can help in surgical planning.

Timing of Reconstructive Surgery

The timing of extensive urethral reconstruction is somewhat dependent on the mechanism of injury. In the case of iatrogenic urethral injury, if recognized at the time of surgery, the repair should be immediate. For example, urethral trocar injury during sling placement recognized at the time of surgery should be primarily repaired and the placement of mesh deferred. However, the majority of severe urethral injuries and urethral loss are more chronic conditions, diagnosed varying amounts of time after the initial insult. Traditionally, reconstructive surgery is performed 3–6 months after injury, to allow resolution of the associated inflammation and edema [31]. However, more recent series have demonstrated successful repair within days or weeks of injury, as long as tissues are healthy and pliable, and there is no concomitant infection present [30–32]. Erosion of a synthetic urethral sling should be removed once diagnosed, as the longer the sling remains in place, the greater the tissue ingrowth and potentially the more severe the erosion [8]. Additionally, traumatic urethral injury after pelvic fracture is also often repaired in the immediate period with either primary catheter realignment or anastomotic repair, although there is up to a 60% incidence of urethral stricture formation and about a 5% risk of subsequent fistula reported in the previously discussed systematic review [24]. However, 47% of the urethral injuries in that review underwent delayed urethral reconstruction, most often due to the delayed nature of diagnosis, and surgeons encountered significant fibrosis and scarring during surgical dissection in those patients. With regard to radiation urethral injuries, repair should not be immediate but occur after a waiting period, sometimes over a year, to allow the tract to mature and stabilization of the ischemic injury [33].

Surgical Management

The goals of female urethral surgical reconstruction after severe urethral injury or urethral loss are to re-establish the two main functions of the native urethra: a conduit for passage of urine and continence. This may be established via reconstruction of a neourethra requiring various local flaps or grafts, with or without concomitant anti-incontinence procedure. In the case of previous failure or lack of viable tissues to aid in a complex reconstruction, urethral continence may be achieved via bladder neck closure or even urinary diversion. It is important in surgical planning to consider the patient's goals and to create a surgical plan using shared decision-making. The principles of urologic reconstructive surgeries are true of complex urethral reconstruction, including clear visualization and exposure of the defect; creation of a tension-free, watertight, multilayer closure with nonoverlapping suture lines; use of well-vascularized tissue flaps; and insuring adequate bladder drainage postoperatively [7, 8]. Herein, we will review the various approaches to manage severe urethral injury or urethral loss, including urethroplasty techniques, urinary diversions and bladder neck closures, urethral repair in the setting of an eroded synthetic mid-urethral sling, and the role for concomitant anti-incontinence procedures.

Techniques for Urethral Reconstruction

Primary Closure or Anastomotic Repair

For small urethral defects with pliable and viable tissue, it is possible to consider closing the defect primarily. Preferably, the urethral closure should occur over at least a 16-French catheter to avoid narrowing of the urethral lumen and future formation of urethral stricture. After primary repair, it is recommended to close another layer of periurethral tissue to cover the mucosal suture line, or to harvest a labial fat pad flap (Martius flap) as needed [31]. Primary anastomotic repair is often advocated for urethral injury after pelvic trauma, especially if discovered immediately at the time of trauma. Management of female pelvic trauma injuries will be discussed in another chapter.

Vaginal Flaps

Anterior Proximal Vaginal Flap Urethroplasty

An anterior proximal vaginal flap can be used to augment a defect in the urethra when the periurethral vaginal tissue is inadequate to perform a tubularized repair (see the following section for this technique) [7, 31]. While often utilized for urethral stricture disease, it can be used for more severe urethral damage as well and can be used to replace large segments of the ventral urethra. As long as there is adequate healthy anterior vaginal wall tissue proximal from the mid-urethra, this technique can be utilized. This technique may also be combined with use of the vaginal wall distal to the urethra meatus to recreate the dorsal urethral plate in cases of complete distal urethral loss, as long as this vaginal tissue is healthy. It is important to remember that before making a vaginal incision, careful planning should take place with an assessment of the viable local tissue present, to determine what can be used for urethral reconstruction and what will be used for coverage of the reconstruction.

The simplest approach is a proximally based ventral vaginal advancement flap. It starts with an inverted "U" incision in the anterior vaginal wall, with the apex at the urethral meatus. After the flap is raised, the apex of the incision is advanced to the proximal extent of the urethral defect such that the vaginal mucosa is inward toward the urethral lumen. The flap is folded over onto itself, and edges are then sutured to the urethral plate. Generally, this technique is more appropriate for distal urethral loss or distal urethral strictures, with a distance of about 2 cm from the meatus [34].

For more extensive urethral loss, a transposed vaginal flap can be created to replace entirely the ventral urethra. A "U"-shaped incision is made on healthy tissue of the anterior vaginal wall (Fig. 1a). The incision should be long enough such that the apex will become the distal neomeatus once the flap is transposed, and generally it is recommended to make the flap about 2 cm wide and 2–3 cm long [34]. The vaginal mucosal flap is raised in the usual fashion. The flap is then flipped up, and the edges sutured to the edges of the dorsal urethral plate with running delayed absorbable suture on either side (Fig. 1b). Lateral vaginal flaps are raised and rotated medially to close a second layer of tissue in the midline over the neourethra. In the case of distal urethral loss, the vaginal wall distal to the meatus can be used as the dorsal plate of the neourethra. In this case, the ends of the "U"-shaped incision can extend distally to the site of the neomeatus to add urethral length. The edges of the distal anterior vaginal wall are raised such that they can be sutured to the flap edges to create the complete neourethra. Additionally, lateral or "C"-shaped vaginal flaps have also been described for reconstruction of the ventral urethra in a similar manner except that the flap is raised on one side laterally to the urethra and sutured over to the other side for urethral coverage [35–37].

Tubularized Vaginal Flap Urethroplasty

In the case of adequate periurethral vaginal wall tissue, lateral vaginal flaps can be used to reconstruct a significant urethral defect. Unlike the vaginal flaps described above, the tubularized vaginal flap urethroplasty never relies on presence of a dorsal urethral plate; as long as there is adequate mobility of the periurethral vaginal tissue, this becomes the entire neourethra. It is good for

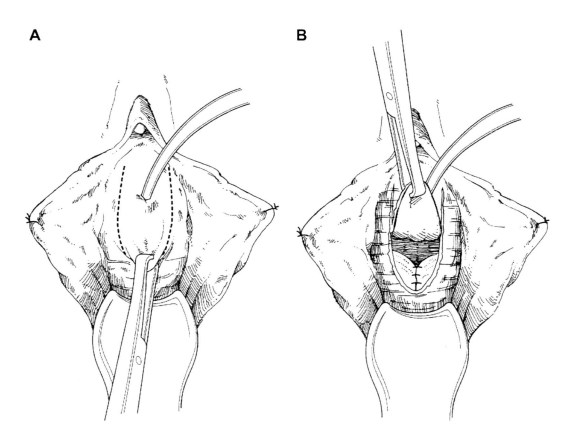

Fig. 1 Technique for vaginal flap urethral reconstruction. (**a**) A "U"-shaped incision is made in the anterior vaginal wall. (**b**) The vaginal wall flap is flipped upward and sutured to the remaining dorsal urethral plate or to the distal vaginal mucosa. (Reprinted with permission [53])

making up urethral length when there has been significant loss.

Two parallel incisions are made in the lateral vaginal wall on either side of the urethral meatus (Fig. 2a). These vaginal flaps are mobilized medially toward the catheter, until they allow for tubularization over a catheter (Fig. 2b). This rectangle or square of the vaginal wall should be about 2 cm wide and 2–3 cm long in order to create an adequate neourethra. An inverted "U" incision is made in the anterior vaginal wall proximally, with the apex at the lower edge of the rectangular tubularized flap (Fig. 2). This serves as an advancement flap for urethral coverage and is sutured to the vaginal wall lateral to the neourethra such that the apex becomes the ventral edge of the neomeatus.

Outcomes of Vaginal Flap Reconstructions

With regard to outcomes, there are numerous series in the literature reporting the use of vaginal flaps for reconstruction of female urethra strictures, although the surgical techniques are roughly the same in the setting of more substantial urethral loss (Table 1). A recent systematic review of surgical repair of female urethral stricture identified nine studies over the last decade on vaginal flap urethroplasty, including 96 cases [38]. Of these patients, four required a concomitant Martius flap for tissue coverage. At a median follow-up of 45.7 months, the pooled success rate from these studies was 90%. Only four patients (4.2%) developed de novo incontinence, and there were no major complications, although two patients developed recurrent urinary tract infections (UTIs) after

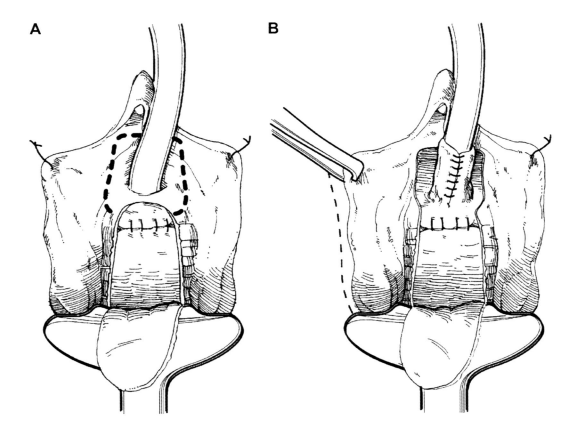

Fig. 2 Technique for tubularized vaginal wall urethroplasty. (**a**) Lateral vaginal wall incisions are made parallel to the urethral meatus. The inverted "U"-shaped incision is made to raise an anterior vaginal wall flap. (**b**) The vaginal epithelium is tubularized over a catheter to create a neourethra. The vaginal flap is then advanced and closed over the neourethra as the last layer of closure. (Reprinted with permission [53])

Table 1 Summary of series on the use of vaginal flaps, labial pedicle grafts, or bladder flaps for urethral reconstruction

	n (no.)	Approach	Concomitant procedures	Cure rate (%)	Mean or median f/u (mo.)	Complications
Vaginal flaps						
Schwender et al. [40]	8	Anterior vaginal advancement flap	Autologous PVS [2] and bulking agent injection [1]	89	30	None
Onol et al. [41]	10	Anterior vaginal advancement flap	None	100 objective, 88 subjective	24	Inward urinary stream [1] – transient
Gormley et al. [46]	12	Anterior vaginal advancement flap	Autologous PVS [2]	92	36	Recurrent UTIs [2]
Blaivas et al. [32]	10	Tubularized vaginal flap	Autologous PVS [5], vaginal needle suspension [4], Martius flap [10]	90	30	Vesicovaginal fistula [1]
Flisser et al. [18]	72	Tubularized vaginal flap	Autologous PVS [56], vaginal needle suspension [6], Martius flap [58], omental flap [3], gracilis myocutaneous flap [1]	93	18	Flap necrosis [5], vesicovaginal fistula [2], iatrogenic obstruction from sling [1]
Lane et al. [47]	30	Anterior vaginal advancement flap	Incontinence procedure [3], other procedure [11]	83	12	At least one postoperative complication [10]
	28	Tubularized vaginal flap				
	2	Labial pedicle grafts				
Simonato et al. [35]	6	Lateral vaginal flap	None	100	58.5	None
Romman et al. [36]	28	Lateral vaginal flap	None	68	52	None
Kowalik et al. [39]	5	Anterior vaginal advancement flap	Autologous PVS [1], laparoscopic nephrectomy [1]	60	47	None
Spilotros et al. [44]	2	Anterior vaginal advancement flap	None	100	31.5	None
Romero-Maroto et al. [37]	9	Lateral vaginal flap	None	89	80.7	None
Hajebrahimi et al. [45]	14	Anterior vaginal advancement flap	None	100	16.6	None
Labial pedicle grafts						
Falandry et al. [49]	56	Single labial pedicle graft [27], tubularized graft [18], double-facing bilateral grafts [11]	Martius flap [56], colposuspension [11]	82	23	–

(continued)

Table 1 (continued)

	n (no.)	Approach	Concomitant procedures	Cure rate (%)	Mean or median f/u (mo.)	Complications
Radwan et al. [50]	10	Tubularized labial graft	TOT sling [10]	66	42	Meatal stenosis [1]
Xu et al. [51]	8	Tubularized labial graft [5], transpubic double-facing bilateral grafts [3]	Rectus muscle interposition flap [8] – all performed via transpubic approach	100	48.3	None
Xu et al. [52]	24	Tubularized labial graft [18], double-facing bilateral grafts [6]	Of all patients in series – bladder neck reconstruction [5], fistula repair [3], colpoplasty [3], vaginoplasty [2], enlargement of vaginal introitus [1]	88	42.3	Of all patients in series – fistula formation [2], stricture [1]
Bladder flaps						
Tanagho [55]	3	Anterior bladder wall flap	–	100	–	–
Hemal et al. [56]	3	Anterior bladder wall flap	–	100	–	–
Radwan et al. [50]	6	Anterior bladder wall flap	None	67	42	None
Elkins et al. [59]	20	Tubularized anterior bladder wall flap	None	90	12	Recurrent vesicovaginal fistula [2]
Xu et al. [52]	2	Anterior bladder wall flap	Of all patients in series – bladder neck reconstruction [5], fistula repair [3], colpoplasty [3], vaginoplasty [2], enlargement of vaginal introitus [1]	100	42.3	Bladder outlet obstruction from mucosal prolapse [1]
Patidar et al. [60]	22	Anterior bladder wall flap [16], posterior bladder flap [6]	Vesicovaginal fistula repair [4]	82	38.4	Wound infection [1], UTIs [2]

f/u follow up, *PVS* pubovaginal sling, *UTI* urinary tract infection

surgery. Although the studies included in this review are quite heterogeneous and are mostly composed of patients with urethral strictures, this demonstrates the overall safety and success of these techniques.

Outcomes regarding the use of the proximal-based advancement vaginal flaps are more often reported in the literature than the transposed vaginal flap urethroplasty (Table 1) [39–45]. One of the initial case series for the proximal-based advancement flap was published in 2006 by Schwender et al., who reported an 89% success rate, defined as no further treatment required in a total of eight women [40]. Several other series have described similarly good outcomes for this technique. In 2011, Onol et al. published a prospective cohort of ten women with urethral strictures who underwent vaginal flap urethroplasty [41]. After 24 months of follow-up, they reported a 100% objective and 88% subjective cure rates. Likewise in a retrospective cohort of 12 women with urethral stricture disease treated with proximal-based vaginal flaps, with a follow-up ranging from 3 months to 9 years, there was a 92% success rate with no de novo incontinence postoperatively [46]. While the outcomes for vaginal flap procedures for urethral strictures are quite good in the literature, outcomes regarding its use in severe urethral defects or complete urethral loss are not well described.

In 1989, Blaivas described the use of the tubularized lateral vaginal wall urethroplasty technique as an alternative to the popularized bladder flap for partial or total urethral loss [32]. Blaivas et al. have written several series on reconstruction after severe urethral injuries in women and describe the use of the tubularized vaginal flap, when feasible, as their preferred technique. In their initial series of ten women, two had complete loss of the urethra and the remaining had significant urethral defects [32]. Of the ten women, six were completely continent, all of whom had a concurrent anti-incontinence procedure performed. Two patients went on to require a fascial sling due to severe persistent SUI, and one patient developed a vesicovaginal fistula that required repair. He subsequently published a series of 74 women who required urethral reconstruction, 72 of whom underwent a tubularized vaginal flap procedure, which is the largest series to date in the literature [18]. They reported successful anatomic repair in a single stage in 93% of women after median follow-up of 1.5 years (maximum 15 years). In this series, 56 patients underwent concomitant pubovaginal sling procedure, due to the initial observation of a high incontinence rate after surgery in women who were continent preoperatively (25%). The higher rate of incontinence here requiring pubovaginal sling is likely a function of the more severe urethral injuries captured in this series. The majority of women underwent a Martius labial fat pad flap as well for tissue coverage. The rate of de novo urge incontinence was 16%, and 3% developed severe vaginal pain postoperatively. Two patients developed recurrent fistulas requiring further repair (2.8%). This is the largest series in the literature on this type of repair and demonstrates the success with careful surgical planning and adjunct procedures for adequate flap coverage and continence.

Overall, the outcomes of vaginal flap urethral reconstructions are quite good. A recent large multi-institutional retrospective cohort study of women who underwent surgical management of urethral strictures demonstrated that of 210 patients who were treated, 83% of patients who underwent local flap reconstruction were cured (no evidence of recurrence or requiring further treatment) at 12 months of follow-up [47]. This large series included mostly patients who had either a transposed or proximal-based vaginal flap (44%) or a tubularized vaginal wall flap (41%). These patients who were treated with vaginal flap surgery had superior outcomes at 12 months as compared to those who underwent endoscopic management or surgery with a free graft (mostly oral mucosa). Evidence from large studies such as this demonstrates the durability and success of using local vaginal tissues for urethral reconstruction. However, in patients where there is significant loss or fibrosis of vaginal tissue, these procedures may not be possible. Therefore, there are numerous other surgical techniques to consider in such situations.

Labial Pedicle Grafts

When there is insufficient viable vaginal tissue to use for urethral repair, the labia minor may be used as an island pedicle graft. The labia minor is harvested and rotated over the urethral defect as a onlay or tubularized graft. Bilateral labial grafts may also be harvested and used as double-facing grafts to reconstruct the urethra circumferentially in the setting of complete urethral loss and/or small labia minora that do not allow for complete tubularization.

An ovoid incision is made in a portion of the labia minora that is hair-free, as close to the urethral repair as possible. Care should be taken to make the size of the graft large enough such that the urethra can be repaired over a 16-French catheter without tension. The graft is dissected, with an anterior or posterior blood supply intact for a robust pedicle. After raising the appropriately sized graft, it is tunneled beneath the vaginal wall into the wound. The graft should be rotated such that the mucosal surface forms the luminal side of the reconstructed urethra. The edges of the graft are then sutured to either the native urethral plate or the vaginal wall distal to the urethra. It is also possible to use the labial graft as a tubularized graft and completely reconstruct the distal urethra.

The outcomes of labial grafts have been reported in a few series with good outcomes (Table 1). The labia minor works well in urethral reconstruction for similar reasons as the vaginal mucosa – the tissue is hairless, elastic, easily obtainable, and easily mobilized to the urethra [48]. In a series of 56 cases with urethral loss after obstetric trauma who were reconstructed using a labial grafts, after mean 23-month follow-up, the authors observed an 82% global success rate in terms of successful surgical reconstruction [49]. In this series, 27 patients required an onlay graft, 18 required a tubularized graft, and double-facing grafts were utilized in 11 patients. All patients also received a Martius flap procedure at the time of surgery, and 11 underwent a colposuspension for concomitant prolapse. They reported a 69% complete continence rate in their series. Similarly, a retrospective cohort describing a single institution's experience with reconstruction of post-traumatic urethral loss described ten patients who underwent labia minor urethroplasty with or without concomitant sling [50]. One patient was lost to follow-up. In the other nine patients after 42 months of follow-up, six were totally continent (66.6%). One patient developed meatal stenosis which required a meatotomy; however, the remainder voided well with a peak urine flow of 19.2 ml/s. Another study reports outcomes after a transpubic approach via a lower midline with a pubectomy in eight women with complex urethral strictures from severe pelvic trauma [51]. In this series, three patients required bilateral grafts, and all patients underwent complete circumferential reconstruction of the urethra. Additionally, all patients underwent rectus muscle interposition flap for coverage of the neourethra. Authors report 100% continence after mean 48.3 months of follow-up, and only one patient who required dilation for meatal stenosis. The same group published a more recent and larger series, including patients who also underwent reconstruction with vaginal flaps, vulvar skin, or anterior bladder flaps for reconstruction of urethrovaginal fistulas after pelvic fracture or other trauma [52]. In this series, they had 24 patients who underwent labial graft reconstructions, 15 of whom had surgery via their initially described transpubic approach, 4 strictly transvaginal, and 5 via a combined approach. Six patients required bilateral grafts. The authors report after follow-up of 42.3 months, 16/24 patients had complete continence, with 2 fistula recurrences and 1 stricture requiring surgical correction. Overall, labial grafts have good outcomes reported in the literature, making it an option to consider in the setting of complex urethrovaginal fistula repair or in the setting of loss of viable vaginal skin.

Bladder Flaps

While local tissue urethroplasties are quite successful, if there is inadequate viable vaginal or labial tissue available due to the extent of the injury, a bladder flap urethroplasty may be utilized. Additionally, this technique can be used for quite proximal or bladder neck injuries, or complete urethral loss. The bladder flap provides a well-vascularized flap made from muscle, which is thought to potentially aid in continence postoperatively [53, 54]. However, it is a more technically demanding procedure and requires more extensive dissection; therefore, it is generally thought it should not be used unless there are no other local tissues available or reconstruction or in the event of a previously failed procedure.

There are two techniques described for bladder flaps, anterior and posterior [8]. The anterior bladder wall flap was initially described by Tanagho in 1976 for the bladder neck and urethral reconstruction in the three female children with congenital absence of the urethra [55]. In this procedure done transvaginally, the bladder is mobilized anteriorly. Starting at the bladder neck, two parallel vertical or oblique incisions in the bladder are made to raise a flap, which is then tubularized over a urethral catheter. Oblique flaps are shorter; however, they are thought to decrease the risk of postoperative fistula formation due to avoiding a midline suture line abutting the anterior vaginal wall as compared to vertical incisions [56]. The anterior vaginal wall is then sharply dissected off the pubic bone, which can be difficult due to scarring depending on the mechanism of injury. This allows for the neourethra to be routed to the vestibule and sutured into place, thus creating the neomeatus. This procedure can also be performed abdominally via retropubic approach

The posterior bladder wall flap, or the Young-Dees-Leadbetter procedure, may also be utilized. This procedure has mostly been described in children with congenital anomalies, and due to the detrusor muscle bolstering the bladder neck, it is often used to provide continence at the level of the bladder neck without the need for catheterization or more morbid urinary diversions. The procedure was initially described by Young in 1922 for bladder neck reconstruction in two patients with epispadias [57] and has undergone several modifications over the years. Most recently, one group reports performing this procedure in a minimally invasive manner using a robotic approach [58].

Through a Pfannenstiel or midline incision, the retropubic space is entered and the anterior bladder is opened over the vesicourethral junction. In the posterior midline, two parallel incisions are made to create the bladder flap. Triangular portions of bladder mucosa are removed on either side of the flap. The mucosal flap is then tubularized over a catheter and brought into the vaginal vestibule. The detrusor flaps on either side of the neourethra are closed over the reconstruction. This wrap of detrusor aids in continence and funnels the bladder neck. Classically, the procedure also required bilateral ureteral reimplantation due to the proximity of the flap to the ureters, which should be performed before creation of the neourethra. In cases of a minimally invasive approach allowing for distal dissection under the pubic bone or in cases where a great deal of urethral length is not required, ureteral reimplantation may be avoided with careful identification of the ureteral orifices throughout the procedure. Due to the abdominal approach and the need for ureteral reimplantation, this procedure is quite a bit more invasive and morbid than even the anterior bladder wall flap.

The literature on outcomes using bladder flaps for urethral or bladder neck reconstruction for women with severe urethral damage is quite scarce (Table 1). In Tanagho's initial description of the anterior bladder wall flap, all patients were continent after surgery [55]. Hemal et al. reported a series of five girls with complete urethral loss from pelvic trauma [56]. In this series, three of the five girls were treated with a Tanagho bladder flap urethroplasty, all of whom had a successful reconstruction and were continent afterward. Finally, in a retrospective series of 16 women who had post-traumatic urethral loss, six patients underwent a bladder flap urethroplasty reconstruction [50]. At a mean follow-up of 42 months, four of the six patients had complete continence (67%), and all patients were able to void with adequate stream after surgery, with a mean peak flow of 19.9 ml/s. The use of tubularized bladder flaps has also been reported in patients with significant urethrovaginal fistulas and urethral loss after obstetric complications [59]. In such patients, due to large fistulas, vaginal flap procedures may not be technically feasible. In a series of 20 women in West Africa who underwent an anterior bladder flap for urethral reconstruction, 18 patients had a successful repair. Complications reported included SUI in four, requiring further surgery (22%). Additionally, two patients in this series had refractory detrusor instability and a small bladder capacity. The patient's bladder capacity should be evaluated preoperatively and deemed adequate such that the loss of volume will not result in capacity or compliance issues [8]. In terms of other unique complications of the procedure, one series reporting on two patients who underwent anterior bladder wall flaps for urethrovaginal fistula repair after pelvic trauma had one patient develop mucosal prolapse at the junction of the neourethra to the bladder, which resulted in internal obstruction of the bladder outlet and voiding difficulties [52]. The authors resected this tissue endoscopically with resolution of obstruction and good urinary flow.

The Young-Dees-Leadbetter-type posterior bladder wall procedure has been generally used in children for bladder neck reconstruction. There are however a few reports of this procedure being used in adult female urethral reconstruction. A recent single institution series describes the use of both anterior and posterior bladder wall flaps in 22 female patients who suffered urethral loss due to pelvic fracture or obstetric trauma [60]. In this series, 16 patients underwent an anterior Tanagho-type reconstruction and 6 had a posterior bladder flap reconstruction. All procedures were performed in a combined abdominal and vaginal approach. After a mean follow-up of 38 months, 18 patients were continent; however, 2 had voiding difficulty (one patient from each group) requiring catheterization. In this series, the decision on whether to pursue anterior or posterior bladder wall flap was not discussed, and outcomes of the two procedures were not directly compared. While bladder flap reconstructions do offer satisfactory outcomes reported in the literature, they can be technically demanding and patients may suffer complications of bladder volume loss. Therefore, they should only really be utilized when local tissue flaps are not viable options.

Flaps for Tissue Interposition or Alternative Vaginal Closures

After urethral reconstruction is complete, other flaps may be utilized to either bolster the repair or for skin coverage. Depending on the assessment of tissue viability in addition to other technical aspects of the completed repair, including blood supply and tension of the closure, a flap may be used in order to support the repair. In the vast majority of women, a labial fat pad or Martius flap works well for this, and in many of the previously mentioned series, Martius flaps are used [8, 53, 61]. Some series report using a Martius flap routinely in all patients [49, 62], while others state they are used in the minority of patients and that local tissue available for a multilayer closure is usually adequate [8]. Likely, this really depends on the extent of the primary injury. A recent retrospective review aimed to assess the subjective and objective outcomes of 159 women after undergoing a Martius flap for any indication, including during female urethral reconstruction [63]. In this series, two women experienced postoperative hematoma that subsequently resolved without further interventions and one woman experienced a wound infection. When surveyed postoperatively regarding the cosmetic outcomes after the procedure, 79% of women reported they felt the labial cosmesis was "good" or "excellent" and only one woman felt it was "unsatisfactory." Rectus abdominis muscle flaps have also been described [64, 65]. This muscle flap is based on the inferior epigastric vessels and has had good outcomes in the literature with no recurrences when used for interposition for urethrovaginal fistulas. There is some limited use of gracilis muscle flaps reported to support the repair as well [66–68]. This can be quite a morbid procedure due to large incision in the inner thigh and has little contemporary literature specifically on its use in female urethral reconstruction. It is however a good technique to keep in the reconstructive urologist's armamentarium. Some studies have shown a decreased recurrence rate or decreased failure rate of complex procedures including vesicovaginal fistula repairs or bladder neck closures with tissue interposition flaps [69, 70]. However, others have shown no differences, although it is likely these retrospective case series are biased such that patients who would have a successful repair without interposition flaps were the ones who did not receive them [16].

Occasionally, after urethral reconstruction, the vaginal mucosa cannot be closed primarily over the neourethra in the midline or an inverted "U" incision. In these instances, other flaps may be utilized to provide skin coverage of the incision. A rotational labial pedicle graft may be utilized and harvested in a similar manner as mentioned above. However, the side of the graft with the skin faces the outside to provide epithelial coverage. Similarly, a Martius flap can be utilized by taking full-thickness labial skin flap. Myocutaneous flaps including gracilis or rectus abdominis have also been described with good results [71, 72]. While the use of different cutaneous flaps for skin coverage of the wound have been described, their use is quite rarely required. Blaivas et al. reported in about 100 cases performed, only requiring a flap for skin coverage three times [8]. Regardless, it is important for reconstructive urologists to be familiar with the options for wound coverage to protect the integrity of their complex reconstructive repairs.

Bladder Neck Closure or Urinary Diversion

In the event that complex urethral reconstruction is not possible, or not in the patient's primary goals, other options can be pursued, including bladder neck closure with suprapubic tube or catheterizable channel or vesicostomy, or complete urinary diversion.

Bladder Neck Closure

Bladder neck closure may be pursued in the event a urethral reconstruction is not possible or desired. In neurogenic patients with urethral erosions who are already dependent on catheterization and therefore volitional urethral voiding would not be restored even with urethroplasty, bladder neck closure with suprapubic catheter or other bladder drainage method can be a good option. If the presenting issue is severe incontinence, an overtight pubovaginal fascial sling should be considered, which allows the preservation of possible urethral access if needed. If a sling has failed or is not possible due to severe tissue loss or fistula, then a bladder neck closure may be pursued. While some surgeons may opt directly for urinary diversion, a benefit of considering bladder neck closure first is that it allows for suprapubic tube for bladder drainage and avoids the need to use bowel segments for reconstruction. It is important that if the bladder is being left in place, it is of adequate compliance; otherwise, bladder augmentation can also be performed.

Transvaginal Approach

Bladder neck closures in female patients can usually be accomplished transvaginally and therefore are often a preferred option over the morbidity of an abdominal surgery such as a urinary diversion for a transabdominal bladder neck closure. The transvaginal technique for bladder neck closure was first described in 1985 by Zimmern et al. [73].

At the start of the procedure, a suprapubic catheter may be placed, unless another form of bladder drainage has already been established (such as a continent stoma or ileovesicostomy). After bladder drainage is established, an inverted "U"-shaped incision is made in the anterior vaginal wall with the apex close to the urethral meatus, and the vaginal flap is raised in the usual fashion. This dissection is continued to the bladder neck and extended laterally through the endopelvic fascia to allow for adequate mobilization of the bladder neck. Any remaining damaged urethra is excised circumferentially and carried back to the bladder neck. The mucosa is closed in one layer (Fig. 3a), followed by another layer of perivesical fascia and detrusor muscle (Fig. 3). The second muscular layer should be sutured from the bladder neck to the bladder behind the pubic bone and thereby roll the bladder neck closure into the retropubic space to decrease the incidence of fistula formation by ensuring the suture lines are not overlapping (Fig. 3b). The anterior vaginal wall flap is advanced and closed (Fig. 4). Other flaps can be used for wound closure as needed depending on tissue viability, including Martius flaps.

Abdominal Approach

The abdominal bladder neck closure performed via a retropubic approach is another option. The patient is placed in a low lithotomy position to allow for vaginal access intraoperatively. The procedure can be performed via either a Pfannenstiel or lower midline incision. The space of Retzius is entered to create an adequate amount of working space. The bladder neck is dissected along the urethra as distally as possible and the pubourethral ligaments should be transected until there is adequate urethral mobility. The urethra is transected to maximize the length of the urethral stump, which may not be much in some patients. The distal urethra should be closed. Next, the bladder is opened anteriorly down through the bladder neck and the ureteral orifices should be identified. The dissection is then continued posteriorly from the bladder neck into the vesicovaginal space,

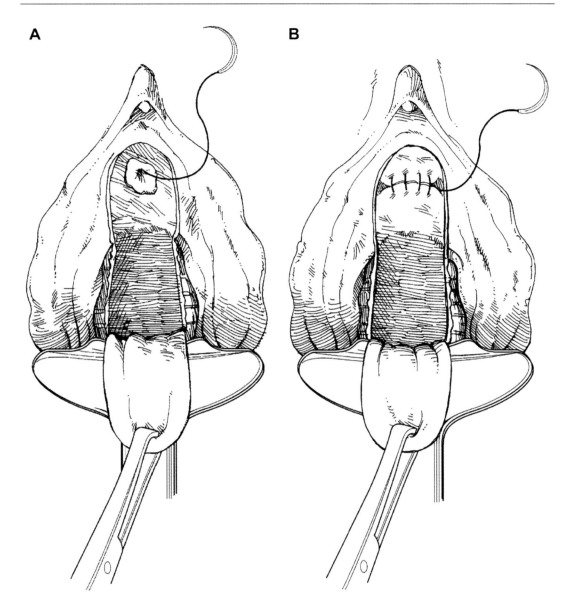

Fig. 3 Technique for transvaginal bladder neck closure. (**a**) After excision of the remaining urethra, the bladder neck mucosa is closed with a vertical running suture. (**b**) The muscular bladder wall and perivesical fascia are closed in a horizontal fashion in a second layer to avoid overlapping suture lines and to rotate the suture line under the pubic bone. (Reprinted with permission [53])

such that the bladder can be mobilized until it is rolled away from the inlet. Prior to bladder closure, a suprapubic tube is usually placed. The bladder neck is then closed in two layers. The first mucosal layer is generally vertical, and the second muscular layer is horizontal and used to roll the closure up and away from the urethra under the pubic bone.

Outcomes of Bladder Neck Closure

Both approaches for bladder neck closure have been used in women with devastated urethras

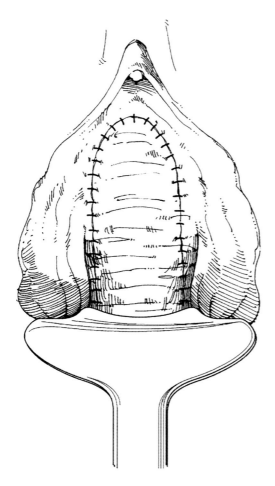

Fig. 4 Technique for transvaginal bladder neck closure. The anterior vaginal wall flap is advanced over the bladder closure and sutured as the third and final layer of the repair. (Reprinted with permission [53])

and are effective. In general, the abdominal approach is considered to have increased morbidity as compared to the vaginal approach due to abdominal entry. However, the vaginal approach has had a higher rate of vesicovaginal fistula formation in some studies [74–77]. There have been several series looking at outcomes of fistula repairs via both approaches.

One case report describes management of a woman with urethral erosion from indwelling catheter for neurogenic bladder with a successful transvaginal bladder neck closure with subsequent Mitrofanoff procedure for bladder drainage [78]. Another single institution retrospective review of 11 women with urethral erosions from long-term urethral catheterization for neurogenic bladder describes using the remainder of the posterior urethral plate to aid in rolling of the bladder under the pubic bone [76]. All women in this series had their bladder managed with suprapubic catheter. The posterior urethral plate at the time of bladder neck closure was not excised, but incorporated the closure to aid in rolling the suture line up under the pubic bone to aid in prevention of postoperative fistula formation. Additionally, the authors state this approach may help ensuring the closure is far from the ureteral orifices. In their series with 9.6 months of follow-up, there were no immediate postoperative complications and patients remained in the hospital only 1.7 days on average. One patient however failed at 6 weeks, but was subsequently salvaged with a transabdominal repair.

With regard to the literature on women undergoing bladder neck closures via an abdominal, there are only a few small series. One series looking at 35 neurogenic patients undergoing bladder neck closure included 12 women [79]. These patients were managed with suprapubic catheters, catheterizable stomas, or ileovesicostomy. Overall, authors reported a 94% success rate; however, 2 of the 12 women in the study failed and required transabdominal repairs. Another series of patients undergoing abdominal bladder neck closure included four women [80]. Patients in this series underwent a continent vesicostomy creation with or without bladder augmentation. Women in this series had neurogenic bladder with catheter erosions and one patient had a vulvectomy for cancer with a devastated urethra. In all patients, an omental flap was used for tissue interposition. They report no recurrent fistula formation, but an overall 82% success rate at 68 months of follow-up. Finally, in one series including 24 women with neurogenic bladder who underwent a bladder neck closure with suprapubic catheter placement, 2 patients had a transvaginal closure versus 22 who underwent a transabdominal procedure [74]. There was a high postoperative complication rate observed in this series of 52%, and both women who had a transvaginal repair failed with a recurrent fistula.

In the short term, the abdominal approach is thought to have more complications due to abdominal entry and longer operative time. This was demonstrated in a recent series that retrospectively looked at 64 women undergoing either a transvaginal or transabdominal bladder neck closure with the objective of comparing outcomes of the two approaches [16]. The most common reason for bladder neck closure again included women with urethral erosion from long-term catheter use, and all patients were managed with a suprapubic catheter. In their study, 35 women underwent a transvaginal repair and 29 a transabdominal repair, with Martius or omental interposition flaps used as needed. After a mean follow-up of 36.8 months (median 21 months), 83.9% of all patients were continent, which was unchanged between the two groups. The transvaginal procedure had a shorter operative time and length of hospital stay (1.5 days vs. 4.9 days in the transabdominal group). Additionally, the short-term complication rate was lower in the transvaginal group (5.7% vs. 31%). Multiple patients in both groups had complications from their suprapubic catheter requiring revision or bladder stones that required intervention, and these rates did not differ based on surgical approach. Therefore, the authors concluded similar outcomes for patients regardless of the approach, aside from the increase in immediate postoperative morbidity with an abdominal surgical approach.

Regardless of the approach, the bladder neck closure is something that can be considered in women with severely damaged urethras that may save them the need to progress to urinary diversion. However, the procedure is complex and can result to numerous complications, in addition to closing off the possibility of urethral bladder access; therefore, we would not advocate for this procedure without first exhausting other reconstructive options.

Urinary Diversion

Finally, patients who have failed other surgical options may undergo a urinary diversion. This is generally performed, if possible, with concomitant supratrigonal cystectomy, as the complication rates for the retained organ can be quite high [81, 82]. Like all urinary diversions, the complication rates can be quite high, with overall complication rate from 11% to 29% in the literature [30]. In many of the series discussed in this chapter regarding other surgical repairs, patients who failed their reconstruction proceeded to urinary diversion as a final option. Urinary diversion and the use of bowel for lower urinary tract reconstruction will be discussed in detail in another chapter.

Repair after Eroded Synthetic Sling

In the event that synthetic sling material has eroded into the urethra, it merits prompt and complete surgical removal. This involves excision of the sling with reconstruction of the urethra. If the mesh perforates the urethra along its diameter, a midline urethrotomy may be performed to completely excise the mesh. If the erosion is small, the urethral defect may be primarily repaired, with care being taken not to narrow the urethral lumen which can cause a urethral stricture. If the erosion is large and excision results in a large urethral defect, any of the aforementioned reconstructive techniques may be utilized for urethral repair. Like all reconstructive surgeries, multilayer closure with nonoverlapping suture lines is advocated to avoid urethrovaginal fistula formation. Complications of synthetic sling surgery and surgical technique for excision will be discussed elsewhere in this book.

Autologous Fascial Pubovaginal Sling for Associated Stress Urinary Incontinence

Given the short length of the female urethra, there is a greater risk of incontinence after surgical reconstruction, due to loss of native continence mechanisms during initial injury or surgical dissection [31]. Simultaneous treatment with an autologous fascial pubovaginal sling with or without Martius flap is advocated at the time of urethral reconstruction by some [8, 83]. Blaivas et al.

reported a high incontinence rate in their early experience with vaginal flap reconstructions (about 50%), and all patients with postoperative incontinence went on to be cured with fascial slings; therefore, these authors advocate for the use of routine autologous fascial pubovaginal sling at the time of initial repair [18, 32]. However, others believe that sling placement should be delayed until the patient has recovered from urethral reconstruction, especially if the repair is in the proximal or mid-urethra [84]. It is agreed upon, however, that placement of a synthetic mid-urethral sling is contraindicated in these patients due to the high risk of urethral exposure in this scenario [12]. If a pubovaginal fascial sling is to be used, it is thought that Stamey needles or other instrument to pass the sling should be passed in the retropubic space prior to complex urethral reconstruction is performed if possible, in order to minimize risk of damaging the neourethra and any local flaps during Stamey needle passage. If a tissue interposition flap, such as a Martius flap, is to be used, this is generally placed over the urethral reconstruction underneath the fascial sling.

Conclusions

Severe damage to the female urethra or complete urethral loss is a rare but serious condition. Diagnosis with careful physical examination and a high clinical suspicion for fistula or other abnormalities is required when evaluating these complex patients in order to provide accurate patient counseling and for surgical planning. The surgical management of these patients is complex and often requires advanced reconstructive techniques. Surgical urethral reconstruction can be accomplished by primary closure, vaginal tissue flaps, labia minora pedicle grafts, or bladder flaps. In the event that urethral reconstruction fails or is not possible, transvaginal or transabdominal bladder neck closure or urinary diversion may be required. There are no studies comparing these techniques; therefore, direct comparison of outcomes is difficult. Generally, the decision regarding surgical reconstructive technique depends on the mechanism of injury, health of local tissues for flaps, and previous reconstructive surgeries. Additionally, all decisions regarding choice of reconstruction should be made with the patient using a shared decision-making model in order to improve each individual patient's quality of life.

The outcome data available for female urethral reconstruction in the devastated urethra are quite limited to single institution retrospective case series, with small sample sizes and no consistent outcome measures. In general, success after reconstruction has been defined as not requiring further interventions. However, the follow-up is generally short, and the series with longer follow-up suggests that nearly 50% of these patients will require some sort of further intervention, whether that is minor or major [31]. Additionally, the need for further interventions in the future does not necessarily mean failure of the initial urethral reconstruction. However, these series do demonstrate that these surgical techniques are safe and often successful procedures. Finally, adherence to the general principles of reconstructive urology including careful planning of surgical incisions, creating a tension-free multilayer urethral closure, and adequate bladder drainage will optimize success of the reconstruction.

Cross-References

- ▶ Bladder Augmentation and Urinary Diversion
- ▶ Complications of Stress-Urinary Incontinence Surgery
- ▶ Female Urethral Reconstruction
- ▶ Indications and Use of Bowel in Female Lower Urinary Tract Reconstruction: Overview
- ▶ Surgical Reconstruction of Pelvic Fracture Urethral Injuries in Females

References

1. Perucchini D, DeLancey JO, Ashton-Miller JA, Peschers U, Kataria T. Age effects on urethral striated muscle I. changes in number and diameter of striated muscle fibers in the ventral urethra. Am J Obstet Gynecol. 2002;186(3):351–5.

2. Pandit M, DeLancey JO, Ashton-Miller JA, Iyengar J, Blaivas M, Perucchini D. Quantification of intramuscular nerves within the female striated urogenital sphincter muscle. Obstet Gynecol. 2000;95(6):797–800.
3. Cardozo L, Staskin DR. Textbook of female urology and urogynecology. Boca Raton: CRC Press/Taylor & Francis Group; 2017.
4. McGuire EJ. The innervation and function of the lower urinary tract. J Neurosurg. 1986;65(3):278–85.
5. Hinman F. Atlas of urosurgical anatomy: development of the female genital tract and urethra. London: Saunders; 1993. p. 393–4.
6. Blaivas JG, Santos JA, Tsui JF, Deibert CM, Rutman MP, Purohit RS, et al. Management of urethral stricture in women. J Urol. 2012;188(5):1778–82.
7. Anast J, Brandes SB, Klutke C. Female urethral reconstruction. Urethral reconstructive surgery. Springer, Totowa, NJ; 2008. p. 303–13.
8. Blaivas JG, Purohit RS. Post-traumatic female urethral reconstruction. Curr Urol Rep. 2008;9(5):397–404.
9. Lee UJ, Goldman H, Moore C, Daneshgari F, Rackley RR, Vasavada SP. Rate of de novo stress urinary incontinence after urethral diverticulum repair. Urology. 2008;71(5):849–53.
10. Kliment J, Berátš T. Urovaginal fistulas: experience with the management of 41 cases. Int Urol Nephrol. 1992;24(2):119–24.
11. Gomes CM, Carvalho FL, Bellucci CHS, Hemerly TS, Baracat F, Bessa J, et al. Update on complications of synthetic suburethral slings. Int Braz J Urol. 2017;43:822–34.
12. Kobashi KC, Albo ME, Dmochowski RR, Ginsberg DA, Goldman HB, Gomelsky A, et al. Surgical treatment of female stress urinary incontinence: AUA/SUFU guideline. J Urol. 2017;198(4):875–83.
13. Ford AA, Rogerson L, Cody JD, Aluko P, Ogah JA. Mid-urethral sling operations for stress urinary incontinence in women. Cochrane Database Syst Rev. 2017;7:CD006375.
14. Partin AW, Peters CA, Kavoussi LR, Dmochowski RR, Wein AJ. Campbell-Walsh-Wein urology twelfth edition review E-book. 2020.
15. McGuire EJ, Savastano J. Comparative urological outcome in women with spinal cord injury. J Urol. 1986;135(4):730–1.
16. Willis H, Safiano NA, Lloyd LK. Comparison of transvaginal and retropubic bladder neck closure with suprapubic catheter in women. J Urol. 2015;193(1):196–202.
17. Johnson D, Ellis H, Standring S, Healy J, Williams A, Collins P, et al. Gray's anatomy: the anatomical basis of clinical practice. Edinburgh: Churchill Livingstone Elsevier; 2008.
18. Flisser AJ, Blaivas JG. Outcome of urethral reconstructive surgery in a series of 74 women. J Urol. 2003;169(6):2246–9.
19. Wall LL, Karshima JA, Kirschner C, Arrowsmith SD. The obstetric vesicovaginal fistula: characteristics of 899 patients from Jos, Nigeria. Am J Obstet Gynecol. 2004;190(4):1011–6.
20. Arrowsmith S, Hamlin EC, Wall LL. Obstructed labor injury complex: obstetric fistula formation and the multifaceted morbidity of maternal birth trauma in the developing world. Obstet Gynecol Surv. 1996;51(9):568–74.
21. Roenneburg ML, Wheeless CR Jr. Traumatic absence of the proximal urethra. Am J Obstet Gynecol. 2005;193(6):2169–72.
22. Battaloglu E, Figuero M, Moran C, Lecky F, Porter K. Urethral injury in major trauma. Injury. 2019;50(5):1053–7.
23. Bjurlin MA, Fantus RJ, Mellett MM, Goble SM. Genitourinary injuries in pelvic fracture morbidity and mortality using the National Trauma Data Bank. J Trauma Acute Care Surg. 2009;67(5):1033–9.
24. Patel DN, Fok CS, Webster GD, Anger JT. Female urethral injuries associated with pelvic fracture: a systematic review of the literature. BJU Int. 2017;120(6):766–73.
25. Venn S, Greenwell T, Mundy A. Pelvic fracture injuries of the female urethra. BJU Int. 1999;83(6):626–30.
26. Patil U, Nesbitt R, Meyer R. Genitourinary tract injuries due to fracture of the pelvis in females: sequelae and their management. Br J Urol. 1982;54(1):32–8.
27. Perry M, Husmann D. Urethral injuries in female subjects following pelvic fractures. J Urol. 1992;147(1):139–43.
28. Hemal A, Singh I, Chahal R, Gupta N. Core through internal urethrotomy in the management of post-traumatic isolated bladder neck and prostatic urethral strictures in adults. A report of 4 cases. Int Urol Nephrol. 1999;31(5):703–8.
29. Podestá ML, Jordan GH. Pelvic fracture urethral injuries in girls. J Urol. 2001;165(5):1660–5.
30. Graham SD, Keane TE, Glenn JF. Glenn's urologic surgery. Philadelphia: Lippincott Williams & Wilkins; 2010.
31. Faiena I, Koprowski C, Tunuguntla H. Female urethral reconstruction. J Urol. 2016;195(3):557–67.
32. Blaivas JG. Vaginal flap urethral reconstruction: an alternative to the bladder flap neourethra. J Urol. 1989;141(3 Part 1):542–5.
33. Pushkar DY, Dyakov VV, Kosko JW, Kasyan GR. Management of urethrovaginal fistulas. Eur Urol. 2006;50(5):1000–5.
34. Smith JA, Howards SS, Preminger GM, Dmochowski RR. Hinman's atlas of urologic surgery revised reprint. Amsterdam: Elsevier Health Sciences; 2019.
35. Simonato A, Varca V, Esposito M, Carmignani G. Vaginal flap urethroplasty for wide female stricture disease. J Urol. 2010;184(4):1381–5.
36. Romman A, Takacs L, Gilleran J, Zimmern P. Vestibular flap urethroplasty in women with recurrent distal intramural urethral pathology. Neurourol Urodyn. 2015;34(3):213–8.
37. Romero-Maroto J, Verdú-Verdú L, Gómez-Pérez L, Pérez-Tomás C, Pacheco-Bru J-J, López-López

A. Lateral-based anterior vaginal wall flap in the treatment of female urethral stricture: efficacy and safety. Eur Urol. 2018;73(1):123–8.
38. Sarin I, Narain TA, Panwar VK, Bhadoria AS, Goldman HB, Mittal A. Deciphering the enigma of female urethral strictures: a systematic review and meta-analysis of management modalities. Neurourol Urodyn. 2021;40(1):65–79.
39. Kowalik C, Stoffel JT, Zinman L, Vanni AJ, Buckley JC. Intermediate outcomes after female urethral reconstruction: graft vs flap. Urology. 2014;83(5):1181–5.
40. Schwender CEB, Ng L, McGuire E, Gormley EA. Technique and results of urethroplasty for female stricture disease. J Urol. 2006;175(3):976–80.
41. Önol FF, Antar B, Köse O, Erdem MR, Önol ŞY. Techniques and results of urethroplasty for female urethral strictures: our experience with 17 patients. Urology. 2011;77(6):1318–24.
42. Bent AE, Foote J, Siegel S, Faerber G, Chao R, Gormley EA. Collagen implant for treating stress urinary incontinence in women with urethral hypermobility. J Urol. 2001;166(4):1354–7.
43. Coburn M, Amling C, Bahnson RR, Dahm P, Kerfoot BP, King L, et al. Urology milestones. J Grad Med Educ. 2013;5(1 Suppl 1):79–98.
44. Spilotros M, Malde S, Solomon E, Grewal M, Mukhtar B, Pakzad M, et al. Female urethral stricture: a contemporary series. World J Urol. 2017;35(6):991–5.
45. Hajebrahimi S, Maroufi H, Mostafaei H, Salehi-Pourmehr H. Reconstruction of the urethra with an anterior vaginal mucosal flap in female urethral stricture. Int Urogynecol J. 2019;30(12):2055–60.
46. Gormley EA. Vaginal flap urethroplasty for female urethral stricture disease. Neurourol Urodyn. 2010;29(S1):S42–S5.
47. Lane GI, Smith AL, Stambakio H, Lin G, Al Hussein Alawamlh O, Anger JT, et al. Treatment of urethral stricture disease in women: a multi-institutional collaborative project from the SUFU research network. Neurourol Urodyn. 2020;39(8):2433–41.
48. Wadie BS, ElHifnawy A, Khair AA. Reconstruction of the female urethra: versatility, complexity and aptness. J Urol. 2007;177(6):2205–10.
49. Falandry L, Xie D, Liang Z, Seydou M, Alphonsi R. Utilization of a pedicled labial flap, single or double face, for the management of post-obstetric urethral damage. J Gynecol Obstet Biol Reprod (Paris). 1999;28(2):151–61.
50. Radwan M, Abou Farha M, Soliman M, El Refai M, Ragab M, Shaaban A, et al. Outcome of female urethral reconstruction: a 12-year experience. World J Urol. 2013;31(4):991–5.
51. Xu YM, Sa YL, Fu Q, Zhang J, Xie H, Jin SB. Transpubic access using pedicle tubularized labial urethroplasty for the treatment of female urethral strictures associated with urethrovaginal fistulas secondary to pelvic fracture. Eur Urol. 2009;56(1):193–200.
52. Xu Y-M, Sa Y-L, Fu Q, Zhang J, Xie H, Feng C. A rationale for procedure selection to repair female urethral stricture associated with urethrovaginal fistulas. J Urol. 2013;189(1):176–81.
53. Rosenblum N, Nitti VW. Female urethral reconstruction. Atlas Urol Clin N Am. 2004;12(2):213–23.
54. Kunisawa Y, Kawabe K, Niijima T, Honda K, Takenaka O. A pharmacological study of alpha adrenergic receptor subtypes in smooth muscle of human urinary bladder base and prostatic urethra. J Urol. 1985;134(2):396–8.
55. Tanagho EA. Urethrosphincteric reconstruction for congenitally absent urethra. J Urol 1976;116(2):237–42.
56. Hemal A, Dorairajan L, Gupta N. Posttraumatic complete and partial loss of urethra with pelvic fracture in girls: an appraisal of management. J Urol. 2000;163(1):282–7.
57. Young HH. An operation for the cure of incontinence associated with epispadias. J Urol. 1922;7(1):1–32.
58. Burns EM, Prasad M, Purves JT, Stec AA. V3-01 robotic young-dees-leadbetter bladder neck reconstruction in the exstrophy-epispadias population: an initial report. J Urol. 2014;191(4S):e421.
59. Elkins TE, Ghosh T, Tagoe G, Stocker R. Transvaginal mobilization and utilization of the anterior bladder wall to repair vesicovaginal fistulas involving the urethra. Obstet Gynecol. 1992;79(3):455–60.
60. Patidar V, Dias S, Prakash S, Kumar L, Dwivedi US, Trivedi S. Results of bladder neck reconstruction using bladder flaps in complex female urethral defects. Int Urogynecol J. 2021;32(3):665–71.
61. Elkins TE, DeLancey J, McGuire EJ. The use of modified Martius graft as an adjunctive technique in vesicovaginal and rectovaginal fistula repair. Obstet Gynecol. 1990;75(4):727–33.
62. Sawant A, Kasat GV, Kumar V, Pawar P, Tamhankar A, Bansal S, et al. Reconstruction of female urethra with tubularized anterior vaginal flap. J Clin Diagn Res. 2016;10(7):PC01.
63. Malde S, Spilotros M, Wilson A, Pakzad M, Hamid R, Ockrim J, et al. The uses and outcomes of the Martius fat pad in female urology. World J Urol. 2017;35(3):473–8.
64. Atan A, Tuncel A, Aslan Y. Treatment of refractory urethrovaginal fistula using rectus abdominis muscle flap in a six-year-old girl. Urology. 2007;69(2):384. e11-. e13.
65. Bruce RG, El-Galley RE, Galloway NT. Use of rectus abdominis muscle flap for the treatment of complex and refractory urethrovaginal fistulas. J Urol. 2000;163(4):1212–5.
66. Ingelman-Sundberg A. An extravaginal technic in the operation for urethro-vaginal and vesico-vaginal fistulas. Gynecol Obstet Investig. 1947;123(6):380–5.
67. Hamlin RH, Nicholson EC. Reconstruction of urethra totally destroyed in labour. Br Med J. 1969;2(5650):147–50.

68. Patil U, Waterhouse K, Laungani G. Management of 18 difficult vesicovaginal and urethrovaginal fistulas with modified Ingelman-Sundberg and Martius operations. J Urol. 1980;123(5):653–6.
69. Kranz J, Anheuser P, Rausch S, Fechner G, Braun M, Müller SC, et al. Continent ileovesicostomy after bladder neck closure as salvage procedure for intractable incontinence. Cent Eur J Urol. 2013;66(4):481.
70. Altaweel WM, Rajih E, Alkhudair W. Interposition flaps in vesicovaginal fistula repairs can optimize cure rate. Urol Ann. 2013;5(4):270.
71. Chun JK, Behnam AB, Dottino P, Cohen C. Use of the umbilicus in reconstruction of the vulva and vagina with a rectus abdominis musculocutaneous flap. Ann Plast Surg. 1998;40(6):659–63.
72. De Lorenzi F, Loschi P, Rietjens M, Sangalli C, Manconi A, Zanagnolo V, et al. Neourethral meatus reconstruction for vulvectomies requiring resection of the distal part of the urethra. Eur J Surg Oncol. 2015;41(12):1664–70.
73. Zimmern PE, Hadley HR, Leach GE, Raz S. Transvaginal closure of the bladder neck and placement of a suprapubic catheter for destroyed urethra after long-term indwelling catheterization. J Urol. 1985;134(3):554–6.
74. Ginger VAT, Miller JL, Yang CC. Bladder neck closure and suprapubic tube placement in a debilitated patient population. Neurourol Urodyn. 2010;29(3):382–6.
75. Andrews H, Shah P. Surgical management of urethral damage in neurologically impaired female patients with chronic indwelling catheters. Br J Urol. 1998;82(6):820–4.
76. Rovner ES, Goudelocke CM, Gilchrist A, Lebed B. Transvaginal bladder neck closure with posterior urethral flap for devastated urethra. Urology. 2011;78(1):208–12.
77. Levy JB, Jacobs JA, Wein AJ. Combined abdominal and vaginal approach for bladder neck closure and permanent suprapubic tube: urinary diversion in the neurologically impaired woman. J Urol. 1994;152(6 Part 1):2081–2.
78. Athanasios Z, Minas P, Aris K, Fotios D, Athanasios Z, Charalampos M, et al. Transvaginal closure of urinary bladder opening and Mitrofanoff technique in a neurologically impaired female with chronic indwelling catheter: a case presentation. BMC Urol. 2021;21(1):1–5.
79. O'Connor R, Stapp E, Donnellan S, Hovey R, Tse V, Stone AR. Long-term results of suprapubic bladder neck closure for treatment of the devastated outlet. Urology. 2005;66(2):311–5.
80. Spahn M, Kocot A, Loeser A, Kneitz B, Riedmiller H. Last resort in devastated bladder outlet: bladder neck closure and continent vesicostomy—long-term results and comparison of different techniques. Urology. 2010;75(5):1185–92.
81. Eigner EB, Freiha FS. The fate of the remaining bladder following supravesical diversion. J Urol. 1990;144(1):31–3.
82. Neulander EZ, Rivera I, Eisenbrown N, Wajsman Z. Simple cystectomy in patients requiring urinary diversion. J Urol. 2000;164(4):1169–72.
83. Faerber G. Urethral diverticulectomy and pubovaginal sling for simultaneous treatment of urethral diverticulum and intrinsic sphincter deficiency. Tech Urol. 1998;4(4):192–7.
84. Webster GD, Sihelnik SA, Stone AR. Urethrovaginal fistula: a review of the surgical management. J Urol. 1984;132(3):460–2.

Vesicovaginal Fistula Repair: Minimally Invasive Approach

42

Caroline A. Brandon and Benjamin M. Brucker

Contents

Introduction	732
Etiology and Epidemiology	733
Evaluation and Diagnosis	734
History	734
Physical Exam	735
Diagnostic Investigations	735
Timing of Repair	737
Conservative Management Options	738
Surgical Repair Options	739
Comparing Laparoscopic and Robotic Approaches to the Open Vesicovaginal Fistula Repair	740
Perioperative Considerations	741
Getting Started: Positioning and Entry	741
Transvesical Approach	744
Extravesical Approach	745
Transvesical Versus Extravesical Approach	747
Bladder Layer Closure	747
Retrograde Filling of the Bladder	748
Vaginal Closure	748
Interposing Tissue Layer	748
Postoperative Catheterization	749
Modified Laparoscopic Approaches	750
Robotic Approach	751
Cost of Robotics: Is It Worth It?	753
Comparing Laparoscopic to Robotic Vesicovaginal Fistula Repair	754

C. A. Brandon · B. M. Brucker (✉)
New York University School of Medicine, New York, NY, USA
e-mail: Caroline.brandon@nyulangone.org; Benjamin.brucker@nyulangone.org

© Springer Nature Switzerland AG 2023
F. E. Martins et al. (eds.), *Female Genitourinary and Pelvic Floor Reconstruction*,
https://doi.org/10.1007/978-3-031-19598-3_43

Other Outcomes 754
Other Urinary Symptoms 754
Long-Term Sexual Function 754

Future Directions 755

Conclusion 755

Cross-References 756

References 756

Abstract

Vesicovaginal fistula is an abnormal connection between the bladder and the vagina that can lead to continuous leakage of urine. The condition can be associated with significant psychosocial stress for women. This chapter focuses on the pre-operative, perioperative, and postoperative considerations surrounding laparoscopic and robot-assisted laparoscopic repairs of vesicovaginal fistula. The evaluation of vesicovaginal fistula, conservative management, and timing of repair are all discussed. Particular attention is paid to examining various surgical techniques that can be performed in a minimally-invasive fashion, as well as the challenges and advantages of each approach. Crucial perioperative components of a minimally-invasive fistula repair, including patient positioning, fistula identification and dissection, bladder closure, use of interposing tissue, and bladder drainage, are all addressed within the context of basic principles of fistula repair. Furthermore, the use of robotic assistance in vesicovaginal fistula repair is also considered given the increasing availability and proficiency in robotic surgery. Current literature surrounding surgical outcomes, lower urinary tract symptoms, and sexual function following these repairs is also reviewed. This chapter serves as a tool for surgeons considering a minimally-invasive approach to vesicovaginal fistula repair

Keywords

Vesicovaginal fistula repair · Laparoscopic · Robotic · Extravesical · Transvesical · Interposing graft · Timing

Introduction

Vesicovaginal fistula is an abnormal connection between the urinary bladder and the vagina (Fig. 1). Some of the earliest scientific evidence of vesicovaginal fistula dates back to remains from ancient Egypt. Published in the 1930s, the cadaveric dissection of the mummified remains of Queen Henhenit, wife of King Menthotep II (circa 2050 BC), revealed a large vesicovaginal fistula [1]. The proposed mechanism at the time of this discovery was obstructed labor based on the mummy's severely narrowed pelvis.

Worldwide, the prevalence of vesicovaginal fistula is unknown given that the majority of vesicovaginal fistula occur in sub-Saharan and South Asian countries, where reporting may be challenging and many do not access medical care at all [2]. However, the World Health Organization (WHO) estimates that over two million women live with obstetric fistula, with 50,000–100,000 new cases annually, making this a major burden on healthcare systems worldwide, as well as a significant source of distress to affected women [3]. If left untreated, urogenital fistula, including vesicovaginal fistula, can be devastating for a woman's physical and mental health, causing social isolation, depression, and physical discomfort, not to mention the financial cost of products to manage the persistent urinary leakage. As such, the diagnosis of a vesicovaginal fistula requires clinical suspicion, a thorough physical examination, and appropriate testing that will help with subsequent management. This chapter will focus on the minimally invasive techniques, particularly laparoscopic and robotic repairs of vesicovaginal fistula.

Fig. 1 A sagittal depiction of a vesicovaginal fistula, which constitutes an abnormal connection between the bladder and the vagina. This schema includes a uterus, which may not always be present. (Reprinted from wiki images: https://commons.wikimedia.org/wiki/Category:Vesicovaginal_fistula#/media/File:Vesicovaginal_Fistula.png)

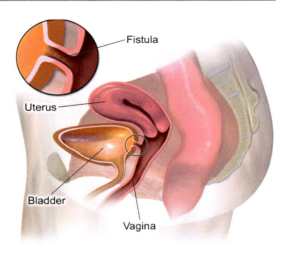

Etiology and Epidemiology

Worldwide, the most common cause of vesicovaginal fistula is obstetrical injury. This usually occurs secondary to prolonged obstructed labor and lack of access to medical care and prompt operative delivery. The "obstructed labor complex," described by Arrowsmith et al., explains the pathophysiology of obstetric fistula and associated multi-organ morbidity [4]. Genitourinary injury is determined by the level at which the fetal head impacts in the pelvis, arresting delivery and results in prolonged pressure on tissue trapped between the fetal head and the boney pelvis. This pressure results in ischemia, then necrosis, and ultimately breakdown of tissue. The result of this is a large devascularized defect. According to Arrowsmith et al., the average obstetric fistula measures 2.5 cm (0.1–10 cm) and is often associated with extensive scarring. Furthermore, depending on the fetal station and extent of necrosis, the bladder trigone, bladder neck, or the urethra (urethrovaginal) may be involved. Also, other urogenital fistula can coexist, such as rectovaginal, compounding the suffering of the patient and complexity of management [5].

Since the advent of operative obstetrics in the developed world, obstetric fistulae are rare, while the majority are iatrogenic, with approximately 75% following a hysterectomy [6, 7]. The incidence of iatrogenic vesicovaginal fistula is estimated at 0.2–2%. Iatrogenic fistula often result from an unrecognized injury to the bladder during pelvic surgery. This can occur from blunt or sharp dissection, delayed thermal injury, or devascularization as a result of crush injury, as well as inadvertent incorporation of the bladder into the vaginal cuff closure during hysterectomy [8–10]. Another cause of iatrogenic vesicovaginal fistula is injury from pelvic radiation used in the treatment of pelvic malignancies such as cervical, uterine, or colorectal cancer. Radiation causes fibrosis in the lamina propria and obliterative arteritis of small and medium arteries, leading to atrophy or necrosis of the bladder epithelium, ulceration, and subsequently a fistula [11]. The estimated rate of vesicovaginal fistula after radiotherapy for cervical cancer is 0.6–2% and quoted as high as 47.8% in one series of women undergoing concomitant chemotherapy with radiation for stage 4 cervical cancer [12, 13].

Bevacizumab is a humanized anti-vascular endothelial growth factor (VEGF) monoclonal antibody that is used in the management of advanced cervical, ovarian, and colorectal cancers, and has also been shown to increase the risk of fistula formation [14–17]. It works by depriving tumors of oxygen and nutrients while improving the delivery of chemotherapy to the tumor. Reports of bevacizumab-induced vesicovaginal fistula exist [15]. Advanced local disease can also result in fistula formation. In one study of 71 locally advanced cervical cancer, 8 (11.3%) women presented with vesicovaginal fistula prior to any treatment, and 15 of the remaining 63 (23.8%) developed a vesicovaginal fistula during their posttreatment follow-up course [18]. Eighty-seven percent (13/15) vesicovaginal fistula occurred within 1 year of radiotherapy, with a median onset of 3.1 months (95% CI, 1.5–11.2 months) following the start of external beam radiotherapy. Of the 15 fistula that formed following treatment, 6 (40%) were associated with local recurrence. As such, in any patient with prior or suspected malignancy, biopsy at the site of fistula is necessary to rule out recurrent disease as this can alter counseling and management.

Mesh implants have been used in anti-incontinence procedures and prolapse repairs. Iatrogenic injury to the urinary bladder during mid-urethral sling insertion or prolapse repair can result in vesicovaginal fistula [19–21]. Though the pathophysiology has never been confirmed, it is suspected that the placement of mesh over an unrecognized iatrogenic injury prevents adequate healing and closure due to foreign body reaction, resulting in a persistent tract. Chronic infection in non-type I mesh implants may also play a role. In one series of 23 surgical mesh excisions of transvaginal mesh used for anterior prolapse with mesh kits, the incidence of concurrent vesicovaginal fistula was 9% [22]. In a systematic review of graft materials for transvaginal pelvic organ prolapse repairs, the rate of fistula formation was 1% [23]. Regardless of the etiology, vesicovaginal fistulae require a methodical evaluation and treatment approach that adheres to the principles of fistula repair [24].

Evaluation and Diagnosis

History

In any woman with a suspected vesicovaginal fistula, the evaluation always begins with a detailed history to assess for likely risk factors, etiology, and prognostic factors pertaining to the fistula. The classic presentation is constant urinary incontinence or vaginal drainage. It is imperative to characterize the presenting symptoms as they can mimic or coexist with more common lower urinary tract conditions. Timing, color, consistency of fluid, onset of leakage, positional variation, and associated symptoms, such as pain or urgency, are important when characterizing the leakage. The presenting symptom can vary with the size, location, and presence of coexisting fistula. The patient's risk factors for fistula, including obstetric, gynecologic, medical, surgical, oncologic, and social history, should be assessed. Whenever possible, prior operative notes and pathology reports should be reviewed to help with future operative planning. A broad differential diagnosis should be maintained for any continuous vaginal drainage (Table 1).

The classical presentation for a vesicovaginal fistula is constant urinary leakage both day and night, including during sleep. Other symptoms, such as blood-tinged vaginal discharge, gross hematuria, dysuria, or recurrent urinary tract infections, can suggest a vesicovaginal fistula. The presence of symptoms such as fever, chills, malaise, nausea, vomiting, ileus, and flank pain should alert to the possibility of a concurrent ureteral injury with a urinoma or obstruction. Concomitant urogenital fistula may add to the symptom complex accordingly, and suspicion

Table 1 Differential diagnosis of vaginal drainage

Vesicovaginal fistula
Ureterovaginal fistula
Urethrovaginal fistula
Vesicouterine fistula
Vesicocervical fistula
Ureterocervical fistula
Ureterofallopian fistula
Peritoneal-vaginal fistula
Pelvic abscess
Lymphocele
Ectopic ureter
Vaginal trapping of urine/vaginal voiding
Urgency urinary incontinence
Stress urinary incontinence
Mixed urinary incontinence
Overflow urinary incontinence
Vaginal discharge

should be maintained for the presence of multiple abnormal connections.

The timing of symptom onset relative to the suspected inciting event is also important. Immediate leakage following pelvic surgery suggests an unrecognized or failed repair of an iatrogenic bladder or ureteral injury. Thermal injury or crush injury may present in a delayed fashion, about 7–10 days after the initial operation. Patients with a history of prior radiation therapy may present immediately following or decades after treatment, and they may also be a harbinger for recurrence.

Physical Exam

A thorough physical exam is crucial in the evaluation of vesicovaginal fistula and should be carried out in a systematic fashion to ensure all signs and sequelae of the fistula are identified and documented. An abdominal exam should be performed to assess for tenderness, distension, flank pain, and assessment of prior incisions. A pelvic examination can identify perineal irritation from chronic incontinence and pad use. A speculum exam should be performed to assess for vaginal canal pooling of fluid. This fluid can be sent off for creatinine to confirm urinary origin. Identification and characterization of the fistula should be performed, including the size, location, and number of fistulous tracts present. The most common location for vesicovaginal fistula following hysterectomy is the vaginal cuff, thus special attention should be paid to the vaginal apex as well as the anterior vaginal wall. Other lesions in the vagina such as granulation tissue or friable mass may signal a fistulous tract and thus should be carefully inspected and noted. This is an opportune time to biopsy any lesion near to the fistula, particularly in women with a history of cancer, in order to rule out a primary lesion or disease recurrence. A small fistula may be difficult to identify on an exam, particularly in women with a stenotic vaginal canal, significant scarring, or difficulty tolerating an exam. As such, further evaluation with an exam under anesthesia or endoscopic or radiologic investigations should be pursued to confirm and characterize the fistulous tract.

Diagnostic Investigations

Several tests have been employed to confirm and better characterize the vesicovaginal fistula and concomitant injuries. A dye test is a simple office-based procedure that can confirm a connection between the bladder and the vagina, with a sensitivity reported up to 100% in one series [25]. The bladder is backfilled with methylene blue-stained saline using a sterile catheter and the vaginal canal is inspected for pooling of blue fluid. A double-dye tampon has been described both to localize a fistulous tract and to discern between a vesicovaginal and a ureterovaginal fistula [26]. The patient is given oral phenazopyridine, which turns the urine orange, approximately 1–2 h before the test. A tampon or a gauze is placed in the vagina. At the time of exam, the bladder is backfilled with methylene-blue saline. The patient is then asked to walk around for several minutes with positional changes that can incite leakage. The tampon is subsequently removed and evaluated for color. If the tampon is stained orange, this suggests a ureterovesical fistula. If the tampon is only blue, this suggests a vesicovaginal fistula or possibly a urethrovaginal fistula if more distal staining is seen. If the tampon demonstrates both colors, this suggests simultaneous fistulous tracts from both the bladder and the ureter.

Endoscopic evaluation is a crucial component of the evaluation of a vesicovaginal fistula. Cystoscopy has a 92–93% sensitivity rate for the diagnosis of vesicovaginal fistula [25, 27]. Flexible cystoscopes are extremely useful for performing both cystoscopic and vaginoscopic evaluations (Fig. 2). An in-office cystoscopy and vaginoscopy can be performed at the same time to locate and characterize the fistulous tract, including size, number, and proximity to adjacent structures such as the ureteral orifices or the bladder neck. This will help with surgical planning, particularly with the route of surgery (abdominal versus vaginal) and likelihood of need for a ureteral implant,

Fig. 2 (**a**) Cystoscopic evaluation demonstrating the right ureteral orifice (blue arrow) and the fistulous tract (red arrow). (**b**) Vaginoscopy demonstrating the fistula located at the right vaginal apex. (Courtesy of B. Brucker & C. Brandon, 2021, reprinted with consent)

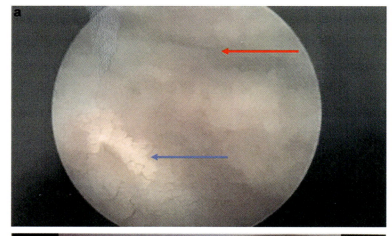

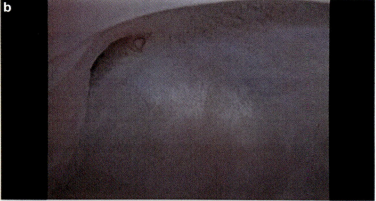

bladder neck reconstruction, autologous pubovaginal sling placement, or less likely, a urinary diversion. Cystoscopy under anesthesia allows for simultaneous retrograde pyelogram to evaluate the ureters and ureteral stenting as required. Vaginoscopy allows for visualization of the vaginal aspect of the suspected fistulous tract and can allow for direct biopsy in anyone with history of prior malignancy. If a fistula is suspected but difficult to visualize, backfilling the bladder with dye-stained saline and visualizing the spill can help to locate smaller tracts. Tandem cystoscopy and vaginoscopy are a useful way to evaluate mesh-related vesicovaginal fistula and identify the extent of mesh involvement.

Upper tract imaging is extremely important for evaluating the involvement of the upper urinary tract. A renal sonogram can evaluate for hydronephrosis and signs of ureteral obstruction. If obstruction is suspected, a retrograde pyelogram should be performed in the operating room to allow for simultaneous stenting of the ureter. If stenting is not possible, a percutaneous nephrostomy tube should be placed to allow for drainage prior to surgical repair. An antegrade nephrostogram can be performed at the same time to evaluate the remaining upper urinary tract. An excretory urogram in the form of an intravenous pyelogram, or more commonly today, a computer tomography urogram, is performed to rule out concomitant ureteral injury and can also evaluate for obstruction. Computer tomography can also allow for characterization of the fistula, including the number and sometimes size of tracts (Fig. 3). It can also evaluate the involvement of adjacent structures such as the uterus, fallopian tube, or cervix. In some clinical scenarios, magnetic resonance urography may also be used. Color Doppler

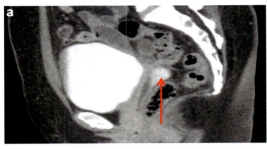 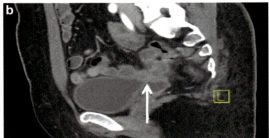

Fig. 3 (**a**) A sagittal view of a post-hysterectomy patient's computer tomography image demonstrating contrast on the bladder as well as the vagina, highlighted by the red arrow. (**b**) The same computer tomography image demonstrating contrast in both the bladder and spilling into the vaginal canal via the fistulous tract indicated by the white arrow. These images differ from the schema above as this patient is post-hysterectomy and no uterus is seen on imaging. (Courtesy of B. Brucker & C. Brandon, 2021, reprinted with consent)

ultrasonography has also been described as a useful imaging study for confirming the diagnosis of vesicovaginal fistula, with sensitivities of 92–100% [25, 27]. Cystography is another imaging option that has been used to confirm a suspected vesicovaginal fistula. A voiding cystogram can also be used to diagnose a urethrovaginal fistula.

Preoperative urodynamics may not be needed in all cases. However, urodynamics can have a role for planning and counseling given that many patients have concomitant lower urinary tract conditions such as stress urinary incontinence or detrusor overactivity [28]. Surgeons may offer a concurrent pubovaginal sling at the time of fistula repair depending on the presence or absence of stress urinary incontinence on testing. In some cases, especially with a larger fistula, maneuvers may be required to ensure the patient is adequately filled for urodynamic assessment. Packing the vagina may help keep fluid from leaking out. The use of simultaneous fluoroscopy at the time of urodynamics can be useful if more anatomical information is desired. Cystogram and voiding cystourethragram can be used independently to identify a fistula from the bladder or urethra. Bladder outlet obstruction can exist in patients with urethrovaginal fistula as there may be scarring, strictures, or foreign material such as a mesh sling that can be addressed at the time of surgery. The use of fluoroscopy (video urodynamics) can help evaluate this in women. In patients with prior radiation, compliance can be evaluated using urodynamics to determine whether a concomitant augmentation cystoplasty or urinary diversion procedure is required. Once a thorough history, examination, and assessment of adjacent structures have been performed, a patient-specific approach to management can be undertaken.

Timing of Repair

The timing of vesicovaginal repair has been debated. Traditionally, it was recommended that surgery be delayed to allow for resolution of acute inflammation from the underlying mechanism of injury. During this time, some patients maintain a Foley catheter for continued drainage and attempted closure of smaller tracts. More recently, some have suggested that delaying repair may result in increased psychosocial stress without improvement in cure rates. The definition of "immediate" varies between publications. Waaldijk defines immediate as less than 3 months from the initial insult [29]. Others report 4 weeks as their cut-off for immediate repairs, citing increasing technical difficulty during the 4–12 week healing period [30]. In an early study evaluating the timing of repair among primary and recurrent vaginal and open abdominal vesicovaginal fistula repairs, those performed within 1–3 months (mean 10.8 weeks) of the inciting injury had comparable closure rates to those who presented in a delayed manner (6–12 months following inciting procedure)

[31]. A comparative study evaluating early (<12 weeks, mean 7.4 weeks) versus late (>12 weeks, mean 75.2 weeks) repair of vesicovaginal fistula found no difference in first attempt cure rates between the two groups (87.8% versus 87.2%, $p = 0.06$) [32]. It should be noted that 95% of these fistulae were a consequence of obstructed labor and measured on average 5 cm in size (0.5–8 cm). Unfortunately, the authors did not discuss surgical approaches to repairs. In a study of 16 patients who underwent transvaginal repair of vesicovaginal fistula, there was no difference in success rates between repairs performed before and after 3 months (100% <3 months vs. 89% <3 months) [33].

Pushkar et al. reported on 210 transvaginal primary repairs of radiation-induced vesicovaginal fistula, noting a delay of 14.8 months (11–18 months) from diagnosis to intervention [11]. A successful closure was noted in 101 (48.1%) patients. Of those who failed the primary attempt, 98 of the 109 patients underwent a secondary operation within approximately 6 months of the initial attempt. The authors note that repair should be considered in a delayed fashion to allow for acute radiation-induced inflammation to subside, suggesting at least 12 months to allow for healing. During this time, they recommend surveillance of the fistula to monitor the evolution of the tract and rule out a recurrence of disease.

Nagraj et al. [34] published a series of 13 laparoscopic iatrogenic supratrigonal vesicovaginal fistula repairs with a mean size of 1.8 cm (1.4–3.1 cm) performed within 4 weeks of initial surgery (mean duration of symptoms 16.7 days) that demonstrated a 91.6% (11/12) success rate with a mean follow-up of 21 months (6–36 months) [34]. In this series, there was one (1/13) conversion to an open abdominal approach due to dense intraperitoneal adhesive disease. Another case series of 5 laparoscopic vesicovaginal fistula repairs performed over a median of 24 days (14–289 days) following initial total abdominal hysterectomy (TAH) reported 100% success without evidence of recurrence during a median follow-up of 56.1 weeks (26.6–74.0 weeks) [35]. The median size of the fistulous tract was 0.6 cm (0.5–0.9 cm) and all were supratrigonal. A series of seven patients with recurrent supratrigonal vesicovaginal fistula measuring a mean of 3 cm (range 2–4 cm) underwent robotic repair at a minimum of 4 months following prior attempts repair [36]. The repairs resulted in a 100% successful closure. With respect to timing of closure, the authors commented that patients presented from outside institutions at least 3 months after prior attempts, accounting for the delay. There was no comparative group to assess the impact of timing on closure success. Furthermore, there is no comparative study evaluating the timing of robotic vesicovaginal fistula repair. In a consensus statement made by the European Association of Urology, there was no minimum amount of time recommended from initial diagnosis to robotic repair [37]. As such, in a patient who desires immediate resolution and is without evidence of active infection or recent irradiation, early repair of a vesicovaginal fistula is a reasonable strategy that may spare women the distress of a prolonged delay without compromising closure rates.

Conservative Management Options

The literature related to the treatment of vesicovaginal fistula includes attempts at conservative management. Conservative management of a vesicovaginal fistula with continuous bladder drainage has been described with varying success [29, 38]. While the success rate of spontaneous closure with continuous bladder drainage varies (~15%), several factors, including size <10 mm, non-radiation, and decreased length of interval from insult to treatment, seem to correlate with a greater chance of success [39, 40]. The European Association of Urology suggests that if a conservative approach with continuous bladder drainage is undertaken, a trial of at least 12 weeks should be attempted [37]. Electrofulguration of the tract to induce fibrosis has also been described with a success rate of 73% when combined with 2 weeks of continuous bladder drainage in fistula smaller than 3.5 mm in diameter [41].

Others have described the use of fibrin glue or tissue sealants as a plug to allow for healing. Based on earlier use of blood products such as plasma, this technique was first described in 1979 in the Lancet, where the surgeons injected lyophilized fibrinogen, calcium, and thrombin into the fistula from a trans-inguinal approach (the Chevassu technique) [42]. A urethral catheter was left in situ for 8 weeks. At 4 month follow-up, the patient was dry. The authors hypothesize that closure of the fistula occurs slowly as the plug disappears by fibrinolysis and is replaced by connective tissue. Fibrin glue has also been instilled endoscopically. Morita and Tokue described the use of bovine collagen and fibrin glue to plug a 5 mm radiation-induced vesicovaginal fistula [43]. They describe electrofulguration of the fistulous tract to destroy the epithelized layer, narrowing the tract using bovine collagen injected transurethrally in the submucosal layer around the tract, and plugging the tract with fibrin glue. The authors then describe injecting more collagen circumferentially around the fistulous tract on the vaginal aspect to ensure retention of the glue. A Foley catheter remained in place for 3 weeks, and at the 11 month follow-up, the patient remained completely dry. Being that this procedure was performed entirely in the outpatient setting and may potentially be performed with only local anesthesia or minimal sedation, this provides a low-morbidity solution for small vesicovaginal fistula. Sharma et al. also describe endoscopic cannulation and injection of fibrin glue into a series of various urologic fistulous tracts, including two vesicovaginal fistula [44]. They note six successful cases (75%) with follow-up ranging from 0 to 34 months, with two cases requiring a second injection. Unfortunately, the sizes of the fistula were never disclosed, thus it remains unclear how useful this technique will be as the tract enlarges. A comparative study between endoscopic fibrin glue and surgical management of iatrogenic vesicovaginal fistula noted a 66% closure rate in six cases treated with endoscopic fibrin glue [45].

Other adhesives, such as cyanoacrylate, have also been used in the endoscopic management of vesicovaginal fistula [46]. Two cases involving recurrent iatrogenic vesicovaginal fistula, 4 mm and 5 mm in size, underwent cystoscopic injection of 0.5 ml of cyanoacrylate, followed by injection of 0.5 ml and 1 ml of cyanoacrylate injected transvaginally into the tract. Catheters were left in place for 8 and 10 days, and patients were dry at follow-up (5 and 3 months post-procedure, respectively). One patient experienced bladder spasms controlled with anticholinergics. The other experienced difficulty with removal of the catheter due to adhesion with the glue to the balloon. In a case series of 13 patients with various urologic fistula, including 3 iatrogenic vesicovaginal fistula, cyanoacrylate was instilled endoscopically [47]. The overall success rate was 85% (11/13) over a median follow-up period of 35 months (6–76 months). Among the three vesicovaginal fistulae included, the size of the tracts were 0.7 cm, 1.0 cm, and 1.5 cm, with failure of closure with transvaginal instillation of cyanoacrylate occurring in the largest of the three cases. Among these patients, the only complication noted was dysuria and hematuria from redundant cyanoacrylate, requiring cystoscopic removal of excess glue within 48 h of application. Stone formation in the bladder at the site of glue instillation was noted in a successfully treated patient with colovesical fistula; this was managed with endoscopic laser lithotripsy. The authors conclude that both the width and length of the fistulous tract are decisive features, explaining that narrower longer tracts are more likely to successfully seal with endoscopic plugging due to the increased surface area of the tract itself. Ultimately, endoscopic instillation of glues/sealants may be an effective conservative treatment option for vesicovaginal fistula less than 1 cm in size, given that they are low-morbidity, cost-effective, and moderately successful alternatives to surgical management. However, data on these techniques is limited to case series.

Surgical Repair Options

For vesicovaginal fistula that persists in spite of conservative management or in cases where conservative options may not be appropriate, surgical repair should be considered. Numerous factors are taken into account when considering the surgical approach of vesicovaginal fistulae: size and number of fistulae, complexity, mechanism of formation, location relative to other structures (e.g., trigone, ureters), the need for concurrent procedures, the tissue quality and need for interposing tissue or flaps, accessibility, patient comorbidities, as well as surgeon comfort and clinical experience. Repairs should follow the basic principles of fistula repair, presented Table 2. The two main approaches to vesicovaginal fistula repair are vaginal and abdominal. Traditionally, vaginal repairs are undertaken when the fistula is lower in the bladder (trigonal or lower), does not appear to involve the ureters or require any concurrent abdominal procedure, and is accessible by a surgeon comfortable with transvaginal surgery. For a more detailed discussion on the vaginal approach to vesicovaginal fistula repair, please refer to the next chapter by Sirls, Hoang Roberts, and Vollstedt.

The abdominal route may be preferred when the fistula is inaccessible vaginally (i.e., supratrigonal), in close proximity to the ureteral orifice, recurrent, and secondary to radiation so that an interposing tissue layer can be utilized [48]. The traditional abdominal procedure, known as the O'Conor technique, takes a transvesical approach to fistula repair by performing an intentional cystotomy to identify and repair the fistulous tract [49]. More recently, an extravesical technique has been described whereby the plane between the posterior bladder and vagina is developed beyond the fistula to allow for tissue mobilization and separate tension-free closure of both the vagina and the bladder [50]. With the emergence of advanced laparoscopy and robotics for deep pelvic surgery, abdominal techniques for vesicovaginal fistula repair have increasingly been performed using minimally invasive surgery. The first laparoscopic repair of vesicovaginal fistula was reported in 1994, followed by the first robotic repair in 2005 [51, 52]. Subsequent non-randomized comparative studies have shown that minimally invasive approaches to vesicovaginal fistula repair confer advantages over open abdominal surgery, including decreased blood loss, decreased length of hospital stay, and decreased postoperative analgesic requirements [48, 53].

Comparing Laparoscopic and Robotic Approaches to the Open Vesicovaginal Fistula Repair

At present, there are no randomized controlled trials comparing laparoscopic or robotic repairs to open vesicovaginal fistula repair, mainly due

Table 2 Basic principles of minimally invasive vesicovaginal fistula repair

Principle	Comment
Evaluate for concomitant injury	Consider upper tract imaging to evaluate the ureters and other necessary investigations to confirm extent of surgical repair
Rule out malignancy	In patients with history of malignancy, radiation, or any suspicious lesion, a biopsy of the tract or lesion should be performed
Adequate exposure	Consider split leg position to allow access to vagina and transurethral route to the bladder Consider displacing bowel away from surgical field Holding sutures may be helpful for manipulation of tissue
Dissection of surrounding tissue	Ensure adequate separation of bladder from vagina with adequate margins for tension-free closure of each layer
Avoid overlapping sutures	Consider perpendicular suture lines on the vagina and bladder Consider use of interposing tissue layer/graft
Watertight closure	Absorbable suture is preferable Confirm integrity of closure with retrograde fill Reinforce areas of leak with suture or tissue glue
Continuous bladder drainage	Adequate bladder drainage (i.e., transurethral and/or suprapubic catheter) Option to confirm integrity of bladder closure with postoperative cystogram prior to removal of catheter

to the challenges with sample size, as well as patient-specific and surgical variability. However, there are a limited number of studies comparing a minimally invasive approach to open procedures in a non-randomized manner. Ghosh et al. retrospectively compared 26 women with primary single supratrigonal vesicovaginal fistula who underwent either open transvesical repair or a laparoscopic transvesical repair [48]. While success rates were 13/13 (100%) in both groups, mean blood loss (58.69 ± 6.48 ml versus 147.30 ± 19.24 ml, $p < 0.0001$), mean hospital stay (4 ± 0.57 days versus 13 ± 1.04 days, $p < 0.0001$), analgesic requirement (261.53 ± 29.95 mg versus 617.30 ± 34.43 mg diclofenac sodium, $p < 0.0001$), and time to catheter removal (11.46 ± 1.66 days versus 27.46 ± 1.61 days, $p < 0.0001$) were all significantly lower in the laparoscopic repair group than the open. Mean operative time did not differ (153 ± 10.27 min versus 156.84 ± 12.96 min, $p = 0.41$). Xiong et al. evaluated 58 women with supratrigonal fistula who underwent laparoscopic ($N = 22$) or open ($N = 36$) transvesical repairs [54]. Among each group, 12/22 (54.5%) and 24/36 (66.7%) were primary fistula, and no one had previously received radiation. The success rates were 95.5% for laparoscopic and 83.3% for open repairs, though not statistically different ($p > 0.05$). Among recurrent fistula, the success rates were 90% for laparoscopic and 75% for open repairs ($p > 0.05$). However, mean blood loss [52 ml (40–75 ml) versus 103 ml (80–180 ml), $p < 0.05$] and mean hospital stay [5.6 days (4–7 days) versus 13.2 days (9–17 days), $p < 0.05$] were significantly lower among laparoscopic repairs. Together, these comparative studies suggest that similarly excellent cure rates can be obtained using conventional laparoscopy while reducing the morbidity associated with traditional open repairs.

Gupta et al. compared 12 women with recurrent vesicovaginal fistula who underwent robotic repair to 20 case controls who underwent open repair in the same time period, both of which were performed in a transvesical manner [53]. Success rates were similar between the robotic and open groups [12/12 (100%) versus 18/20 (90%), respectively, $p > 0.05$], although follow-up time was not explicitly stated. Importantly, length of stay [3.1 days (2–5 days) versus 5.6 days (4–10 days), respectively, $p < 0.05$] and blood loss [88 ml (50–200 ml) versus 170 ml (110–400 ml), respectively, $p < 0.05$] were both significantly less in the robotic group than the open group, mimicking the advantages of conventional laparoscopy. There were no differences in overall complication rates between groups. While there remains a gap in the literature regarding the direct comparison of minimally invasive and open vesicovaginal fistula repair, the current data suggests that success is not compromised with a minimally invasive approach, and given the reduction in morbidity and thus potential reduction in healthcare costs (at least with conventional laparoscopy), a minimally invasive approach should be considered whenever feasible so long as the surgeon is competent in this approach.

Perioperative Considerations

Getting Started: Positioning and Entry

Prior incision, institutional and regional guidelines should be consulted when determining antibiotic prophylaxis. Antibiotics should be administered within 60 min of incision [55, 56]. Choice of antibiosis may also be influenced by prior urine culture results. Venous thromboembolism prevention in the form of intermittent pneumatic compression should be initiated. Chemoprophylaxis should be considered based on risk factors, which can be assessed preoperatively using a validated risk-stratification tool [57]. Whether for traditional laparoscopic or robotic repair of vesicovaginal fistula, positioning is typically the same. Following administration of general anesthesia, it is advisable to place the patient in the dorsal lithotomy position (Fig. 4). This is done to maintain access to the vagina and bladder from below. Attention should be paid to avoid injury to the peroneal nerve, the femoral nerve, or the sciatic nerve when positioning the patient. Arms may or may not be tucked alongside the body for ease of bedside surgeon positioning.

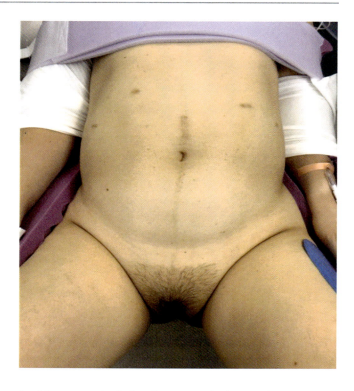

Fig. 4 Patient in dorsal lithotomy position for robot-assisted vesicovaginal fistula repair in order to allow exposure of the abdomen, transurethral access to the bladder, and access to the vagina simultaneously. (Courtesy of B. Brucker & C. Brandon, 2021, reprinted with consent)

Abdominal skin preparation is performed with a 70% alcohol-based solution; however, 10% povidone-iodine can be used if there is a contraindication to alcohol-based skin antiseptics. Vaginal antiseptics include 4% chlorhexidine gluconate or povidone-iodine should be used as the vaginal canal will be encountered intraoperatively [55].

Following surgical preparation of the field and sterile draping that allows simultaneous access to the abdomen as well as the vagina, urethra, and bladder. A cystoscopy is usually repeated to identify the ureteral orifices and their proximity to the fistulous tract. In some cases, due to the close relationship between the ureters and the fistula, the ureters can be stented with ureteral support stents (i.e., open-ended or Pollack catheter). These can be removed at the end of the case if appropriate. If there is suspicion for the need to leave stents in place longer term, the surgeon may elect to stent with double J-stents (or double pigtail catheters). In order to help identify the fistula tract during repair, the fistula can be intubated, possibly with a different color ureteral stent to aid in manipulation intraoperatively. At times, only a wire will be able to cannulate the tract, but having something through and through can aid in the identification and dissection to ensure that the entire fistula is dissected. This stent or wire can be externalized cystoscopically and secured vaginally with a clamp to prevent dislodging (Fig. 5).

Next, intraperitoneal entry can be obtained in any standard fashion, usually left to surgeon preference. If a urinary catheter not already in situ, the bladder should be drained to prevent inadvertent cystotomy. Prior surgical history should be considered when planning entry, and use of alternative access points other than the umbilicus, such as Palmer's point, should be considered in patient with prior pelvic or abdominal surgery. Following confirmed intraperitoneal access, placement of ports should again be placed according to surgeon preference and consideration of all steps of the surgery must be incorporated into planning, including potential need to harvest an omental J-flap or the need to suture deep in the pelvis. Most often at least one 8 mm or larger trocar is placed laterally for ease of suture transfer (Fig. 6).

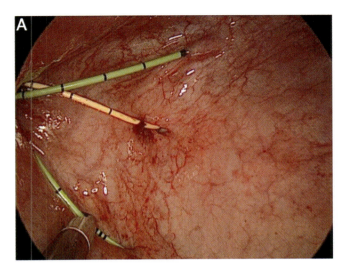

Fig. 5 The ureteral orifices are cannulated with green ureteral catheters and the fistula is cannulated with a yellow ureteral catheter, enabling easy identification of the tract. (Reprinted from Videosurgery and Other Miniinvasive Techniques, 7 [4], M. Roslan, M. Markuszewski, Baginska, K. Krajka, Suprapubic transvesical laparoendoscopic single-site surgery for vesicovaginal fistula repair: a case report, 307–310., Copyright (2012) with permission from Termedia Publishing House [58])

Fig. 6 Example of port placement in a robot-assisted vesicovaginal fistula repair. A 10 mm supraumbilical Hasson port was placed during the open entry, with a robotic trocar inserted for docking. Two additional 8 mm robotic trocars are placed on the left lateral aspect approximately 8 cm apart in a straight configuration. A third additional 8 mm robotic trocar was inserted, approximately 8 cm lateral to the Hasson port on the right side, and an 8 mm assistant port was placed 8 cm lateral to the last port in the right flank, again in a line configuration. An 8 mm assist port allows for safe and facile suture transfer. (Courtesy of B. Brucker & C. Brandon, 2021, reprinted with consent)

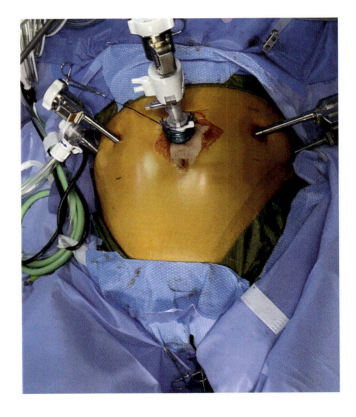

The patient should be placed in a Trendelenburg position, usually between 15 and 30 degrees, to encourage cranial displacement of the small bowels out of the pelvis for improved visualization and access.

Transvesical Approach

There are two main approaches to laparoscopic vesicovaginal fistula repair: transvesical (also known as the O'Conor technique) or extravesical [50, 51]. The transvesical approach was initially described by O'Conor and Sokol in their 1951 case series of open abdominal vesicovaginal fistula repair [49]. The procedure involves an intentional bivalving of the bladder to visualize the fistula tract. A cystotomy is made in the posterior wall of the bladder and extends down to the fistula that is found connecting the vagina to the bladder (Fig. 7). The epithelized fistula tract can be excised leaving a fresh edge of the bladder that promotes healing. If there are multiple fistula present, assuming bladder capacity allows for it, all tracts can be incorporated into the cystotomy, creating a solitary suture line. Next, a wide dissection of the vesicovaginal plane surrounding the tract is undertaken to ensure adequate mobilization of the bladder and vagina to perform a tension-free watertight closure. Vaginal stents such as lucite stents or even an end-to-end anastomosis (EEA) sizer in the vagina can also help with traction and visualization when dissecting in the vesicovaginal plane. When adapted for laparoscopy and robotic-assisted laparoscopy, this procedure has the advantage of easy visualization of the fistula to ensure adequate resection. This technique also allows for excellent visualization of the ureteral orifices throughout the entire repair, which is helpful to ensure they are not incorporated into the bladder closure. Furthermore, the ureters can easily be cannulated via the cystotomy if needed and not already performed cystoscopically earlier in the case.

Sotelo et al. published a series of 15 patients who underwent laparoscopic transvesical repair of vesicovaginal fistula [59]. Ninety-three percent (14/15) of fistulae were following a TAH, 11/15 (73.3%) were primary repairs, and the majority (93.3%) were supratrigonal. After performing a cystotomy in the posterior bladder with a harmonic scalpel to the posterior aspect of the fistula, the edges of the tract are excised until viable tissue is exposed. The bladder was separated from the vagina circumferentially around the opening using laparoscopic scissors without energy. Subsequently, the cystotomy is closed in a running continuous caudal to cranial fashion and reinforced with a serosal imbricating layer. The vaginal opening was closed in a transverse continuous fashion, adhering to the principle of avoiding overlapping suture lines and limiting

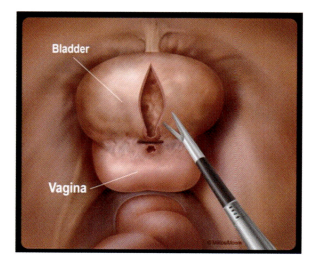

Fig. 7 A controlled cystotomy is performed on the posterior aspect of the bladder until it connects with the fistulous tract and incorporates it into the cystotomy following resection of the epithelialized edges. (Reprinted from J. R. Miklos & R. D. Moore. Laparoscopic extravesical vesicovaginal fistula repair: our technique and 15-year experience. Int Urogynecol J. 2015;26(3):441–6. Copyright (2014) with permission from Springer Nature [64])

narrowing of the vaginal canal. In this series, they also utilize an interposing tissue layer between the vagina and the bladder, usually originating from omentum, sigmoid epiploic fat appendages, or peritoneum. Of the 15 cases, 1 failure was noted over a median follow-up of 26.2 months (3–60 months).

Zhang et al. also describe a similar operation performed in 18 consecutive women found to have a supratrigonal fistula with a mean size of 19.7 mm (12–30 mm) [60]. A mean operative time of 135 min (75–175 min), mean blood loss of 95 ml (50–200 ml), and a 100% cure rate after a mean follow-up of 22.7 weeks (3–45 weeks) was described. In a series of 25 patients undergoing transvesical repair, Shah describes a very similar technique to Sotelo's and Zhang's, other than subtle differences such as the use of the laparoscopic scissors for creation of the cystotomy [61]. Of the 25 patients initially included, 3 were converted to open procedures due to significant adhesive disease. At 6 weeks following surgery, 3 of 22 patients were found to have persistent leakage consistent with a failed repair, resulting in a success rate of 86%. Ghosh et al. describe the use of a "limited cystotomy" rather than the traditional bivalving of the bladder, while the remainder of the operation is similar to above [62]. They report a 100% success rate at a mean follow-up of 15.6 months (±8.6 months). Similarly, others have also noted excellent success rates with a "limited cystotomy," often described as 2 cm in length [63]. Some have used light from the cystoscopy to help guide the intentional cystotomy, minimizing disruption to the bladder wall during this approach [59].

Extravesical Approach

The extravesical laparoscopic vesicovaginal fistula repair was first described in a 49 year-old woman with a supratrigonal 5 mm fistula secondary to recognized and repaired iatrogenic bladder injury at the time of benign TAH [50]. Unlike the transvesical approach, there is no intentional cystotomy performed, minimizing any suture lines on the bladder that could ultimately result in a new fistula or irritative symptoms postoperatively. The extravesical approach is described as a careful dissection of the bladder off the anterior vaginal wall in the vesicovaginal plane. The separation of the posterior bladder from the anterior vaginal is facilitated by the use of a vaginal stent or packing to provide tension on the tissue and minimize leakage through the tract itself. The dissection is carried out until the fistula is identified, often with the help of cannulation using a ureteral stent or wire for visual or haptic feedback. If the bladder is backfilled or the catheter intentionally clamped, urine will also spill out into the field once the fistulous tract is encountered. Once the tract is identified, de-epithelialization of the edges can be performed on both the bladder and vaginal side. The dissection within the vesicovaginal plane should extend wide enough beyond the fistula edge to allow for tension-free closure of the bladder wall. Effort should be made to avoid overlapping suture lines of the vagina and the bladder, which can be achieved by varying the direction of closure or interposing tissue or graft material between the layers. As with all cystotomies, the integrity of the bladder closure should be evaluated to ensure it is watertight. While in the transvesical approach the ureteral orifices are easily visualized through the cystotomy, identification of the ureters can be more challenging in the extravesical approach. As such, various options for ureteral identification can include simultaneous cystoscopic guidance during laparoscopic closure or the use of lighted ureteral stents [65]. In robotic surgery, indocyanine green (ICG) can be injected through ureteral stents, and the ureters can be visualized as a fluorescent green tubular structure when the near infrared fluorescence filter is used, minimizing the risk of iatrogenic injury at the time of repair [66]. Simply using intravenous sodium fluorescein or indigo carmine to confirm ureteral patency cystoscopically at the end of the closure is also an option, but it does not assist in the primary prevention of ureteral injury.

In subsequent series of extravesical repair, it is often noted that the bladder is backfilled with saline (~150–300 ml) to enable identification of the vesicovaginal junction. In a prospective study of 15 women, Abdel-Karim et al. describe incision of the peritoneum using cautery and subsequent sharp dissection between the posterior bladder and vagina with the laparoscopic scissors and gentle traction [67]. In addition, they note backfilling of the bladder with saline to assist with dissection and eventual identification of the fistula through observed spillage from the tract. They also note mobilization of the bladder off the vagina to allow for tension-free closure with 3–0 polyglactin suture (delayed absorbable suture) in a cranio-caudal manner, while the vagina was closed transversely with 2–0 polyglactin suture in a single continuous fashion to minimize suture overlap. In this series, fistulae were all described as supratrigonal, ranging from 0.5–2.5 cm in size, and required 171.6 min (range 145–210 min) to repair. All 15 patients were cured after mean follow-up time of 18.9 ± 8.6 months (range 10–26 months). Similarly, 100% cure rate was noted in another series of 5 iatrogenic supratrigonal vesicovaginal fistula after a median 56.1 weeks (26.6–74.0 weeks) using a laparoscopic extravesical approach [35]. Importantly, this series demonstrated successful closure without complication or recurrence despite the fact that there was no debriding of the fistulous tract or interposing tissue layer used between the bladder and the vagina. However, the median size of fistula was smaller than the prior series (range 0.5–0.9 cm), possibly accounting for their success.

A retrospective series of 44 patients, the largest of its kind, demonstrated a success rate of 43/44 (98%) when both primary and recurrent vesicovaginal fistulae are closed using the laparoscopic transperitoneal extravesical approach [64]. The authors describe the use of a ureteral stent for fistula tract identification during surgery (Fig. 8) and approach their vesicovaginal dissection similar to that of a sacrocolpopexy dissection using laparoscopic scissors. They note the use of an end-to-end anastomosis (EEA) sizer for vaginal traction and a backstop during dissection. Similarly, an interposing omental flap was not used in 43/44 repairs. In this particular series, patients underwent suprapubic tube placement to allow for early removal of the transurethral catheter. Similar to most studies published on vesicovaginal fistula repair, continuous bladder drainage was maintained for approximately 14–21 days postoperatively, and suprapubic catheters were removed following confirmation of the integrity of the bladder closure by cystoscopic and vaginal evaluation.

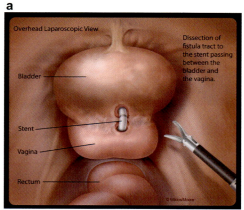 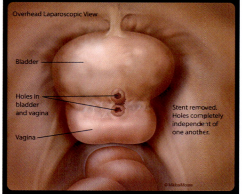

Fig. 8 (**a**) Use of a ureteral catheter passed cystoscopically through the fistulous tract, as seen from a laparoscopic view, helps to identify the tract during the extravesical dissection of the bladder away from the anterior vagina. (**b**) Following identification of the fistulous tract, the ureteral catheter can be removed and the dissection continued to ensure adequate mobilization for tension-free closure. (Reprinted from J. R. Miklos & R. D. Moore. Laparoscopic extravesical vesicovaginal fistula repair: our technique and 15-year experience. Int Urogynecol J. 2015;26(3):441-6. Copyright (2014) with permission from Springer Nature [64])

Transvesical Versus Extravesical Approach

A systematic review of minimally invasive vesicovaginal fistula repairs demonstrated no difference in success rates between the transvesical (O'Conor) and extravesical approaches [RR 0.98 (95% CI, 0.94–1.02)] among pooled data from 260 repairs [68]. In a retrospective cohort study of 64 patients undergoing either laparoscopic transvesical ($N = 33$) or extravesical ($N = 31$), similar success rates were demonstrated between both techniques (97.0% versus 96.8%, respectively) over the follow-up period of 12–36 months [69]. Most operative outcomes were similar between groups, including estimated blood loss (55.3 ± 10.8 ml versus 60.2 ± 14.6 ml, $p = 0.136$) and length of stay (7.4 ± 1.8 days versus 6.9 ± 1.3 days, $p = 0.21$), but authors noted significantly decreased operative time for the transvesical approach compared to extravesical (137 ± 22.7 min versus 178 ± 17.8 min, respectively, $p < 0.001$). It is worth mentioning that while the baseline characteristics of the patients were similar, these were not randomized populations, but calculated and individualized decisions made by the surgeon. The authors remark that a transvesical approach is advantageous due to the rapid manner in which the fistulous tract can be identified with a bivalved bladder and the avoidance of adhesiolysis in the vesicovaginal plane of patients with prior hysterectomy. Furthermore, they note that time saved was most notable on lower-lying fistulae, although they do not provide any specific definitions for how they defined high versus low-lying fistulae. The extravesical approach is ideal for supratrigonal vesicovaginal fistula to minimize risk of ureteral injury at the time of repair. Ultimately, the current data does not identify a superior technique but highlights the persistent principle that the best technique is the one that the surgeon deems most appropriate for the patient they are treating and are most comfortable performing.

Bladder Layer Closure

There is no established gold standard for bladder closure in the setting of vesicovaginal fistula repair. Principles of bladder closure include tension-free, watertight, and avoid overlapping suture lines with the vaginal closure. A tension-free closure is ensured with a wide mobilization of the posterior bladder off the anterior vaginal wall within the vesicovaginal plane, typically described as 1–2 cm wide (Fig. 9). A watertight

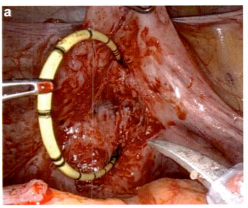
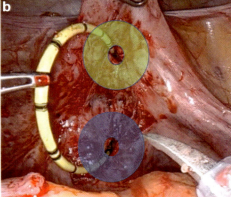

Fig. 9 (**a**) Extravesical dissection of the vesicovaginal plane demonstrating a wide dissection around the fistula tract (cannulated by a yellow open-ended ureteral catheter) to ensure adequate mobilization of the posterior bladder off the anterior vagina, which is crucial for tension-free closure. (**b**) The same dissection with a 1–2 cm periphery highlighted by the blue circle around the fistula on the anterior vaginal wall and the green circle around the fistula on the posterior bladder wall. (Courtesy of B. Brucker & C. Brandon, 2021, reprinted with consent)

closure can be obtained in any number of ways but is most commonly described using a single- or double-layer continuous closure using absorbable suture, classically polyglactin [35, 62, 63]. Others have described a figure-of-eight technique [64]. However, traditional laparoscopic knot-tying can be tedious and time-consuming, with robotic assistance facilitating this component of the procedure. In response to this limitation, absorbable barbed suture has been described for bladder closure, with good success [70, 71]. To date, only Miklos et al. have evaluated the impact of a single- versus double-layer closure on repair success and noted no difference between the two [80–100% versus 93.3–100%, respectively; RR 0.98 (95%CI, 0.94–1.03)] [68].

Retrograde Filling of the Bladder

To confirm the integrity of the bladder repair intraoperatively, most studies describe retrograde filling the bladder to observe leakage from the suture line and perform directed reinforcement of the suture line wherever required. Miklos et al. evaluated the impact of testing the bladder at the time of repair and found that, according to pooled data, patients who underwent retrograde fill of the bladder for testing had a higher success rate compared to those who did not [99.25% versus 93.64%, respectively; RR 1.06 (95% CI: 1.01–1.12)].

Vaginal Closure

There are a few principles that should be considered when closing the vaginal opening at the time of a vesicovaginal fistula repair. Care should be taken to avoid narrowing the vaginal canal if a patient is sexually active and there is adequate tissue for closure. It is also preferable if the vaginal suture line is non-overlapping with the closure with the bladder. This can be achieved by ensuring a perpendicular closure to that of the bladder closure (Fig. 10), as well as the use of an interposing tissue flap between layers. In some cases, no vaginal closure was performed if an interposing layer was placed in order to allow for drainage of peritoneal fluid and blood, preventing hematoma and abscess formation [50, 72]. The majority of studies describe a horizontal (transverse) single layer full-thickness vaginal closure with absorbable (i.e., polyglactin) suture. According to a systematic review of laparoscopic and robotic vesicovaginal fistula repairs, there is no difference in the success of repairs based on zero (93.7%), single (96.4%), or double layer (100%) closure of the vaginal layer of the fistula [single layer as reference group, zero-layer: RR 0.97 (95% CI: 0.85–1.11); double layer: RR 0.94 (95% CI: 0.83–1.06)] [68].

Interposing Tissue Layer

Interposing tissue flaps are thought to reinforce repairs, fill dead-space, and improve neo-vascularization and lymph drainage by importing vital vascular tissue to the region [40]. Since Kiricuta and Goldstein were the first elucidated the usefulness of an interposing omental flap in the abdominal repair of postradiation vesicovaginal repair, many other surgeons have reported on the integration of this adjunct technique with various other flaps [73]. Evans et al. reported on the importance of including an interposing flap on the success of repairing vesicovaginal fistula of benign or malignant origin, demonstrating a 100% (2/2) cure rate in the setting of a flap, while only 66.7% (4/6) were cured without a flap among repaired fistula of malignant origin [74]. Of note, the majority (7/8) had previously undergone radiotherapy. While the use of interposing tissue in postradiation fistula is relatively widely accepted, the use of interposing flaps in fistula of benign origin is more widely debated. In the same study, differences in cure rates between those where an interposing tissue layer was used and those where one was not were also reported (10/10, 100% versus 12/19, 63.2%, respectively). In a retrospective study investigating prognostic factors associated with recurrence after vesicovaginal fistula repair, it was found that use of an interposing flap was associated with lower odds of recurrence [OR 0.3 (95% CI: 0.1–0.7)] [75]. However, none of these cases were performed using conventional or robotic-assisted laparoscopy.

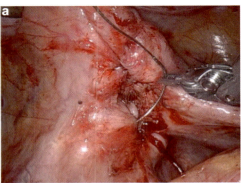 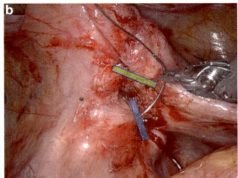

Fig. 10 (**a**) The bladder defect is closed in a horizontal fashion, while the vaginal tract is closed in a vertical fashion using barbed dissolvable suture. (**b**) The green bar highlights the direction of the vesical closure while the blue bar highlights the direction of the vaginal closure, demonstrating non-overlapping suture lines. (Courtesy of B. Brucker & C. Brandon, 2021, reprinted with consent)

The first reported case of laparoscopic closure of a vesicovaginal fistula in 1994 employed a peritoneal flap obtained superior and lateral to the bladder dome was utilized as an interposing graft between the bladder and vagina [51]. Several studies have since reported the use of interposing tissue layers, including omentum, sigmoid epiploic fat appendages, and peritoneal flaps (Fig. 11) [50, 59, 72, 76]. Erdogru et al. also published their positive experience with a fleece-bound sealing system that incorporates human coagulation factor as a tissue barrier [77]. Dehydrated amniotic membrane has also been described as an interposing patch in a woman with a vesicovaginal fistula secondary to an irradiated pelvis, with success noted out to 5 months follow-up [78]. Melamud et al. describe the use of fibrin glue injected between the bladder and vaginal closures with the purpose of separating the suture lines [52]. However, other groups report successful fistula repairs without the use of any interposing layer [35, 79, 80].

When the impact of using an interposing tissue layer on the success of minimally invasive vesicovaginal fistula repair was evaluated by Miklos et al., there was no association between the use of a flap and success of repair [RR 0.98 (95% CI: 0.94–1.03)] [68]. While anecdotally many would agree that a vascular tissue layer may be helpful when repairing complex fistulae, including those secondary to irradiation, it remains less clear whether the added morbidity of an interposing layer, albeit often minimal, is necessary for successful closure.

Postoperative Catheterization

Continuous bladder drainage is a crucial component of successful outcomes after vesicovaginal fistula repair. Early data from bladder trauma literature suggest that following bladder repair, a transurethral catheter left in situ for an average of 13 days was sufficient for healing [81]. While there have been no clinical trials evaluating minimum drainage time, the majority of studies describe 14 days or longer for drainage and will often perform a cystogram to evaluate the integrity of the closure prior to catheter removal. In one study evaluating the use of cystograms after lower urinary tract repairs ($N = 245$), including 49 vesicovaginal fistula, cystograms were performed a median of 11 days (10–12 days) following closure [82]. Of the 49 vesicovaginal fistula repairs, one demonstrated an abnormal cystogram on postoperative day 11, prompting replacement of the catheter for an additional 7 days, with follow-up cystogram demonstrating no leak on postoperative day 18. Of the 245 cystograms performed for various lower urinary tract repairs, only 7 (2.9%) were abnormal, resulting in a change in management such as prolongation of catheter drainage. In regions where resources are scarce, cystograms can be

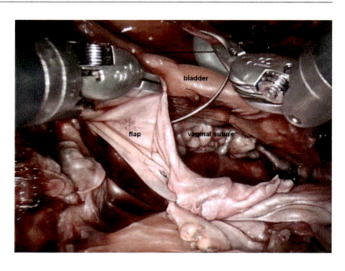

Fig. 11 A peritoneal flap harvested from the right iliac fossa to lay above the vaginal suture between the vagina and the bladder. (Reprinted from European Urology, 61, M. Kurtz, M. Horstmann, & H. John, Robot-Assisted Laparoscopic Repair of High Vesicovaginal fistulae with peritoneal inlay, 229–230., Copyright (2012) with permission from Elsevier)

replaced with dye tests, where the bladder is back-filled with methylene blue-instilled saline, or the patient can consume phenazopyridine orally to dye urine orange. In patients with a positive dye test after the initial 14-day postoperative catheterization period, an extension of 7 days of catheterization resulted in negative dye tests in greater than half the population (29/52, 55.7%), suggesting conservative management with catheterization is a reasonable step when attempting to avoid another surgical re-intervention [83]. The type of catheter material was often not mentioned, and no studies have been performed to evaluate the superiority of one material over another. While the majority of continuous bladder drainage employed 16-20Fr urethral catheters, a small proportion of studies reported suprapubic catheter placement for ease of drainage [64]. Several groups note the use of anticholinergic bladder medications to prevent bladder spasms during the healing process [54, 84, 85]. Though no studies mention the use of a beta-3-agonist for this purpose, it is presumed to provide similar antispasmodic relief.

Modified Laparoscopic Approaches

Several groups have published on the use of laparoendoscopic single-site surgery (LESS) to repair vesicovaginal fistula [84]. The first report of a vesicovaginal fistular repair using a LESS approach included 5 patients with iatrogenic supratrigonal fistula ranging from 1 cm to 2.5 cm in size [86]. Abdel-Karim et al. describe the use of a 2 cm infraumbilical incision and a single port with pre-bent instruments and a 5 mm 0 degree deflectable camera, as well as the addition of a 5-mm side port for triangulation and extracorporeal suturing. An extravesical route was used to identify the fistulous tract as well as perform the necessary mobilization dissection. The vagina was closed in a single layer and the bladder was closed in two layers, both with absorbable suture. Furthermore, they describe the use of an omental flap for tissue interposition. The operative time ranged from 170 to 240 min, with a mean blood loss of 90 ± 25 ml and no perioperative complications. Complete resolution was noted at 8 ± 3.2 months follow-up. Mahadevappa et al. reported on their experience involving 10 post-hysterectomy patients who underwent vesicovaginal fistula repair with single-site skin incision and three separate conventional ports (10 mm x1, 5 mm x2) placed at varying levels that allowed for the use of traditional laparoscopic instruments [87]. Their surgical technique was otherwise similar to those previously described above, including the use of an omental flap for tissue interposition. The mean operative time was 182 ± 32 min, with an estimated blood loss of 100 ml or less, requiring 2.6 ± 0.7 admission days, and no major peri- or postoperative complications. All patients were cured over the course of a mean 13.2 month follow-up (range 6–30 months). While this technique does suggest the advantage of fewer abdominal incisions for the patient, it demands advanced technical competency, particularly with respect to suturing when loss of triangulation is encountered. As such, its use is not widespread and no comparative studies have been performed.

A percutaneous transvesical LESS approach directly through a 1.5 cm skin incision made 2 cm cranial to the pubic symphysis has also been described by Roslan et al. [58]. At the start, the ureters as well as the fistula are catheterized under cystoscopic guidance. Subsequently, the multichannel port is inserted through the direct suprapubic cystotomy and the bladder was insufflated with carbon dioxide to a pressure of 14 mmHg. A 10 mm 30° rigid laparoscope was used, while three additional 5 mm instrument channels are employed for standard laparoscopic instruments. They also noted use of the urethra as an added channel of access for suction. The fistulous tract was excised with cautery and the defect was closed with 3–0 unidirectional barbed absorbable suture. The integrity of the bladder was checked with a retrograde fill of 200 ml of saline. The skin incision was sutured closed, and an 18Fr Foley catheter was inserted for continuous drainage for 2 weeks. The operative time was 170 min with negligible blood loss and no perioperative complications. At 4 month follow-up, the patient did not show any signs of recurrence.

Other retroperitoneal transvesical approaches have also been described. Nerli and Reddy [88] report their experience with extraperitoneal transvesical conventional laparoscopy with cystoscopic guidance in four patients with post-hysterectomy vesicovaginal fistula [88]. Initial cystoscopy was performed with gas insufflation. Following fixation of the bladder to the anterior abdominal wall under direct visualization, a 5 mm endoscopic port was inserted halfway between the umbilicus and pubic symphysis in the midline, as were two additional 5 mm ports 5 cm inferolateral on either side. Pneumovesical pressure was maintained with a betadine-socked vaginal pack. The fistulous tract was circumferentially excised and the surrounding bladder was dissected off the underlying vagina. The vaginal defect was closed vertically, while the bladder closure was performed horizontally with 4–0 synthetic absorbable suture. Subsequently, the ureters were catheterized, as was the bladder, which were removed 1 and 2 weeks later, respectively. The authors noted various challenges that were ultimately overcome with a learning curve: fixation of the bladder to the anterior abdominal wall, maintenance of insufflation pressure during port placement and suction, suturing with continuous urine drainage, and narrow operative field. The operative time ranged from 175 to 235 min, with minimal blood loss and no complications. One patient suffered an upper respiratory tract infection while another suffered from an ileus, though oral feeding commenced 48 h postoperatively. No recurrences were noted over the follow-up time of 8–17 months. This approach evades peritoneal entry and potential damage to intraabdominal structures but does require proficiency of laparoscopic skills in a narrow field.

Robotic Approach

As previously noted, the benefits of conventional laparoscopy over an open approach include improved cosmesis, lower surgical site infections, decreased blood loss, shorter length of stay, and reduced analgesic requirements [53]. However, limitations of laparoscopy include a slower learning curve, counterintuitive hand movements, two-dimensional visualization, limited haptic feedback, limited range of motion, and challenging ergonomics for the surgeon [89]. One study from general surgery compared the subjective surgeon experience between laparoscopic and robotic biliary-enteric anastomoses in surgeons naïve to either approach using pig models and found that while conventional laparoscopy provided improved tactile feedback compared to the robotic-assisted technique, image quality, depth perception, comfort, eye fatigue, fluidity of motion, speed of motion, range of motion, precision, dexterity, and the overall degree of difficulty were rated significantly better with robot-assisted laparoscopy compared to the traditional technique

[90]. As such, from a surgeon's perspective, there may be many advantages to the robot, including a faster learning curve in part due to the above findings.

Melamud et al. were the first to report their experience with robot-assisted laparoscopic repair using a transvesical approach [52]. They describe the use of a 12 mm camera port 20 cm from the pubis in the midline, as well as 2 × 8 mm ports lateral to the rectus muscle on either side, an additional 12 mm port in the right iliac fossa, and a 5 mm assist port for 7 cm lateral and superior to the camera port. Steps of the procedure were similar to those described with conventional laparoscopy; the posterior bladder is incised and an intentional cystotomy is carried down to a previously catheterized fistulous tract. The tract is excised, and the bladder is further dissected away from the underlying vagina to allow for a tension-free closure using two-layers of 3–0 absorbable suture. The vagina was closed in a single layer. The team chose to use fibrin glue as an interposing layer separating the suture lines. The bladder was tested for integrity and an 18Fr catheter was left in situ. The case required 280 min of operative time, resulted in 50 ml of blood loss, and went without reported complication. The patient was discharged home on postoperative day 1 and was symptom-free at 16 weeks follow-up.

Similar technique was reported by Sundaram et al., where 5 women with iatrogenic fistula averaging 3.1 cm were operated on for an average of 233 min [91]. The basic principles of fistula repair were adhered to, with a tension-free watertight closure without overlapping suture lines, reinforced by an interposing omental flap. Postoperatively, a catheter remained in place for 10 days and was removed after confirmation of bladder integrity with voiding cystourethrogram. All patients were noted to be voiding normally at 6 months follow-up.

Schimpf et al. describe the first extravesical robot-assisted laparoscopic vesicovaginal fistula repair, relying on sigmoid epiploic fat for interposing tissue between suture lines [92]. Cure was noted at 3 month follow-up. Kidd et al. describe a series of 34 patients with vesicovaginal ($N = 22$) and ureterovaginal ($N = 12$) fistula who undergo robotic repair [93]. Of the 22 vesicovaginal fistulae, 21 were sequelae of surgery, one was radiation-induced, and 4 patients had prior attempted closures. The mean console time was 187 min (151–219 min), blood loss was always less than 100 ml, and the length of stay was 1 day (range 1–2 days). 21 of 22 patients received an interposing flap, of which the omentum was the most common tissue flap (13/21, 62%). Two (9%) postoperative complications were noted: a urinary tract infection requiring antibiotics and an exacerbation of preexisting restrictive lung disease requiring critical level care. At 28.8 months follow-up, 20/22 (90%) were symptom free, and 2 patients requiring a subsequent repair, one performed robotically and the other via transvaginal route. Both patients were subsequently cured.

Similar to modifications made with conventional laparoscopy, single-port robotic vesicovaginal repair has been reported [94]. In this solitary report, they describe the placement of a central gel port with multiple channels through a periumbilical incision. Their set up consists of placing a camera at 12 o'clock, bipolar forceps at 9 o'clock, monopolar curved scissors at 6 o'clock, and Cadiere forceps at 3 o'clock. An assistant port may also be placed alongside the single-port trocar in the gel port or placed as an additional trocar inferolateral on the right or the left of the single central port. This can be useful for suctioning, retraction, or efficient exchange of suture. When suturing, the needle drivers replace instruments at 6 and 9 o'clock. This set up enables the wrist to be held laterally and eversion of the needle drivers allows the sutures to be pulled and the knot to be secured. The authors chose an extravesical approach, excision of the fistulous tract, following closure of the bladder and vagina individually, they interpose omentum or peritoneum, depending on availability. Unfortunately, they did not receive internal review board approval and consent to report the outcomes of the repairs at the time of publication.

With the rise in use of robot-assisted techniques in urology and gynecology, the European Association of Urology produced a best practices consensus report on robotic-assisted repair of vesicovaginal fistula [37]. However, given that traditional and robotic-assisted laparoscopy have not been compared in the setting of vesicovaginal fistula repair, it is not clear at this time whether there is an objective improvement in outcomes between the two approaches. With similar operative times, blood loss, length of stay, and success rates, the decision to use robotic assistance may be distilled down to surgeon preference, availability, and cost.

Cost of Robotics: Is It Worth It?

At present, a cost-effectiveness analysis comparing robotic-assisted to conventional laparoscopic repairs of vesicovaginal fistula are lacking. However, sacrocolpopexies are urogynecologic procedures that require similar technical proficiencies, including delicate dissection of tissue planes as well as suturing. A study by Paraiso et al. comparing robotic and laparoscopic sacrocolpopexy noted significantly higher cost for robotic sacrocolpopexy (+US $1667, 95% CI: $448–2885, $p = 0.008$), which was primarily driven by increased operative times and operating room use [95]. Importantly, operative time decreases with surgical volume, as demonstrated Geller and colleagues, who compared the first 20 cases with the subsequent 127 cases [96]. They noted significantly shorter operative times across all key components of the procedure, including decreased skin-to-skin time of >55 min, among the latter 127 compared to the first 20 cases. Importantly, when assessing the relationship between efficiency and procedures performed, they noted an improvement in performance time after 20 sacrocolpopexies and considerable reduction in operative times after 60 cases performed. These findings, while not specific to vesicovaginal fistula repair, illustrate the need for high surgical volume, whenever possible, to improve efficiency and decrease operative times, thereby resulting in decreased costs. However, this does not factor in the cost of purchasing a robot, as well as the annual maintenance fees. Given the relative rarity of vesicovaginal fistula, it may be difficult to justify the cost if surgeons are already proficient and laparoscopic repairs given similar outcomes and the widespread availability of straight-stick laparoscopic equipment. However, surgeon proficiency with one route over another may drive individual surgeons more than cost, particularly as robotic surgery becomes more ubiquitous and available to trainees.

Work-related musculoskeletal disorders have a huge impact on work absenteeism and decreased productivity, costing the United States an estimated US $20 billion annually [97]. As such, surgeon ergonomics is necessary to consider when comparing the cost of laparoscopic and robotic surgery to the surgeon as well as a healthcare system. According to several survey-based studies evaluating work-related musculoskeletal disorders among conventional laparoscopists, the prevalence of injury was between 73 and 100% [98]. Potential advantages from robotic assistance include the use of wristed instruments with 7 degrees of freedom that reduce the need for awkward body positioning, intuitive fine motor movements that mimic open surgery principles, three-dimensional optics, and the ability to sit with a monitor below eye level, minimizing neck strain. One study compared ergonomic strain and workload between traditional laparoscopic and robot-assisted laparoscopic sacrocolpopexy [99]. The study uses two validated questionnaires, the body part discomfort (BPD) scale and the National Aeronautics and Space Administration task load index (NASA-TLX), of which higher scores correlate with greater musculoskeletal discomfort. 16 healthy surgeons, with median age 33 years (27–54 years) performed a total of 33 robotic and 53 laparoscopic sacrocolpopexies. There was no appreciable difference in operative time, estimated blood loss, mean patient BMI, or rate of concomitant hysterectomy between laparoscopic and robotic cases. Robotic surgery was associated with lower neck/shoulder as well as back discomfort compared with laparoscopy. Knee/ankle/foot discomfort also increased with operative time, with a trend toward greater discomfort in laparoscopic cases compared with robotic assistance. These ergonomic concerns are not exclusive to vesicovaginal fistula repair but do contribute to a surgeon's decision to pursue one technique over another.

Comparing Laparoscopic to Robotic Vesicovaginal Fistula Repair

To date, there are no comparative studies evaluating the success outcomes or secondary quality-of-life outcomes between traditional straight-stick laparoscopy and robot-assisted laparoscopy. Based on the available literature, success rates are comparable and the decision to pursue one over the other appears to be influenced more by surgeon preference and experience, availability of equipment, and cost.

Other Outcomes

Other Urinary Symptoms

While the majority of studies focus on resolution of the fistula as the outcome of interest, a small number do address other urinary symptoms that either coexist or result from the vesicovaginal fistula repair. Hilton reported on the urodynamic findings associated with urogenital fistula, noting a 47% (14/30) concurrence of stress incontinence prior to repair, particularly in women with bladder neck and urethral involvement, as well as 40% (12/30) with detrusor overactivity [28]. Follow repair using an unspecified approach, 10 patients reported persistent urinary symptoms (1 stress urinary incontinence and 9 urgency/urgency incontinence) despite anatomic resolution of the fistula. In another study looking at urinary and sexual function following open and transvaginal repairs, 15 (18.5%) of women had urinary symptoms, with 7 (8.6%) and 8 (9.9%) noting urgency- and stress urinary incontinence, respectively [100]. Higher rates of urgency urinary incontinence were noted in the open repair group compared to the transvaginal repair group (17.9% versus 3.8%, $p = 0.04$), which may be attributed to the bivalving and long suture lines associated with the transvesical approach. Using validated patient-reported outcome questionnaires evaluating urinary symptoms, scores improved significantly following abdominal or transvaginal repair of the vesicovaginal fistula [101].

Mohr et al. compared transvaginal (Latzko procedure) and abdominal vesicovaginal fistula repairs and noted no difference in OAB and SUI rates, which were overall low in both groups [102]. While the majority of data comes from open and vaginal repairs, one comparative study noted a 4.5% (1/22) and 5.6% (2/36) incidence of postoperative stress urinary incontinence among the laparoscopic and open vesicovaginal repairs, respectively [54]. All were treated successful with transobturator slings. They also noted similar rates of bladder spasms between laparoscopic and open repairs (4.5% versus 8.3% respectively, $p > 0.05$), all of which were managed with anticholinergics for 3–4 weeks. Symptoms subsequently resolved in all patients. The majority of urinary outcomes are reported on a case-by-case basis and are often limited in their assessment. There also remains a paucity of data in the laparoscopic and robotic literature. The International Continence Society did publish a paper regarding the role of pelvic floor physical therapy in women who suffered obstetrical fistula of all kinds and remarked on the utility of therapy for persistent urinary symptoms following repair [103]. While they do acknowledge challenges to access these services, when available, there is little risk to pursuing pelvic floor physical therapy prior to and following the repair of vesicovaginal fistula.

Long-Term Sexual Function

It is well accepted that urinary incontinence of any kind has a negative effect on sexual function [104]. However, little is known regarding the sexual function outcomes of women undergoing vesicovaginal fistula repair. In one study focusing on sexual function outcomes following transvaginal and transabdominal vesicovaginal fistula repair, Mohr et al. noted that using the female sexual function index (FSFI), a 19-item validated questionnaire on sexual function, overall sexual function improved following repair of either approach [102]. However, some domains did not improve significantly across both groups, including pain, arousal, and orgasm. The authors surmised that while overall improvement may reflect improvement in urinary incontinence, vaginal pain and dyspareunia may account for the lack of improvement in pain, arousal, and orgasm domains. These suppositions are supported by findings reported by Pope and colleagues [105]. Among 115 Malawian women who underwent 6- and 12 month follow-up after transvaginal repair of vesicovaginal fistula, 14 (12.2%) noted problems with intercourse, half attributed to pain and half attributed to persistent incontinence. While sexual function according to the revised female sexual distress scale (FSDS-R) improved after surgery across the entire group [before: 27.1 (24.6–29.6) versus after: 4.9 (2.9–7.0), $p < 0.01$)], 19 (16.5%) continued to score in the sexual dysfunction range (score >11). They noted that decreased vaginal caliber (as assessed by dilator size) and fistula size >3 cm were associated with sexual dysfunction. Grewal et al. reviewed several quality-of-life outcomes following transvaginal and abdominal repair, including return to sexual function. They noted that two-thirds (23/36) of patients returned to sexual activity following repair, while 13/36 remained sexually inactive [101]. Despite the interview-style data collection, the authors did not determine the reason for sexual inactivity. While they captured pelvic organ prolapse/urinary incontinence sexual questionnaire (PISQ-12) scores among sexually active women at a median 40.5 months follow-up [PISQ-12: 14 (range 3–30)], however, a preoperative score for comparison was not obtained, making it difficult to interpret their findings. In another study of 63 sexually active women who underwent either transvaginal or transabdominal repair, 17 (27%) women scored <26.5 on the FSFI, suggesting female sexual dysfunction at mean 2.5 years follow-up [100]. On multivariate analysis, only parity >2 was associated with female sexual dysfunction. There were no differences in FSFI scores between transvaginal and transabdominal repairs. No preoperative scores were captured to assess improvement or deterioration in sexual function. Unfortunately, to date, there are no studies evaluating sexual function following laparoscopic or robotic closure of vesicovaginal fistula, nor are there comparative studies evaluating differences between surgical routes of repair with respect to sexual function. The International Continence Society's Physiotherapy Committee also suggests utility in pelvic floor relaxation for women suffering from dyspareunia, vaginismus, and pelvic floor hypertonicity following fistula repair [103].

Future Directions

Currently, there is no consensus on the optimal approach for surgical management of vesicovaginal fistula. Comparative studies, albeit limited, have demonstrated comparable success rates among open, vaginal, and minimally invasive approaches, while maintaining the peri- and postoperative advantages ascribed to vaginal, laparoscopic, and robotic surgery, including lower blood loss, shorter length of stay, and decreased analgesia requirements. Despite these advantages, many questions remain to be answered regarding laparoscopic and robotic repairs, including but not limited to the transvesical versus extravesical approach, the bladder and vaginal closure techniques, suture material, the need for and interposing tissue layer in a non-radiated fistula, the ideal tissue graft for such a purpose, and postoperative bladder drainage. Furthermore, there is limited data surrounding longer-term functional outcomes aside from closure rates, including lower urinary tract symptoms such as overactive bladder or stress urinary incontinence, as well as sexual function following repair. Given the paucity of data in the minimally invasive repair cohort, more research is needed to close these gaps in our knowledge.

Conclusion

It is often felt that the greatest chance of success of a vesicovaginal fistula repair occurs with the first attempt. Accomplishing this is thought to be more likely when the principles of fistula closure are respected and the surgeon is conversant in the procedures required. The decision to pursue one route over another will depend on a number of patient- and surgeon-specific factors: size, location, and complexity of the fistula; concomitant injury requiring concurrent procedures such as ureteral reimplantation; a history of radiation; as well as surgeon comfort and expertise. As the number of surgeons proficient in laparoscopic and robotic surgery increases, one would expect these techniques to replace open repairs in the majority of cases. Conventional laparoscopy, while comparable to open surgery in cure rates, does present with some technical challenges, particularly with suturing. The difficult learning curve of laparoscopy may be offset by the more ergonomic robot that allows for instrument handling that mimics open surgery and requires a shorter learning curve. The downside to robotics at present is cost and availability. Ultimately, a laparoscopic or robotic approach to vesicovaginal fistula repair demonstrates excellent cure rates and is a viable option for any surgeon proficient in this technique.

Cross-References

▶ Vesicovaginal Fistula Repair: Abdominal Approach
▶ Vesicovaginal Fistula Repair: Vaginal Approach

References

1. Derry D. Note on five pelves of women in the eleventh dynasty in Egypt. J Obstet Gynaecol Br Emp. 1935;42:490–5.
2. Adler AJ, Ronsmans C, Calvert C, Filippi V. Estimating the prevalence of obstetric fistula: a systematic review and meta-analysis. BMC Pregnancy Childbirth. 2013;13:246.
3. De Bernis L. Obstetric fistula: guiding principles for clinical management and programme development, a new WHO guideline. Int J Gynecol Obstet. 2007;99: S117–S21.
4. Arrowsmith S, Hamlin EC, Wall LL. Obstructed labor injury complex: obstetric fistula formation and the multifaceted morbidity of maternal birth trauma in the developing world. Obstet Gynecol Surv. 1996;51 (9):568–74.
5. Wall LL. Obstetric vesicovaginal fistula as an international public-health problem. Lancet. 2006;368 (9542):1201–9.
6. Goodwin WE, Scardino PT. Vesicovaginal and ureterovaginal fistulas: a summary of 25 years of experience. J Urol. 1980;123(3):370–4.
7. Symmonds RE. Incontinence: vesical and urethral fistulas. Clin Obstet Gynecol. 1984;27(2):499–514.
8. Dallas KB, Rogo-Gupta L, Elliott CS. Urologic injury and fistula after hysterectomy for benign indications. Obstet Gynecol. 2019;134(2):241–9.
9. Harkki-Siren P, Sjoberg J, Tiitinen A. Urinary tract injuries after hysterectomy. Obstet Gynecol. 1998;92 (1):113–8.
10. Eilber KS, Kavaler E, Rodriguez LV, Rosenblum N, Raz S. Ten-year experience with transvaginal vesicovaginal fistula repair using tissue interposition. J Urol. 2003;169(3):1033–6.
11. Pushkar DY, Dyakov VV, Kasyan GR. Management of radiation-induced vesicovaginal fistula. Eur Urol. 2009;55(1):131–8.
12. Perez CA, Grigsby PW, Lockett MA, Chao KS, Williamson J. Radiation therapy morbidity in carcinoma of the uterine cervix: dosimetric and clinical correlation. Int J Radiat Oncol Biol Phys. 1999;44(4): 855–66.
13. Moore KN, Gold MA, McMeekin DS, Zorn KK. Vesicovaginal fistula formation in patients with stage IVA cervical carcinoma. Gynecol Oncol. 2007;106(3):498–501.
14. Ganapathi AM, Westmoreland T, Tyler D, Mantyh CR. Bevacizumab-associated fistula formation in postoperative colorectal cancer patients. J Am Coll Surg. 2012;214(4):582–8. discussion 8–90
15. Lin HY, Kuo WT, Hsu CW. Laparoscopic repair of bevacizumab-induced vesicovaginal fistula in metastatic colon cancer – a video vignette. Color Dis. 2019;21(1):123.
16. Tewari KS, Sill MW, Long HJ 3rd, Penson RT, Huang H, Ramondetta LM, et al. Improved survival with bevacizumab in advanced cervical cancer. N Engl J Med. 2014;370(8):734–43.
17. Gogineni V, Morand S, Staats H, Royfman R, Devanaboyina M, Einloth K, et al. Current ovarian cancer maintenance strategies and promising new developments. J Cancer. 2021;12(1):38–53.
18. Sun R, Koubaa I, Limkin EJ, Dumas I, Bentivegna E, Castanon E, et al. Locally advanced cervical cancer with bladder invasion: clinical outcomes and predictive factors for vesicovaginal fistulae. Oncotarget. 2018;9(10):9299–310.
19. Starkman JS, Meints L, Scarpero HM, Dmochowski RR. Vesicovaginal fistula following a transobturator midurethral sling procedure. Int Urogynecol J Pelvic Floor Dysfunct. 2007;18(1):113–5.
20. Yamada BS, Govier FE, Stefanovic KB, Kobashi KC. Vesicovaginal fistula and mesh erosion after

Perigee (transobturator polypropylene mesh anterior repair). Urology. 2006;68(5):1121 e5–7.
21. Margulies RU, Lewicky-Gaupp C, Fenner DE, McGuire EJ, Clemens JQ, Delancey JO. Complications requiring reoperation following vaginal mesh kit procedures for prolapse. Am J Obstet Gynecol. 2008;199(6):678.e1–4.
22. Firoozi F, Ingber MS, Moore CK, Vasavada SP, Rackley RR, Goldman HB. Purely transvaginal/perineal management of complications from commercial prolapse kits using a new prostheses/grafts complication classification system. J Urol. 2012;187(5):1674–9.
23. Sung VW, Rogers RG, Schaffer JI, Balk EM, Uhlig K, Lau J, et al. Graft use in transvaginal pelvic organ prolapse repair: a systematic review. Obstet Gynecol. 2008;112(5):1131–42.
24. Cohen BL, Gousse AE. Current techniques for vesicovaginal fistula repair: surgical pearls to optimize cure rate. Curr Urol Rep. 2007;8(5):413–8.
25. Volkmer BG, Kuefer R, Nesslauer T, Loeffler M, Gottfried HW. Colour Doppler ultrasound in vesicovaginal fistulas. Ultrasound Med Biol. 2000;26(5):771–5.
26. Raghavaiah NV. Double-dye test to diagnose various types of vaginal fistulas. J Urol. 1974;112(6):811–2.
27. Sohail S, Siddiqui KJ. Trans-vaginal sonographic evaluation of vesicovaginal fistula. J Pak Med Assoc. 2005;55(7):292–4.
28. Hilton P. Urodynamic findings in patients with urogenital fistulae. Br J Urol. 1998;81(4):539–42.
29. Waaldijk K. The immediate management of fresh obstetric fistulas. Am J Obstet Gynecol. 2004;191(3):795–9.
30. Hillary CJ, Chapple CR. The choice of surgical approach in the treatment of vesico-vaginal fistulae. Asian J Urol. 2018;5(3):155–9.
31. Blaivas JG, Heritz DM, Romanzi LJ. Early versus late repair of vesicovaginal fistulas: vaginal and abdominal approaches. J Urol. 1995;153(4):1110–2. discussion 2–3
32. Melah GS, El-Nafaty AU, Bukar M. Early versus late closure of vesicovaginal fistulas. Int J Gynaecol Obstet. 2006;93(3):252–3.
33. Wang Y, Hadley HR. Nondelayed transvaginal repair of high lying vesicovaginal fistula. J Urol. 1990;144(1):34–6.
34. Nagraj HK, Kishore TA, Nagalaksmi S. Early laparoscopic repair for supratrigonal vesicovaginal fistula. Int Urogynecol J Pelvic Floor Dysfunct. 2007;18(7):759–62.
35. Lee JH, Choi JS, Lee KW, Han JS, Choi PC, Hoh JK. Immediate laparoscopic nontransvesical repair without omental interposition for vesicovaginal fistula developing after total abdominal hysterectomy. JSLS. 2010;14(2):187–91.
36. Hemal AK, Kolla SB, Wadhwa P. Robotic reconstruction for recurrent supratrigonal vesicovaginal fistulas. J Urol. 2008;180(3):981–5.
37. Randazzo M, Lengauer L, Rochat CH, Ploumidis A, Kröpfl D, Rassweiler J, et al. Best practices in robotic-assisted repair of vesicovaginal fistula: a consensus report from the European Association of Urology Robotic Urology Section Scientific Working Group for reconstructive urology. Eur Urol. 2020;78(3):432–42.
38. Tayler-Smith K, Zachariah R, Manzi M, van den Boogaard W, Vandeborne A, Bishinga A, et al. Obstetric fistula in Burundi: a comprehensive approach to managing women with this neglected disease. BMC Pregnancy Childbirth. 2013;13(1):1–8.
39. Bazi T. Spontaneous closure of vesicovaginal fistulas after bladder drainage alone: review of the evidence. Int Urogynecol J Pelvic Floor Dysfunct. 2007;18(3):329–33.
40. Hillary CJ, Osman NI, Hilton P, Chapple CR. The aetiology, treatment, and outcome of urogenital fistulae managed in well- and low-resourced countries: a systematic review. Eur Urol. 2016;70(3):478–92.
41. Stovsky MD, Ignatoff JM, Blum MD, Nanninga JB, O'Conor VJ, Kursh ED. Use of electrocoagulation in the treatment of vesicovaginal fistulas. J Urol. 1994;152(5 Pt 1):1443–4.
42. Pettersson S, Hedelin H, Jansson I, Teger-Nilsson AC. Fibrin occlusion of a vesicovaginal fistula. Lancet. 1979;313(8122):933.
43. Morita T, Tokue A. Successful endoscopic closure of radiation induced vesicovaginal fistula with fibrin glue and bovine collagen. J Urol. 1999;162(5):1689.
44. Sharma SK, Perry KT, Turk TM. Endoscopic injection of fibrin glue for the treatment of urinary-tract pathology. J Endourol. 2005;19(3):419–23.
45. Schneider JA, Patel VJ, Hertel E. Closure of vesicovaginal fistulas from the urologic viewpoint with reference to endoscopic fibrin glue technique. Zentralbl Gynakol. 1992;114(2):70–3.
46. Sawant AS, Kasat GV, Kumar V. Cyanoacrylate injection in management of recurrent vesicovaginal fistula: our experience. Indian J Urol. 2016;32(4):323–5.
47. Muto G, D'Urso L, Castelli E, Formiconi A, Bardari F. Cyanoacrylic glue: a minimally invasive non-surgical first line approach for the treatment of some urinary fistulas. J Urol. 2005;174(6):2239–43.
48. Ghosh B, Wats V, Pal DK. Comparative analysis of outcome between laparoscopic versus open surgical repair for vesico-vaginal fistula. Obstet Gynecol Sci. 2016;59(6):525.
49. O'Conor VJ, Sokol JK. Vesicovaginal fistula from the standpoint of the urologist. J Urol. 1951;66(4):579–85.
50. von Theobald P, Hamel P, Febbraro W. Laparoscopic repair of a vesicovaginal fistula using an omental J flap. BJOG Int J Obstet Gynaecol. 1998;105(11):1216–8.
51. Nezhat CH, Nezhat F, Nezhat C, Rottenberg H. Laparoscopic repair of a vesicovaginal fistula: a case report. Obstet Gynecol. 1994;83(5):899–901.

52. Melamud O, Eichel L, Turbow B, Shanberg A. Laparoscopic vesicovaginal fistula repair with robotic reconstruction. Urology. 2005;65(1):163–6.
53. Gupta NP, Mishra S, Hemal AK, Mishra A, Seth A, Dogra PN. Comparative analysis of outcome between open and robotic surgical repair of recurrent supratrigonal vesico-vaginal fistula. J Endourol. 2010;24(11):1779–82.
54. Xiong Y, Tang Y, Huang F, Liu L, Zhang X. Transperitoneal laparoscopic repair of vesicovaginal fistula for patients with supratrigonal fistula: comparison with open transperitoneal technique. Int Urogynecol J. 2016;27(9):1415–22.
55. ACOG Practice Bulletin No. 195: prevention of infection after gynecologic procedures. Obstet Gynecol. 2018;131(6):e172–e89.
56. Van Eyk N, van Schalkwyk J, Yudin MH, Allen VM, Bouchard C, Boucher M, et al. Antibiotic prophylaxis in gynaecologic procedures. J Obstet Gynaecol Can. 2012;34(4):382–91.
57. Bartlett MA, Mauck KF, Stephenson CR, Ganesh R, Daniels PR. Perioperative venous thromboembolism prophylaxis. Mayo Clin Proc. 2020;95:2775.
58. Roslan M, Markuszewski MM, Bagińska J, Krajka K. Suprapubic transvesical laparoendoscopic single-site surgery for vesicovaginal fistula repair: a case report. Wideochir Inne Tech Maloinwazyjne. 2012;7(4):307–10.
59. Sotelo R, Mariano MB, García-Segui A, Dubois R, Spaliviero M, Keklikian W, et al. Laparoscopic repair of vesicovaginal fistula. J Urol. 2005;173(5):1615–8.
60. Zhang Q, Ye Z, Liu F, Qi X, Shao C, He X, et al. Laparoscopic transabdominal transvesical repair of supratrigonal vesicovaginal fistula. Int Urogynecol J. 2013;24(2):337–42.
61. Shah SJ. Laparoscopic transabdominal transvesical vesicovaginal fistula repair. J Endourol. 2009;23(7):1135–7.
62. Ghosh B, Biswal DK, Bera MK, Pal DK. Laparoscopic vesicovaginal fistula repair with limited cystotomy: a rewarding treatment option. J Obstet Gynaecol India. 2016;66(1):370–6.
63. Giannakopoulos S, Arif H, Nastos Z, Liapis A, Kalaitzis C, Touloupidis S. Laparoscopic transvesical vesicovaginal fistula repair with the least invasive way: only three trocars and a limited posterior cystotomy. Asian J Urol. 2020;7(4):351–6.
64. Miklos JR, Moore RD. Laparoscopic extravesical vesicovaginal fistula repair: our technique and 15 year experience. Int Urogynecol J. 2015;26(3):441–6.
65. Lee Z, Kaplan J, Giusto L, Eun D. Prevention of iatrogenic ureteral injuries during robotic gynecologic surgery: a review. Am J Obstet Gynecol. 2016;214(5):566–71.
66. Lee Z, Simhan J, Parker DC, Reilly C, Llukani E, Lee DI, et al. Novel use of indocyanine green for intraoperative, real-time localization of ureteral stenosis during robot-assisted ureteroureterostomy. Urology. 2013;82(3):729–33.
67. Abdel-Karim AM, Mousa A, Hasouna M, Elsalmy S. Laparoscopic transperitoneal extravesical repair of vesicovaginal fistula. Int Urogynecol J. 2011;22(6):693–7.
68. Miklos JR, Moore RD, Chinthakanan O. Laparoscopic and robotic-assisted vesicovaginal fistula repair: a systematic review of the literature. J Minim Invasive Gynecol. 2015;22(5):727–36.
69. Zhou P, Deng W, Li J, Pan H, Wang Y, Song C, et al. Transvesical versus extravesical approach to laparoscopic posthysterectomy vesicovaginal fistula repair: a retrospective study from two medical centers. Neurourol Urodyn. 2021;40:1593.
70. Javali TD, Katti A, Nagaraj HK. A simplified laparoscopic approach to repair vesicovaginal fistula: the M.S. Ramaiah technique. Urology. 2015;85(3):544–6.
71. Mallikarjuna C, Nayak P, Reddy KP, Ghouse SM, Ragoori D, Bendigeri MT, et al. The AINU technique for laparoscopic vesico-vaginal fistula repair: a preliminary report. Urol Int. 2015;95(3):357–60.
72. Das Mahapatra P, Bhattacharyya P. Laparoscopic intraperitoneal repair of high-up urinary bladder fistula: a review of 12 cases. Int Urogynecol J Pelvic Floor Dysfunct. 2007;18(6):635–9.
73. Kiricuta I. Use of the greater omentum in the treatment of vesicovaginal and rectovesicovaginal fistulae after radiotherapy and cystoplasties. J Chir (Paris). 1965;89(4):477–84.
74. Evans DH, Madjar S, Politano VA, Bejany DE, Lynne CM, Gousse AE. Interposition flaps in transabdominal vesicovaginal fistula repairs: are they really necessary? Urology. 2001;57(4):670–4.
75. Ayed M, El Atat R, Hassine LB, Sfaxi M, Chebil M, Zmerli S. Prognostic factors of recurrence after vesicovaginal fistula repair. Int J Urol. 2006;13(4):345–9.
76. Kurz M, Horstmann M, John H. Robot-assisted laparoscopic repair of high vesicovaginal fistulae with peritoneal flap inlay. Eur Urol. 2012;61(1):229–30.
77. Erdogru T, Sanli A, Celik O, Baykara M. Laparoscopic transvesical repair of recurrent vesicovaginal fistula using with fleece-bound sealing system. Arch Gynecol Obstet. 2008;277(5):461–4.
78. Price DT, Price TC. Robotic repair of a vesicovaginal fistula in an irradiated field using a dehydrated amniotic allograft as an interposition patch. J Robot Surg. 2016;10(1):77–80.
79. Miklos JR, Moore RD. Laparoscopic transperitoneal extravesical approach to vesicovaginal fistula repair without omental flap: a novel technique. Int Urogynecol J. 2015;26(3):447–8.
80. Martini A, Dattolo E, Frizzi J, Villari D, Paoletti MC. Robotic vesico-vaginal fistula repair with no omental flap interposition. Int Urogynecol J. 2016;27(8):1277–8.

81. Thomae KR, Kilambi NK, Poole GV, Eddy VA, et al. Method of urinary diversion in nonurethral traumatic bladder injuries: retrospective analysis of 70 cases/discussion. Am Surg. 1998;64(1):77–80. discussion −1
82. Bochenska K, Zyczynski HM. Utility of postoperative voiding cystourethrogram after lower urinary tract repair. Female Pelvic Med Reconstr Surg. 2016;22(5):369–72.
83. Chang OH, Ganesh P, Wilkinson JP, Pope RJ. Extended bladder catheterization for women with positive dye tests after obstetric vesicovaginal fistula repair surgery. Int J Gynaecol Obstet. 2020;149(1):61–5.
84. Abdel-Karim A, Elmissiry M, Moussa A, Mahfouz W, Abulfotooh A, Dawood W, et al. Laparoscopic repair of female genitourinary fistulae: 10 year single-center experience. Int Urogynecol J. 2020;31(7):1357–62.
85. Chandna A, Mavuduru RS, Bora GS, Sharma AP, Parmar KM, Devana SK, et al. Robot-assisted repair of complex vesicovaginal fistulae: feasibility and outcomes. Urology. 2020;144:92–8.
86. Abdel-Karim AM, Moussa A, Elsalmy S. Laparoendoscopic single-site surgery extravesical repair of vesicovaginal fistula: early experience. Urology. 2011;78(3):567–71.
87. Mahadevappa N, Gudage S, Senguttavan KV, Mallya A, Dharwadkar S. Laparoendoscopic single site surgery for extravesical repair of vesicovaginal fistula using conventional instruments: our initial experience. Urol Ann. 2016;8(3):305–11.
88. Nerli R, Reddy M. Transvesicoscopic repair of vesicovaginal fistula. Diagn Ther Endosc. 2010;2010:760348.
89. Advincula AP, Song A. The role of robotic surgery in gynecology. Curr Opin Obstet Gynecol. 2007;19(4):331–6.
90. Van Koughnett JA, Jayaraman S, Eagleson R, Quan D, van Wynsberghe A, Schlachta CM. Are there advantages to robotic-assisted surgery over laparoscopy from the surgeon's perspective? J Robot Surg. 2009;3(2):79–82.
91. Sundaram BM, Kalidasan G, Hemal AK. Robotic repair of vesicovaginal fistula: case series of five patients. Urology. 2006;67(5):970–3.
92. Schimpf MO, Morgenstern JH, Tulikangas PK, Wagner JR. Vesicovaginal fistula repair without intentional cystotomy using the laparoscopic robotic approach: a case report. JSLS. 2007;11(3):378–80.
93. Kidd LC, Lee M, Lee Z, Epstein M, Liu S, Rangel E, et al. A multi-institutional experience with robotic vesicovaginal and ureterovaginal fistula repair after iatrogenic injury. J Endourol. 2021;35:1659.
94. Billah MS, Stifelman M, Munver R, Tsui J, Lovallo G, Ahmed M. Single port robotic assisted reconstructive urologic surgery-with the da Vinci SP surgical system. Transl Androl Urol. 2020;9(2):870–8.
95. Paraiso MFR, Jelovsek JE, Frick A, Chen CCG, Barber MD. Laparoscopic compared with robotic sacrocolpopexy for vaginal prolapse: a randomized controlled trial. Obstet Gynecol. 2011;118(5):1005–13.
96. Geller EJ, Lin FC, Matthews CA. Analysis of robotic performance times to improve operative efficiency. J Minim Invasive Gynecol. 2013;20(1):43–8.
97. Bernard BP, Putz-Anderson V. Musculoskeletal disorders and workplace factors; a critical review of epidemiologic evidence for work-related musculoskeletal disorders of the neck, upper extremity, and low back. Cincinnati: NIOSH; 1997.
98. Catanzarite T, Tan-Kim J, Whitcomb EL, Menefee S. Ergonomics in surgery: a review. Female Pelvic Med Reconstr Surg. 2018;24(1):1–12.
99. Tarr ME, Brancato SJ, Cunkelman JA, Polcari A, Nutter B, Kenton K. Comparison of postural ergonomics between laparoscopic and robotic sacrocolpopexy: a pilot study. J Minim Invasive Gynecol. 2015;22(2):234–8.
100. Panaiyadiyan S, Nayyar BU, Nayyar R, Kumar N, Seth A, Kumar R, et al. Impact of vesicovaginal fistula repair on urinary and sexual function: patient-reported outcomes over long-term follow-up. Int Urogynecol J. 2021;32:2521.
101. Grewal M, Pakzad MH, Hamid R, Ockrim JL, Greenwell TJ. The medium- to long-term functional outcomes of women who have had successful anatomical closure of vesicovaginal fistulae. Urol Ann. 2019;11(3):247–51.
102. Mohr S, Brandner S, Mueller MD, Dreher EF, Kuhn A. Sexual function after vaginal and abdominal fistula repair. Am J Obstet Gynecol. 2014;211(1):74.e1–6.
103. Brook G. Obstetric fistula: the role of physiotherapy: a report from the Physiotherapy Committee of the International Continence Society. Neurourol Urodyn. 2019;38(1):407–16.
104. Shaw C. A systematic review of the literature on the prevalence of sexual impairment in women with urinary incontinence and the prevalence of urinary leakage during sexual activity. Eur Urol. 2002;42(5):432–40.
105. Pope R, Ganesh P, Chalamanda C, Nundwe W, Wilkinson J. Sexual function before and after vesicovaginal fistula repair. J Sex Med. 2018;15(8):1125–32.

Vesicovaginal Fistula Repair: Vaginal Approach

Annah Vollstedt, Ly Hoang Roberts, and Larry T. Sirls

Contents

Etiology and Incidence	762
Classification Systems	762
Clinical Presentation and Evaluation	763
Risk Factors	765
Physical Examination	765
Preoperative Management	766
Timing of Repair	767
Surgical Approach	768
Transvaginal Approaches	768
Vaginal Flap/Flap-Splitting Technique	768
Latzko Technique	771
Radiation-Associated and Complex VVF Repair	772
Martius Flap	772
Peritoneal Flap	774
Omental Flap	774
Gracilis Flap	775
Amniotic Membrane	776

A. Vollstedt
Department of Urology, University of Iowa Hospitals and Clinics, Iowa City, IA, USA

L. Hoang Roberts
William Beaumont School of Medicine, Beaumont Hospital, Oakland University, Royal Oak, MI, USA

L. T. Sirls (✉)
Oakland University William Beaumont School of Medicine, Beaumont Hospital, Royal Oak, MI, USA

Postoperative Management	776
Surgical Outcomes	782
Summary	783
Cross-References	783
References	783

Abstract

A vesicovaginal fistula (VVF) is an abnormal connection between the bladder and the vagina. This is a devastating and often debilitating disorder affecting up to 0.3–2% of women worldwide. In the developed world, VVF is most often due to injury to the genitourinary tract at the time of pelvic surgery, with pelvic cancer and radiation being less common causes. In the developing world, prolonged and obstructed labor is the most common cause. Evaluation with a physical exam, cystoscopy, and imaging is key in deciding surgical planning. The same principles of fistula repair apply to both abdominal and vaginal approaches. Though there are no prospective, randomized trials on the vaginal and the abdominal approaches to repair, the vaginal approach for VVF repair is the preferred approach for most vaginal surgeons and has high success rates.

Keywords

Vesicovaginal fistula · Transvaginal approach

Etiology and Incidence

A vesicovaginal fistula (VVF) is an abnormal connection between the bladder and the vagina. VVF account for most genitourinary fistulae and have devastating physical and psychosocial consequences. The incidence of VVF in the developed world is estimated between 0.3% and 2.0% [1, 2], most forming after trauma to the genitourinary tract from pelvic surgery, such as an unrecognized cystotomy at the time of hysterectomy. Advanced pelvic cancer and radiation are less common causes. In a recent review of 5698 hysterectomies by Duong et al., larger uterine size, longer operative time, and more severe bladder injuries were associated with a higher risk of VVF formation [3].

In contrast, in developing countries, most VVF are a consequence of childbirth, often a combination of prolonged and obstructed labor due to cephalopelvic disproportion (from reduced pelvic dimensions of early childbearing), poor nutritional status, and lack of healthcare resources [4, 5]. Figure 1 shows an example of a large obstetric-related VVF. It is estimated that over three million women in the developing world are living with a VVF, with an incidence of 30,000–130,000 per year [6–8]. It is important to note that, for those with access to healthcare, the transvaginal approach to repair VVF is the standard of care in developing countries with good success rates.

Classification Systems

Several classification systems for VVF are reported in the literature. In general, VVF can be divided into two categories: simple or complex. Simple VVF has been defined as ≤2 cm, solitary, and not associated with radiated tissue. Complex VVF are >2 cm, involve the ureter, are recurrent after failed repair, or are associated with radiation [9]. Agnoli et al. have proposed a more nuanced classification system as follows: simple fistula defined as small (<0.5 cm), nonradiated tissue and solitary versus complex fistula defined as medium (0.6–2.4 cm), or large (≥2.5 cm), radiated, multiple, or recurrent [10]. Similarly, the World Health Organization has defined a simple

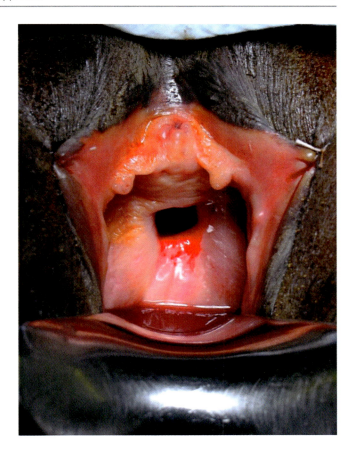

Fig. 1 Example of a large obstetric-related vesicovaginal fistula. (Courtesy of Michael Breen, FRCOG)

fistula as being midvagina in location with minimal scarring and < 3 cm [11].

The Goh and Waaldjik are the two most commonly used classification systems to describe the complexity of VVF related to obstetric trauma. Described in 2004, the Goh classification divides genitourinary fistulae into four main types, depending on the distance of the distal edge of the fistula from the external urinary meatus, as well as a subtype for the size of the fistula itself [12]. Similar to the Goh classification, the Waaldjik system described three types of VVF based on relation to the "closing mechanism," which is described as the urethra and the bladder neck. Comparison of the two systems is outlined in Table 1. In a recent analysis, the Goh classification was better at predicting fistula closure, compared to the Waaldjik system [13].

Clinical Presentation and Evaluation

Patients with VVF classically present with continuous leakage of urine. In the developing world, this is often associated with severe social isolation due to abandonment by their loved ones because of the odor and the continuous wetness. In some countries, women with VVF carry a bucket with them at all times to catch the urine, as in Fig. 2.

In contrast, in developed countries, a VVF should be suspected with continuous incontinence following a hysterectomy or other pelvic surgery. The degree of incontinence is associated with the

Table 1 Goh and Waaldjik classifications systems for obstetric-related VVF

Goh classification [12]		Waaldjik classification [13]	
Type		Type	
1	Distal edge of fistula >3.5 cm from external urinary meatus	1	Fistula not involving the closing mechanism

2	Distal edge of fistula 2.5–3.5 cm from external urinary meatus	2	Fistula involving the closing mechanism
			A Without (sub) total involvement of the urethra
			  a Without circumferential defect
			  b With circumferential defect
			B With (sub)total involvement of the urethra
			  a Without circumferential defect
			  b With circumferential defect

3	Distal edge of fistula 1.5–<2.5 cm from external urinary meatus		
4	Distal edge of fistula <1.5 cm from external urinary meatus		
Subtype modifiers			
a	Size <1.5 cm, in the largest diameter		
b	Size 1.5–3 cm, in the largest diameter		
c	Size >3 cm, in the largest diameter	3	Miscellaneous, e.g., ureterovaginal or other exceptional fistulas

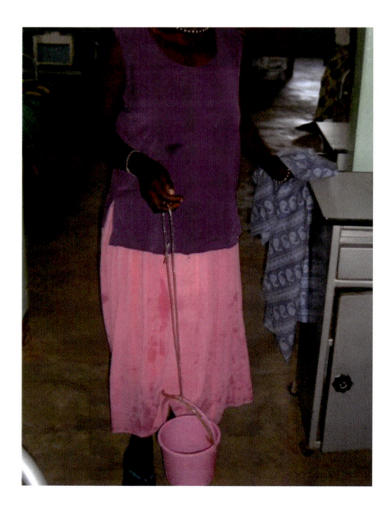

Fig. 2 Woman carries a bucket to catch large amount of continuous urinary leaking from the VVF. (Courtesy of Michael Breen, FRCOG)

size of the VVF. For instance, the only symptom of a small VVF may be minimal watery vaginal discharge associated with a normal voiding pattern. Leakage may worsen with positional changes, such as moving from supine to upright. Other symptoms can include vaginal discharge, hematuria, and recurrent cystitis.

Risk Factors

Review of the index operative note is essential. The clinician should note if there is a previous history of cesarean section, as this can be a risk factor for VVF at the time of hysterectomy [14]. Bladder injury with devascularization usually is the underlying cause of VVF. Suture erosion, hematoma formation, and infection may also contribute to the development of VVF [15]. Oncologic and radiation therapy history should also be noted. Radiation-induced VVF may occur many years after treatment, secondary to hypoperfusion of the irradiated tissue and subsequent tissue necrosis. Medical comorbidities that negatively affect vascular health such as diabetes mellitus, chronic steroid use, increased blood loss, and tobacco use can all increase the risk of VVF [15, 16].

Physical Examination

A detailed pelvic examination with a speculum and adequate lighting should be performed. Upon speculum pelvic exam, urine may be present on the vulva and may be seen as a fluid collection in the posterior vagina. The size, location, severity, and number of tracts should be noted. The quality of the surrounding tissue should be assessed, looking specifically for signs of infection, necrosis, foreign body-like vaginal mesh, and radiation change. Inspect the vulva for skin irritation from constant contact with urine. Vaginoscopy using a flexible cystoscope may also aid in the assessment of the VVF. Some authors describe the classic "double-dye tampon test" [17], in which a tampon is placed in the vagina and a methylene blue solution is instilled into the bladder via a catheter. The patient is also given oral pyridium which is excreted renally. After ambulation, the tampon is removed and inspected. If the tampon is stained blue, a VVF should be suspected. If the tampon is stained orange, a ureterovaginal fistula should be suspected. In lieu of this test, the authors prefer to assess the presence of a VVF by placing 300 mL of blue-colored saline into the bladder. After 10 min, a vaginal exam is performed to assess for the presence of the VVF. If this examination is negative, the patient is brought to the operating room for cystoscopy and examination under anesthesia, with possible retrograde pyelograms depending on any prior upper tract imaging, such as a CT urogram.

The physical examination is critical to inform the surgeon of three important issues, especially in cases of iatrogenic postoperative fistula. First, the surgeon must clearly see the fistula before operating to repair. Second, the surgeon is evaluating the location of the fistula with respect to the depth of the vagina and whether the fistula can be reached. Experienced vaginal surgeons can reach the majority of fistulae from a vaginal approach. Finally, the surgeon must assess whether there is sufficient introital opening to provide access to the fistula or if a vaginal relaxing incision (episiotomy) is needed.

Obstetric fistulas in developing countries may be much larger with more scarring and associated organ involvement like the urethra, the uterus, or rectum. Examination of these patients is more complex as is their planned reconstruction. Reconstruction of large, complex, obstetric fistula is beyond the scope of this chapter.

Cystourethroscopy should be performed to determine the anatomic location of the fistula in the bladder and its relation to the ureteral orifices [17]. The viability of the surrounding tissues can be evaluated cystoscopically, as well. Figure 3 shows a discrete fistula on cystoscopic exam. A voiding cystourethrogram (VCUG) with lateral views can also confirm the presence of a VVF, as in Fig. 4.

Upper tract imaging with a computed tomography (CT) urogram, intravenous pyelogram, or retrograde pyelogram is recommended for all cases of VVF, as 10–12% of postsurgical VVF are associated with ureteral injury, as well as all suspected cases of ureterovaginal fistulae [17, 18] (Fig. 5).

It should be noted that a negative CT urogram does not exclude a ureterovaginal fistula. If a ureterovaginal fistula is suspected, a retrograde pyelogram should be performed at the time of cystoscopy. This can be performed in the operating room at the time of exam under anesthesia, to assess the fistula more thoroughly than what may be allowed in the office. If malignancy is suspected, a biopsy should be performed.

Preoperative Management

Initial management of a VVF is continuous bladder drainage via a Foley catheter. The diversion of the urine away from the fistula may allow it to close spontaneously [19]. If a VVF is very small, catheterization may be all that is required for the VVF to close. It has been suggested to wait 3–7 days to assess the initial response to catheterization. If very little urine drains through the VVF, the catheter may be removed. If most of the urine drains through the catheter, then it is left in place for up to 6 weeks or more [19]. In addition to size of the defect, other factors such as the presence of malignancy, history of radiation, and the time-period between diagnosis and catheter placement will determine the rate of cure from catheterization alone. If catheter placement is delayed, the fistulous tract will epithelialize, preventing spontaneous closure. In one study of postsurgical VVF, if the catheter was inserted less than 3 weeks following the index surgery, 39% (22/57) of women had spontaneous closure of their VVF. If the catheter was inserted more than 6 weeks after the injury, only 3% (1/32) of VVF spontaneously closed.

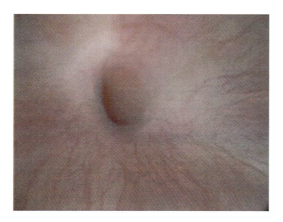

Fig. 3 Cystoscopic evaluation can reveal the fistulous tract. (Permission from Complications of Female Incontinence and Pelvic Reconstructive Surgery, 2nd Edition. Springer. Chapter 21. Vesicovaginal and Urethrovaginal Fistula Repair)

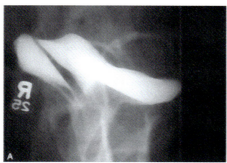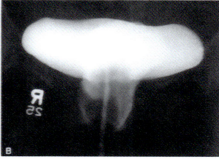

Fig. 4 Cystogram demonstrating a vesicovaginal fistula (VVF): (**a**) Lateral image demonstrates a posthysterectomy VVF; (**b**) anteroposterior view. The contrast agent is seen opacifying and outlining the vagina superimposed on the bladder. (Permission from Campbell-Walsh Urology, 10th edition. Chapter 77)

Fig. 5 Retrograde pyelogram showing extravasation of contrast from the ureter to the vagina. (Permission from Complications of Female Incontinence and Pelvic Reconstructive Surgery, 2nd Edition. Springer. Chapter 21. Vesicovaginal and Urethrovaginal Fistula Repair)

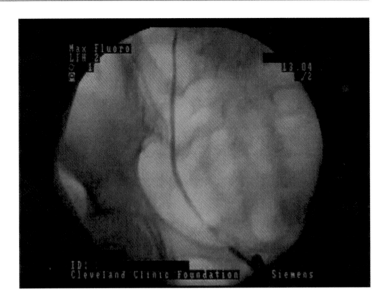

The need for proper nutrition, smoking cessation, and good glucose control prior to VVF repair should be discussed with the patients. Preoperative vaginal estrogen may be beneficial in postmenopausal patients with vaginal atrophy [20], as this may improve local tissue quality and increase vascularity.

In the developing world, patients are often times asked to continue to drink large amounts of water up until 4 hours prior to surgery for VVF. This is because, in many cases, patients tend to restrict their water intake in an effort to decrease their amount of wetness, which can lead to hypotension during anesthesia, as well as make identification of the ureteric orifices difficult intraoperatively [21].

Sexual activity should be documented prior to VVF repair, especially given the potential for sexual dysfunction and dyspareunia after a transvaginal approach.

Timing of Repair

The timing of VVF repair is a controversial topic. While there are no guidelines or literature to support a specific timeline, most experts agree that 10–12 weeks after the index surgery is the most appropriate time for postsurgical VVF repair [22, 23]. Prior to 10 weeks, the tissues may still by friable and inflamed, making a successful repair more difficult. The caveat is if the VVF is diagnosed within a few days of the index surgery, an immediate repair may be performed, as the inflammation and tissue edema are still minimal at that time [19, 26]. Some authors recommend waiting up to 6 months, especially for larger defects [24]. In a recent systematic review, a waiting period of 3 months was typically recommended [25]. In cases of VVF following prolonged labor, the general rule is to wait 12 weeks after delivery, again, to allow the tissues to become less friable. For radiation-induced VVF, waiting 12 months after completion of the radiation treatments is recommended [19].

The dramatic decrease in patient's quality of life is one reason why a surgeon may consider definitive repair sooner rather than later. Some argue that a vaginal approach, especially after a recent abdominal surgery which caused fistula, can be done as soon as the fistula is recognized postoperatively, and this is typically the authors approach. However, as pointed out by Dr. Michael Breen, one of the world's leading experts in surgical fistula repair and who practices in a high-volume center in Africa, "one should never sacrifice success of surgery by operating too early, as the best chance of closure is at the first attempt" [19].

Surgical Approach

There is no consensus regarding the most successful surgical approach. Vaginal or abdominal, open or laparoscopic/robotic, and with/without interpositional flap are all viable options. The best surgical approach, however, should be based on the size and location of the fistula, as well as the surgeon's experience [27]. Regardless of the approach, the basic principles of fistula repair should be performed: treatment of infection, removal of foreign bodies/nondissolving material or malignancy, tissue mobilization for a tension-free and watertight repair, multilayer closure with nonoverlapping suture lines, continuous bladder drainage, and hemostasis [14, 28].

Currently, there are no randomization control trials examining the best surgical route. In one recent meta-analysis, the most common surgical technique was the transvaginal approach (535/1379, 39%), followed by transabdominal (493/1379, 36%), and laparoscopic/robotic (207/1379, 15%) [29]. In one study by Gedik et al., the success rates for patients who have failed conservative treatment for their VVF (15–20 mm in size) were comparable between transvaginal and transabdominal repair (25/25, 100% vs 27/28, 96.4%, $p = 1.00$). However, the length of stay was longer and the complication rate higher for the transabdominal approach [23]. Recently, Panaiydiyan et al. analyzed the sexual and urinary dysfunction of women undergoing transabdominal and transvaginal repair of VVF and found that the mean Female Sexual Function Index and International Consultation of Incontinence Questionnaire-Short Form for both repairs was comparable at a mean follow-up of 30 months [30].

Generally, the abdominal approach is best when there is ureteric involvement requiring reimplantation, the fistula is high and the vagina deep, or if vaginal access is limited such as with vaginal stenosis. Some argue for abdominal repair after a failed vaginal approach; however, the authors are comfortable with a repeat vaginal approach in selected patients based on complexity of the VVF. The abdominal approach also allows for easier access to the omentum, peritoneum, or rectus muscle for creation of an interpositional flap, if needed.

The advantages of the transvaginal approach include its minimally invasive nature, shorter hospital stay (oftentimes performed on an outpatient basis), less postoperative pain, lower intraoperative blood loss, and faster return to normal activities [28]. In patients who have had multiple abdominal surgeries, the transvaginal approach can be advantageous by avoiding another intra-abdominal procedure. The vaginal approach lends itself to various interpositional tissue options, such as the peritoneum, Martius fat pad, and a gracilis muscle flap [10]. In addition, the transvaginal approach can be performed in limited-resource areas around the world. Disadvantages to the transvaginal approach include potential for vaginal shortening with apical fistula (especially the Latzko technique) and difficulty in exposing high fistulae near the vaginal cuff, especially in a narrow vagina, and the deep vagina in the absence of any degree of apical prolapse. Table 2 shows the differences between transvaginal and transabdominal approaches.

The fistula surgeon should be familiar with both transabdominal and transvaginal approaches. For instance, a difficult transvaginal case may need to be converted to transabdominal in order to access the entire fistula or repair adjacent structures.

Transvaginal Approaches

Vaginal Flap/Flap-Splitting Technique

The vaginal flap approach was first described by Raz and colleagues in the 1980s [31, 32]. In this approach, a three-layer closure is performed, or four-layer if an interpositional flap is used. This is

Table 2 Comparison of transvaginal and transabdominal approaches

Variable	Transvaginal	Transabdominal
Indication	Simple	Complex: ureter involvement, high fistula/deep vagina, narrow introitus, and prior failed vaginal repair in select patients
Blood loss	Less	More
Invasiveness	Less	More
Vaginal shortening	Possible	No
Flap options	Martius, peritoneum, and gracilis	Peritoneum, omentum, and rectus
Operative time	Less	More
Postoperative pain	Mild	Moderate/severe

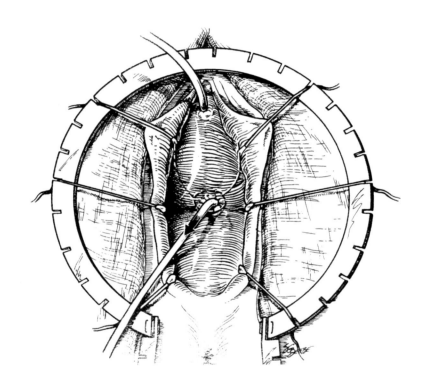

Fig. 6 A small catheter is placed in the fistula tract to aid in dissection. Urethral catheter is placed. LoneStar® retractor provides optimal exposure. Here, an inverted-U vaginal skin incision is planned with the base distally. (Permission from Traumatic and Reconstructive Urology, McAnnich, Carroll, Jordan (Eds). Chapter 23. Vesicovaginal Fistulas: Reconstructive Techniques. Ganabathi, Sirls, Zimmern, Leach. WB Saunders. Philadelphia)

the transvaginal technique preferred by the authors. The following are the surgical steps:

1. The patient is placed in a dorsal lithotomy position. The lower abdomen and perineum are prepped. Some surgeons choose to use a betadine-soaked rectal packing for easy identification of the rectum during the repair. Vaginal exposure is achieved with a LoneStar® retractor. A weighted vaginal speculum may be used. In rare cases, a posterolateral relaxing incision at the 5 or 7 o'clock position is performed to aid in vaginal access in patients with a narrow introitus. A headlight is critical.

2. Cystoscopy is performed first, and a ureteral catheter may be placed if the fistula tract is in close proximity to the ureteral orifice(s). For maximal postoperative drainage, a suprapubic catheter may be placed but is uncommon in the authors experience.

Fig. 7 The anterior vaginal wall is dissected, and lateral vaginal wall flaps are developed between bladder and vagina. (Permission from Traumatic and Reconstructive Urology, McAnnich, Carroll, Jordan (Eds). Chapter 23. Vesicovaginal Fistulas: Reconstructive Techniques. Ganabathi, Sirls, Zimmern, Leach. WB Saunders. Philadelphia)

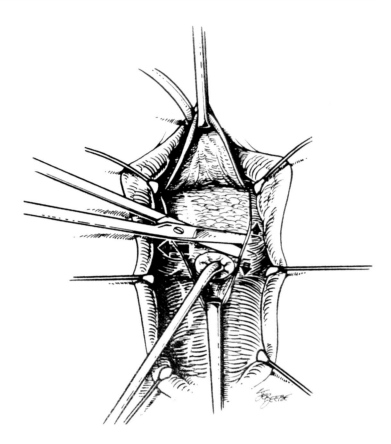

3. The pediatric catheter (8–10 French) or Fogarty catheter is placed in the fistulous tract. Sometimes, if the fistulous tract is difficult to discern, a wire can be placed cystoscopically through the fistula tract and then the catheter advanced retrograde over this (Fig. 6). Gentle traction on this catheter helps bring the VVF down toward the introitus for better access.

4. A U-shaped incision is made in the vaginal skin, incorporating the opening of the fistula, with the limbs of the U extending either toward the apex of the vagina or along the anterior vaginal wall toward the introitus. The authors make this decision intraoperatively depending on the fistula location and the patient's anatomy. In this example, the vaginal wall flap is based distally. This vaginal wall flap will eventually be mobilized as the final layer over the fistula repair, which helps prevent vaginal shortening and overlapping suture lines.

5. The vaginal wall flap is mobilized proximally, distally, and laterally from the fistula tract. Wide mobilization of the vaginal wall flap from the underlying perivesical fascia, at least 2 cm from the fistula, is a critical process to allow the mobility to create a tension-free repair (Fig. 7). When dissecting along the posterior vaginal wall, care must be taken not to injure the rectum (Fig. 8).

It should be noted here that the authors prefer not to excise the fistulous tract. This minimizes the size of the defect, avoids encroachment toward the ureter, and avoids bleeding edges of the fistula tract.

6. The catheter within the fistulous tract is now removed in preparation for closure of the defect. 3–0 or 4–0 absorbable suture is used to close the first layer. This layer incorporates the fistulous tract and the healthy bladder mucosa by starting about 0.5 cm away from the defect (Fig. 9).

Fig. 8 The posterior vaginal wall flap is created, taking care not to enter the rectum. (Permission from Traumatic and Reconstructive Urology, McAnnich, Carroll, Jordan (Eds). Chapter 23. Vesicovaginal Fistulas: Reconstructive Techniques. Ganabathi, Sirls, Zimmern, Leach. WB Saunders. Philadelphia)

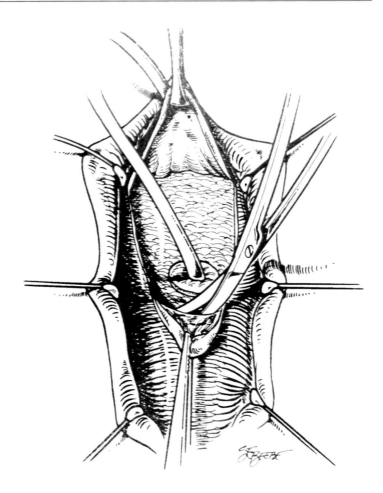

7. The second layer is an imbricating layer of the perivesical fascia and detrusor muscle over the first layer, perpendicular to the first layer closure (Fig. 10). At this point, the repair should be tested by filling the catheter with 200 mL of saline. Some surgeons may stain with methylene blue to aid visualization.
8. An interpositional flap may be placed at this point, if necessary.
9. Lastly, the vaginal flap is inspected, making sure that it is mobilized at least 2–3 cm beyond the repair for complete coverage. The flap is advanced and reapproximated to the vaginal skin with running, locking absorbable suture (Fig. 11). A vaginal pack may be placed overnight. The authors prefer to keep the urethral catheter in place for at least 10–14 days for simple fistula, and 14–21 days for more complex fistula, with a cystogram confirming successful repair prior to removal of the catheter.

Depending on the location of the fistula and the patient's anatomy, an apically based inverted U- or J-shaped incision can also be utilized, as in Fig. 12.

Latzko Technique

Described in 1942, the Latzko technique is in effect a partial colpocleisis and can be used to repair small, uncomplicated apical fistulae [33]. This is a simple procedure that has yielded high success rates, ranging from 89 to 100% [33–35]. The main disadvantage to this technique is the shortening of the vagina with resulting sexual

Fig. 9 The first layer of horizontal closure of the fistula is performed using running absorbable sutures at the fistula margins without excising the fistula. (Permission from Traumatic and Reconstructive Urology, McAnnich, Carroll, Jordan (Eds). Chapter 23. Vesicovaginal Fistulas: Reconstructive Techniques. Ganabathi, Sirls, Zimmern, Leach. WB Saunders. Philadelphia)

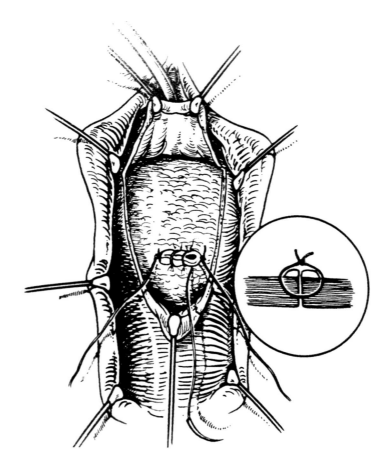

dysfunction. In this technique, an elliptical or spherical portion of vaginal skin is mobilized and denuded around the fistulous tract about 1–2 cm in all directions, Fig. 13.

The pubovesical fascia is first closed and then the vaginal skin as the second layer, using interrupted sutures (Fig. 14). The bladder defect is not disturbed, meaning the sutures are not placed into the bladder wall or mucosa.

Radiation-Associated and Complex VVF Repair

A well-vascularized interpositional tissue layer is recommended for postradiation VVF repair [10] in order to enhance healing. The most commonly used interpositional flap is the Martius flap. Other flaps that may be used for a transvaginal technique include the peritoneum, omental, and the gracilis muscle.

Martius Flap

Henirich Martius first described the use of a fibrofatty labial flap in 1928 [36]. This flap contains adipose and connective tissue and is most commonly used for distal or low fistulae. The Martius flap is used for other reconstructive surgeries, such as urethrolysis, urethrovaginal fistula, and rectovaginal fistula. The blood supply to the flap is the external pudendal artery superiorly, obturator artery laterally, and the inferior posterior labial vessels off the internal pudendal artery

Fig. 10 The second layer of closure incorporates the perivescial fascia using interrupted Lembert-type sutures at right angles to the first layer of closure. The watertightness of the fistula closure is then verified with intravesical instillation of diluted methylene blue. (Permission from Traumatic and Reconstructive Urology, McAninch, Carroll, Jordan (Eds). Chapter 23. Vesicovaginal Fistulas: Reconstructive Techniques. Ganabathi, Sirls, Zimmern, Leach. WB Saunders. Philadelphia)

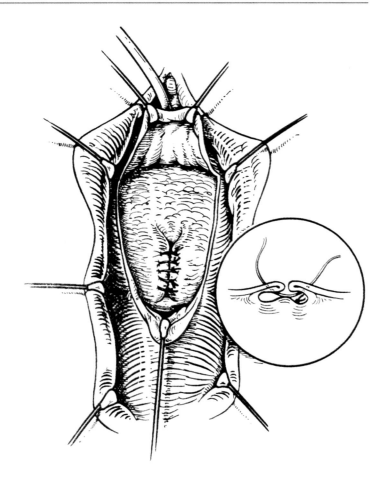

inferiorly (Fig. 15). In addition to lateral blood supply, the superior or inferior blood supply is also sacrificed, depending on where the flap will be transferred [37].

Prior to closing the vaginal skin flap, the Martius is harvested. A vertical incision is made over the labia majora (Fig. 16).

The incision is carried down to the level of the labial fat pad. The borders of the dissection are the labiocrural fold laterally, the labia minora and bulbocavernosus muscle medially, and Colles fascia covering the urogenital diaphragm posteriorly [37]. A Penrose drain can be used for gentle traction to facilitate mobilization before sacrificing the superior or inferior blood supply. After clamping and transecting either the superior or inferior blood supply, a tunnel is created from the labial incision to the site of the fistula (Fig. 17). The tunnel should be widened to accept about 2 fingers to prevent compression of the blood supply of the flap [14].

A hemostat can be used to transfer the flap to the fistula repair, Fig. 18.

Once the flap is positioned over the repair, it is secured using interrupted absorbable sutures, Fig. 19.

The vaginal skin flap is then advanced over the flap and closed as previously described. A small drain can be left in the labial incision. The labial incision is closed in two layers, and a gentle pressure dressing is applied (Fig. 20).

In a recent review by Malde et al., 43 patients had a Martius flap at the time of transvaginal VVF repair with a cure rate of 95%. Eilber et al.

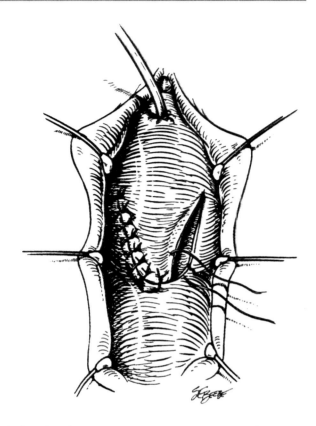

Fig. 11 The third layer of closure is performed by advancing the U-shaped anterior vaginal wall flap over the fistula to avoid overlapping suture lines. (Permission from Traumatic and Reconstructive Urology, McAnnich, Carroll, Jordan (Eds). Chapter 23. Vesicovaginal Fistulas: Reconstructive Techniques. Ganabathi, Sirls, Zimmern, Leach. WB Saunders. Philadelphia)

also showed a 97% success rate [38] in 34 patients, and Lee et al. also showed a 97% success rate and minimal long-term morbidity and complication rate in 122 patients who underwent Martius flap at a mean follow-up time of 7 years [39]. However, in a recent retrospective review of 440 VVF repairs at a high-volume center in Ethiopia, the use of a Martius flap did not show a benefit and, in fact, was associated with a high rate of persistent incontinence and risk of surgical site complication [40].

Peritoneal Flap

First described in 1993 by Raz and colleagues, the posterior peritoneal flap lends itself for high-riding apical VVF. After closure of the first two layers, dissection is carried beyond the posterior wall of the bladder to expose an edge of the peritoneum in the anterior cul-de sac [31]. Care is taken to not enter the peritoneum. After mobilization of the peritoneal flap, it is advanced over the repair and secured in a tension-free manner using interrupted absorbable sutures [37]. Eliber et al. described a 96.4% (80/83) success rate after transvaginal VVF repair with a peritoneal flap [38].

Omental Flap

More commonly used for transabdominal VVF, omentum may be used if it has previously been brought down to the pelvis during a previous surgery [37]. The advantages to the omentum as an interpositional flap are its well-vascularized pedicle and inherent lymphatic properties. During a transvaginal approach, a tongue of omentum may be accessed via peritoneal window and advanced over the fistula repair site and secured with absorbable interrupted sutures.

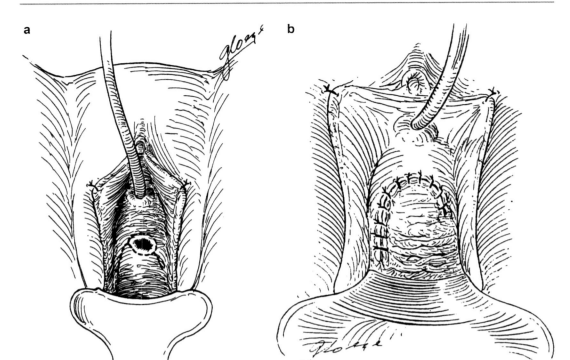

Fig. 12 (**a**) Diagram showing the incision for VVF repair. The incision is made to circumscribe the fistulous tract and extends in an inverted J shape toward the vaginal cuff; the base of the flap is apical. (Permission from Raz S, Little NA, Juma S. Female urology. Chapter 46. Vesicovaginal Fistulae. In Walsh PC, Retik AB, Stamey TA, Vaughn ED Jr [eds]: Campbell's Urology, 6th edition. Philadelphia, WB Saunders, 1992, pp. 2782–2828); (**b**) the use of an inverted J incision with advancement of the flap over the first two layers of fistula closure voids overlapping suture lines. (Permission from Raz S, Little NA, Juma S. Female urology. Chapter 46. Vesicovaginal Fistulae)

Gracilis Flap

The gracilis flap was first described by Garlock in 1928 and is used for vaginal reconstruction after a pelvic exenteration or if a fistula is associated with radiation. The blood supply is derived from a branch of the profunda femoris entering the upper one-third of the muscle [14]. This is a long flap that can cover the medial portion of the groin, vulva, perineum and lower abdomen. Plastic surgery involvement may be needed for these complex situations. In these situations, a combination of a transvaginal and transabdominal approach may be necessary. Figure 21 shows the anatomical landmarks that guide the dissection of the gracilis flap. The pubic symphysis and the medial condyle of the tibia are marked, and a line is drawn between them [41]. The approximate location of the dominant neurovascular bundle of the gracilis flap can be identified ≈10 cm inferior to the pubic symphysis along the marked line. Either one long incision can be made along this mark, or a series of skin incision, as seen in Fig. 22.

In a study of 35 patients with very large VVF (all >3.5 cm, average 7 cm), a tissue flap was used in 23 patients: 13 gracilis flap, 5 omental, 2 peritoneal, and 3 Martius. Though the authors did not comment specifically on the success rate of the gracilis flap patients alone, they did report a success rate of 91% (21/23) altogether in the interpositional flap patients, compared to a success rate of 83% (10/12) in patients who did not receive a flap [41].

Fig. 13 With a small catheter in the fistula tract to aid in dissection, vaginal skin around the margins of the fistula is excised. In this illustration, a relaxing incision has been made at the 5 o'clock position to help exposure of the fistula and create space for dissection. (Permission from Reconstructive Urology. Volume 2. Webster, Kirby, King, Goldwasser (Eds). Blackwell Scientific Publications. Boston. 1993. Chapter 42. Lower Urinary Tract Fistulae. Chapple)

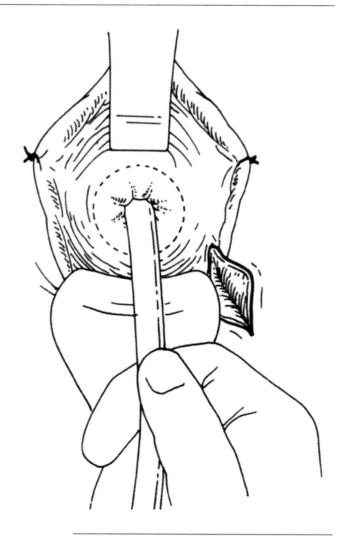

Amniotic Membrane

Used for decades for complex wound dressings, such as burns, researchers have proposed using an amniotic membrane as a patch over the repair for complex VVF [42, 43]. Amniotic membranes act as a biological barrier and release peptide growth factors required for tissue growth, collagen deposition, and angiogenesis, while also functioning as a scaffold for tissue ingrowth [43]. This is a technique that warrants further clinical study.

Postoperative Management

Adequate, continuous bladder drainage is of utmost importance postoperatively. Controlling bladder spasms is important not only for patient comfort, but also to promote healing of the repair. Anticholinergic medications to manage bladder spasms due to the suture lines and/or catheter balloons can be used. The authors prefer to use short-acting oxybutynin three times per day. Constipation should be treated aggressively. The addition of belladonna (B&O) suppositories may also be needed if bladder spasms continue despite oral anticholinergic medication. Sirls et al. reported

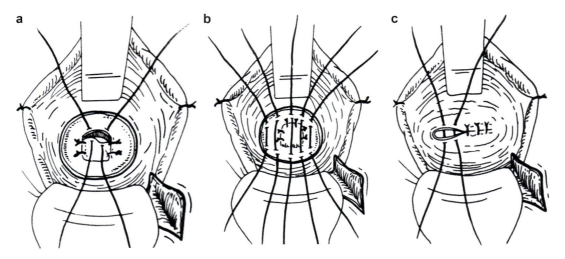

Fig. 14 (**a–c**) Closure of the fistula tract in two layers. (Permission from Reconstructive Urology. Volume 2. George Webster, Roger Kirby, Lowell King, Benad Goldwasser (Eds). Blackwell Scientific Publications. Boston. 1993. Chapter 42. Lower Urinary Tract Fistulae. Chistopher R. Chapple): (**a**) Closure of the fistula tract; (**b**) closure of the pubovesical fascia; and (**c**) closure of the vaginal skin

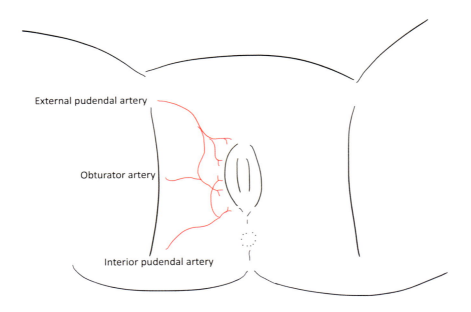

Fig. 15 Schematic of the blood supply of the Martius flap. The blood supply to the flap is the external pudendal artery superiorly, obturator artery laterally, and the inferior posterior labial vessels off the internal pudendal artery inferiorly

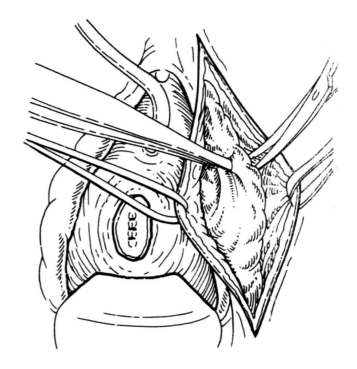

Fig. 16 Incision along the left labia majora and dissection of the fibrofatty graft. (Permission from Reconstructive Urology. Volume 2. George Webster, Roger Kirby, Lowell King, Benad Goldwasser (Eds). Blackwell Scientific Publications. Boston. 1993. Chapter 42. Lower Urinary Tract Fistulae. Christopher R. Chapple)

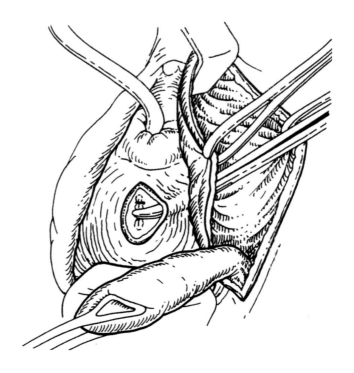

Fig. 17 The posterior attachment of the pedicle is preserved and a tunnel formed through to the vaginal dissection. (Permission from Reconstructive Urology. Volume 2. George Webster, Roger Kirby, Lowell King, Benad Goldwasser (Eds). Blackwell Scientific Publications. Boston. 1993. Chapter 42. Lower Urinary Tract Fistulae. Christopher R. Chapple)

Fig. 18 The flap is drawn through the tunnel. (Permission from Reconstructive Urology. Volume 2. George Webster, Roger Kirby, Lowell King, Benad Goldwasser (Eds). Blackwell Scientific Publications. Boston. 1993. Chapter 42. Lower Urinary Tract Fistulae. Christopher R. Chapple)

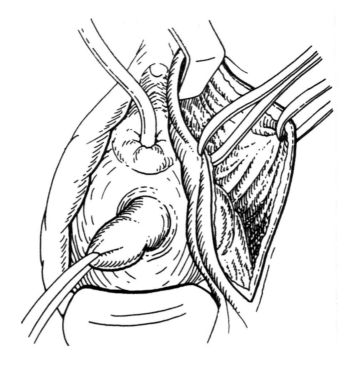

Fig. 19 The flap is sutured in place over the fistula. (Permission from Reconstructive Urology. Volume 2. George Webster, Roger Kirby, Lowell King, Benad Goldwasser (Eds). Blackwell Scientific Publications. Boston. 1993. Chapter 42. Lower Urinary Tract Fistulae. Chapple)

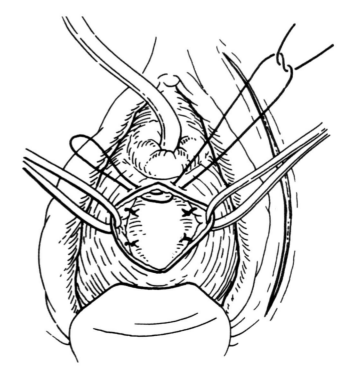

Fig. 20 Closure is completed. (Permission from Reconstructive Urology. Volume 2. George Webster, Roger Kirby, Lowell King, Benad Goldwasser (Eds). Blackwell Scientific Publications. Boston. 1993. Chapter 42. Lower Urinary Tract Fistulae. Christopher R. Chapple)

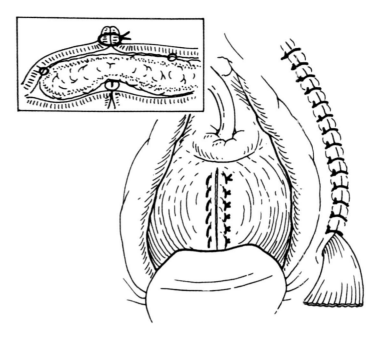

the successful use of intradetrusor onabotulinum toxin A for control of severe bladder spasms in women who failed prior VVF repair [44]. Low-dose prophylactic antibiotics may be used while the catheters are in place.

A cystogram with lateral images is performed prior to removal of the urethral catheter, usually 10–14 days postoperatively. Historically, both a suprapubic catheter and a urethral catheter were left in place at the time of transabdominal approach, but the authors do this only in higher-risk patients [45]. For transvaginal repairs, usually only a urethral catheter is needed, unless the VVF repair was more complex. If the cystogram is negative for a leak, the catheter can be removed. At the time of catheter removal, the authors recommend a dose of prophylactic antibiotics. If a suprapubic catheter is in place, it can be kept in place to monitor postvoid residuals and then be removed as soon as adequate bladder emptying has returned [14]. Sexual activity is avoided for 2–3 months after surgery. In cases of a radiation-associated VVF, catheterization is recommended for at least 28 days [19].

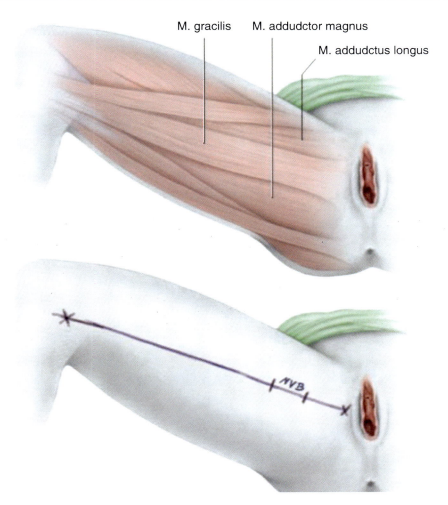

Fig. 21 The gracilis flap harvest begins by delineating the anatomical landmarks. The pubic symphysis and the medial condyle of the tibia are marked, and a line is drawn between them. The approximate location of the dominant neurovascular bundle (NVB) of the gracilis flap can be identified ≈10 cm inferior to the pubic symphysis along the marked line. (Permission from Tran VQ, Ezzat M, Aboseif SR. Repair of giant vesico-vaginal fistulae using a rotational bladder flap with or without a gracilis flap. BJU Int. 2010 Mar;105(5):730–9. doi: https://doi.org/10.1111/j.1464-410X.2009.09177.x. PMID: 20149210)

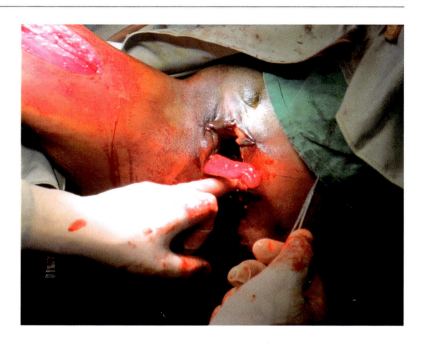

Fig. 22 One long or two separate incisions are made along the medial thigh, over the gracilis muscle. Here, the distal tendinous attachment that has ligated the gracilis muscle flap has been tunneled to the vaginal/perineal defect

Table 3 Post-transvaginal VVF repair outcomes: recent studies

Study	N	Follow-up (years)	Tissue graft used	Cure/success rate %
Eilber, 2003 [38]	207	10	Peritoneal/Martius/full-thickness skin[a]	97[b]
Kochakarn, 2007 [46]	19	8	Martius	89.5
Hadzi-Djoki, 2009	59	Not reported	None	94.9
Hilton, 2012 [22]	201	Not reported	Martius	96.1
Pshak, 2013 [47]	49	1	N/A[c]	100
Lee, 2014 [48]	50	4.5	Martius, peritoneal, perirectal fat, and none	97
Gedik, 2015 [23]	25	1	None	100
Malde, 2017 [49]	43	3.2	Martius	95

[a]Tissue interposition was used for complex (greater than 2 cm. and/or radiation induced) fistulas and/or failed previous repairs. Peritoneal flap was used for proximal fistulas. Martius flap was used for distal fistulas. A full-thickness labial flap used for cases of insufficient vaginal epithelium
[b]Cure rate after initial repair with a peritoneal, Martius, and labial flap was 96%, 97%, and 33%, respectively
[c]Patients were divided into primary VVF (25) and recurrent VVF (24). Primary VVF patients had mean follow-up of 16 months +/− 15 months. Recurrent VVF patients had a follow-up of 32 months +/− 26 months

If a urinary leak is seen on cystography, the catheter should remain for another 2–4 weeks, which may allow the fistula to heal.

Surgical Outcomes

Given the lack of randomized control trials, most of the data regarding outcomes of transvaginal repair is from retrospective reviews. The nonstandardization of surgical technique and heterogeneity of the VVF qualities and patient population makes it difficult to perform meta-analyses. However, the estimated success rate of the transvaginal repair ranges from 83% to 100%. Table 3 summarizes the outcomes of transvaginal VVF repair.

Summary

The transvaginal approach for vesicovaginal fistula repair is the preferred approach for most vaginal surgeons and has success rates from 83% to 100%. Interposition flaps are critical for postradiation VVF and may be needed for recurrent VVF after prior repair. Pelvic reconstructive surgeons should be familiar with the transvaginal approach to VVF repair.

Cross-References

▶ Options for Surgical Reconstruction of the Heavily Irradiated Pelvis
▶ Reconstruction of the Absent or Severely Damaged Urethra
▶ Urethrovaginal Fistula Repair
▶ Vesicovaginal Fistula Repair: Abdominal Approach
▶ Vesicovaginal Fistula Repair: Minimally Invasive Approach

References

1. Thompson JC, Rogers RG. Surgical management for pelvic organ prolapse and its impact on sexual function. Sex Med Rev. 2016;4(3):213–20.
2. Härkki-Sirén P, Sjöberg J, Tiitinen A. Urinary tract injuries after hysterectomy. Obstet Gynecol. 1998;92(1):113–8.
3. Duong TH, Taylor DP, Meeks GR. A multicenter study of vesicovaginal fistula following incidental cystotomy during benign hysterectomies. Int Urogynecol J. 2011;22(8):975–9.
4. Wall LL. Obstetric vesicovaginal fistula as an international public-health problem. Lancet. 2006;368(9542):1201–9.
5. Tebeu PM, et al. Risk factors for obstetric vesicovaginal fistula at University Teaching Hospital, Yaounde, Cameroon. Int J Gynecol Obstet. 2012;118(3):256–8.
6. Tancer ML. Observations on prevention and management of vesicovaginal fistula after total hysterectomy. Surg Gynecol Obstet. 1992;175(6):501–6.
7. Armenakas NA, Pareek G, Fracchia JA. Iatrogenic bladder perforations: long-term follow-up of 65 patients. J Am Coll Surg. 2004;198(1):78–82.
8. Raghavaiah NV. Double-dye test to diagnose various types of vaginal fistulas. J Urol. 1974;112(6):811–2.
9. Stamatakos M, et al. Vesicovaginal fistula: diagnosis and management. Indian J Surg. 2014;76(2):131–6.
10. Angioli R, et al. Guidelines of how to manage vesicovaginal fistula. Crit Rev Oncol Hematol. 2003;48(3):295–304.
11. World Health Organization. WHO guidelines approved by the guidelines review committee. In: WHO recommendation on duration of bladder catheterization after surgical repair of simple obstetric urinary fistula. Geneva: World Health Organization; 2018.
12. Goh JT. A new classification for female genital tract fistula. Aust N Z J Obstet Gynaecol. 2004;44(6):502–4.
13. Capes T, et al. Comparison of two classification systems for vesicovaginal fistula. Int Urogynecol J. 2012;23(12):1679–85.
14. Lee D, Zimmern P. Vaginal Approach to Vesicovaginal Fistula. Urol Clin North Am. 2019;46(1):123–33.
15. Goodwin TM, et al. Management of common problems in obstetrics and gynecology. Fifth ed. Wiley-Blackwell; 2010.
16. Duong TH, Gellasch TL, Adam RA. Risk factors for the development of vesicovaginal fistula after incidental cystotomy at the time of a benign hysterectomy. Am J Obstet Gynecol. 2009;201(5):512e1–4.
17. Goodwin MT, Montoro MN, Muderspach LI. Management of Common Problems in obstetrics and gynecology. Wiley-Blackwell: Chichester; 2010.
18. Goodwin WE, Scardino PT. Vesicovaginal and ureterovaginal fistulas: a summary of 25 years of experience. J Urol. 1980;123(3):370–4.
19. Breen M, Ingber M. Controversies in the management of vesicovaginal fistula. Best Pract Res Clin Obstet Gynaecol. 2019;54:61–72.
20. Massee JS, et al. Management of urinary-vaginal fistula; ten-year survey. JAMA. 1964;190:902–6.
21. Hancock B. Preoperative preparation. In: First steps in vesico vaginal fistula repair. Lewisville: Royal Society of Medicine Press; 2005. First steps in vesico vaginal fistula repair.
22. Hilton P. Urogenital fistula in the UK: a personal case series managed over 25 years. BJU Int. 2012;110(1):102–10.
23. Gedik A, et al. Which surgical technique should be preferred to repair benign, primary vesicovaginal fistulas? Urol J. 2015;12(6):2422–7.
24. Lee JH, et al. Immediate laparoscopic nontransvesical repair without omental interposition for vesicovaginal fistula developing after total abdominal hysterectomy. Jsls. 2010;14(2):187–91.
25. El-Azab AS, Abolella HA, Farouk M. Update on vesicovaginal fistula: a systematic review. Arab J Urol. 2019;17(1):61–8.

26. Blandy JP, et al. Early repair of iatrogenic injury to the ureter or bladder after gynecological surgery. J Urol. 1991;146(3):761–5.
27. Akman RY, et al. Vesicovaginal and ureterovaginal fistulas: a review of 39 cases. Int Urol Nephrol. 1999;31(3):321–6.
28. Moses RA, Ann Gormley E. State of the art for treatment of vesicovaginal fistula. Curr Urol Rep. 2017;18(8):60.
29. Bodner-Adler B, et al. Management of vesicovaginal fistulas (VVFs) in women following benign gynaecologic surgery: a systematic review and meta-analysis. PLoS One. 2017;12(2):e0171554.
30. Panaiyadiyan S, et al. Impact of vesicovaginal fistula repair on urinary and sexual function: patient-reported outcomes over long-term follow-up. Int Urogynecol J. 2021;32(9):2521–8.
31. Raz S, et al. Transvaginal repair of vesicovaginal fistula using a peritoneal flap. J Urol. 1993;150(1):56–9.
32. Zimmern PE, et al. Genitourinary fistulas: vaginal approach for repair of vesicovaginal fistulas. Clin Obstet Gynaecol. 1985;12(2):403–13.
33. Latzko W. Postoperative vesicovaginal fistulas; genesis and therapy. Am J Surg. 1942;58:211–28.
34. Dorairajan LN, et al. Latzko repair for vesicovaginal fistula revisited in the era of minimal-access surgery. Int Urol Nephrol. 2008;40(2):317–20.
35. Ansquer Y, et al. Latzko operation for vault vesicovaginal fistula. Acta Obstet Gynecol Scand. 2006;85(10):1248–51.
36. Martius H. The repair of vesicovaginal fistulas with interposition pedicle graft of labial tissue. Zentralbl Gynakol. 1928;52:480.
37. Rovner ES. Urinary tract fistulae. In: Kavoussi LR, Wein AJ, Novick AC, editors. Campbell-Walsh urology. Philadephia: Elsevier; 2012.
38. Eilber KS, et al. Ten-year experience with transvaginal vesicovaginal fistula repair using tissue interposition. J Urol. 2003;169(3):1033–6.
39. Lee D, Dillon BE, Zimmern PE. Long-term morbidity of Martius labial fat pad graft in vaginal reconstruction surgery. Urology. 2013;82(6):1261–6.
40. Browning A. Lack of value of the Martius fibrofatty graft in obstetric fistula repair. Int J Gynaecol Obstet. 2006;93(1):33–7.
41. Ezzat M, et al. Repair of giant vesicovaginal fistulas. J Urol. 2009;181(3):1184–8.
42. Barski D, et al. Repair of a vesico-vaginal fistula with amniotic membrane – step 1 of the IDEAL recommendations of surgical innovation. Cent European J Urol. 2015;68(4):459–61.
43. Price DT, Price TC. Robotic repair of a vesicovaginal fistula in an irradiated field using a dehydrated amniotic allograft as an interposition patch. J Robot Surg. 2016;10(1):77–80.
44. Evan Sirls RP, Sirls LT. Intradetrusor Onabotuliniumtoxina injection for refractory bladder spasms before vesicovaginal fistula repair. In: SUFU. Florida: Miami; 2019.
45. O'Conor VJ Jr. Review of experience with vesicovaginal fistula repair. J Urol. 1980;123(3):367–9.
46. Kochakarn W, Pummangura W. A new dimension in vesicovaginal fistula management: an 8-year experience at Ramathibodi hospital. Asian J Surg. 2007;30(4):267–71.
47. Pshak T, et al. Is tissue interposition always necessary in transvaginal repair of benign, recurrent vesicovaginal fistulae? Urology. 2013;82(3):707–12.
48. Lee D, et al. Long-term functional outcomes following nonradiated vesicovaginal repair. J Urol. 2014;191(1):120–4.
49. Malde S, et al. The uses and outcomes of the Martius fat pad in female urology. World J Urol. 2017;35(3):473–8.

Vesicovaginal Fistula Repair: Abdominal Approach

44

F. Reeves and A. Lawrence

Contents

Introduction	786
Etiology	787
Classification	788
Clinical Evaluation	788
Preoperative Workup	790
Management	791
Conservative Management	792
Transabdominal Versus Transvaginal Approach	793
Outcomes	793
Transabdominal Repair: A Step-by-Step Guide	793
Excision of the Fistula Tract	795
Interposition Tissue Flap	796
Omental Pedicle Flap	798
Closure	798
Leak Testing	798
Drains	798
Minimally Invasive Approach (Laparoscopic/Robotic)	799
Postoperative Care	800
Special Considerations	800
Radiation-Induced Fistulae	800
Palliative Procedures	801

F. Reeves
Department of Urology, The Royal Melbourne Hospital, Melbourne, Australia

A. Lawrence (✉)
Counties Manukau and Auckland Hospital, Auckland, New Zealand
e-mail: annala@adhb.govt.nz

© Springer Nature Switzerland AG 2023
F. E. Martins et al. (eds.), *Female Genitourinary and Pelvic Floor Reconstruction*,
https://doi.org/10.1007/978-3-031-19598-3_45

Conclusion	801
Cross-References	801
References	801

Abstract

Vesicovaginal fistulae have enormous worldwide impact. This chapter provides an evidence-based review of abdominal repair for vesicovaginal fistulae (VVF). Effective management is underpinned by an appreciation of the underlying pathophysiology of VVF and performance of a thorough clinical evaluation prior to embarking on repair. This is particularly important as the first repair is generally the most successful.

Aetiology is varied, with different patterns seen in lower resourced countries (predominantly obstetric related) compared with well-resourced countries (primarily iatrogenic). Abdominal repair is a versatile approach that is suitable for many fistulae. It can be performed via an open or minimally invasive technique and allows for concomitant adjunct procedures where required, such as ureteric reimplant. Guiding principles and a step-by-step guide for transabdominal repair are provided here.

Keywords

Vesicovaginal fistula · Fistula · VVF · Abdominal repair · Female urology · Urogenital · Transvesical

Introduction

Vesicovaginal fistula (VVF) is an abnormal communication between the bladder and vagina and is the most common urogenital fistula (Fig. 1). It has been described in the literature as early as 1550 BC, and its relationship to obstructed labor was recognized as early as 1037 AD [1].

Its clinical manifestation is continuous urinary incontinence, which can have devastating psychological, social, economic, and physical consequences [2–5]. Its worldwide impact is immense, particularly in low-resourced countries (LRC), where obstetric fistulae are the most common, and those who are affected often find themselves marginalized.

It is estimated that approximately two million women are living with unrepaired VVF [6, 7] with the greatest burden of disease in developing counties and 30,000–130,000 new fistulae a year [8]. This number is thought to be an underestimate as the data remains difficult to collect and collate across different counties and health systems. Across Africa, rates of VVF range from 1.16 to 3.2 fistulae per 1000 women of reproductive age [9], accumulating into a lifetime prevalence of

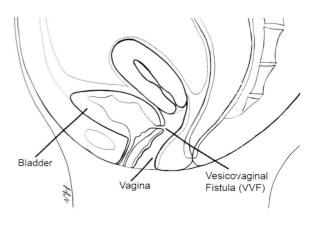

Fig. 1 Vesicovaginal fistula (VVF). (Figure courtesy of Dr. Vanessa Young, BSc, MBChB, Auckland, NZ)

VVF symptoms in sub-Saharan Africa of 3.0 per 1000 women of reproductive age [10].

In contrast, the estimated number of repairs carried out per year in the UK is 120 [11].

There are no standardized management algorithms for the management of VVF. The approach to VVF repair most commonly relies on clinician experience. However, the relatively few numbers of cases in well-resourced countries (WRC) result in limited per clinician experience. Similarly, although the numbers are significantly higher in LRC, often charitable organizations are involved in setting up dedicated programs, which lead to centralization of care with relatively few specialists involved [12]. The consequence of this is that, apart from a small number of highly experienced specialists, most clinicians will not frequently encounter fistula management in their career.

This chapter presents evidence-based insights into the etiology, evaluation, and transabdominal management of VVF.

Etiology

Both the incidence and etiology vary greatly between well-resourced and low-resourced countries. Traditionally, obstetric-related fistula relating to prolonged obstructed labor is the main etiology of VVF in LRC, while in WRC, it is most commonly related to pelvic surgery [13] (Table 1). Of note, surgical birthing injuries have been listed in Table 1 as iatrogenic injuries as they are not a result of obstructed labor but relate to the surgical intervention undertaken to assist in the birth [14].

In LRC, 80.2–95.2% of VVF are obstetric related [12, 15]. The majority are associated with prolonged neglected obstructed labor, which leads to sustained pressure necrosis [16]. Obstetric fistula is a result of a "field injury" to a broad area, and as such, there may be various related injuries. Understanding this is instrumental in appreciating that one must not simply focus on the "hole" between the bladder and vagina when planning for repair. Multifaceted injuries may include urethral loss, stress urinary incontinence (SUI), ureteric fistula, pelvic inflammatory disease (PID), secondary infertility, vaginal stenosis, and osteitis pubis [17]. More recently, there has been an increased number of iatrogenic VVF in the LRC [13, 14], with increased VVF associated with surgical interventions for deliveries, in what is noted as a concerning trend [13].

In the WRC, fistulae are more commonly the result of pelvic surgery or malignancy

Table 1 Etiology of VVF

Etiology		
Iatrogenic	Post-surgery	Hysterectomy – abdominal or vaginal
		Vascular, benign or oncological pelvic surgery
		Continence procedures including vaginal and abdominal approaches
		Anterior vaginal wall prolapse procedures
		Mesh-related erosions
		Vaginal biopsies
		Vaginal laser surgeries
	Obstetric related	Caesarean section injury to bladder
		Forceps laceration
	Radiation therapy	Pelvic malignancies
Non-iatrogenic	Obstetric related	Obstructed labor
		Uterine rupture
	Malignancy	Advanced pelvic malignancy
	Trauma	Pelvic fractures
		Sexual assault
	Vaginal foreign bodies	Including pessaries
	Infection/inflammation	
	Congenital	

management [18]. In the United States, the true incidence of VVF is not known but has previously been reported to be about 0.3–4%, with some studies reporting an overall incidence of 0.5% after simple hysterectomy and 10% after radical hysterectomy [19, 20].

The number of hysterectomy procedures undertaken in the UK has been falling over the last decade, with increasing availability and acceptability of nonsurgical treatments for menorrhagia in particular. However, with the number of surgically treated urogenital fistulae remaining fairly constant over the same period, this suggests that the risk of urogenital fistula following hysterectomy may be increasing [11]. In a review of NHS cases of female urogenital fistulae between 2000 and 2008, there was a 46% rise in rate of fistula formation [21].

Iatrogenic fistulae tend to be supratrigonal as they are located higher in the pelvis.

Mechanisms of iatrogenic fistula formation include unrecognized cystotomy during dissection, insufficiently repaired or breakdown of cystotomy repair, inadvertent incorporation of the bladder with surrounding tissue while suturing, devascularization injuries due to extensive dissection, and thermal injuries [22] VVF related to pelvic radiation is caused by obliterative arteritis, which leads to atrophy or necrosis of the bladder epithelium and the development of ulceration or the formation of fissures [23].

Other causes include foreign bodies, infection, inflammation, sexual assault, and trauma [24–27].

Classification

The classification of VVF can be traced back to Sims in 1852 [28]. Although more than 12 different classifications have been developed since then, there remains no standardization, and only a few systems are associated with outcome-based studies that allow for prediction of success [29]. Comparative assessment of surgical technique is therefore particularly difficult due to the significant variability in VVF classification, making it impossible to recommend one technique over another based on current research. Large multicenter prospective studies are required to facilitate the development of a clinically meaningful standardized classification that can be used for triage, prognostication, and appropriate patient counselling and consent.

The World Health Organization has devised a classification that divides fistula into simple (good prognosis) and complex (uncertain prognosis) (Table 2). This assesses not only size and location but compounding factors such as previous repairs and radiation, which decrease the likelihood of success of a repair. It is a simple reference that surgeons with limited experience in VVF can use to guide when a patient should be considered for referral to a tertiary center.

Clinical Evaluation

As the first attempt at repair is often the most successful, it is imperative that a thorough clinical evaluation and preoperative workup be completed prior to embarking on surgery.

When evaluating a potential VVF, it is important to establish the number of fistulae (beware of hidden fistula), size, location, anatomical relations (e.g., distance from ureteric orifice, bladder neck), previous surgical inventions, pelvic or vaginal scarring, and any associated injuries.

The etiology of the VVF is essential to establish, as those associated with radiation, malignancy, or other organ involvement will require a different surgical approach and a larger

Table 2 WHO classification of urogenital fistulae

Simplex fistula (good prognosis)	Complex fistula (uncertain prognosis)
Single fistula < 4 cm	Fistula > 4 cm
Vesicovaginal fistula	Multiple fistula
Closing mechanism not involved	Rectovaginal, mixed, cervical fistula
No circumferential defect	Closing mechanism involved
Minimal tissue loss	Scarring
Ureters not involved	Circumferential defect
First attempt to repair	Extensive tissue loss
	Intravaginal ureters
	Failed previous repair
	Radiation fistula

armamentarium of repair techniques and adjuvants, including potential urinary diversion, when compared to a simple post-benign surgery fistula, which may be less surgically challenging. Consideration should also be given to referral to experienced clinicians or teams once the diagnosis is established, especially in the case of complex fistula, as outcomes are reported to be better in units that perform more than three operations per year [30].

VVF usually present day 7–12 post benign gynecological or obstetric surgery. At this time, patients may complain of persistent urinary incontinence, requiring multiple continence pads to manage. It is vital to ensure you have an exhaustive history regarding previous abdominal and pelvic surgeries, cancers, radiation treatments, previous continence, trauma, labors, and/or deliveries. The leakage volume should be established as a base line. It is critical to differentiate urogenital fistula-related symptoms from other possible causes of urinary incontinence.

Once suspicious of VVF, traditionally, dye testing can be completed in the outpatient setting to establish the location of the fistula and confirm the diagnosis. This involves placing three sponges/ gauzes in the vagina and then filing the bladder with a colored dye (e.g., Indigo carmine, methylene blue, or sterile infant formula) via a Foley catheter. Once bladder is filled, the catheter is removed and patient is asked to mobilize for approximately 30 min. After this time, the sponges are removed and inspected for dye staining; if present, it indicates a fistula. If there is concern that there is a potential concurrent ureterovaginal (UVF) fistula, then the patient could be instructed to take oral phenazopyridine just before coming into the office. This would cause the sponges to turn orange if a concurrent UVF was present. While this may help with establishing a diagnosis, this study would not be sufficient, however, to complete surgical planning, and further studies, including cystoscopy and MRI/CT urogram, should be undertaken.

Cystoscopy under general anesthesia (GA) is a vital step in the clinical assessment (Images 1 and 2). Cystoscopy allows clarification of the location of the VVF, distance from bladder neck and UOs, as well as identification of other potential pathologies such as bladder stones, sutures, and diverticulum. It allows for the assessment of bladder capacity, which is particularly important in the irradiated patient, informing the decision regarding possible need to augment the bladder or consider urinary diversion. The health of the bladder tissues is also assessed. If edema and necrosis are present, it indicates a delay is required to allow for resolution before undertaking a surgical repair. In these cases, the cystoscopy should be repeated later to reassess.

If a small tract is noted during cystoscopy, you can also attempt to cannulate with a ureteric catheter to help locate the vaginal end of the fistula. Additionally, retrograde ureterograms can be

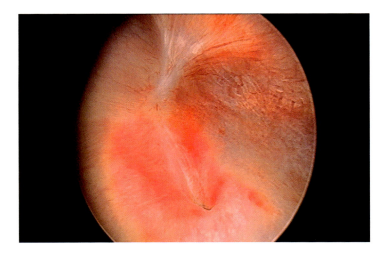

Image 1 Cystoscopic view of a previous vesicovaginal fistula repair location. (Images courtesy of Prof. Judith Goh AO Griffith University School of Medicine, Greenslopes Private Hospital, Australia)

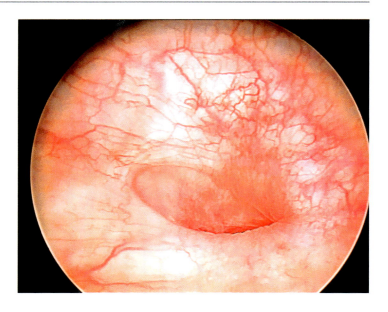

Image 2 Cystoscopic view of VVF after an abdominal hysterectomy. (Images courtesy of Prof. Judith Goh AO Griffith University School of Medicine, Greenslopes Private Hospital, Australia)

completed to ensure no concurrent ureteric injuries, as these are reportedly present in up to 5–12% of VVF [31–33].

While under a GA for cystoscopy, a physical examination can be completed looking at the rigidity of the vagina, any shortening of the vagina, and a general assessment of the health of surrounding tissues, including evidence of post-irradiation involvement of the rectum, which could all require a change in surgical approach (Image 3).

Additional imaging is required in the majority of cases, especially in the situation where cystoscopy and vaginoscopy did not reveal the fistula tract. Current radiological imaging that can be utilized includes transvaginal ultrasound and MRI and CT urogram (Images 4 and 5) [34]. The advantage of a reconstructed CT or MRI is their ability to localize the fistula in three dimensions and identify the underlying etiology, allowing for easier surgical planning [35]. Contrast-enhanced CT with multiplanar reconstruction has been considered the gold standard in the detection of fistulae and evaluation of the underlying pathological conditions, especially in patients with pelvic malignancy, and has previously demonstrated a diagnostic accuracy of 100% [36, 37]. More recently, though, MRI has superseded CT as the modality of choice for the detection and evaluation of VVF. MRI has higher soft-tissue contrast compared to CT, which aids in the identification of the fistula and damage or disease in surrounding tissues [38].

Transvaginal ultrasound is a well-tolerated investigation that allows the evaluation of the site, size, and course of the fistula [39, 40]. Like all ultrasound scanning techniques, it is an operator-dependent procedure, and if experienced operators are not available, the results must be interpreted with caution.

At the conclusion of your clinical evaluation, you should feel confident that you have the correct diagnosis, with sufficient information about the location, size, number of fistulae, etiology such that detailed surgical planning can occur.

Preoperative Workup

Prior to undertaking any repair, the patient must be stable. All clinical elevations and investigations should be complete, and patient should be appropriately counselled regarding the predicted outcome of intervention. At the time of surgery, the patient should be free of infection. If there is evidence of infection, urosepsis, or a urinoma, then the repair should be deferred until resolution

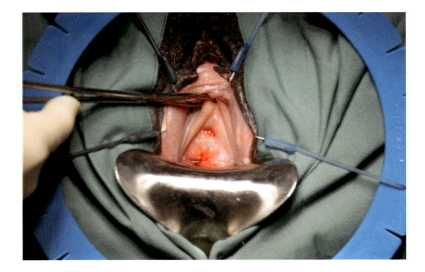

Image 3 Vaginal examination under anesthetic: for surgical planning. Vaginal examination under anesthetic allowing assessment of the fistula, its location, the health of surrounding tissues, and therefore appropriate surgical planning. (Images courtesy of Prof. Judith Goh AO Griffith University School of Medicine, Greenslopes Private Hospital, Australia)

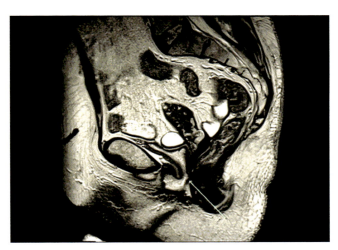

Image 4 MRI, T2 sagittal view. MRI: T2 weighted completed for VVF workup: Arrow indicates the site of the vesicovaginal fistula

[41]. Additionally, in the setting of a postpartum VVF, the repair should be delayed until the uterus involutes.

The timing of the repair remains the most controversial part of VVF repair, and there remains no consensus. However, most experts agree that it should not be done until the tissues are healthy and well vascularized, and any edema, inflammation, and necrosis has resolved [42]. This may take up to 12 weeks for most patients, and this delay then increases the likelihood of success. Longer waits may be required in certain situations, in particular post-radiation [23] (Table 3).

This period of incontinence and waiting related to the VVF can be difficult for patients, and reassurance is often required. It is important for them to understand that the first attempt at repair is likely to be the most successful, therefore all steps to ensure a successful outcome, including the timing of the repair, should not be rushed.

Management

The primary focus of this chapter is abdominal repair of VVF. However, for all VVF operative planning, one should consider conservative management as well as all alternative surgical options. It is important to be familiar with a large array of surgical techniques so that unforeseen

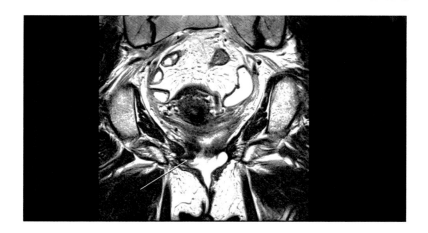

Image 5 MRI, T2 coronal view. MRI, T2 weighted completed for VVF workup for surgical planning. Arrow indicates the site of the VVF

Table 3 General guidelines for timing of VVF repair

	General approach	Caveat
Post-benign surgery	Wait until tissues are well vascularized and healthy Approximately 12 weeks	Early diagnosis up to 3 days after surgery Possibly that tissue is not inflamed or edematous and therefore likely good prognosis
Postpartum: post prolonged labor	Wait till uterus involutes (approximately 12 weeks) Consideration to catheter drainage over this time should be given as a trial of conservative management. Once involution is complete, if VVF is still present, surgery can be completed	If concurrent ureteric injury, consider nephrostomy tube placement to decrease risk of sepsis, renal injury, or pain from urine leak
Post-radiation	Irradiated fistulae tend to evolve over time. Therefore, an extended time is needed to ensure evolution complete, prior to assessment for surgical options This can take 12 months post-completion of radiation treatment	

intraoperative difficulties do not impact the likelihood of a successful outcome. Multiple techniques for VVF repair are now described: conservative, endoscopic furgation with plasma products, transvaginal, Latzko technique, laparoscopic, robotic, and open.

Conservative Management

The probability of spontaneous closure is low in most series (7–12.5%). However, reported rates vary, with some studies painting a more optimistic picture with success rates of up to 28%. Furthermore, success rates may also be underestimated, as these cases do not get referred for further treatment [14].

The key to conservative management is continuous bladder drainage with a catheter to divert urine away from the fistula. For most studies, a 6-to-8-week period of diversion is described. The European Association of Urology Robotic Urology Section (ERUS) panel recommends trial with catheter for attempting conservative management of up to 12 weeks [43].

Favorable variables that may indicate suitability for conservative management include recent onset (less than 3 weeks), if urine leak decreases with IDC and small fistula size. Unfavorable characteristics where conservative management should not be recommended include large fistula size (greater than 3 cm), radiation induced, extensive surrounding scarring, and a delay from fistula onset (greater than 6 weeks) [44].

Transabdominal Versus Transvaginal Approach

The choice of surgical approach is often determined primarily by surgeon familiarity and preference, as well as available resources (availability of general anesthetic, postoperative care) [45, 46]. While the vaginal approach is commonly used and does offer a cost-effective alternative compared to transabdominal surgery, it is not suited to the management of all VVF^x. The benefit of the transabdominal approach is that it provides maximal space for dissection, which provides a good basis for complete excision and tension-free closure.

Factors that necessitate an abdominal approach include:

- Small capacity, fixed, inaccessible vagina making exposure inadequate
- Close proximity of fistula to ureter (possibility of need for reimplant)
- High in vagina making difficult access
- Need for concurrent reconstructive procedures injuries (e.g., bladder augmentation, ureteric reconstruction)
- Complex fistula involving another intrabdominal organ (ureter or bowel)
- Multiple fistula

A previously failed transvaginal repair does not preclude a new transvaginal approach, as good results may still be achieved [47].

Contraindications to surgery abdominally and vaginally include active infection/sepsis or urinoma. It is best to manage these contraindications initially and then reassess for surgery.

Outcomes

Variability in the definition of success across publications makes it difficult to compare studies and should be taken into account when interpreting results. Definitions used include "anatomical closure of fistula," "need for repeat procedure," "failed repair," and "residual leakage." In WRC, often a cystogram is done prior to the removal of catheter. In contrast, LRC may be more likely to use a clinical parameter of success such as residual leakage. Clinicians need to beware that the presence of leakage following surgery may also be from stress or urge urinary incontinence and does not necessarily represent failure of closure of the fistula.

With these caveats in mind, the systematic review reported overall success rates of surgical closure of urogenital fistulae in WRC at 94.6%. Studies with highest failure rate had the highest proportion of radiation-induced fistulae [13].

There are no randomized trials that directly compare transvaginal and transabdominal outcomes. In Hillary's systematic review, closure was more likely to be achieved using a transvaginal approach (90.8% vs. 83.9%, $p = 0.0176$); however, this was most likely due to bias associated with case selection. In a more recent publication, a 50-year single institution experience out of Italy reported a success rate of 94.1% for the first attempt, which increased to 100% after excluding women who were previously unsuccessfully treated in other institutions [48].

Transabdominal Repair: A Step-by-Step Guide

The transabdominal approach to VVF repair was reported as early as 1893 (von Dittel). However, O'Conor published a seminal description of a transabdominal extraperitoneal approach in 1980, which has formed the basis for contemporary open VVF surgery [49].

The abdominal approach to VVF repair can be either transvesical or extravesical, and the same reconstructive principles that apply to an open abdominal approach apply to laparoscopic or robotic repairs (Table 4).

Each fistula is unique and requires a nuanced repair; however, the fundamental surgical steps of VVF repair to ensure the best possible outcome for the patient remain the same (Table 5).

Table 4 Reconstructive principles of VVF repair: abdominal approach

Repair principle	Rationale
Good exposure of fistula and surrounding tissues	It is vital to have good visualization, and this allows all other principles to be followed with ease
Complete excision of fistula tract and scar	Removing surrounding fibrosis scar and ensuring tissue is healthy and pliable will ensure better healing This also allows a tension-free repair Send sample for histology
Avoid ureteric orifice (UO) movement/dissection	If the UO's are not involved, avoid any dissection or movement to avoid damage. Placing ureteric catheters identifies the UO and helps avoid unintentional harm
Continuous bladder drainage	Until postoperative imaging is completed and results demonstrate a success repair If this a repeat repair, we recommend bladder drainage via both a urethral and suprapubic catheter
Watertight closure	Ensuring no major deficits in closure that may result in a failure This can be tested intraoperatively Tension-free repair and good drainage also ensure this principle is adhered to
Non overlapping suture lines	
Suitable suture material	Sutures that will dissolve so that they are not a nidus for stones or failure of repair
Interposition of tissue	This requires the separation of the bladder and vagina Placement of tissue in between, which can be omentum, peritoneum flap, or abdominal muscle, to improve tissue integrity and reduce chance of failure

Patient Positioning

The patient should be positioned in a low lithotomy position to facilitate cystoscopy prior to abdominal access. This enables the surgeon to access the vagina for an abdominal-perineal approach should it be required [50].

Table 5 Steps of VVF repair

Careful preoperative evaluation using radiology and cystoscopy
Biopsy where appropriate to exclude malignancy
Cystoscopy and localization of VVF with catheter/wire
+/−placement of ureteric catheters with cystoscopy
Localization of VVF with catheter or wire
Separation of involved organs (bladder/vagina)
Excision/debridement of fibrous tissue +/− fistulous tract
Multilayer, tension-free, watertight closure with nonoverlapping suture lines
Consideration of interposition tissue
Appropriate bladder drainage with catheter/s postoperatively

TED stockings and sequential calf compressors should be used for DVT prophylaxis.

Prophylactic antibiotics are administered prior to commencement, ensuring that preoperative urine is sterile.

Cystoscopy

The first step is to complete a cystoscopy and EUA, identifying the fistula tract(s) and inspecting the vaginal tissues. This should always be completed even if already done in your preoperative clinical evaluation, as fistula tracts can evolve, creating a different fistula than previously planned for.

The tract is then marked with a guide wire, ureteric catheter, or Fogarty catheter across the fistula from bladder to vagina (Fig. 2). The benefit of a Fogarty catheter is that it can be used to lift the fistula anteriorly as dissection occurs helping create a plan for cystotomy with a transvesical approach. Occasionally, it is easier to cannulate the vaginal opening of the VVF and have the wire/catheter move from the vagina to the bladder; however, as the vagina is unable to be sterilized during the preparation for the surgery, this is not the preferred route for catheter/wire placement.

This catheter/wire placement allows easier identification of the fistula tract once the abdomen is opened. If there are multiple tracts, cannulation of all those seen on cystoscopy allows for easier visualization in the abdomen and therefore complete excision of all fistula tracts, associated scar, and fibrotic tissue. When cannulating multiple

Fig. 2 Placement of Fogarty catheter into the fistula. (Figure courtesy of Dr. Vanessa Young, BSc, MBChB, Auckland, NZ)

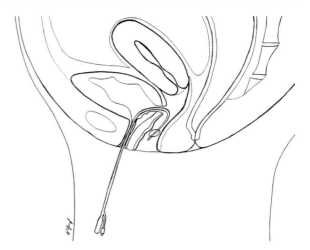

fistulae tracts, it is advisable to use only one color or type of catheter for the fistula tracts so as not to confuse them with the ureteric catheters used to identify the UOs.

The recommendation of placing ureteric catheters is dependent on the position of the fistula, if it is close to the ureteric orifices catheters should be placed. Particularly in the situation of repeat repair, a radiation fistula, or a complex fistula, ureteric catheters allow easy recognition of UOs and therefore avoidance of harm to them. These ureteric catheters can be removed before leaving the operation room.

A gauze swab stick can then be inserted into the vagina to assist identification during dissection.

Abdominal Incision

Attention is then turned to the abdominal approach. The incision depends on the complexity of the fistula and surgeon's experience. Either a Pfannenstiel/lower transverse incision or infraumbilical midline incision can be utilized and are well described, but benefits and risk of should be considered. The benefit of an infraumbilical midline incision is that it allows easier access to the omentum for an interposition flap and, if needed, access to the ureters for reimplantation. The Pfannenstiel/transverse incision, however, is more comfortable postoperatively for patients, allowing for a faster recovery. Once abdomen is open, the use of packing and self-retaining retractors allows for adequate expose.

Generally, the preferred approach is extraperitoneal, with exposure of the anterior bladder wall. Transperitoneal is preferred when managing a recurrent fistula, multiple previous abdominal operations, additional abdominal or ureteric procedures are required concurrently, or if a robotic approach has been undertaken.

Excision of the Fistula Tract

Either a transvesical or extravesical approach can be used to expose and excise fistula tract. The approach should be based on surgeon experience and fistula characteristics.

Extravesical

With this approach, attention is turned to creating the vesicovaginal plane and locating and dissecting fistula tract from here.

Transvesical

The bladder can then be bivalved as initially described by O'Conor, down to the fistula tract or a posterior cystotomy/anterior cystotomy can be undertaken (Fig. 3). A smaller posterior or anterior cystotomy reduces the morbidity of bivalving the bladder. After completing an anterior cystotomy [48, 51] stay sutures can be placed to allow increased access to the posterior wall of

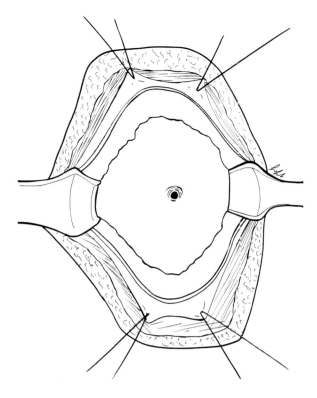

Fig. 3 Cystotomy revealing fistula track. (Figure courtesy of Dr. Vanessa Young, BSc, MBChB, Auckland, NZ)

bladder and catheter/wire through the fistula tract. If no catheter is placed to use to lift the fistula tract when dissecting, then sutures for traction should be placed through the fistula tract at this time.

A circular incision should then be made around the fistula opening (Fig. 4). The stay sutures or catheter can then be used to help lift the fistula tract to allow sharp dissection and excision of the fistula tract (Fig. 5). This should leave well-vascularized pliable tissue to allow for a tension-free closure.

The bladder and vaginal walls should then be carefully dissected to create free edges that will allow for a tension-free closure.

Interposition Tissue Flap

At this stage, consideration should be given to whether any interposition tissue flap is required. The rationale for interposition tissue flap is that it provides a physical barrier and introduces vascular tissue and potentially lymphatic vessels that improve tissue growth and maturation [19]. Peritoneum, omentum, epiploic tissue, Martius flap, and rectus abdominus muscle have all been described as an interposition tissue. Non-autologous grafts of small intestine mucosa and human dura graft have also been used. Despite no randomized trials to evaluate the use of interposition tissue, its use allows the reconstruction complex and irradiated fistulae that otherwise would not have been treatable [52, 53]. As such, the decision of whether to use an interpositional tissue flap and, if so, what type of tissue flap, is largely down to surgeon's preference, experience, and individual case assessment. It should be noted that peritoneum and omentum may not be available in patients who have previously had extensive surgery, particularly for malignancy, and hence a plan for alternative tissues should be put in place.

The omentum may be long enough to be placed in between the vagina and bladder without dissection; if not, a formal pedicle omental flap is required so the interpositional flap can be placed without tension.

Fig. 4 Encircling incision about fistula track. (Figure courtesy of Dr. Vanessa Young, BSc, MBChB, Auckland, NZ)

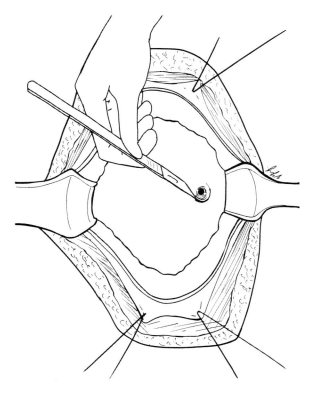

Fig. 5 Lifting the fistula for excision of tract. (Figure courtesy of Dr. Vanessa Young, BSc, MBChB, Auckland, NZ)

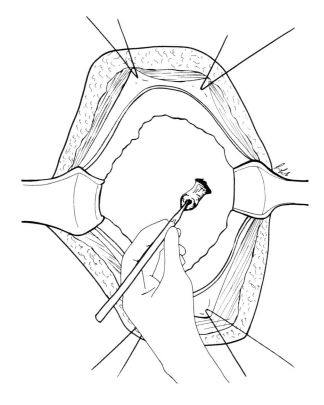

Omental Pedicle Flap

If unfamiliar with omental anatomy, having a general surgeon to assist in the mobilization and creation of the omental flap will decrease the complications and ensure a healthy flap for the repair. This pedicle is based on the right gastroepiploic vessels, thereby requiring the dissection of the omentum from the greater curvature of the stomach and the transverse colon.

If access to the omentum is limited, the infraumbilical incision can be extended cranially. A lower transverse incision can be manipulated into a J shape; however, access can grossly limited, and consideration for another interpositional flap should be given.

Once the omentum is located, mobilizing it superiorly allows attachments to the transverse colon to be identified and incised, ligating and dividing perforating vessels as you go. Once this is complete, the omentum is now attached only on the greater curvature of the stomach; at this time, the flap can then be dissected off the greater curvature of the stomach commencing on the left side and ligating vessels entering the omentum. The entire flap is based on the pedicle from the right gastroepiploic vessels, so care should be taken as you near these not to damage them. Once the flap is freed, it can then be brought down to the pelvis and placed as an interpositional flap. It should be secure in place with 3/0 multifilament suture. Avoid placing these sutures in line with the suture line of the bladder or vagina, in keeping with the principle of nonoverlapping suture lines.

Closure

Vaginal Closure

The vagina should first be closed in a transverse fashion, so as to create nonoverlapping suture lines with the bladder closure. Different sutures are recommended by different authors, from a 2/0 mono filament to a 3/0 multifilament [51, 54]. The principle to adhere to is suitable suture that will absorb within 3 months, so a 3/0 monofilament is our preferred suture. If interposition tissue is being utilized, it should now be fixed between the bladder and vagina.

Bladder Closure

The bladder should be closed after interposition tissue is secured in place. This can be either a multilayer closure or single layer but should be performed in a vertical manner to avoid overlapping suture lines with the vaginal closure. An absorbable monofilament 3/0 with interrupted sutures is the most common practice.

If fistula is quite large and in close proximity to the ureteric orifice, a Z-form bladder closure or V-Y plasty can be used to provide tension-free closure [55].

After fistula excision site is closed, the initial anterior cystotomy should be closed, again using a double layer closure with an absorbable monofilament 3/0 with interrupted or continuous sutures lines.

Leak Testing

Once satisfied with the cystotomy closures, leak testing should be undertaken. This allows any hidden leaks that may cause a delay in healing to be located and closed before abdominal closure.

This can be completed with filling the bladder with saline and methylene blue to approximately 200 ml. At the time of filling, ensuring good visualization of the repair is recommended so any leak of blue can be seen early before staining of tissues makes it difficult to locate. Alternatives to this include using indigo carmine, sterilized infant formula, or completing it with a cystoscope. Using a cystoscope allows light and fluid to be seen at the site of leakage, and the urothelium can be directly inspected for any defects/potential leaks.

Drains

A suction drain should be placed in the pelvis and a urethral IDC should be left in post-procedure for continuous bladder drainage and decompression

Fig. 6 Port placement for Laparoscopic/Robotic approach to VVF repair (Figure courtesy of Dr. Vanessa Young, BSc, MBChB, Auckland, NZ)

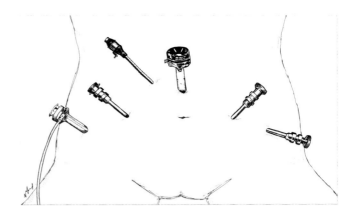

of the bladder while it is healing. A suprapubic catheter is not considered necessary in most cases; however, in the case of a complex repair, repeat repair, or radiation fistula, it should be considered for complete bladder decompression in the postoperative period.

Minimally Invasive Approach (Laparoscopic/Robotic)

The first reported laparoscopic VVF repair was by Nezhat in 1994, followed nearly a decade later by the first robotic repair in 2005 [56]. Although laparoscopic repair has been used with similar success to open with lower associated morbidity, the technical challenges of laparoscopy in the pelvis, in particular reconstructive suturing, have meant that the robotic approach has gained increasing popularity. The success rate in a recently published robotic series is 100% [46].

Robotic approach to transabdominal VVF repair in essence replicates the open approach already described in this chapter. Additional considerations include patient positioning, port placement, and tricks to maintaining pneumoperitoneum.

After cystoscopy, to identify and mark the fistula tract, and place ureteric stents (if needed), the patient should be positioned in Trendelenburg, with 25-degree tilt. A gauze swab stick may be inserted into the vagina to assist with identification during dissection later in the procedure and to ensure pneumoperitoneum is maintained after this space is opened.

Once pneumoperitoneum is established, ports should be placed as per a radical prostatectomy (Fig. 6).

After any necessary adhesiolysis is undertaken, to clear off bowel loops from the underlying bladder exposing the rectovaginal (Douglas) pouch, the rest of the dissection and repair can proceed in the same fashion as the open transabdominal approach described above. As in the open technique, a transvesical or retrovesical approach may be taken. Dissecting straight down onto the fistula in the retrovesical space can be very challenging. As such, a transvesical approach akin to a modified O'Conor technique may be preferable.

Once the bladder surface is clear, it is important to localize the fistula in order to plan the cystotomy carefully to minimize its size. Pulling on the localizing catheter through the fistula may suffice. Sotelo also describes an alternate method that involves using concurrent cystoscopy, performed with the laparoscopic/robotic light off, and the cystoscope light pointing at the fistula tract [56]. The cystoscope light can then be seen transilluminating the bladder wall near the site of the fistula.

After opening the bladder, the fistula tract is excised, and the bladder and vagina are dissected to allow for interposition and closure as in the open approach. Of note, if using omentum for interposition, it is often helpful to return the patient to a flat position to allow it to reach more easily. A 3-0 V-Loc can be used for both the vaginal and bladder closure. Suture lines should not overlap; the vagina is closed transversely and the bladder vertically.

At completion, a drain should be placed and an indwelling urethral catheter left in situ. Trocars should be removed under vision to ensure no bleeding. The fascia of the camera and assistant ports should be closed to prevent hernia.

Postoperative Care

Patients should be encouraged to mobilize early. Low-molecular-weight heparin should be administered for DVT prophylaxis until patients are fully ambulatory. In most cases, oral fluids can be resumed immediately postoperatively with a gradual increase in diet as tolerated.

Depending on surgeon experience and individual case selection, in uncomplicated cases, ureteric catheters may be able to be removed at the end of the case or on day 1 post-procedure. For cases where ureteric stents have been placed, these can be removed at 4 weeks to allow ample time for recovery prior to embarking on cystoscopy.

Generally, the drain can be removed on day 1 or 2 postoperatively if there is no evidence of a leak.

The duration of postoperative catheterization is surgeon-dependent and ranges from 10 to 26 days. There is some evidence that 7 days is non-inferior [43], although due to the nature of VVF repairs, the risk of early catheter removal for patient comfort should not outweigh the risk of VVF repair breakdown [57]. Once again, based on the premise that the first attempt at repair is the most likely to be successful, no shortcuts should be considered, even in the postoperative period.

In the postoperative period, many patients have increased bladder spasm due to bladder irritation from surgery and catheter/s in place, this should be aggressively managed with anticholinergics to avoid any breakdown of repair. It is also important to ensure that the catheter is well supported and not moving excessively as the movement of the catheter tip may cause disruption in the suture line.

At day 14 post simple repair, a limited cystogram should be completed to ensure successful repair prior to removal of catheter/s. Consider a cystogram at longer interval in the complex or radiation fistula repair. If at the initial cystogram there is still a fistula/leak, then leave the catheter in place for another 14–21 days and repeat the study.

Some authors advocate the use of antibiotic prophylaxis until all tubes are removed; however, there is little in the way of evidence to guide the use of antibiotics beyond the time of surgery.

Patients should be advised to refrain from sexual intercourse and the use of tampons for a minimum of 4 weeks, with some authors recommending 2 months [56, 57].

Special Considerations

Radiation-Induced Fistulae

After radiotherapy, many surgeons will opt to avoid entering the potentially hostile abdomen. This is certainly reflected in the fact that 97% of VVF managed in the largest published series of radiation-induced VVF were managed via a vaginal approach. However, the abdominal approach is still sometimes needed, particularly where there has been significant vaginal scarring and shrinkage. In these cases, interposition tissue is often advocated, with omental flaps being described.

In the series published by Pushkar, only half of the radiation-induced VVF were cured after a single surgical procedure [23]. Failure was mainly due to continuing tissue reaction caused by radiation. Therefore, they recommend that subsequent repairs can be considered as "primary" surgery, with high cumulative rate of cure (primary repair 48.1%, overall efficacy 80.4%). With this in mind, patients with radiation-induced fistulae should be warned of the high probability of needing multiple procedures before embarking on surgery.

There are limited studies that report outcomes specific to radiation-induced fistulae. In a recent retrospective series out of London, 70% of patients required primary or secondary diversion.

Many of the cases in this cohort were associated with compromised bladder function as well as ureteric involvement, highlighting the importance of identifying associated injuries when planning fistula management.

Palliative Procedures

It may not always be in the patient's best interest to embark on surgical repair of a VVF. Either patient fitness for reconstructive surgery or fistula-related factors (including complexity and etiology) may lead the clinicians to conclude on a case-by-case basis that palliative management may be more suitable.

This may include urinary diversion with an ileal conduit for patients who are fit. For others, a bilateral nephrostomy may relieve symptoms of leakage. Sometimes in larger fistulae, nephrostomies alone may not be adequate to make the patient dry, and consideration of ureteric occlusion is required. In these extreme cases, a multidisciplinary team discussion or review at a high-volume center is extremely beneficial before committing a patient to a palliative procedure.

Conclusion

The guiding reconstructive principles presented in this chapter underpin successful VVF repair. As the first repair generally has the best chance of success, it is essential that any intervention be carefully planned.

A thorough clinical workup is imperative. Cystoscopy with examination under anesthetic to assess the fistula, associated injuries, as well as tissue integrity in planning for repair is essential. Imaging with an MRI or CT urogram provides invaluable information.

Consideration of suitability for conservative management or vaginal approach should also be made prior to settling on abdominal approach. Open or minimally invasive abdominal repair may be undertaken depending on the expertise of the operating surgeon and local resources.

Many clinicians only have limited experience with VVF management. Particularly for complex fistulae where there is a higher probability of an uncertain prognosis, consideration of referral to a tertiary center should be made.

The current level of published evidence regarding VVF is low, with most being retrospective studies. Prospective studies are warranted to help drive improvement in management globally.

Cross-References

▶ Complications of Stress-Urinary Incontinence Surgery
▶ Complications of the Use of Synthetic Mesh Materials in Stress Urinary Incontinence and Pelvic Organ Prolapse
▶ Transvaginal Repair of Cystocele
▶ Urethrovaginal Fistula Repair

References

1. Zacharin RF. A history of obstetric vesicovaginal fistula. Aust N Z J Surg. 2000;70:851–4.
2. Tebeu PM, Fomulu JN, Khaddaj S, et al. Risk factors for obstetric fistula: a clinical review. Int Urogynecol J. 2012;23:387–94.
3. Mulete M, Rasmussen S, Kiserud T. Obstetric fistula in 14,928 Ethiopian women. Acta Obstet Gynecol Scand. 2010;89(7):945–51.
4. Wilson SM, et al. Psychological symptoms among obstetric fistula patients compared to gynecology outpatients in Tanzania. Int J Behav Med. 2015;22 (5):605–13.
5. Gharoro EP, Agholor KN. Aspects of psychosocial problems of patients with vesico-vaginal fistula. J Obstet Gynaecol. 2009;29(7):644–7.
6. Olukemi Bello O, et al. Nigeria, a high burden state of obstetric fistula: a contextual analysis of key drivers. Pan African Medical Journal. 2020;36:22.
7. USAID. United States Agency International Development (USAID). USAID'S Fistula Program. 2015; p. 1–3.
8. Lewis L, Wall. Obstetric vesicovaginal fistula as an international public-health problem. Lancet. 2006;368: 1201–9.
9. Adler AJ, Ronsmans C, et al. Estimating the prevalence of obstetric fistula: a systematic review and meta-analysis. BMC Pregnancy Childbirth. 2013;13:246.
10. Gouda HN, Charlson F, Sorsdahl K, Ahmadzada S, et al. Burden of non-communicable diseases in sub-Saharan Africa, 1990–2017: results from the

Global Burden of Disease Study. Lancet Global Health Oct. 2019;7:1375–87.
11. Cromwell D, Hilton P. Retrospective cohort study on patterns of care and outcomes of surgical treatment for lower urinary-genital tract fistula among English National Health Service hospitals between 2000 and 2009'. BJU Int. 2013;111:E257–62.
12. Hillary CJ, Osman NI, Hilton P, Chapple CR. The aetiology, treatment, and outcome of urogenital fistulae managed in well- and low-resourced countries: a systematic review. Eur Urol. 2016;70:478–92.
13. Hilton P. Trends in the aetiology of urogenital fistula: a case of retrogressive evolution. Int Urogynecol J. 2016;27:831–7.
14. Bangash K, Amin O, Luqman S, Hina H. Rising trends in iatrogenic urogenital fistula: a new challenge. Int J Gynaecol Obstet. 2020;148(Suppl 1):33–6.
15. Raassen TJIP, Ngongo CJ, Mahendeka MM. Iatrogenic genitourinary fistula: an 18-year retrospective review of 805 injuries. Int Urogynecol J. 2014;25:1699–706.
16. Rogers RG, Jeppson PC. Current diagnosis and management of pelvic fistulae in women. Obstet Gynecol. 2016;128:635–50.
17. Arrowsmith S, Hamlin EC, Wall LL. Obstructed labor injury complex: obstetric fistula formation and the multifaceted morbidity of maternal birth trauma in the developing world. Obstetrics Gynaecology Survey. 1996;51:568–74.
18. Angioli R, Penalver M, Muzii L, et al. Guidelines of how to manage vesicovaginal fistula. Crit Rev Oncol Hematol. 2003;48(3):295–304.
19. Bora GS, Singh S, Mavuduru RS, Devana SK, et al. Robot-assisted vesicovaginal fistula repair: a safe and feasible technique. Int Urogynecol J. 2017;28:957–62.
20. Forsgren C, Altman D. Risk of pelvic organ fistula in patients undergoing hysterectomy. Current Opinion Obstetrics Gynaecology. 2010;22(5):404–7. https://doi.org/10.1097/GCO.0b013e32833e49b0. PMID: 20739885
21. Hilton P, Cromwell DA. The risk of vesicovaginal and urethrovaginal fistula after hysterectomy performed in the English National Health Service--a retrospective cohort study examining patterns of care between 2000 and 2008. Br J Obstet Gynaecol. 2012;119(12):1447–54.
22. Thayalan K, Parghi S, Krause H, Goh J. Vesicovaginal fistula following pelvic surgery: our experiences and recommendations for diagnosis and prompt referral. Aust N Z J Obstet Gynaecol. 2020;60:449–53.
23. Pushkar DY, Dyakov VV, Kasyan GR. Management of radiation-induced vesicovaginal fistula. Eur Urol. 2009;55:131–7.
24. Massinde A, Kihunrwa A. Large vesico-vaginal fistula caused by a foreign body. Ann Med Health Sci Res. 2013;3(3):456–7.
25. Puppo A, Naselli A, Centurioni MG. Vesicovaginal fistula caused by a vaginal foreign body in a 72-year-old woman: case report and literature review. Int Urogynecol J Pelvic Floor Dysfunct. 2009;20:1387–9.
26. Chapman GW. An unusual intravaginal foreign body. J Natl Med Assoc. 1984;76:811–2.
27. Ichihara K, Masumori N, Takahashi S. et al. Bladder neck rupture and vesicovaginal fistula associated with pelvic fracture in female. Low Urin Tract Symptoms. 2015;7(2):115–7.
28. Sims JM. On the treatment of vesico-vaginal fistula. 1852. Int Urogynecol J Pelvic Floor Dysfunct. 1998;9: 236.
29. Streit–Ciećkiewicz D, Nowakoski L. Predictive value of classification systems and single fistula-related factors in surgical management of vesicovaginal fistula. Neurourol Urodyn. 2021;40(1):529–37.
30. Cromwell D, Hilton P. Retrospective cohort study on patterns of care and outcomes of surgical treatment for lower urinary-genital tract fistula amoung English National Helath Service hospitals between 2000 and 2009. BJU Int. 2013;111:E257–62.
31. Seth J, Kiosoglous A, Pakzad M, Hamid R, Shah J, Ockrim J, Greenwell T. Incidence, type and management of ureteric injury associated with vesicovaginal fistulas: report of a series from a specialized center. Int J Urol 2019. 2019;26(7):717–23.
32. Goodwin WE, Scardino PT. Vesicovaginal and ureterovaginal fistulas: a summary of 25 years experience. J Urol. 1980;123:370–4.
33. Rovner E. Urinary tract fistulae. In: Wein AJ, Kavoussi LR, Novick AC, editors. Campbell-Walsh urology, vol. 3. Philadelphia: Saunders Elsevier; 2012 p. 2223–61.
34. Yu NC, Raman SS, Patel M, Barbaric Z. Fistulas of the genitourinary tract: a radiologic review. Radiographics. 2004;24:5.
35. Outwater E, Schiebler ML. Pelvic fistulas: findings on Mr. images. AJR Am J Roentgenol. 1993;160:327–30.
36. Narayanan P, Nobbenhuis M, Reynolds KM, Sahdev A, Reznek RH, Rockall AG. Review fistulas in malignant gynecologic disease: etiology, imaging, and management. Radiographics. 2009;29(4):1073–83.
37. Mandava A, Koppula V, Sharma G, Kandati M, Raju KVVN, Subramanyeshwar RT. Evaluation of genitourinary fistulas in pelvic malignancies with etiopathologic correlation: role of cross-sectional imaging in detection and management. Br J Radiol. 2020;93(1111):20200049. https://doi.org/10.1259/bjr.20200049. Epub 2020 Jun 15. PMID: 32539548; PMCID: PMC7336052.
38. Hyde BJ, Byrnes JN, Occhino JA, Sheedy SP, VanBuren WM. MRI review of female pelvic fistulizing disease. J Magn Reson Imaging. 2018;48:1172–84.
39. Volkmer BG, Kuefer R, Nesslauer T, Loeffler M. Colour Doppler ultrasound in vesicovaginal fistulas. Study Ultrasound Med Biol. 2000;26(5):771–5.
40. Sohail S, Siddiqui KJ. Trans-vaginal sonographic evaluation of vesicovaginal fistula. J Pak Med Assoc. 2005;55(7):292–4.
41. Lee D, Zimmern P. Vaginal approach to vesicovaginal. Urol Clin N Am. 2019;46:123–33.
42. Persky L, Herman G, Guerrier K. Non delay in vesicovaginal fistula repair. Urology. 1979;13(3):273–5.

43. Randazzo M, Lengauer L, Rochat CH, Ploumidis A, Kropfl D, Rassweiler J, Buffi NM, Wiklund P, Mottrie A, John H. Best practices in robotic-assisted repair of vesicovaginal fistula: a consensus report from the European Association of Urology Robotic Urology Section Scientific Working Group for Reconstructive Urology. Eur Urol. 2020;78:432–42.
44. Rajaian S, Pragatheeswarane M, Panda A. Vesicovaginal fistula: review and recent trends. Indian J Urol. 2019;35:250–8.
45. Warner R, Beardmore-Gray A, Pakzad M, Hamid R, Ockrim J, Greenwell T. The cost effectiveness of vaginal versus abdominal repair of vesicovaginal fistulae. Int Urogynecol J. 2020;31:1363–9.
46. Frajzyngier V, Ruminjo J, Asiimwe F, Barry T, Bello A. Factors influencing choice of surgical route of repair of genitourinary fistula, and the influence of route of repair on surgical outcomes: findings from a prospective cohort study. BJOG. 2012;119:1344–53.
47. Blaivas JG. Early versus late repair of vesicovaginal fistulas: vaginal and abdominal approaches. J Urol. 1995;153:1110–3.
48. Mancini M, Righetto M, Modonutti D, Morlacco A, Dal Moro F, Zattoni F. et al. Successful treatment of vesicovaginal fistulas via an abdominal transvesical approach: a single-center 50-yr experience. Eur Urol Focus. 2020;7(6):1485–92.
49. O'Conor VJ Jr. Review of experience with vesicovaginal fistula repair. J Urol. 1980;123:367–9.
50. Chapple C, Turner-Warwick R. Vesicovaginal fistula. BJU Int. 2005;95:193–214.
51. Hellenthal NJ, Nanigian DK, Ambert L, Stone AR. Limited anterior cystotomy: a useful alternative to the vaginal approach for vesicovaginal fistula repair. Urology. 2007;70(4):797–8.
52. Shak TP, Nikolavsky D, Terlecki R, Flynn BJ. Is tissue interposition always necessary in transvaginal repair of benign, recurrent vesicovaginal fistulae? Urology. 2013;82(3):707–12.
53. Altaweel W, Rajih E, Alkhudair W. Interposition flaps in vesicovaginal fistula repairs can optimize cure rate. Urol Ann. 2013;5(4):270–2.
54. Kumar S, Kekre NS, Gopalakrishnan G. Vesicovaginal fistula: an update. Indian Journal of Urology. 2007;23(2):187–91. https://doi.org/10.4103/0970-1591.32073.
55. Sotelo R, Moros V, et al. Robotic repair of vesicovaginal fistula. BJUI. 2012;109; 9:1416–34.
56. Melamud O, Eichel L, et al. Laparoscopic vesicovaginal fistula repair with robotic reconstruction. Urology. 2005;65(1):163–6.
57. WHO recommendation on duration of bladder catheterization after surgical repair of simple obstetric urinary fistula.

Rectovaginal Fistula

Christine A. Burke, Jennifer E. Park, and Tamara Grisales

Contents

Introduction	806
Background/Statistics	806
Causes of Rectovaginal Fistula	806
Obstetric	806
Inflammatory Bowel Disease	807
Infectious	807
Surgical	807
Cancer and Radiation	808
Miscellaneous	808
Classification	808
Size	808
Location	808
Etiology	809
Other	809
Presentation	809
Workup/Diagnosis	809
Physical Exam	809
Imaging	811
Conservative Treatment (Non-primary Repair)	812
Expectant Management	812
Medical Management	812
Seton Placement	813
Miscellaneous	813
Surgical Repair	814
Introduction	814
Optimization Prior to Surgical Repair	814
Methods of Rectovaginal Fistula Repair	815
Tissue Flaps	816

C. A. Burke · J. E. Park · T. Grisales (✉)
University of California Los Angeles, Los Angeles, CA, USA
e-mail: tgrisales@mednet.ucla.edu

Abdominal Approach	817
Novel and Future Approaches	817
Postsurgical Considerations and Complications	817
Postsurgical Care and Expectations	817
Postoperative Complications	817
Conclusion	818
Cross-References	818
References	818

Abstract

A rectovaginal fistula (RVF) is an abnormal communicating tract between the epithelialized surfaces of the rectum and vagina that is formed as a consequence of injury or inflammation. The etiologies are vast, ranging from obstetric trauma to inflammatory bowel disease; therefore, several modalities exist for both workup and treatment. Given the inherent diversity in RVF pathophysiology, this chapter will review various considerations and tools to utilize in approaching individualized cases. Diagnosis should comprise of a thorough history and targeted physical exam, along with imaging and/or direct visualization. Though the treatment is primarily surgical, this chapter will review expectant and medical management as well as the clinical contexts in which these options can be. Significant emphasis is placed on the careful and thoughtful extent of multidisciplinary planning to diagnosis and address rectovaginal fistulas and their underlying etiology.

Keywords

Rectovaginal fistula · Fecal incontinence · Obstetric injury

Introduction

Rectovaginal fistulas (RVF) pose a significant quality of life burden on affected patients. Though overall rare, there can be wide variation in etiologies, presentation, and treatment, making it difficult to standardize workup and management. Understanding the unique challenges to surgical and medical management of rectovaginal fistulas is crucial in the overall treatment of genital fistulas.

Background/Statistics

A rectovaginal fistula is an abnormal communicating tract between the epithelialized surfaces of the rectum and vagina that is formed as a consequence of injury or inflammation. The overall incidence of rectovaginal fistula is unknown, although a rare finding in developed countries. Obstetric fistulas in general are thought to occur in estimates as high as 4 in 1000 deliveries, but there is a paucity of population data looking at non-obstetric causes or data specifically for rectovaginal fistulas [1]. Given that the etiology and presentation of RVF worldwide are extremely varied, the prevalence and incidence have been difficult to characterize.

Causes of Rectovaginal Fistula

Obstetric

Outside of the United States, obstetric causes are thought to account for as many as 88% of fistulas. The most likely pathophysiology of obstetric-related rectovaginal fistula worldwide is trauma from the presenting fetal part, causing prolonged pressure on vaginal tissue with subsequent ischemia and necrosis. This often presents in situations where obstetric care is limited or delayed. Direct delivery trauma, most commonly seen with operative vaginal delivery, midline episiotomy, obstetric anal sphincter injury (OASIS), and shoulder dystocia, has also been attributed to obstetric RVF [2, 3]. In the United States, obstetric injury accounts for about 9% of all rectovaginal fistulas, which occur after 0.1% of spontaneous vaginal deliveries [4, 5]. Obstetric risk factors that contribute to complex lacerations and thus risk of RVF include advanced maternal age, teen pregnancy, large for gestational age infants, prolonged labor, primiparity, Asian race, home delivery, and precipitous delivery [4, 6]. A population-based observational study of over seven million women between 1998 and 2010 noted that obstetric injury occurrence is still significant, with 3.3% of deliveries sustaining a third-degree perineal laceration and 1.1% with fourth-degree laceration after vaginal delivery between [2]. The risk of RVF development especially increases when the obstetric injury is unrepaired or as a consequence of repair breakdown or infection.

An increase in public awareness of these risk factors has led to changes in obstetric practices and consequently lower rectovaginal fistula rates. Between 1979 and 2006, data pooled from the National Hospital Discharge Survey demonstrated that RVF repair declined from 7.8 to 4.8 per 100,000 women, in the setting of decreasing operative delivery and episiotomy and rising rates of cesarean section [3]. In the United States, rectovaginal fistulas most often present within 7–10 days of vaginal delivery [4].

Inflammatory Bowel Disease

Ten to 20% of RVF in the United States can be attributed to Crohn's disease due to chronic transmural inflammation in patients with perianal or rectal involvement. Crohn's disease poses an overall lifetime risk of up to 35% for developing RVF [4, 6]. Presence of RVF may be high as 50% within the first 10 years of Crohn's diagnosis [7]. Though rectovaginal fistulas occur less frequently in ulcerative colitis, since its etiology does not span the full mural thickness of the rectal tract, the risk is still present. A thorough gastrointestinal history should be obtained in all patients with rectovaginal fistulas.

Infectious

Chronic inflammation is another etiology of rectovaginal fistulas. One proposed theory is that impaired tissue healing and damage at a microvascular level prevent normal tissue epithelization and allow a communicating tract to persist. Etiologies associated with rectovaginal fistula formation in the literature include anal gland/crypt abscess extending into the vagina and sigmoid diverticulitis, especially in patients who have had prior hysterectomy [4]. Gynecologic etiologies with chronic inflammation, such as pelvic inflammatory disease with tubo-ovarian abscesses, Bartholin gland abscesses, endometriosis with bowel involvement, and ulcerative diseases like Behcet's syndrome, have been associated with genital and bowel fistula formation.

Surgical

Rectal and gynecologic surgeries for all indications are risk factors for rectovaginal fistula development. Surgical procedures may cause direct vaginal or rectal injury, result in insufficient tissue between these epithelialized surfaces, or subsequently cause ischemia or necrosis of the surgical sites which may result in a fistulous tract. Risks of iatrogenic RVF after gynecologic surgery are overall quite low and vary on the viscera involved and the surgical indication. Gynecologic surgery involving hysterectomy carries more risk than gynecologic surgery performed without hysterectomy. The overall risk occurs after 0.8–3 in 1000 hysterectomies in the United States, but can vary depending on the method or cause for hysterectomy [4]. Radical hysterectomy carries slightly more risk than simple hysterectomy, and a minimally invasive approach may pose more risk than abdominal or vaginal hysterectomy [4, 8]. Endometriosis surgery with bowel manipulation or dissection has also been cited as a gynecologic surgical cause.

Postsurgical sequelae, like anastomotic leaks or intraabdominal abscesses, may also indirectly lead to fistula formation. Additionally, the increasing utilization of staples or other foreign materials areas, especially with hemorrhoid surgery, may be associated with a slight increase in RVF occurrence [9]. The rate of rectovaginal fistula occurrence after pelvic organ prolapse repair has seen a declination since mesh placement has fallen out of practice.

Cancer and Radiation

Colorectal, bladder, and gynecologic cancers are associated with RVF formation. This etiology is multifactorial and can be from the disease process itself or as sequelae of treatment (surgery, chemotherapy, and/or radiation). Anastomotic leaks, perforations, pelvic abscess, hematoma drainage, rectal strictures, and anastomosis <5 cm from the anal verge have been shown to be risk factors for formation after rectal cancer resection [10, 11]. As many as 10% of women after low anterior resection for cancer may develop fistulas from their anastomosis [12].

Radiation is an independent risk factor for the development of RVFs due to its sequelae of chronic inflammation and obliteration of native tissue. Fistula formation at the time of radiation therapy is secondary to tumor necrosis, whereas fistula formation in the months and sometimes years following therapy is caused by recurrent malignancy, chronic injury with inflammation and poor wound healing, and ischemic necrosis [13]. Rectovaginal fistula formation after radiation for cervical, endometrial, and vaginal cancer occurs in about 3% of patients and tends to present on average 2 years after treatment, within a range of 5–40 months. Risk factors for formation after radiation for gynecologic malignancies may include prolonged radiation treatment, treatment >70 Gy, and stage of cancer at the time of initial treatment [14]. Radiation is also an independent risk factor for RVF formation after rectal cancer resection [10]. Subsequent pelvic trauma after radiation, like repeat surgeries and biopsies, adds additional risk to rectovaginal fistula formation [15].

Miscellaneous

Many rectovaginal fistulas – up to 20% in some retrospective studies – are unable to be characterized by the descriptors discussed previously [16]. This includes spontaneous RVF, congenital or acquired RVF, those caused by trauma, and chronic inflammation from indwelling objects in the vagina like pessaries or colpotomy cup. The treatment of these otherwise unspecific RVF causes is individualized due to the wide variation of presentation and etiology.

Classification

There is no universally utilized classification or grading system for rectovaginal fistulas. Descriptors in the literature vary, but most generally tend to utilize size, location, and etiology as descriptors of RVF severity. As such, it is imperative to document a carefully taken history and physical exam findings of a fistula thoroughly in order to comprehensively depict its pathology. In the table below, you may appreciate the several classification systems. Within each classification type, there is no universally accepted or standardized methodology (Table 1).

Size

Most RVFs are <2 cm and can be further classified by location [17]. Other proposed size categories have included a tiny (pinpoint to <0.5 cm), large (>3 cm), and middle size option [6, 16]. Again, given the lack of standardization, several sizing classifications can be found in the literature.

Location

RVF can be characterized based on anatomic landmarks, with "low" indicating below dentate line, "high" indicating near the cervix or apex, and "mid" corresponding between the hymen and cervix [6]. Others describe the communicating vaginal location in location by halves or thirds. When classified by location, RVFs are categorized by appropriate treatment and specialty of surgical team. A high RVF typically requires a transabdominal approach by colorectal surgery specialists, whereas a middle or low RVF can be corrected vaginally by urogynecology specialists.

Table 1 Various classification systems

Classification type	Subtype	Description
Location	Low	Between the vaginal fourchette and below the dentate line
	Middle	Between low and high
	High	Between the vaginal fornix and above the dentate line
Size	Small	<0.5 cm
	Medium	0.5–2.5 cm
	Large	>2.5 cm
Complexity	Simple	Low, <2.5 cm, resulting from obstetric injury or infection
	Complex	Higher, >1 cm, resulting from radiation, cancer, or surgical complications
Relationship to anal sphincter	Superficial	Does not involve anal sphincters or intersphincteric plane
	Intersphincteric	Passes through intersphincteric plane
	Transsphincteric	Passes through portion of IAS and EAS
	Suprasphincteric	Passes through entire sphincter complex, encompassing IAS and EAS
	Extrasphincteric	Primary opening in rectum that travels to encompass sphincter complex

Etiology

Some specialists classify RVF by etiology – most commonly obstetric, trauma, cancer, or Crohn's/inflammatory. However, as mentioned above, categorizing by cause may not capture the wide range of contributing factors when listed as "other." Additionally, characterization is not always consistent, i.e., some characterize obstetric fistulas under "trauma," or inflammatory bowel diseases under "infectious."

Other

Additionally, some use combined classifications to describe "simple" vs "complex" RVF. This most commonly characterizes "simple" RVF as due to infection/trauma, and "complex" due to inflammatory bowel diseases or based on size/location or recurrence [6].

Presentation

Flatulence or stool passage through the vagina is often the most commonly associated symptom of RVF. Other presentations arise from the sequelae of stool in the vagina like recurrent vaginitis or genitourinary infection. Perianal or rectal pain with sensitivity to external irritation or with intercourse may also be present. A history of vulvovaginal abscesses, particularly if recurrent, should prompt further questions regarding bowel symptoms since perianal abscesses may be an initial presentation of Crohn's disease. Young women may be more likely to see gynecologists for vulvovaginal/perineal symptoms while attributing bowel symptoms to a benign etiology. Patients may also be asymptomatic depending on the size and cause of RVF. The emotional and physical distress that symptomatic RVF has on quality of life and social factors, however, can be unimaginable.

As previously discussed, the timing of rectovaginal fistula presentation varies with etiology. A thorough medical and surgical history should be obtained on initial evaluation to assist with identification.

Workup/Diagnosis

Physical Exam

An initial physical exam should be performed with the patient in dorsal lithotomy. Begin with a thorough perineum and perianal skin assessment. Evaluate for any defects, depressions, and indurations, especially if draining any abnormal discharge. A gaping introitus may be noted on exam [6].

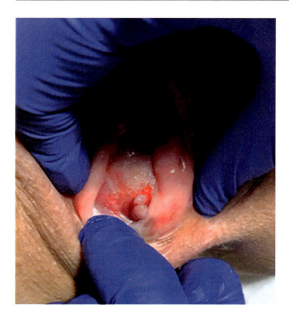

Fig. 1 Vaginal exam of rectovaginal fistula showing puckering and erythema at the vaginal entrance

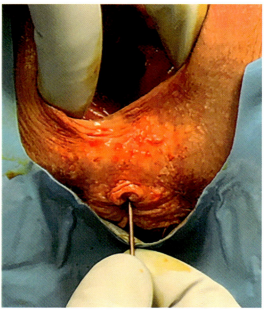

Fig. 2 Fistulous tract identification using a lacrimal duct

An internal visual examination is recommended with placement of the speculum to assess the cervix or vaginal cuff and lateral vaginal walls. A split speculum exam should be used to visualize the anterior and posterior vaginal walls. If available, a transparent speculum may offer more optimal visualization. All efforts should be made to visualize areas between rugae, as fistulas may be small and easily missed. Findings may include granulation tissue, puckering, and surrounding erythema/irritation. There may be darker vaginal mucosa of the fistula contrasting normal pink vagina tissue (Fig. 1) [13, 18]. Additionally, an endoanal speculum can be considered for further visualization.

Digital bimanual exam and rectal exam should carefully assess for palpable masses or strictures; however, digital exams are often unremarkable. If performing an exam under anesthesia, probes can be utilized to trace the fistula from the vagina to the rectum, or vice versa (Fig. 2).

Tampon dye test with methylene blue enema and air bubble test are tests that can be utilized if rectovaginal exam is unable to confirm fistula (Table 2, Fig. 3).

Table 2 Physical examination tests to evaluate rectovaginal fistulas [13]

Test	Instructions
Tampon dye test	Instill dilute methylene blue into the rectum and place a tampon in the vagina. After 15 min, remove the tampon and evaluate for staining and take note of its location if possible. Additionally, a digital rectal exam with methylene stained gel with concurrent transparent vaginal speculum exam can be performed
Air bubble test	Place patient in Trendelenburg position and fill the vagina with water. Use a syringe with a Foley catheter tip to insert air in the rectum. Presence of bubbles in the vagina confirms the diagnosis
Direct visualization with scope	Vaginoscopy, anoscopy, proctoscopy, colonoscopy
Fistulous tract identification	Pass material to track area of fistulous openings. Tools like tonsil, lacrimal duct probes (skinny and malleable), Foley catheter, or Foley with wire can be used

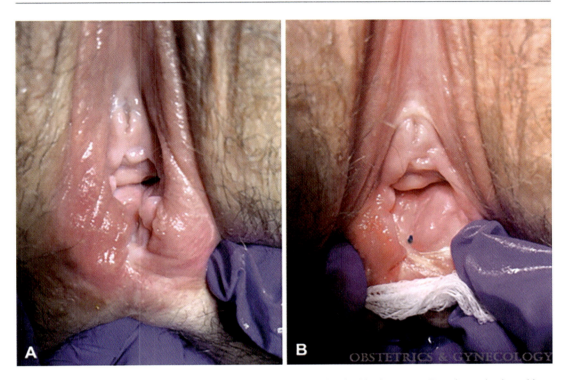

Fig. 3 Small fistula visualized after the insertion of methylene blue-dyed gel in the rectum. Rectal examination without methylene blue (**a**); rectal examination with methylene blue (**b**) [19]

Imaging

Vaginoscopy has considerable benefit in identifying rectovaginal fistulas, with up to 87% sensitivity and 100% specificity [4]. Other modalities of visualization include colonoscopy or proctosigmoidoscopy, often used in conjunction with vaginoscopy. MRI is also commonly used, as it is valuable for evaluating other fistulas or abscesses. CT scan with or without contrast may pose some initial benefit as well [4]. IV and rectal contrasts are recommended. Evidence of contrast in the vagina confirms the diagnosis of RVF even if the fistula is not visualized [17].

Endoanal and transperineal ultrasounds have been utilized in identifying, classifying, and characterizing fistulas. Endoanal ultrasound (EAU) has the advantage of visualizing the entire sphincter complex and intersphincteric plane. One study showed it can correctly classify sphincter defects in as high as 92% of known RVF [19, 20]. Endoanal ultrasound has been shown to have up to 84% accuracy for identification for fistula-in-ano comparable to barium and CT studies, with peroxide enhancement increasing the sensitivity to 89%, and has the added benefit of distinguishing perianal from perineal disease [21, 22]. However, its sensitivity for identifying rectovaginal fistulas specifically can be quite low, regardless of etiology. One early study specifically looking at EUS for RVF showed that an RVF was only identified in 28% of cases, and these were limited to smaller fistula sizes (<5 cm) and mid- to high RVF [19]. Additionally, endoanal ultrasound cannot distinguish inflammation from scarring, delineate spaces outside of the endoanal sphincters, and assess fistula spread [20].

Transperineal ultrasound is another option for imaging which is favorable in terms of patient discomfort or for patients with anal or rectal strictures. One study looking at perianal and

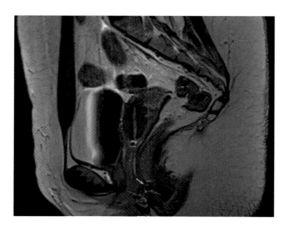

Fig. 4 MRI images of recurrent RVF. Patient initially presented with a history of Crohn's colitis and development of RVF who represented with subsequent wound breakdown after transvaginal repair

rectovaginal fistulas associated with Crohn's disease saw that detection rates and sphincter classification of fistula location are comparable between transperineal and endoanal ultrasound [23]. Transperineal ultrasound may have the advantage of identifying smaller abscesses than endoanal ultrasound. It can also identify fistula openings on the vaginal side that may otherwise be compressed by the endoanal ultrasound probe [22]. However, the transperineal ultrasound is limited in its depth of penetration of up to 7 cm, so it should not be utilized as the sole imaging for classification of more complex or higher fistulas [23].

Vaginography or anal manography may be considered, especially if evaluating for defecatory dysfunction. Barium enemas can be utilized to help identify fistulous tracts in the upper rectum, but does not rule out presence of genital fistulas if negative. Rarely are small bowel series utilized for primary diagnostic method of rectovaginal fistulas. The best imaging approach has found to be the utilization of multiple imaging modalities in combination (endoanal ultrasound, MRI, exam under anesthesia); this has been shown to have the greatest sensitivity and specificity for detection of fistulas [24] (Fig. 4).

Conservative Treatment (Non-primary Repair)

Expectant Management

Treatment of rectovaginal fistulas often is directed by patient symptoms and clinical status. Expectant management can be considered; one recent retrospective review of current rectovaginal fistula management reports about 18% of cases are treated initially with expectant management [16]. There are no formal trials or guidelines for qualifications for expectant management, aside from asymptomatic status. Rectovaginal fistulas that are generally pinpoint size and not associated with infectious cause or radiation may respond better, with healing in potentially up to 50% of patients, although this is likely an overestimate [24]. There have been few case reports of spontaneous resolution of rectovaginal fistulas, although these cases have been more often driven by patient preference for limited intervention.

Methods of expectant management aim to limit irritation and trauma to the affected area. This can range from treatments as conservative as bowel rest and total parenteral nutrition to more patient-guided approaches like low residue diet, stool bulking, sitz baths, self-directed irrigation, and 5-ASA enemas [12, 25]. Additionally, estrogen cream has to be used to facilitate healing in limited case reports, though larger-scale support of efficacy is lacking.

Medical Management

Medical management of rectovaginal fistulas also varies based on etiology. There are few cases where medical management alone aids in resolution of RVF, but primary medical management may help with initial symptomatic therapy or optimization before surgery. Antibiotics are often a common mainstay of medical management regardless of RVF cause, with metronidazole as monotherapy or in combination with cephalosporins or ciprofloxacin [7]. Care for patients with rectovaginal fistula of inflammatory bowel disease etiology should be coordinated with a multidisciplinary team that includes a gastroenterologist. For RVF associated with Crohn's disease, medication treatment has low success as monotherapy but aids in disease optimization prior to surgical repair. The efficacy of corticosteroids, sulfasalazine, tacrolimus, TNF-alpha, methotrexate, and azathioprine has been evaluated in the literature for rectovaginal fistula treatment, but successful fistula closure is limited [25, 26]. Infliximab for Crohn's disease has been shown to have some short-term benefits, like lengthening time of RVF closure compared to placebo, but has not yet been proven as efficacious monotherapy [12]. There have been some preliminary studies showing potential for RVF treatment in ulcerative colitis patients as well.

Seton Placement

A seton is often placed for initial conservative treatment. Most commonly made of a thin piece of rubber or plastic such as a vessel loop, the seton is threaded through the fistulous tract to ensure that continuous drainage occurs to prevent the risk of abscess formation (Fig. 5). According to a recent retrospective review of current practices, seton placement is used as initial or concurrent treatment in almost 50% of rectovaginal fistula cases of all etiologies, primarily in those involving the lower vagina [27]. Though its use as primary treatment of RVF has not been shown to be significantly efficacious, with success rates as low as 5%, seton placement has multiple advantages. It can be utilized for symptomatic relief for patients who are poor candidates for repair or awaiting primary repair. Their purpose is twofold – allow for spontaneous drainage to reduce inflammation, infection, and incidence of sepsis as well as for the fistula to mature (loose seton) or allowing it to create fistulotomy for it to close (tight seton) [4, 24]. Setons can potentially improve the success of future repair for patients undergoing medical optimization, especially in patients with active anorectal disease or acute perianal sepsis [24, 25]. Patients who may benefit the most are those with smaller-sized fistulas, especially on the vaginal opening side, or with multiple tracts, although exact qualifications for seton placement have not been determined. The maximum amount of time that a seton can be utilized has not yet been determined, although its use for long-term management of complex fistulas associated with Crohn's disease has been considered (evidence grade 1C) [24]. Further investigation is needed to determine the benefit of seton use in conjunction with medical or immunotherapies or with its continuation after fistula repair to prevent fecal incontinence or preserve surgical outcomes.

Miscellaneous

Prosthetic insertions are available in sheets, plugs, or fibrin glue form. These can be made of synthetic material or animal-derived material, commonly porcine intestinal mucosa. Examples available currently include Gore BIO-A© tissue reinforcement or fistula plug, BioGlue©, and Cook Biotech© Biodesign Fistula Plug sets. The treatment utilization for these inserts is limited and often restricted by fistula size and complexity.

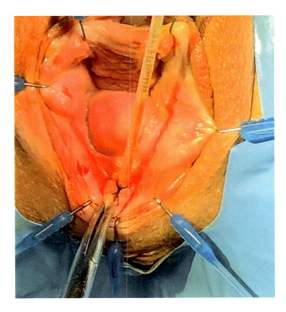

Fig. 5 Foley catheter placement through the vaginal opening to delineate the fistulous tract

Risk factors for treatment failure are longer length of fistulous tract, preexisting abscesses, and other communicating fistulas [28]. The data is more prevalent for treatment in fistula-in-ano; however, there are case reports of successful prosthetic utilization for rectovaginal fistulas in varying positions in relation to the vaginal wall. Overall, the treatment success on a larger scale is thought to be minimal, especially long term, and is more often accompanied by dislodgement or infection rather than clinical improvement [24].

The utilization of stem cells is a novel concept that may be promising for treatment in the near future. Mesenchymal-derived cells from the bone marrow or adipose tissue, either autologous or from donors, can be injected directly into the fistulous tract or coated onto a prosthetic plug [29, 30]. Injection of other autologous materials like adipose tissue is being investigated. Current limited trials have demonstrated varying success in treatment-refractory Crohn's-associated rectovaginal fistulas, but further research is underway.

Surgical Repair

Introduction

Successful healing after RVF repair is highest after initial surgical repair. Guidelines for timing, method, and optimization for repair however are lacking, due to the varied nature of presentation and causes for rectovaginal fistulas. In practice, the abovementioned conservative approaches are often utilized simultaneously while awaiting surgical repair as an indirect staged approach. Extensive counseling and consideration should be geared toward patient risk factors for wound breakdown or surgical failure, like prior pelvic radiation, active inflammatory bowel disease, or malignancy. As previously discussed, there are several imaging modalities that assist in not only identifying fistulas but also characterizing sphincter dysfunction, fistula location to sphincter, and the presence of any abscesses or strictures. All of these considerations should guide surgical counseling and treatment.

Optimization Prior to Surgical Repair

Given the risk of repair breakdown and fistula reoccurrence, preoperative surgical planning and optimization is imperative. For obstetric or surgical trauma related, repair as early as 72 h after injury can be performed to minimize surrounding tissue damage; otherwise, delayed repair up to 12 weeks later can be performed [4]. Minimal differences in surgical outcomes have been cited between early and delayed repairs for other vaginal fistulas. The recommendations for optimal timing of other etiologies of RVF are less well defined, but an average of 3–6 months from medical management of etiology is often quoted [18]. Regardless of the etiology, there is recent preliminary evidence across multiple specialties arguing for earlier and more aggressive surgical repair in comparison to older data.

For patients with Crohn's disease, there are currently no standardized recommendations for length of recurrence-free interval before surgical repair. The extent of anorectal disease and overall health status often dictates timing and method of surgical repair. Any abscesses noted on initial exam, regardless of RVF etiology but especially in Crohn's-related RVF, should be drained to assist with healing and outcomes for future surgical intervention. Preoperative anemia and nutrition optimization is crucial prior to repair for malignancy-associated or radiation-associated RVF.

The argument has been made for fecal diversion, either as a treatment to allow for RVF healing without any other primary repair or prophylactically to preserve surgical integrity after repair. No large randomized trials have been performed, but diversion may improve 1-year recurrence rates in both conservative and surgical repairs [11]. One recent retrospective review of RVF repair across several specialties has shown that this practice is becoming widely adopted. Intestinal diversion, either concomitant or prior to primary repair, is currently performed in up to 80% of cancer-related RVF repairs and 46% of inflammatory bowel disease RVF repairs [27]. Fecal diversion has been considered for primary treatment of radiation-related RVF as well [12].

Prophylactic diversion may also help reduce development of RVF after deep endometriosis surgery involving the bowel and rectum [31].

Antibiotic prophylaxis is commonly given as a single dose perioperatively. Most surgeons utilize at least cefazolin and metronidazole, or other antibiotics geared toward targeting infectious cause or abscess cultures if present and known at the time of repair. There is currently no recommendation for preoperative or prolonged postoperative antibiotics in the abscess of infection or immunosuppression.

Preoperative bowel evacuation can be considered and vary based on surgeon preference from no bowel preparation to mechanical, chemical, or enema preparation. However, there is currently no recommendation for preoperative or prolonged postoperative bowel preparation.

Methods of Rectovaginal Fistula Repair

Overall, a local repair is thought to be the best first surgical method. This can be completed through a transvaginal, transperineal, transrectal, or abdominal approaches. Many surgeons utilize location of the rectovaginal fistula to guide surgical planning, although etiology and extent of disease are also important contributing factors. Primary fistulotomy can be considered, as it is often performed during surgical repair for other fistulous types, but there is not yet consensus about its role in RVF repair. Performing fistulotomy involves expanding the area around the fistula during mobilization where there is less tissue in-between the vaginal and rectal fistulous tracts, minimizing potential surgical space and increasing surgical risk. Regardless of surgical approach, the ideal distance of circumferential mobilization has not been identified. Trimming or resecting RVF edges to improve healing after re-approximation is left to surgeon discretion and intraoperative findings.

Vaginal repairs are most common in gynecologic and pelvic surgery literature. For fistulas involving the perineal tissue and sphincter, an episioproctotomy is commonly performed to remove the fistula and repair and reconstruct perineal tissue and sphincter, if involved [4, 6, 12].

Successful repair rates may be as high as 64–78%. The rate of fecal incontinence improvement (minimal to none) may be even higher [12, 24]. If the sphincter is intact, a primary repair can be done by incising around the fistulous tract vaginally to mobilize the posterior vagina from the rectum. After excision of fibrotic tissue if deemed necessary, the rectum is closed in a two-layer approach with plication of the anal sphincters or levator ani if needed, followed by closure of the vaginal mucosa. Vaginal flap advancement has been described to aid in surgical repair. For transvaginal repair for rectovaginal fistulas associated with Crohn's disease, the surgical outcomes may be comparable to endorectal flap, although more research is warranted [12]. Complete fistula excision with flapless repair can be considered as well.

The initial incision is dependent on the location of the fistula. Many distal fistulas can be approached utilizing a U-shaped incision at the perineum. This allows wide mobilization of the tissues and access to the anal sphincter and perineal muscles. If the anal sphincter is intact, it can be preserved. The surgeon can use a nondominant finger in the rectum to guide the dissection of the vaginal tissue away from the rectum. This dissection is continued widely, creating a margin of 1.5–2 cm surrounding the fistulous opening. Once the rectal and vaginal walls are separated, the rectal wall edges are typically refreshed, which enlarges the size of the fistula. The rectal wall is closed with 4–0 delayed absorbable suture, typically placed extramucosally. A second layer of 3–0 or 4–0 delayed absorbable suture is placed such as to imbricate the first layer. If available, a third layer of 3–0 or 2–0 absorbable suture is placed plicating the perirectal fascia and lastly the vaginal epithelium is reapproximated. Anal sphincteroplasty and perineal repair is performed as indicated (Fig. 6).

A transanal or transrectal repair is often the preferred method of approach for colorectal specialists. Primary repair with or without endorectal advancement flap (ERAF) is commonly described. In instances where the fistula passes through the anal sphincter and primary fistulotomy cannot be performed, a LIFT procedure can be performed.

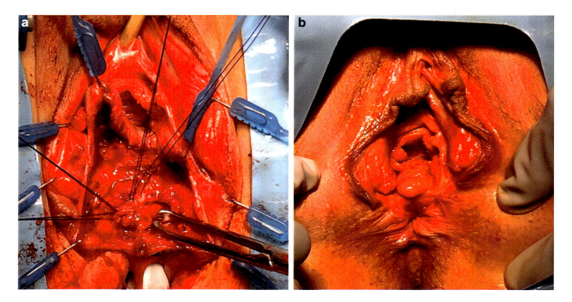

Fig. 6 (**a**) Transvaginal repair of rectovaginal fistula. The anal sphincter is reapproximated with overlapping sutures. (**b**) Completed transvaginal repair

The intersphincteric tract can be identified between the internal and external anal sphincter and then divided and repaired with native tissue or with the inclusion of bioprosthetic material [4]. For intersphincteric fistulas, both LIFT and ERAF procedures may have similar short-term outcomes for high anal fistulas, but the benefit for RVF specifically has not yet been investigated [32]. Another type of transrectal repair is a rectal sleeve advancement, which involves resection of the distal diseased rectum and advancement of the proximal healthy rectum, in patients who otherwise are looking at permanent fecal diversion or total proctocolectomy [12]. The advantage of a transrectal approach is repair from the high pressure side of the fistulous tract, which may help improve success rates [6].

Successful cases with transperineal approaches have been described in the literature. The advantages include preservation of the anal sphincters, greater allowance for tissue mobilization, and opportunity for reconstruction of the anovaginal septum and the perineum if desired [9]. One retrospective study looking at transperineal approaches showed failure rates ranging from 11% to 40% across multiple RVF etiologies and fistula sizes [33].

Tissue Flaps

Current guidelines from the American Society of Colon and Rectal Surgeons (ASCRS) strongly endorse ERAF advancement as the primary surgical management for simple RVF (grade 1C evidence) [24]. Successful repair rates range as high as 43–93% [12]. This repair is most ideal in a patient with disease involvement of the distal rectum but with presence of healthy, viable rectal mucosa and muscle more proximally. A multi-tissue flap from the viable area is mobilized and reapproximated over the fistulous tract after its excision. The vaginal mucosa is often not repaired to allow for drainage for healing. Concomitant sphincteroplasty and fecal diversion can be considered, although the efficacy at the time of ERAF advancement warrants further investigation.

Another common tissue flap utilized in RVF repair is the Martius flap. Adipose tissue from the labia majora, utilizing blood supply from external and internal pudendal artery, is mobilized and sutured in between the fistulous vaginal and rectal openings. The bulbocavernosus and ischiocavernosus muscle can be included in this flap as well. This technique has success rates of up to

50–90% for low and middle third RVF with excellent healing and minimal postoperative complications [12]. Repairs have been described across a variety of rectovaginal fistula sizes and etiologies.

Omentum, peritoneum, and gracilis flaps have also been described for rectovaginal fistula repair. However, most of the literature supporting RVF flap repair do not include large percentage of Crohn's or inflammatory causes, so their overall success rate is unknown.

Abdominal Approach

An abdominal approach is often utilized for larger fistulas or fistulas located in the middle third and upper third of the rectum and the posterior vaginal fornix. This is the more common approach in the literature for repair after Crohn's disease, cancer, and overall more complex etiologies (i.e., after colorectal anastomosis). Traditionally, an open approach has been utilized, although laparoscopic and robotic techniques have been described. Previous anastomosis and surgical repair with distortion of anatomy and pelvic adhesive disease poses unique surgical challenges with an abdominal approach. Once abdominal access is obtained, one repair technique involves a primary excision with omental flap if otherwise surrounded by healthy tissue [12]. Anastomosis after excision may be considered but also poses its own risk for anastomotic leak and further risks for fistulization. Benefits of abdominal repair include ability to perform concomitant bowel diversion, resection of diseased bowel, and muscle transposition to prevent abdominal organ displacement [4, 34]. Additionally, in one of the larger retrospective studies of rectovaginal fistula repair, abdominal repairs had a 1-year recurrence-free survival rate that was threefold higher than local repairs [27].

Novel and Future Approaches

The fistula-tract laser closure (FiLaC) procedure is a promising new minimally invasive surgical technique using laser probes and energy to obliterate the fistulous tracts in transsphincteric or perianal fistulas [35, 36]. Success rates are quoted as high as 66.8%, with factors limiting success being curved tract or > 5 mm [28]. Additionally, video-assisted fistula repair, where cautery is used to obliterate fistulous tracts under video guidance, has been gaining traction for treatment of anorectal fistulas [28]. Though the healing rate seems promising, both of these novel techniques have yet to prove efficacy in rectovaginal fistulas as well as patients with prior Crohn's, malignancy, radiation, or surgery.

Postsurgical Considerations and Complications

Postsurgical Care and Expectations

Care after rectovaginal fistula surgery often depends on the method, etiology, and extent of the repair. Postoperative antibiotics can be considered but are not routinely used or recommended. Primary local repairs, especially when done transvaginal or transrectal, often do not require prolonged hospitalization nor significant dietary restrictions besides the utilization of stool softener or mineral oil to lubricate the stool [12]. There is currently no consensus on routine vaginal packing postoperatively. Patients should be extensively counseled on risks of postoperative dyspareunia and pelvic pain. Additionally, expectations for postsurgical bowel function should be discussed. Postoperative change in bowel function is common and can include de novo fecal incontinence or persistence of preexisting incontinence [34]. Defecation difficulties may exist separate from the rectovaginal fistula or its concomitant sphincter damage, and patients should be counseled that these can persist even after RVF repair.

Postoperative Complications

Infections requiring antibiotic treatment, blood transfusions, and utilization of total parental nutrition are all complications following fistula repair [27]. Common associated risk factors for postoperative complications are smoking, obesity, and age [33]. Modifiable risks should be well optimized prior to surgical repair. Recovery and healing may be prolonged especially in the setting of significant bowel disease, immunocompromised state, or malnutrition depending on RVF etiology. The most frustrating complication that patients should be extensively counseled on is risk of fistula recurrence, which can occur in up to 30% of patients 1 year after surgical repair [27]. It can be difficult to identify what is most predictive of recurrence: the etiology of the fistula or the treatment itself. Obstetric-related fistulas may be prone to less breakdown and higher success regardless of method of management.

RVF due to Crohn's disease has a higher risk of recurrence that other fistula types, with up to 25–50% recurrence rate. Additionally, failure rate is higher after Crohn's-associated RVF repair compared to repairs for other RVF etiology [33]. Even when treatment success is achieved, there is a higher risk of Crohn's-related RVF undergoing malignant transformation [25]. One proposed etiology is the implantation of cancer cells in injured mucosa of the fistula, with subsequent healing or inflammatory responses promoting cancer proliferation [37]. Though the overall incidence is rare, the presence does seem to correlate with length of disease. Long-term surveillance should be discussed and initiated with these patients. Other risk factors for failed RVF repair include prior radiation, malignancy, and number of prior repairs [24].

Conclusion

Rectovaginal fistulas are a medically and surgically complex dilemma that transcends multiple specialties and treatment modalities. The widely variable etiologies and presentations make it difficult to conduct large patient studies and trials, and much of the current evidence is based on limited case studies, retrospective cohorts, and surgeon experience. Based on current literature and practices, the future of RVF treatment may show better characterization of RVF presentation, earlier surgical management, and more advanced medical or prosthetic options for conservative management or preoperative optimization.

Cross-References

▶ Management of Vaginal Posterior Compartment Prolapse: Is There Ever a Case for Graft/Mesh?

References

1. Cowgill KD, Bishop J, Norgaard AK, Rubens CE, Gravett MG. Obstetric fistula in low-resource countries: an under-valued and under-studied problem – systematic review of its incidence, prevalence, and association with stillbirth. BMC Pregnancy Childbirth. 2015;15:1–7.
2. Friedman AM, Ananth CV, Prendergast E, D'Alton ME, Wright JD. Evaluation of third-degree and fourth-degree laceration rates as quality indicators. Obstet Gynecol. 2015;125:927–37.
3. Pergialiotis V, Vlachos D, Protopapas A, Pappa K, Vlachos G. Risk factors for severe perineal lacerations during childbirth. Int J Gynecol Obstet. 2014;125:6–14.
4. Chen CCG, Long JB. Vesicovaginal and rectovaginal fistula repair. In: Van LL, Handa VL, editors. Te Linde's operative gynecology. 12th ed. Philadelphia: Elsevier; 2020. p. 578–605.
5. Brown HW, Wang L, Bunker CH, Lowder JL. Lower reproductive tract fistula repairs in. In: Urogynecol J. 2012;23:403–10.
6. Karram MM. Rectovaginal fistula and perineal breakdown. In: Walters MD, Karram MM, editors. Urogynecology and reconstructive pelvic surgery. 4th ed. Philadelphia, PA: Elsevier Saunders; 2007. p. 331–9.
7. De la Poza G, López-Sanroman A, Taxonera C, Marín-Jimenez IP, Gisbert J, Bermejo F, Opio V, Muriel A. Genital fistulas in female Crohn's disease patients. Clinical characteristics and response to therapy. J Crohns Colitis. 2012;6:276–80.
8. Forsgren C, Altman D. Risk of pelvic organ fistula in patients undergoing hysterectomy. Curr Opin Obstet Gynecol. 2010;22:404–7.
9. Pata G, Pasini M, Roncali S, Tognai D, Ragni F. Iatrogenic rectovaginal fistula repair by trans-perineal approach and pubo-coccygeus muscle interposition. Int J Surg Case Rep. 2014;5:527–31.
10. Kazi MK, Gori J, Engineer R, Ankathi SKK, Bhuta P, Patel S, Sukumar V, Desouza A, Saklani AP. Incidence and treatment outcomes of rectovaginal fistula after rectal cancer resection. Female Pelvic Med Reconstr Surg. 2022;28:115–9.
11. Corte H, Maggiori L, Treton X, Lefevre JH, Ferron M, Panis Y. Rectovaginal fistula: what is the optimal strategy? Ann Surg. 2015;262:855–61.

12. Gurland BH, Vogel JD. Rectovaginal fistula. In: The ASCRS textbook of colon and rectal surgery. 4th ed. Cham: Springer; 2022. p. 281–91.
13. Rogers RG, Jeppson PC. Current diagnosis and management of pelvic fistulae in women. Obstet Gynecol. 2016;128:635–50.
14. Zelga P, Tchórzewski M, Zelga M, Sobotkowski J, Dziki A. Radiation-induced rectovaginal fistulas in locally advanced gynaecological malignancies – new patients, old problem? Langenbeck's Arch Surg. 2017;402:1079–88.
15. Feddock J, Randall M, Kudrimoti M, Baldwin L, Shah P, Weiss H, DeSimone C. Impact of post-radiation biopsies on development of fistulae in patients with cervical cancer. Gynecol Oncol. 2014;133:263–7.
16. Oakley SH, Brown HW, Yurteri-Kaplan L, et al. Practice patterns regarding management of rectovaginal fistulae: a multicenter review from the fellows' pelvic research network. Female Pelvic Med Reconstr Surg. 2015;21:123–8.
17. Tuma F, McKeown DG, Al-Wahab Z. Rectovaginal fistula. Treasure Island: StatPearls; 2022.
18. Debeche-Adams TH, Bohl JL. Rectovaginal fistulas. Clin Colon Rectal Surg. 2010;23:99–103.
19. Yee LF, Birnbaum EH, Read TE, Kodner IJ, Fleshman JW. Use of endoanal ultrasound in patients with rectovaginal fistulas. Dis Colon Rectum. 1999;42:1057–64.
20. Engin G. Endosonographic imaging of anorectal diseases. J Ultrasound Med. 2006;25:57–73.
21. Nevler A, Beer-Gabel M, Lebedyev A, Soffer A, Gutman M, Carter D, Zbar AP. Transperineal ultrasonography in perianal Crohn's disease and recurrent cryptogenic fistula-in-ano. Color Dis. 2013;15:1011–8.
22. Denson L, Shobeiri SA. Peroxide-enhanced 3-dimensional endovaginal ultrasound imaging for diagnosis of rectovaginal fistula. Female Pelvic Med Reconstr Surg. 2014;20:240–2.
23. Maconi G, Ardizzone S, Greco S, Radice E, Bezzio C, Bianchi Porro G. Transperineal ultrasound in the detection of perianal and rectovaginal fistulae in Crohn's disease. Am J Gastroenterol. 2007;102:2214–9.
24. Vogel JD. Johnson EK, Morris AM, Paquette IM, Saclarides TJ, Feingold DL, Steele SR. Clinical practice guideline for the management of anorectal abscess, fistula-in-ano, and rectovaginal fistula. Dis Colon Rectum. 2016;59:1117–33.
25. Hannaway CD, Hull TL. Current considerations in the management of rectovaginal fistula from Crohn's disease. Color Dis. 2008;10:747–55.
26. Zhu YF, Tao GQ, Zhou N, Xiang C. Current treatment of rectovaginal fistula in Crohn's disease. World J Gastroenterol. 2011;17:963–7.
27. Byrnes JN, Schmitt JJ, Faustich BM, Mara KC, Weaver AL, Chua HK, Occhino JA. Outcomes of rectovaginal fistula repair. Female Pelvic Med Reconstr Surg. 2017;23:124–30.
28. Hong Y, Xu Z, Gao Y, Sun M, Chen Y, Wen K, Wang X, Sun X. Sphincter-preserving fistulectomy is an effective minimally invasive technique for complex anal fistulas. Front Surg. 2022; https://doi.org/10.3389/fsurg.2022.832397.
29. Lightner AL, Dozois EJ, Dietz AB, Fletcher JG, Friton J, Butler G, Faubion WA. Matrix-delivered autologous mesenchymal stem cell therapy for refractory rectovaginal Crohn's fistulas. Inflamm Bowel Dis. 2020;26:670–7.
30. García-Arranz M, Herreros MD, González-Gómez C, Quintana P de la, Guadalajara H, Georgiev-Hristov T, Trébol J, Garcia-Olmoa D. Treatment of Crohn's-related rectovaginal fistula with allogeneic expanded-adipose derived stem cells: a phase I–IIa clinical trial. Stem Cells Transl Med. 2016;5:1441–6.
31. Roman H, Bridoux V, Merlot B, Noailles M, Magne E, Resch B, Forestier D, Tuech JJ. Risk of rectovaginal fistula in women with excision of deep endometriosis requiring concomitant vaginal and rectal sutures, with or without preventive stoma: a before-and-after comparative study. J Minim Invasive Gynecol. 2022;29:56–64.e1.
32. Vergara-Fernandez O, Espino-Urbina LA. Ligation of intersphincteric fistula tract: what is the evidence in a review? World J Gastroenterol. 2013;19:6805–13.
33. Karp NE, Kobernik EK, Berger MB, Low CM, Fenner DE. Do the surgical outcomes of rectovaginal fistula repairs differ for obstetric and nonobstetric fistulas? A retrospective cohort study. Female Pelvic Med Reconstr Surg. 2019;25:36–40.
34. Hauch A, Ramamoorthy S, Zelhart M, Dobke M. Refining approaches to surgical repair of rectovaginal fistulas. Ann Plast Surg. 2020;84:S250–6.
35. Garg P, Singh P. Video-Assisted Anal Fistula Treatment (VAAFT) in cryptoglandular fistula-in-ano: a systematic review and proportional meta-analysis. Int J Surg. 2017;46:85–91.
36. Zulkarnain FM, Soeselo DA, Suryanto SGG. Case report: complex perianal fistula treated with fistula laser closure (FILAC) and suction catheter. Int J Surg Case Rep. 2021; https://doi.org/10.1016/j.ijscr.2021.106085.
37. Takahashi R, Ichikawa R, Ito S, et al. A case of metastatic carcinoma of anal fistula caused by implantation from rectal cancer. Surg Case Reports. 2015; https://doi.org/10.1186/s40792-015-0125-2.

Ureterovaginal Fistula Repair

Kelsey E. Gallo, Michael W. Witthaus, and Jill C. Buckley

Contents

Introduction	822
Definition and Etiology	822
Diagnosis	822
Clinical Features	822
Exam Findings	822
Imaging Studies	823
Management	824
Endoscopic Management	824
Surgical Management	825
Conclusion	827
References	827

Abstract

Ureterovaginal fistulae most commonly occur after ureteral injury during pelvic surgery. Risk factors for the development of ureterovaginal fistulae include endometriosis, radiation therapy, and malignancy, though most reported ureterovaginal fistulae occurred in patients after uncomplicated hysterectomy for benign disease. The most common complaint in patients with ureterovaginal fistula is constant drainage of fluid per the vagina. The diagnosis can be confirmed with either intravenous pyelogram, antegrade nephrostogram or CT/MRI urography. Ureterovaginal fistula will rarely resolve without intervention. Treatment goals include the return of normal urinary and genital function, avoidance of urinary tract infection and preservation of renal function. In some situations, patients can under go trial of ureteral stenting, as this may resolve the fistula. Surgical management is required in cases of failed endoscopic management. Transabdominal ureteroneocystostomy with or without psoas hitch is the most common surgical approach for ureterovaginal fistula, although each case should be approached on an individual basis. Successful fistula repair is expected in more than 90% of cases with appropriate management.

K. E. Gallo · M. W. Witthaus · J. C. Buckley (✉)
UC San Diego Health, San Diego, CA, USA
e-mail: kgallo@health.ucsd.edu;
miwitthaus@health.ucsd.edu; jcbuckley@health.ucsd.edu

Keywords

Fistula · Ureteral injury · Urinary leakage · Ureterovaginal fistula

Introduction

Ureterovaginal fistula is most often a complication of ureteral injury during pelvic surgery. While this is an uncommon complication, it causes significant distress for both patients and physicians. Prompt diagnosis and management are therefore critical. Patients can expect excellent results with appropriate management.

Definition and Etiology

A ureterovaginal fistula is an abnormal connection between the ureter and the vagina. Most ureterovaginal fistulae are iatrogenic, caused by ureteral injury during pelvic surgery [26]. The distal ureter courses in close proximity to the rectum and gynecologic organs, making it susceptible to injury during pelvic surgery. Hysterectomy is specifically implicated in most cases of ureterovaginal fistula [14, 26]. Contemporary series show that ureteral injury ranges from 0.9% to 1.3% of women undergoing hysterectomy [3, 11]. Ureteral injury results in the formation of a fistula when urinary extravasation occurs and preferentially drains through the vaginal cuff suture line or opening. When a ureteral injury is recognized in a delayed fashion, the risk of fistula formation is significantly higher than when an injury is recognized at the time of surgery [3]. Immediate corrective surgery (ureteral repair or reimplantation into the bladder) or urinary stenting (with consideration of proximal urinary diversion) may prevent fistula formation. A prior history of radiation, advanced malignancy, diabetes, pelvic inflammatory disease, and postoperative surgical infection are associated with a higher risk of fistula formation due to their poor wound healing characteristics ([11]; Gerber and Schoenberg [4]).

Other surgical causes of ureterovaginal fistula include Cesarian section, anterior colporrhaphy, retropubic bladder neck suspensions, and vascular and colon surgery. Rarely, a ureterovaginal fistula is due to a congenital condition resulting from ectopic insertion of the ureter into the vagina. Other reported causes include malignancy, infection, radiation, and pelvic trauma (Gerber and Schoenberg [4]).

Diagnosis

Clinical Features

The most common complaint in patients with ureterovaginal fistula is constant drainage of fluid per the vagina. Leakage of fluid must be distinguished from other causes of vaginal discharge, as well as other forms of urinary incontinence. In the setting of recent pelvic surgery, leakage typically starts between 1 and 4 weeks postoperatively [14]. This presentation may be preceded by flank pain or low-grade fever from urinoma formation or ureteral obstruction, although incontinence is the main presenting symptom in most cases ([14]; Gerber and Schoenberg [4]). The degree of urinary leakage may vary depending on the size of the fistula tract. Patients will have normal voiding function when the contralateral ureter is unaffected, except in the case of concurrent vesicovaginal fistula. Careful and systematic staging of the injury will ensure a concurrent fistula to another organ is not missed. Patients may also report skin breakdown and irritation from wetness, vaginal infections, or urinary tract infections. It is essential to address these concerns while performing additional workup to reduce associated patient distress.

Exam Findings

A speculum exam should be performed to assess the location, size, and number of fistulae. Vaginoscopy can be used as an adjunct for better visualization and to assess surrounding tissue quality. A double dye test can be used to distinguish between vesicovaginal and ureterovaginal fistulae [19]. The test is performed by administering phenazopyridine orally, instilling methylene blue intravesically, and placing a tampon or packing in the vagina. Orange staining on the tampon or packing confirms a ureteral fistula, while blue staining confirms a vesical fistula. If both colors are seen, the patient may have a concurrent ureterovaginal and vesicovaginal fistulae, occurring in 6% of ureterovaginal fistula cases [3]. Cystoscopy can be used to support the diagnosis. If no staining is seen, peritoneal fluid, vaginitis, lymphatic fistula, and fallopian tube fistula should be considered as alternative diagnoses [28]. Vaginal fluid can be collected and sent for creatinine to confirm a urinary source, recognizing that the fistula site to the urinary tract still needs to be determined.

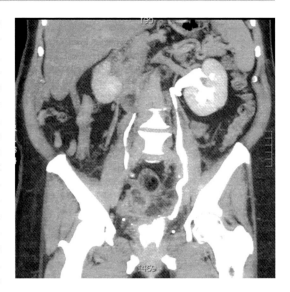

Fig. 1 CT Urogram with pyelogram images of a left ureterovaginal fistula diagnosed 5 weeks after a left distal ureteral injury during total abdominal hysterectomy for uterine carcinosarcoma

Imaging Studies

The diagnosis of a ureterovaginal fistula can be confirmed with either intravenous pyelogram, antegrade nephrostogram, or CT/MRI urography (Figs. 1 and 2). Even if the index of suspicion is very high based on history and exam, imaging studies should be obtained to thoroughly assess the location and extent of ureteral injury prior to intervention. Historically, an intravenous pyelogram with lateral films was used to assess for drainage of contrast into the vagina. The most common 2D imaging is an antegrade nephrostogram via a nephrostomy which has often been placed in the setting of a ureteral injury with urinary extravasation. Cross-sectional imaging with CT or MRI urography is commonly performed as well (if readily available), which provides a more detailed anatomical survey of surrounding tissue and can easily diagnose a urinoma or abscess. Caliectasis and ureteral dilation proximal to the fistula may be observed when a ureteral narrowing is associated with an ongoing urinary leakage. In the case of a large ureteral injury, hydroureteronephrosis may not occur [14]. Cystography, either X-ray or CT, can be performed in cases of suspected concurrent vesicovaginal fistula and to assess bladder capacity.

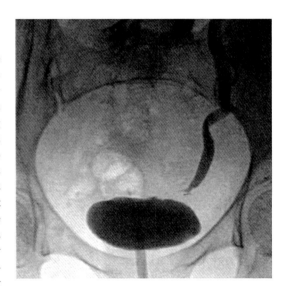

Fig. 2 Concurrent cystogram and antegrade nephrostogram showing the location of a ureteral injury

Management

Treatment goals include the return of normal urinary and genital function, avoidance of urinary tract infection, and preservation of renal function [18]. Ureterovaginal fistula will rarely resolve without intervention. Historically, all ureterovaginal fistulas were treated with open ureteroneocystostomy (Goodwin and Scardino [7, 21]). Beginning in the 1980s, advances in endourologic equipment made antegrade or retrograde placement of a ureteral stent more common. Contemporary series show that some ureterovaginal fistulas will heal with stenting alone [23]. With the advent of laparoscopic and robotic surgery, early reconstruction yields excellent outcomes with less morbidity than traditional open surgeries (Shelbaia and Hashish [25]). Regardless of ultimate management strategy, the upper urinary tract of the affected side should be decompressed with a ureteral stent or percutaneous nephrostomy tube as soon as the diagnosis of a ureterovaginal fistula is confirmed. Decompression will relieve urinary obstruction and prevent infection if surgical intervention is not immediately considered (Morey et al. [16]).

Endoscopic Management

Most advocate that all patients diagnosed with a ureterovaginal fistula undergo initial evaluation with retrograde pyelogram, as this can be both diagnostic and therapeutic. In very select cases when the ureter is in continuity on retrograde pyelogram and the infralesional ureter appears normal, the fistula may close spontaneously [2]. In these cases, stent placement is often feasible with minimal added morbidity and therefore is preferred to observation (Morey et al. [16]). Several studies have shown that when stenting is feasible and straightforward, that alone may be enough to prevent or allow closure of the fistula [2, 20, 23, 27]. Success is more likely if stenting is performed within 2 weeks of the index surgery or within 2 weeks of leakage onset [20]. Ureteroscopy can be utilized for stent placement when routine cystoscopic guided placement is unsuccessful. Direct visualization and using a hydrophilic coated guide wire may also increase the chance of successful passage. However, this should be approached cautiously as to not traumatize the ureter. As with any acute ureteral injury, prolonged endoscopic manipulation can convert a minor or partial injury into a complete ureteral injury. In patients for whom retrograde stent placement is not technically feasible or are too ill to undergo general anesthesia, percutaneous nephrostomy tube may be placed instead. Percutaneous nephrostomy drainage has rarely been reported to resolve the fistula successfully but can allow future attempts at antegrade stent placement [2].

In patients that successfully have a ureteral stent placed, fistula resolution has been reported between 63% and 100% (case series) though these patients are at risk of developing future ureteral stricture with an unknown incidence [2, 9, 23]. Selzman et al. reported success in a small case series of seven patients who underwent stenting for 4–8 weeks, one of whom developed a ureteral stricture at 2 months. In another small case series, Kumar et al. reported fistula resolution in eight patients with stenting, three of whom developed a ureteral stricture at 6 months. A combined retrograde and antegrade approach to establish ureteral continuity has been reported in cases of distal ureteral occlusion, though this technique results in a high ureteral stricture rate of 30–55% [13, 27].

In series that recommended ureteral stenting as primary management, duration is commonly recommended for 6–8 weeks prior to assessment for resolution. Symptom assessment and repeat ureteral imaging will confirm the resolution of the fistula prior to stent removal. Depending on the imaging modality available, this could include a retrograde pyelogram, antegrade nephrostogram (if a nephrostomy is present), or CT/MRI urography. If the fistula has resolved and the stent is removed, follow-up imaging can be obtained at regular intervals to assess for the development of a ureteral stricture. If the fistula remains, surgical reconstruction must be considered.

Surgical Management

Depending on the extent and timing of the recognition of the ureteral injury, immediate surgical repair may be indicated. If the injury is diagnosed intraoperatively or in the acute postoperative period (less than 10–12 days), immediate surgical repair can be carried out in an otherwise uncomplicated situation. Those that have failed or could not undergo endoscopic management will also require ureteral reconstruction.

Patients with delayed ureteral reconstruction should be optimized prior to repair by eliminating infection, ensuring adequate nutrition, and relieving urinary obstruction with either stent or nephrostomy tube. Relevant history should be noted, including prior abdominal and pelvic surgeries, to inform options for an operative approach. Vaginal anatomy including depth, tissue quality, and presence of prolapse or mesh may also affect the surgical plan. Transabdominal ureteroneocystostomy with or without psoas hitch is the most common surgical approach for ureterovaginal fistula, although each case should be approached on an individual basis (Fig. 3). The surgeon should be prepared to enlist a variety of techniques depending on intraoperative findings and assessment.

Ureterovaginal fistula repair can be done open or via minimally invasive techniques. Open surgery has historically been the gold standard approach; however, multiple groups have shown excellent results with minimally invasive techniques and when available is the preferred approach. Laparoscopic-/robotic-assisted surgery results in shorter hospital stays and less perioperative pain compared to open surgery with enhanced visualization and magnification [15]. Robotic-assisted techniques provide additional advantages, including 3D tissue magnification, precision dissection, and suturing in small anatomic spaces without compromising operative time [5, 8].

The principles of fistula repair and intraoperative decision-making are the same regardless of whether an open or minimally invasive technique is used. The patient should be positioned in dorsal lithotomy to allow access to the vagina. For an open approach, a Pfannenstiel or lower midline incision may be employed. For a laparoscopic or robotic approach, ports can be placed parallel about 1 cm above the umbilicus. The ureter is identified at the location of the crossing iliac vessels, as ureterovaginal fistulae occur almost exclusively in the distal ureter. Ureteral mobilization is performed caudally, careful to preserve periureteral blood supply. VessiLoop may be used to aid in counter tension to ensure adequate ureteral mobilization [12]. The tissue often becomes more fibrotic as the area of the fistula is approached. An abscess cavity or loculated urinoma may need to be evacuated [8]. Vaginal apex inspection either prior to surgery or intraoperatively should ensure no foreign body is in the vaginal closure. If a long-standing fistula tract is present, it can be excised with vaginal closure [12]. In the case of a ureterovaginal fistula occurring after a hysterectomy, the resolution of continuous urine leakage with a ureteral reimplantation will allow the fistula to close spontaneously without additional vaginal cuff sutures.

The ureter and surrounding tissue should then be assessed. The ureter should be transected just proximal to the area of the fistula and widely spatulated [12]. A 10 French catheter can be passed proximally into the ureter to ensure sufficient ureteral diameter. Indocyanine green (ICG) fluorescence may be used if tissue quality is of

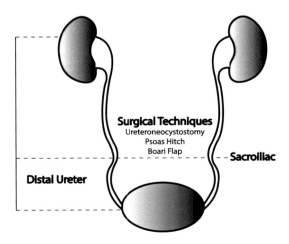

Fig. 3 Diagram of distal ureteral reconstructive techniques

concern to assess for ureteral perfusion. The gold standard reconstructive technique for a distal ureteral injury is a ureteroneocystostomy. Success rates are above 95% when the principles of this surgery are carried out well regardless of the technique.

If the distal ureter is not viable or a tensionless ureteric reimplantation is not achievable, a psoas hitch will need to be performed. Under these circumstances, the bladder is mobilized and secured to the psoas tendon, avoiding the genitofemoral nerve. A tension-free anastomosis may be achieved with bladder mobilization alone or may require a psoas hitch and Boari flaps in rare cases.

To perform the ureteroneocystostomy, a small cystotomy is made on the posterior lateral aspect of the bladder. Some series describe performing a non-refluxing anastomosis, though evidence does not support that this is superior to a refluxing anastomosis. The ureteral mucosa is anastomosed to the bladder mucosa with absorbable sutures in a tension-free, watertight fashion. The ureter is anastomosed over a ureteral stent. Retrograde filling of the bladder can confirm the integrity of the anastomosis.

Table 1 Summary of minimally invasive surgical outcomes of ureterovaginal fistula repair

Reference	Surgical UVF cases	Repair type	Mean follow-up	Complications	Success rate
Abdel-Karim et al. [1]	7	Laparoscopic ureteroneocystostomy	6.5 years		7/7, 100%
Gellhaus et al. [5]	10 of 37 ureteral injury cases	Robotic-assisted ureteroneocystostomy with or without psoas hitch; Ureteroureterostomy	14 months		35/37
Ghosh et al. [6]	9	Laparoscopic non-refluxing ureteroneocystostomy with psoas hitch	15 months	1 patient with poorly functioning kidney on DMSA	8/9, 89%
Kidd et al. [8]	12	Robotic-assisted ureteroneocystostomy with or without psoas hitch (10 patients); ureteroureterostomy (2 patients)	29 months		12/12, 100%
Laungani et al. [10]	3	Robotic-assisted ureteroneocystostomy	6 months	None	3/3, 100%
Linder et al. [12]	1	Robotic-assisted ureteroneocystostomy	3 months	None	1/1, 100%
Modi et al. [15]	18	Laparoscopic non-refluxing ureteroneocystostomy with psoas hitch	26 months	1 patient with intraoperative cardiac arrhythmia requiring conversion to open	18/18, 100%
Patil et al. [17]	2 of 12 ureteral stricture cases	Robotic-assisted non-refluxing ureteroneocystostomy	16 months	2 patients with mild hydronephrosis	12/12, 100%
Sharma et al. [22]	31	Laparoscopic non-refluxing ureteroneocystostomy with or without psoas hitch	34 months		Not specified
Shaw et al. [24]	14	10 open ureteroneocystostomy; 1 laparoscopic- and 3 robotic-assisted ureteroneocystostomy with or without psoas hitch	4 months	1 patient with extrusion of vaginal mesh requiring excision at 5 years	14/14, 100%

Based on intraoperative findings, flap interposition between the reconstructed ureter and the vagina can be achieved with omentum or peritoneum. A pelvic drain may be placed, depending on the surgeon's preference. Postoperative urinary drainage is achieved with urethral catheterization for 7–14 days and ureteral stenting for 4–8 weeks.

Multiple contemporary series have confirmed high success rates of minimally invasive surgical repair of ureterovaginal fistula (Table 1). Modi et al. performed laparoscopic ureteroneocystostomy with psoas hitch in 17 patients with ureterovaginal fistula after hysterectomy. All patients failed endourologic management with stenting and had a nephrostomy tube placed. A non-refluxing anastomosis was performed, and no stent was left at the time of surgery. No patient had stricture or leak after 23 months of follow-up. In 2008, Laungani et al. published on the feasibility and benefits of performing the repair with robotic assistance. The three patients in this series underwent repair within 2 h on the robotic console. At a mean follow-up of 6 months, there was no leak or residual hydronephrosis. Additional series of robotic ureterovaginal fistulae repair include 3 patients by Linder et al. and 12 patients by Kidd et al. who had 100% successful repair at 6 weeks and 29 months, respectively. In a larger multi-institutional study of 37 patients who had robotic-assisted repair after ureteral injury, including 10 patients with ureterovaginal fistula, 95.9% of patients had a successful repair at 16.6 months [5].

Conclusion

Ureterovaginal fistula most often results from iatrogenic ureteral injury and can therefore be distressing for both patients and physicians. A careful and systematic staging of the injury will ensure prompt diagnosis and appropriate management. For patients in whom endoscopic management is not feasible or has failed, surgical repair provides excellent and durable results. Surgeons should be familiar with basic reconstructive principles of ureteral surgery as well as special considerations for ureterovaginal fistula to provide optimal care.

References

1. Abdel-Karim A, Elmissiry M, Moussa A, Mahfouz W, Abulfotooh A, Dawood W, Elsalmy S. Laparoscopic repair of female genitourinary fistulae: 10-year single-center experience. Int Urogynecol J. 2020;31(7):1357–62. https://doi.org/10.1007/s00192-019-04002-y. Epub 2019 Jun 29. PMID: 31256224
2. Al-Otaibi KM. Ureterovaginal fistulas: the role of endoscopy and a percutaneous approach. Urol Ann. 2012;4(2):102–5. https://doi.org/10.4103/0974-7796.95556. PMID: 22629006; PMCID: PMC3355691
3. Dallas KB, Rogo-Gupta L, Elliott CS. Urologic injury and fistula after hysterectomy for benign indications. Obstet Gynecol. 2019;134(2):241–9. https://doi.org/10.1097/AOG.0000000000003353. PMID: 31306326
4. Gerber GS, Schoenberg HW. Female urinary tract fistulas. J Urol. 1993;149(2):229–36. https://doi.org/10.1016/s0022-5347(17)36045-7. PMID: 8426392
5. Gellhaus PT, Bhandari A, Monn MF, Gardner TA, Kanagarajah P, Reilly CE, Llukani E, Lee Z, Eun DD, Rashid H, Joseph JV, Ghazi AE, Wu G, Boris RS. Robotic management of genitourinary injuries from obstetric and gynaecological operations: a multi-institutional report of outcomes. BJU Int. 2015;115(3):430–6. https://doi.org/10.1111/bju.12785. Epub 2014 Oct 23. PMID: 24750903
6. Ghosh B, Biswal DK, Bera MK, Pal DK. Laparoscopic extravesical lich-gregoir ureteroneocystostomy with psoas hitch for the management of ureterovaginal fistula in post-hysterectomy patients. Urol Int. 2016;96(2):171–6. https://doi.org/10.1159/000434727. Epub 2015 Aug 19. PMID: 26303766
7. Goodwin WE, Scardino PT. Vesicovaginal and ureterovaginal fistulas: a summary of 25 years of experience. J Urol. 1980;123(3):370–4. https://doi.org/10.1016/s0022-5347(17)55941-8. PMID: 7359641
8. Kidd LC, Lee M, Lee Z, Epstein M, Liu S, Rangel E, Ahmed N, Sotelo R, Hemal A, Eun DD. A multi-institutional experience with robotic vesicovaginal and ureterovaginal fistula repair after iatrogenic injury. J Endourol. 2021;35(11):1659–64. https://doi.org/10.1089/end.2020.0993. Epub 2021 Aug 13. PMID: 33787314
9. Kumar A, Goyal NK, Das SK, Trivedi S, Dwivedi US, Singh PB. Our experience with genitourinary fistulae. Urol Int. 2009;82(4):404–10. https://doi.org/10.1159/000218528. Epub 2009 Jun 8. PMID: 19506406
10. Laungani R, Patil N, Krane LS, Hemal AK, Raja S, Bhandari M, Menon M. Robotic-assisted ureterovaginal fistula repair: report of efficacy and feasiblity. J Laparoendosc Adv Surg Tech A. 2008;18(5):731–4. https://doi.org/10.1089/lap.2008.0037. PMID: 18699746

11. Likic IS, Kadija S, Ladjevic NG, Stefanovic A, Jeremic K, Petkovic S, Dzamic Z. Analysis of urologic complications after radical hysterectomy. Am J Obstet Gynecol. 2008;199(6):644.e1–3. https://doi.org/10.1016/j.ajog.2008.06.034. Epub 2008 Aug 22. PMID: 18722569
12. Linder BJ, Frank I, Occhino JA. Extravesical robotic ureteral reimplantation for ureterovaginal fistula. Int Urogynecol J. 2018;29(4):595–7. https://doi.org/10.1007/s00192-017-3459-4. Epub 2017 Sep 7. PMID: 28884348
13. Lingeman JE, Wong MY, Newmark JR. Endoscopic management of total ureteral occlusion and ureterovaginal fistula. J Endourol. 1995;9(5):391–6. https://doi.org/10.1089/end.1995.9.391. PMID: 8580939
14. Mandal AK, Sharma SK, Vaidyanathan S, Goswami AK. Ureterovaginal fistula: summary of 18 years' experience. Br J Urol. 1990;65(5):453–6. https://doi.org/10.1111/j.1464-410x.1990.tb14785.x. PMID: 2354309
15. Modi P, Gupta R, Rizvi SJ. Laparoscopic ureteroneocystostomy and psoas hitch for post-hysterectomy ureterovaginal fistula. J Urol. 2008;180(2):615–7. https://doi.org/10.1016/j.juro.2008.04.029. Epub 2008 Jun 12. PMID: 18554656
16. Morey AF, Broghammer JA, Hollowell CMP, McKibben MJ, Souter L. Urotrauma guideline 2020: AUA guideline. J Urol. 2021;205(1):30–5. https://doi.org/10.1097/JU.0000000000001408. Epub 2020 Oct 14. PMID: 33053308
17. Patil NN, Mottrie A, Sundaram B, Patel VR. Robotic-assisted laparoscopic ureteral reimplantation with psoas hitch: a multi-institutional, multinational evaluation. Urology. 2008;72(1):47–50. https://doi.org/10.1016/j.urology.2007.12.097. discussion 50. Epub 2008 Apr 2. PMID: 18384858
18. Rabani SM, Rabani S. Early detection and endoscopic management of post cesarean section ureterovaginal fistula: a case series study. Int Urogynecol J. 2021;32(9):2537–41. https://doi.org/10.1007/s00192-020-04589-7. Epub 2020 Nov 11. PMID: 33175224
19. Raghavaiah NV. Double-dye test to diagnose various types of vaginal fistulas. J Urol. 1974;112(6):811–2. https://doi.org/10.1016/s0022-5347(17)59857-2. PMID: 4436904
20. Rajamaheswari N, Chhikara AB, Seethalakshmi K. Management of ureterovaginal fistulae: an audit. Int Urogynecol J. 2013;24(6):959–62. https://doi.org/10.1007/s00192-012-1959-9. Epub 2012 Oct 24. PMID: 23093322
21. Ramesh B, Paliwal S. Ureteroneocystostomy for ureterovaginal fistula. J Obstet Gynaecol India. 2020;70(2):176–8. https://doi.org/10.1007/s13224-019-01298-0. Epub 2020 Jan 13. PMID: 32255959; PMCID: PMC7109246
22. Sharma S, Rizvi SJ, Bethur SS, Bansal J, Qadri SJ, Modi P. Laparoscopic repair of urogenital fistulae: a single centre experience. J Minim Access Surg. 2014;10(4):180–4. https://doi.org/10.4103/0972-9941.141508. PMID: 25336817; PMCID: PMC4204260
23. Selzman AA, Spirnak JP, Kursh ED. The changing management of ureterovaginal fistulas. J Urol. 1995;153(3 Pt 1):626–8. https://doi.org/10.1097/00005392-199503000-00020. PMID: 7861500
24. Shaw J, Tunitsky-Bitton E, Barber MD, Jelovsek JE. Ureterovaginal fistula: a case series. Int Urogynecol J. 2014;25(5):615–21. https://doi.org/10.1007/s00192-013-2272-y. Epub 2013 Dec 18. PMID: 24346812
25. Shelbaia AM, Hashish NM. Limited experience in early management of genitourinary tract fistulas. Urology. 2007;69(3):572–4. https://doi.org/10.1016/j.urology.2007.01.058. PMID: 17382171
26. Symmonds RE. Ureteral injuries associated with gynecologic surgery: prevention and management. Clin Obstet Gynecol. 1976;19(3):623–44. https://doi.org/10.1097/00003081-197609000-00012. PMID: 954253
27. Tsai CK, Taylor FC, Beaghler MA. Endoscopic ureteroureterostomy: long-term followup using a new technique. J Urol. 2000;164(2):332–5. PMID: 10893578
28. Wein AJ, Kavoussi LR, Campbell MF. Campbell-Walsh urology. 11th ed. Philadelphia: Elsevier Saunders; 2016.

Female Urethral Reconstruction

Ignacio Alvarez de Toledo

Contents

Introduction	830
Diagnosis	831
Anatomy	832
Management	833
Urethral Diverticulum	833
Urethral Stricture	833
Vesico-Vaginal Fistula	834
Preoperative Planning	834
Prep and Patient Positioning	835
Procedural Approach (Our Techniques)	835
Urethral Diverticulum	835
Urethral Stricture	836
Vesico-Vaginal Fistula	836
Recovery and Rehabilitation	837
Outcomes	837
Urethral Diverticulum	837
Urethral Stricture	837
Vesico-Vaginal Fistula	838
Summary	838
Conflicts of Interest	839
Cross-References	839
References	839

Abstract

Female urethral reconstruction encompasses a variety of different entities including female urethral stricture (FUS), female urethral diverticulum (FUD), and vesicovaginal fistula

I. Alvarez de Toledo (✉)
Buenos Aires British Hospital, University of Buenos Aires, Buenos Aires, Argentina

© Springer Nature Switzerland AG 2023
F. E. Martins et al. (eds.), *Female Genitourinary and Pelvic Floor Reconstruction*,
https://doi.org/10.1007/978-3-031-19598-3_48

(VVF). Although very different in their etiologies, they all have in common a vague and nonspecific onset of symptoms and, usually, a delayed diagnosis. Once identified and evaluated, urologists must review management options with the patient which range from minimally invasive procedures to complex reconstructive surgeries. In complicated cases, we recommend referral to an experienced specialized center for definitive management.

Keywords

Female urethral stricture · Female urethral diverticulum · Vesicovaginal fistula · Urethroplasty · Urethral diverticulectomy · Buccal mucosa graft · Vaginal flap

Introduction

Much has been written regarding female pelvic reconstruction. Moreover, many of the early advances that were made in female pelvic dysfunction and reconstruction were later extrapolated to male patients and to urologic diseases in general. The opposite situation can be found when describing urethral diseases. It took some time for the urologic scientific community to remind us that *females have urethras too*.

For many years, female urethral diseases have been overlooked and, oftentimes, underdiagnosed. Although most female lower urinary tract symptoms (LUTS) can be attributed to multiple etiologies, bladder outlet obstruction (BOO) accounts for 8.3–29% of the cases [1, 2]. Within these patients, it is important to differentiate between functional versus anatomic causes of BOO. Anatomical causes of BOO include a wide variety of pathologic entities such as FUS, FUD, VVF, pelvic organ prolapse (POP), post-anti-incontinence procedure, and malignancy, among others. FUS disease accounts for a considerable proportion ranging from 4–18% of women with BOO [3], whereas the prevalence of FUD ranges between 0.6% and 4.7% according to the literature [4] and the real incidence of VVF is unknown although it has been reported to be between 0.3% and 2.0% [5].

Finding a suitable definition for FUS remains controversial. It has been proposed that a urethral lumen too narrow to admit a 17Fr flexible cystoscope or that has the feel of scar tissue by cystoscopic haptic feedback is diagnostic for stricture [3], whereas others define FUS as a fixed anatomical narrowing of the urethra such that the lumen will not accommodate instrumentation without disruption of the urethral mucosal lining [6]. On the contrary, FUD is well defined as a variably sized urine-filled periurethral cystic structure adjacent to the urethra within the confines of the pelvic fascia, connected to the urethra via an ostium [7]. Finally, VVF is defined as a pathologic connection between the bladder and the vagina.

A majority of female urethral disease can be attributed to four etiologies: idiopathic, iatrogenic, inflammatory, or traumatic. There is a small proportion of rare etiologies which include: urethral tuberculosis, urethral carcinoma, locally advanced cervical carcinoma, fibroepithelial polyps, and infection [8–10]. Most patients with FUS disease will have an unknown etiology (51.3%). Another large proportion (32.8%) will have a history of past surgical interventions in the form of urethral dilations, anti-incontinence surgery, transurethral bladder surgery, or other types of urethral surgery. A smaller percentage will occur due to inflammation (9.2%) or trauma (6.6%) [11]. Regarding FUD, the most accepted etiopathogenic theory relies on a history of chronic inflammation of peri-urethral ducts which ultimately result in sacculation and diverticulum formation [12]. Finally, it is important to discriminate between VVF diagnosed in developing versus developed countries. Most VVF's in developing countries occur as a result of obstructed labor during childbirth [13], whereas in developed countries VVFs are rare and often encountered after hysterectomies or as a consequence of complex pelvic surgery, malignancies, and/or radiation [14].

The purpose of this chapter is to describe complex female urethral diseases such as FUS, FUD, and VVF as well as to review the available reconstructive surgical techniques for these entities. Step-by-step videos of urethral stricture reconstruction and urethral diverticulectomy are included. For instructive videos of VVF repair, we strongly recommend the Lee et al. (vaginal approach) and McKay et al. (abdominal approach) articles from prior issues of this journal [5, 15].

Diagnosis

Diagnosing female urethral pathology can be challenging. Frequently, these patients will see several specialists before a definitive diagnosis is made. Some authors reported that it can take up to 5 years between the onset of symptoms and the definitive diagnosis of FUD [16]. Clinicians should have a high index of suspicion in order to avoid a delay in treatment. Thorough investigation regarding past medical history, surgical history, voiding and sexual habits, and history of malignancies or radiation is crucial to differentiate urethral anatomic pathologies from functional ones.

Physical examination (PE) is mandatory. It is very important to perform a complete PE as it may provide the clinician with key information not only to arrive at a definitive diagnosis but also for surgical planning. Observation of poor tissue quality, meatal stenosis, or lichen sclerosus may guide our diagnosis toward a FUS, whereas a paraurethral bulging mass will be diagnostic of FUD in more than 80% of cases [17]. On the other hand, continuous vaginal leakage after a pelvic surgical procedure is suspicious for VVF. In every case, PE should be performed thoroughly, including bimanual pelvic, vaginal, and speculum exams.

Regarding lower urinary tract symptoms (LUTS), there are vague and generally non-pathognomonic signs. Classically, a 3D triad (dysuria, dyspareunia, and post-void dribbling) has been described associated with FUD but studies have shown that only 23% of patients have all three and, even more, 23% of the patients did not present with any of those symptoms [18, 19]. Patients with FUS might have a variety of symptoms ranging from minor discomfort to a wide spectrum of voiding and storage symptoms. Inconsistently, the classic obstructive picture with a weak urinary stream, sensation of incomplete voiding, and straining will suggest FUS. However, as Kuo demonstrated, the differential diagnosis of lower urinary tract dysfunction in women cannot be based on LUTS alone [20].

Patients with voiding dysfunction and suspicion for obstruction should have a uroflow and a post-void residual (PVR) checked as it contributes important initial information. While there are no specific cutoffs for uroflowmetry or PVR volumes, a curve that reaches a plateau, flow less than 12–15 ml/s, or PVRs >100, may suggest obstruction [21]. Cystourethroscopy (CU) is very useful in assessing tissue quality, an area of maximal stricture and/or finding anomalous communication between the urinary tract and the genitalia. When available, we encourage the use of pediatric cystoscopes in cases with a narrow lumen. We generally do not perform an office CU in suspected UD cases as it will not change our management. Simple urethral calibration with bougie-à-boule can also provide important information regarding urethral diameter and stricture location as well as tissue quality although we should not rely on urethral diameter itself to completely rule out FUS [22]. In cases where we want to assess bladder function, a urodynamic study (UDS) might be indicated. In obstructed patients, it will show a classic high-pressure low flow pattern. To maximize the information provided by UDS, we recommend adding fluoroscopy and performing a video-UDS, as it will provide critical anatomical information regarding bladder neck function as well as the location of any obstruction. It has been proposed that a detrusor contraction at a maximum of >25 cm H_2O, with a flow <12 cc/s, could be diagnostic of BOO, although there is no consensus regarding cutoff values [23]. Other fluoroscopic studies such as retrograde urethrogram or voiding cystourethrogram (RUG/VCUG) may be helpful in diagnosing an outpouching diverticulum or an anomalous communication in patients with suspected VVF. These studies may not be as helpful as in male patients as it can often be challenging to distinguish between a primary bladder neck obstruction, a urethral sphincter obstruction, a pelvic floor obstruction, or a urethral stricture itself. Cystoscopy with bilateral retrograde

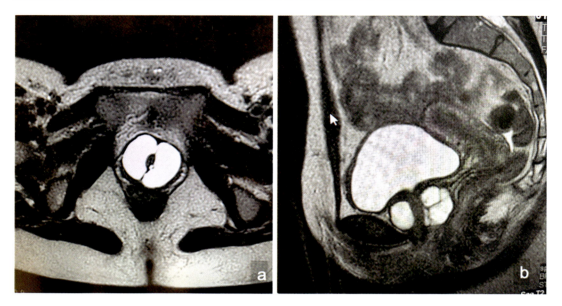

Fig. 1 Complex urethral diverticulum on MRI (**a**: axial; **b**: sagittal)

pyelography is often recommended to rule out ureteral involvement in the case of VVF.

Finally, pelvic magnetic resonance imaging (MRI) plays a central role in the diagnosis and management of patients with urethral dysfunction, particularly FUD and VVF. In recent years, there has been an increasing interest in utilizing this diagnostic tool not only for diagnosis but also to rule out other pathologies such as malignancy, concomitant calculus, abscesses, or other findings. MRI's superiority relies on its multiplanar scanning capability, superior soft tissue differentiation, noninvasive nature, and overall excellent contrast resolution [24]. Additional features such as the ability to provide functional imaging make the MRI the gold standard diagnostic test for diagnosing periurethral entities [25]. (Fig. 1: **FUD seen on MRI**).

Anatomy

Female urethral surgery requires a great understanding of anatomy and surgical planes. The goal in performing urethral reconstructive surgery is to alleviate symptoms while preserving and hopefully improving voiding and sexual function.

The normal female urethra is a musculofascial tube approximately 3–4 cm in length, extending from the bladder neck to the external urethral meatus. The urethra is suspended by the urethropelvic ligament, which is a bilayered connective tissue. It is between these two layers that FUD usually develops [7].

The urethral lumen is lined proximally by urothelial tissue, and distally by nonkeratinized stratified squamous epithelium. The female urethra is lined by a longitudinal inner smooth muscle layer and outer circular smooth muscle layer. Its striated skeletal muscle component is omega-shaped and located in the mid-urethra, thinner in the dorsal aspect. This sphincteric mechanism is not completely described and it has been hypothesized that the inner longitudinal layer not only helps with micturition but also acts as a plug while contracted to help with the overall continence mechanism [26].

Beyond the lamina propria, there are a series of periurethral glands. These are located posterolaterally and have a central role in the pathophysiologic development of FUD. It has been proposed that chronic inflammation and obliteration of these glands may ultimately result in UD formation. The majority of these glands are located in the distal one-third of the urethra. The Skene glands (SG) are the largest and most distal of these glands. These glands drain outside the urethral lumen and this is why when they obliterate, they have a similar presentation to FUD, but represent a different entity as SG are more distal, almost sub-meatal, and do not communicate with the urethra [7]. Finally, the neurovascular clitoral structures are located cephalad and lateral to the dorsal aspect of the external urethral meatus, so the risk of injury and compromising sexual function is low.

Management

Urethral Diverticulum

Female urethral diverticulum has been described as one of the most challenging diagnostic and reconstructive problems in female urology and we agree with that statement [7]. Its wide variety of clinical presentations and its surgical approach make it a unique challenge. In their series, Pincus et al. found that 21% of patients with a UD were asymptomatic, and only 51% of them needed a surgical excision [27]. In patients who do not undergo treatment, it is advisable to monitor the diverticulum. Alternatives to surgical reconstruction can be minimally invasive approaches such as endoscopic coagulation, marsupialization, fulguration, or endoscopic or open incision and drainage, although these might have high recurrence rates [28]. Bodner-Adler and colleagues reported their surgical management as follows: transvaginal resection of the UD ± reconstruction (84%), marsupialization (3.8%), transurethral endoscopic unroofing (2.0%), and various other techniques (9.7%) [4]. Furthermore, some authors propose a robotic approach for proximal dorsal FUD, reporting satisfactory results and feasibility with this technique [29]. Finally, there is a current debate on whether a concomitant stress urinary incontinence procedure should be done along with the urethral diverticulectomy. Juang et al. suggest that meticulous suture of the urethral defect left by the diverticulectomy with reconstruction of the periurethral fascia might enhance urethral resistance and thus overcome the problem of stress urinary incontinence, therefore a combined anti-incontinence procedure should not be mandatory [30]. If done, a bladder neck suspension or autologous fascial pubovaginal sling has proven to be safe and successful [31].

Urethral Stricture

We like to separate treatment options into conservative versus definitive management. Conservative management includes urethral dilation, which is the most utilized treatment modality by urologists [32]. The other minimally invasive option is a direct vision internal urethrotomy (DVIU), although it is not as popular as urethral dilation, and is only anecdotally reported. Urethral dilation is easy to do and has relatively low morbidity and complication rates.

Within definitive management, options include augmented urethroplasty using either flaps or grafts, and, very rarely, excision and primary anastomosis (EPA). Once considered as a second-line treatment, recently it has become more popular due to improved knowledge and training, and has made primary reconstruction a first-line treatment option, as suggested by Önol et al. [33].

Urethral reconstruction using flaps remains a valid option when considering approaches for urethroplasty in women. Flaps can be obtained from vaginal (U-shaped or C-shaped), labial, or vestibular tissue. They are relatively easy to obtain, with low donor site morbidity. One should take into consideration the health of local tissue before deciding to use a flap. In patients with lichen sclerosus or a history of radiation, the use of local flaps is discouraged and, in this case, we strongly recommend the use of grafts.

Within urethral reconstruction utilizing grafts, local grafts or oral mucosa grafts may be used. Local grafts can be obtained from the vagina as well as from the labia minora. As with local flaps, these grafts are contraindicated in patients with unhealthy tissues. Another aspect to take into consideration is treatment with local estrogens when considering local flaps or grafts. This type of adjuvant local treatment has proven to be safe and efficacious by Romero-Maroto et al. [34]. As mentioned above, our preferred surgical technique is a urethral reconstruction using a buccal mucosa graft (BMG). As with male patients, BMG is popular because of its versatility and relatively low morbidity. Some authors presented their work using lingual mucosa grafts with acceptable results compared to the available literature [35]. In our experience, we only use lingual mucosa grafts when we have no available healthy buccal mucosa to harvest.

Vesico-Vaginal Fistula

VVF diagnosis includes a heterogeneous number of patients that range from minorly symptomatic to life-devastating cases and, because of this, it can be difficult to determine management options and treatment algorithms. Principles of VVF repair should include: treatment of infection, anemia, and malnutrition; ensure no foreign non-dissolving material or malignancy; tension-free watertight repair; and uninterrupted bladder drainage [5]. These repairs can be classified into simple or complex. Simple fistulas are small (<0.5 cm) and single in nonradiated patients with no associated malignancy. Complex fistulas are large (≥2.5 cm), those that failed previous fistula repair, or are associated with chronic disease or post-radiation. A fistula sized between 0.5 and 2.5 cm is considered intermediate [36].

Conservative management can be attempted when we encounter a simple fistula. The first and simplest option is to insert a Foley catheter, drain the bladder, and prescribe an anticholinergic. This strategy alone has proven to be effective up to 39% of the time [37]. Many other minimally invasive treatments have also been reported such as injection of fibrin sealant/cyanoacrylic glue and/or electrocautery with laser or coagulation diathermy, all showing acceptable results although practiced in a small number of patients and with short follow-up.

Finally, if conservative measures do not resolve the VVF or if the fistula is not suitable for conservative management, a formal surgical repair is indicated. In these cases, the surgeon will have to sort through a series of dichotomies: immediate repair versus delayed repair; vaginal approach versus abdominal approach; open procedure or laparoscopic/robotic; interposition of tissue versus no interposition; and removal of fistulous tract versus no removal. All of these are still open controversies and there is a lack of sufficient data to recommend one over the other. In summary, we agree with Malik et al. who opined that VVF can be best managed following basic surgical principles, such as adequate exposure, identification of structures, wide mobilization, tension-free closure, good hemostasis, and uninterrupted bladder drainage [38]. Additional discussion can be found in the next heading.

Preoperative Planning

After a diagnosis is made, the reconstructive surgeon must consider additional imaging or studies, if necessary, to adequately plan intervention. Some authors suggest that performing UDS in patients with FUD is helpful as it may diagnose BOO in up to 50% of the cases [39]. Reeves et al. propose that in cases where MRI is needed, it should be done sagittal and post-void, in order to allow the UD to fill with urine and provide better imaging [31]. In patients where a cystourethroscopy might be needed, it may be beneficial to perform under sedation to avoid patient discomfort. Cystoscopy with bilateral retrograde pyelography may be indicated for patients with VVF to rule out ureteral involvement.

There is no consensus on whether or not to perform a preoperative urine culture. If the patient has a history of recurrent UTIs, it is beneficial to obtain one in order to adjust therapy according to the antibiogram. Some authors advocate the idea that a urine culture should be done for every patient before surgery [40]. In cases with VVF where urinoma or urosepsis is present, it is advised to delay the definitive repair for at least 6 weeks after drainage, if possible. This is also the case in a postpartum event since the uterus takes some time to return to its involute state [5]. In postmenopausal women, intravaginal estrogens may be administrated preoperatively to treat vaginal mucosal atrophy [34].

In patients with suspected malignancy, a biopsy should be done before undergoing a reconstructive procedure, as this would likely change management. It is in these cases where an MRI is potentially useful as well. Malignancies can present as part of a stricture, diverticulum, or fistula, so in every case the surgeon should be aware of this possibility and patients properly counseled.

As with male patients, the reconstructive surgeon must be ready to change the plan if intraoperative findings differ from the preoperative plan. It is highly recommended to be precise and clear with the patient before consenting to avoid misunderstandings. It is also of the utmost importance to manage patients' expectations appropriately before performing these procedures as, sometimes, resolving one urethral problem (FUS, FUD, and VVF) may bring on an additional urethral problem and more than one procedure may be needed.

Prep and Patient Positioning

Patients with urethral pathology are widely variable and ultimately each treatment option should be adjusted to each particular need. In general, we use the low lithotomy position as it provides us with access to the urethral meatus, vaginal introitus, and the vestibule as well as the abdomen. Interestingly, Reeves et al. propose a novel prone position stating it can provide better access in these patients, especially in complex high VVF [31]. We prep and drape our patients in the usual sterile fashion, using 2% chlorhexidine gluconate (CHG) or povidone-iodine solution according to the surgeon's preference. It is very important to carefully pad all pressure points to avoid nerve injury.

To help with retraction we use the Lonestar-Scott retractor with 4–6 blue (sharp) hooks, although labia minora could also be retracted with sutures. Oftentimes, the FUD ostium is difficult to encounter so in these cases we find it very useful to instill diluted methylene blue to help find the ostium and dye the diverticulum which is helpful during dissection. The same retractor is utilized in cases where a Martius flap is harvested.

Finally, in cases where we will need to harvest a buccal mucosa graft, the patient's mouth is also prepped and draped. Typically, we harvest our own grafts, however, it is acceptable to have a separate team harvest if desired. There is no need for nasotracheal intubation as this procedure can be done with an orotracheal tube in place carefully secured to one side, while we harvest from the opposite inner cheek.

Procedural Approach (Our Techniques)

Urethral Diverticulum

We start with 17 Fr rigid cystoscopy to assess the entire urethra and bladder. We look for the FUD ostium, which is not always found. If found it is usually in the posterolateral position. As mentioned prior, we use a Scott retractor and blue hooks for better visualization and instill dilute methylene blue. A 14 or 16 Fr catheter is then placed with 10 cc in the balloon. The bladder neck is marked for reference. A vaginal incision is made in an inverted-U fashion with a wide based flap and into the lateral sulci to permit the later use of a Martius flap, if needed. Further dissection is done sharply with Metzenbaum scissors. It is critical for the dissection to leave enough tissue to avoid thinning the flap and cause devascularization as well as to avoid entering the diverticulum. Bipolar cautery can be judiciously used to control small bleeders. Dissection continues until the level of the bladder neck. Once the diverticulum is identified, a transverse incision is made just through the endopelvic and endocervical fascia, and flaps are created in both cranial and caudal directions. The diverticulum is visible with a light blue hue and dissected circumferentially until it is defined in all planes. At this point, the diverticulum is opened in order to better appreciate its borders and avoid entry into the urethra. A lacrimal duct probe can be used to identify the os. Manipulating the Foley catheter can bring fluid into the diverticulum to assist in locating the position of the os. If the os is noted to be in a challenging position, consideration can be made to placing a stay suture to better identify the location for later closure. Once the diverticulum is traced back to the os, it is truncated at that point. We always send the diverticulum as a specimen for pathologic analysis. Interrupted 4/0 absorbable sutures are placed to close the os. The flaps created previously can be closed with 4/0 absorbable sutures with a vest over pants, or pants over vest technique. Care needs to be taken when placing these sutures to avoid devascularization of the flaps. Over this flap, a Martius flap can be rotated in from either labia majora if the patient has a history of radiation or notably poor tissue quality. The vaginal closure is performed with 2/0 interrupted absorbable sutures and a vaginal packing is left in place overnight. The catheter is left in for 2–3 weeks.

Urethral Stricture

We prefer the dorsal onlay buccal mucosal graft although some might argue it is a more difficult approach. The risk of sexual dysfunction with this dissection is low, as the plane of dissection is well away from neurovascular clitoral structures. Leaving the ventral plane untouched is useful for a possible continence procedure in the future if indicated. In addition, a dorsal fixation helps prevent sacculation of the graft. We harvest, clean, and fenestrate a 4 × 2 cm buccal mucosal graft in the standard fashion. Urethral length is relatively constant, so these graft dimensions are generally sufficient even if the stricture is panurethral. A semilunar, suprameatal incision is made. Careful dissection is carried outside the corpus spongiosum until healthy urethra is encountered. We typically open the meatus, however, an alternate meatus-sparing technique is also acceptable. The dissection may be carried out to the bladder neck when necessary without fear of de novo stress urinary incontinence. The graft is sewn in with delayed absorbable suture; we favor 4-0 PDS. Several quilting sutures of 5-0 Vicryl are placed. We ensure patency to 30 Fr with intraoperative bougie-à-boule. A 14 French silicone catheter is left in place for 3 weeks.

Vesico-Vaginal Fistula

For most fistula, we prefer the vaginal approach. When possible the fistula is cannulated with either a 5 Fr ureteral catheter, a wire, or ideally a Fogarty balloon or small foley to aid in identification and manipulation. We start with an U-shaped incision the apex of which is at the fistula and develops a vaginal flap, taking care to preserve the periurethral fascia. Once we encounter the fistula we dissect and widely mobilize it. Typically, we will excise the tract and send it for pathology. The bladder is then closed in two layers, and inner running and outer interrupted layer with 4-0 absorbable suture. Based on the quality of the surrounding tissues and fistula etiology, a Martius flap may or may not be utilized. Typically, in radiated patients or redo cases we recommend the interposition of a Martius flap, which is almost always available. The Martius flap is raised based on the upper or lower vascular pedicle depending on the position of the fistula and the patient's anatomy. If the Martius flap is insufficient or not available, other flaps such as peritoneal, omental, or a gracilis interposition flap may be utilized. The repair is leak tested. The vaginal incision is then closed interrupted 2-0 Vicryl. A 14 Fr silicone catheter is left in place for 2–4 weeks. If a suprapubic catheter was present, this is also left in situ for maximal bladder drainage.

For complex, high, or recurrent fistula, an abdominal approach may be utilized. We prefer a minimally invasive robotic-assisted transvesical approach in these cases. Similar to the vaginal approach, the fistula is cannulated whenever possible. Temporary external ureteral catheters may be placed if the fistula is near the ureteral orifices. The bladder is opened at the posterior dome and the fistula is identified. It is widely mobilized and the tract is sent for pathology. The vagina is closed with 3-0 or 4-0 absorbable suture, and the bladder is similarly closed, in one or two layers avoiding overlapping suture lines. The cystotomy is finally closed with running 3-0 or 4-0 suture. The repair is leak tested. A 14 Fr silicone catheter is left in place for 2–4 weeks.

Excellent videos of both the vaginal [5] and abdominal approach to VVF [15] is available in a prior volume of *Urologic Clinics of North America (Volume 46, Issue 1)*.

Recovery and Rehabilitation

Recovery from urethroplasty for FUS is generally brief. Minor stress incontinence may be encountered initially, however, this generally resolves. In our institution, this is an outpatient surgery. We do leave a small labial drain for 1–2 days if a Martius flap was harvested. We usually leave a vaginal packing in place, which will be removed within the first 24 hours post-op. We discharge patients with pain medication as needed and also anticholinergic medication to help with bladder spasms. Unless the patient had recurrent UTI, we do not provide antibiotics during the catheterization period.

Most patients are seen in the office for a wound check within 1 week, and the catheter is removed between 2 and 4 weeks depending on the procedure performed. Any relevant pathology results are reviewed.

Outcomes

Urethral Diverticulum

Interestingly, some authors propose classification of urethral diverticulum into simple or complex in order to predict their postoperative outcomes. Complex FUD are those extending partially or circumferentially around the urethra. In their series, Nickles et al. showed that patients with complex FUD were most likely to present postoperatively with urinary tract symptoms (27% vs 3%) compared to patients following reconstruction for simple FUD [41]. In a different study, Ko et al. published an overall cure rate with surgery of 77.9% but when the different UD were broken down into simple, U-shaped, and circumferential, their cure rates were 100%, 75.0%, and 64.0%, respectively [42]. This demonstrates that successful surgical outcomes in these patients have a direct correlation with anatomical complexity. This is important for patient counseling.

Regarding complications, the most commonly reported are urethrovaginal fistula, de novo stress urinary incontinence, urethral strictures, recurrent UTIs, and recurrence of the diverticulum [4]. One study showed that the most common pathology was squamous metaplasia (31%) and also reported a 2.5% malignancy rate (adenocarcinoma) within their UD specimens [27], which is consistent with other malignancy reports (2%) found in the literature [31].

Finally, there is currently no existing data showing a well-documented comparison regarding different surgical approaches for UD. In the future, a proper randomized controlled trial comparing success and complication rates with each treatment would be useful to help guide practice.

Urethral Stricture

The goals for female urethral reconstruction are to restore function, urinate without obstruction, maintain continence, prevent vaginal voiding, and maintain sexual function. Although these goals are considered an ideal scenario, there is a dearth of literature considering all five variables when analyzing outcomes. Much of the available literature regarding FUS has been published within the last 5 years. The most common management is urethral dilation although its success rate ranges between 47% and 49% [11, 43], with success defined as the lack of need for further intervention. The mean time to failure was 12 months [44]. In our practice, we follow the same principle as in male patients with no more than one attempt at UD given the poor outcomes of repeated dilations (30%), unless the patient is not a surgical candidate [45].

There is no statistical difference in terms of success rate among reconstructive options. Both reconstructive surgeries using flaps or grafts have proven to be equally safe and efficacious [46]. Success rates using flap urethroplasty were 92% with a mean follow-up of 42 months, whereas success rates with BMG graft urethroplasty were 89% with a mean follow-up of 19 months and 87% with vaginal graft urethroplasty with a mean follow-up of 15 months according to the most recent systematic review [11].

Acceptable complication rates were reported with flap procedures, with only 3.7% de novo SUI noted [11]. Furthermore, in patients with concomitant SUI, a pubovaginal sling could be placed without major morbidity. Where to place the graft still remains a controversy, with some authors advocating to place it dorsally while others opine it should be placed ventrally. There is no data available supporting one over the other, so, ultimately, it remains at the surgeon's discretion. Finally, de novo SUI was found to be similar in both approaches (3.6% with a dorsal approach versus 5.8% with a ventral approach) [11].

Vesico-Vaginal Fistula

Traditionally, the classic strategy has always been to repair within 1 week of injury or after a delay of 3–6 months to allow for healing of the traumatized tissue. Studies have shown that early repairs have similar rates of success as delayed ones [47]. When a delayed approach is selected, the surgeon must optimize preoperative patient factors such as nutrition, urinary drainage, and skincare. If there is a recurrence, data suggests that a revision VVF repair is less successful, highlighting that, generally, the best chance of fistula closure is at the time of the first operation [13].

VVF can be repaired via a vaginal approach or an abdominal approach. To date, there are no randomized controlled trials comparing the route of repair, so the decision is up to the surgeon's preference. Typically, simple VVF will be approached vaginally first, as the vaginal approach has demonstrated significantly shorter operative times, decreased blood loss, and a shorter duration of hospitalization [15]. Another advantage to the vaginal approach is that it can be done as an outpatient. On the other hand, in complex VVF or redo cases, an abdominal approach may be preferred. The estimated success rate of transvaginal repair ranges from 83–100%, whereas the overall success rate of laparoscopic/robotic VVF repairs was 80–100% [5]. Tissue interposition is advantageous in some cases. In our practice, we use a Martius flap if approached vaginally when necessary, but other tissue such as omentum or a peritoneal flap have been described as well. The utilization of minimally invasive techniques has significantly improved recovery times in these cases.

We agree with Lee et al. that heterogeneity of the fistula (size and location) and the occasional use of an interposition graft make treatment standardization very difficult [5].

Summary

Female urethral reconstruction is an evolving art that bases its principles on excellent knowledge of vaginal, urethral, and pelvic anatomy. Reconstructive surgeons eager to manage this type of pathology require the right skillset and armamentarium in order to find an appropriate solution for their patients. Oftentimes, the diagnosis will be delayed and in the context of a suffering patient with truly bothersome symptoms such as urinary leakage, recurrent UTIs, dyspareunia, dysuria, and voiding and storage symptoms. Managing patient expectations is crucial. The most important consideration when approaching these patients is to follow basic reconstructive surgical principles such as adequate exposure, broad mobilization, gentle handling of tissue, tension-free closure, and satisfactory hemostasis. Finally, in complex cases, it is always a wise option to refer these patients to an experienced specialized center for definitive management.

Conflicts of Interest

Dr. Alvarez de Toledo has no conflicts to report.

Cross-References

▶ Vesicovaginal Fistula Repair: Abdominal Approach
▶ Vesicovaginal Fistula Repair: Minimally Invasive Approach
▶ Vesicovaginal Fistula Repair: Vaginal Approach

References

1. Nitti VW, Tu LM, Gitlin J. Diagnosing bladder outlet obstruction in women. J Urol. 1999;161:1535.
2. Blaivas JG, Groutz A. Bladder outlet obstruction nomogram for women with lower urinary tract symptomatology. Neurourol Urodyn. 2000;19:553.
3. Blaivas JG, Santos JA, Tsui JF, Deibert CM, Rutman MP, Purohit RS, et al. Management of urethral stricture in women. J Urol. 2012;188(5):1778–82.
4. Bodner-Adler B, Halpern K, Hanzal E. Surgical management of urethral diverticula in women: a systematic review. Int Urogynecol J. 2016;27:993–1001.
5. Lee D, Zimmern P. Vaginal approach to vesicovaginal fistula. Urol Clin N Am. 2019;46:123–33.
6. Smith AL, Ferlise VJ, Rovner ES. Female urethral strictures: successful management with long-term clean intermittent catheterization after urethral dilatation. BJU Int. 2006;98(1):96–9.
7. Rovner ES. Bladder and female urethral diverticula. 11th ed. Campbell-Walsh Urology; 2016. p. 2140–68.
8. Keegan KA, Nanigian DK, Stone AR. Female urethral stricture disease. Curr Urol Rep. 2008;9(5):419–23.
9. Desai S, Libertino JA, Zinman L. Primary carcinoma of the female urethra. J Urol. 1973;110(6):693–5.
10. Indudhara R, Vaidyanathan S, Radotra BD. Urethral tuberculosis. Urol Int. 1992;48(4):436–8.
11. Sarin I, Narain TA, Panwar VK, Bhadoria AS, et al. Deciphering the enigma of female urethral strictures: a systematic review and meta-analysis of management modalities. Neurourol Urodyn. 2021;40:65–79.
12. Huffman JW. The detailed anatomy of the paraurethral ducts in the adult human female. Am J Obstet Gynecol. 1948;55:86–101.
13. Wall LL. Obstetric vesicovaginal fistula as an international public-health problem. Lancet. 2006;368:1201–9.
14. Goodwin WE, Scardino PT. Vesicovaginal and ureterovaginal fistulas: a summary of 25 years of experience. J Urol. 1980;123:370–4.
15. McKay E, Watts K, Abraham N. Abdominal approach to vesicovaginal fistula. Urol Clin N Am. 2019;46: 135–46.
16. Romanzi LJ, Groutz A, Blaivas JG. Urethral diverticulum in women: diverse presentations resulting in diagnostic delay and mismanagement. J Urol. 2000;164(2):428–33.
17. Blaivas JG, Flisser AJ, Bleustein CB, Panagopoulos G. Periurethral masses: etiology and diagnosis in a large series of women. Obstet Gynecol. 2004;103 (5 Pt 1):842–7.
18. Ockrim JL, Allen DJ, Shah PJ, Greenwell TJ. A tertiary experience of urethral diverticulectomy: diagnosis, imaging and surgical outcomes. BJU Int. 2009;103 (11):1550–4.
19. Baradaran N, Chiles LR, Freilich DA, Rames RA, Cox L, Rovner ES. Female urethral diverticula in the contemporary era: is the classic triad of the "3Ds" still relevant? Urology. 2016;94:53–6.
20. Kuo HC. Clinical symptoms are not reliable in the diagnosis of lower urinary tract dysfunction in women. J Formos Med Assoc. 2012;111:386–91.
21. Agochukwu-Mmonu N, Srirangapatnam S, Cohen A, Breyer B. Female urethral strictures: review of diagnosis, etiology, and management. Curr Urol Rep. 2019;20 (11):74.
22. Kalra S, Gupta P, Dorairajan L, Hota S, et al. Does successful urethral calibration rule out significant female urethral stenosis? Confronting the confounder-an outcome analysis of successfully treated female urethral strictures. Int Braz J Urol. 2021;47:829–40.
23. West C, Lawrence A. Female urethroplasty: contemporary thinking. World J Urol. 2019;37:619–29.
24. Itani M, Kielar A, Menias CO, Dighe MK, Surabhi V, Prasad SR, O'Malley R, Gangadhar K, Lalwani N. MRI of female urethra and periurethral pathologies. Int Urogynecol J. 2016;27(2):195–204.
25. Crescenze IM, Goldman HB. Female urethral diverticulum: current diagnosis and management. Curr Urol Rep. 2015;16(10):71.
26. Mistry MA, Klarskov N, DeLancey JO, Lose G. A structured review on the female urethral anatomy and innervation with an emphasis on the role of the urethral longitudinal smooth muscle. Int Urogynecol J. 2020;31 (1):63–71.
27. Pincus JB, Laudano M, Leegant A, Downing K. Female urethral diverticula: diagnosis, pathology, and surgical outcomes at an academic, urban medical Center. Urology. 2019;128:42–6.
28. Aldamanhori R, Inman R. The treatment of complex female urethral pathology. Asian J Urol. 2018;5(3): 160–3.
29. Mozafarpour S, Nwaoha N, Pucheril D, De EJB. Robotic assisted proximal dorsal urethral diverticulectomy. Int Urogynecol J. 2021;32(10):2863–6.
30. Juang CM, Horng HC, Yu HC, Chen CY, Chang CM, Yu KJ, Yen MS. Combined diverticulectomy and anti-incontinence surgery for patients with urethral diverticulum and stress urinary incontinence: is anti-

incontinence surgery really necessary? Taiwan J Obstet Gynecol. 2006;45(1):67–9.
31. Reeves FA, Inman RD, Chapple CR. Management of symptomatic urethral diverticula in women: a single-center experience. Eur Urol. 2014;66(1):164–72.
32. Heidari F, Abbaszadeh S, Ghadian A, Tehrani KF. On demand urethral dilatation versus intermittent urethral dilatation: results and complications in women with urethral stricture. Nephrourol Mon. 2014;6(2): e15212.
33. Önol FF, Antar B, Köse O, Erdem MR, Önol ŞY. Techniques and results of urethroplasty for female urethral strictures: our experience with 17 patients. Urology. 2011;77(6):1318–24.
34. Romero-Maroto J, Verdú-Verdú L, Gómez-Pérez L, Pérez-Tomás C, Pacheco-Bru JJ, López-López A. Lateral-based anterior vaginal wall flap in the treatment of female urethral stricture: efficacy and safety. Eur Urol. 2018;73(1):123–8.
35. Sharma GK, Pandey A, Bansal H, et al. Dorsal onlay lingual mucosal graft urethroplasty for urethral strictures in women. BJU Int. 2010;105(9):1309–12.
36. Stamatakos M, Sargedi C, Stasinou T, Kontzoglou K. Vesicovaginal fistula: diagnosis and management. Indian J Surg. 2014;76:131–6.
37. Fouad LS, Chen AH, Santoni CJ, Wehbe C, Pettit PD. Revisiting conservative management of vesicovaginal fistula. J Minim Invasive Gynecol. 2017;24(4):514–5.
38. Malik MA, Sohail M, Malik MT, Khalid N, Akram A. Changing trends in the etiology and management of vesicovaginal fistula. Int J Urol. 2018;25(1):25–9.
39. Lin KJ, Fan YH, Lin AT. Role of urodynamics in management of urethral diverticulum in females. J Chin Med Assoc. 2017;80(11):712–6.
40. Waterloos M, Verla W. Female urethroplasty: a practical guide emphasizing diagnosis and surgical treatment of female urethral stricture disease. Biomed Res Int. 2019;2019:6715257.
41. Nickles SW, Ikwuezunma G, MacLachlan L, El-Zawahry A, Rames R, Rovner E. Simple vs complex urethral diverticulum: presentation and outcomes. Urology. 2014;84(6):1516–9.
42. Ko KJ, Suh YS, Kim TH, Lee HS, Cho WJ, Han DH, Lee KS. Surgical outcomes of primary and recurrent female urethral diverticula. Urology. 2017;105:181–5.
43. Osman NI, Mangera A, Chapple CR. A systematic review of surgical techniques used in the treatment of female urethral stricture. Eur Urol. 2013;64(6):965–73.
44. Romman AN, Alhalabi F, Zimmern PE. Distal intramural urethral pathology in women. J Urol. 2012;188: 1218–23.
45. Popat S, Zimmern PE. Long-term management of luminal urethral stricture in women. Int Urogynecol J. 2016;27(11):1735–41.
46. Kowalik C, Stoffel JT, Zinman L, Vanni AJ, Buckley JC. Intermediate outcomes after female urethral reconstruction: graft vs flap. Urology. 2014;83(5):1181–5.
47. Blandy JP, Badenoch DF, Fowler CG, Jenkins BJ, Thomas NW. Early repair of iatrogenic injury to the ureter or bladder after gynecological surgery. J Urol. 1991;146(3):761–5.

Surgical Reconstruction of Pelvic Fracture Urethral Injuries in Females

48

Pankaj M. Joshi, Sanjay B. Kulkarni, Bobby Viswaroop, and Ganesh Gopalakrishnan

Contents

Introduction	842
Evaluation	842
Treatment	844
Anastomotic Urethroplasty for Female Pelvic Fracture Urethral Injury	844
Total Urethral Loss in Female Pelvic Fracture Urethral Injury	848
Conclusion	853
References	854

Abstract

Pelvic fracture urethral injury in females is regarded as rare and, therefore, has received sporadic attention. The female urethra seems relatively resistant to injury. Generally, milder injuries eventually associated with damage of the urethral innervation, and even more severe injuries resulting in a longitudinal tear of the urethra, may present mainly with symptoms related to urinary incontinence. Complete urethral distraction usually results from an avulsion injury. Generally, a more severe injury is necessary to damage the female urethra as compared to the male urethra. This chapter will review the literature available on female urethral injuries associated with pelvic fracture as well as include the authors' experience in their two high-volume institutions. Mechanisms of injury, diagnostic evaluation, specifically careful vaginal examination, endoscopic and imaging evaluations, and optimal management of this rare entity are discussed in detail according to two distinct clinical scenarios in female patients following pelvic fracture: 1) urethral injury (distraction), and 2) total urethral loss. In the urethral distraction scenario, three injury levels were typically identified, including proximal urethral avulsion, mid-urethral avulsion, and bladder neck-urethra avulsion. Meatal stenosis, concomitant urethrovaginal fistula, and vaginal stenosis were additionally present in some patients. In the total urethral loss scenario, the reconstructive urologist will deal with total absence of the urethra, either due to a primary initial traumatic

P. M. Joshi (✉) · S. B. Kulkarni
UROKUL, Pune, India

B. Viswaroop · G. Gopalakrishnan
Vedanayagam Hospital, Coimbatore, India

© Springer Nature Switzerland AG 2023
F. E. Martins et al. (eds.), *Female Genitourinary and Pelvic Floor Reconstruction*,
https://doi.org/10.1007/978-3-031-19598-3_49

injury, or resulting from iatrogenic intervention. In the former case, anastomotic urethroplasty is usually the treatment of choice, whereas in the latter more complex scenario reconstructive options involving different types of flaps, grafts, and intestinal interposition are commonly necessary. The female pelvic fracture urethral injury is usually more difficult to treat both anatomically and functionally in terms of restoring urinary continence.

Keywords

Female urethroplasty · PFUI · Fistula · Urethra · Stricture · Pelvic fracture · Injury · Traumatic

Introduction

Urethral injuries in females with pelvic fractures are rare [1–8]. Consequently, the literature on the management of female pelvic urethral injuries is scarce and unclear. This is due to limited experience across the world. The main reason could be that this patient population represents a wide spectrum ranging from young girls to adult females generating referral problems in terms of Pediatric Urology, Gynecology, and Adult Urology.

Although the association between pelvic fractures and male urethral injuries resulting from road traffic accidents is well recognized, blunt trauma resulting in pelvic fractures and injury to the female urethra has received less attention. The incidence of female traumatic urethral injury, even with pelvic fracture, is very low. In a report of the National Trauma Data Bank for the period 2001–2005, it was shown that, although male and female populations experienced similar rates of bladder injury associated with pelvic fracture (3.41% in males vs. 3.37% in females), males had a higher propensity for urethral injury than female counterparts (1.54% vs. 0.15%, respectively) [9]. A potential explanation for this disparity might be the flexibility provided by the vagina and the exceptional inherent elasticity of the female urethra [4]. The earliest report of such injury was by Perry and Hussmann in 1992 [5]. These authors reviewed the literature before 1985 and concluded that the entity was so rare that it essentially could be ignored. The earlier injuries reported were longitudinal injuries and those perhaps go unnoticed. The injuries that are seen in the current practice are usually avulsion injuries. Historically, female urethral injuries have been grouped into two types: complete- or transverse-type injuries that present as transection of the urethra, and partial- or longitudinal-type injuries that present as lacerations within the urethra. Both types of injuries can have concomitant vaginal and/or bladder injuries [8]. Most of these injuries have been reported in girls [1, 3, 4, 10–14] rather than adult women suggesting a lesser vulnerability pattern or a higher tendency to die from other associated severe injuries in adults [1, 3, 4, 6, 15–19]. In a systematic review by Patel et al. among 158 urethral injuries that were identified, 99 (63%) occurred in children and 59 (37%) in adults [20].

Generally, there are two types of surgical reconstruction for this spectrum of female urethral injuries: 1) anastomotic urethroplasty, and 2) urethral substitution. In the interest of better schematic exposure and clarification of the subject, the management of the female pelvic fracture urethral injury will be described in two sections according to two distinct clinical scenarios: 1) urethral injury (distraction) associated with pelvic fracture, and 2) total urethral loss associated with pelvic fracture. The first half of the chapter is written by Joshi and Kulkarni. Viswaroop and Gopalakrishnan discuss the management of total urethral loss in the second half of this chapter.

Evaluation

Initial assessment includes a detailed medical history followed by pelvic examination, including vaginal exam, which may be challenging in girls. Prior to surgical reconstruction, all patients should undergo retrograde urethrogram and voiding cystourethrogram, cystourethroscopy under general anesthesia to achieve an accurate evaluation of the anatomic characteristics of the urethral and bladder neck injuries, such as the exact location and length of the urethral injury, as well as involvement of the rectum. Other very useful auxiliary investigations including MRI of the pelvis have also been used in the evaluation of the female pelvic trauma involving the lower urinary tract (Fig. 1) [21]. The female urethra is about 4 cm in length, and even smaller in young women and girls. Retrograde and antegrade cystourethrograms are considered critical for assessment of the urethral injury, and all patients should undergo pelvic MRI, in which the bladder and urethra are filled with saline solution and jelly to enhance the lumen and the level of the urethral distraction. Preoperative endoscopy is also a critical part of the evaluation. Urethra is best visualized with a 0-degree endoscope. Endoscopic evaluation should begin at the meatus to assess the distal urethra. Next, vaginoscopy is performed, which usually demonstrates three possible findings:

1. Normal vagina, exhibiting the cervix and meatal injury (Fig. 2).
2. A transverse vaginal septum (traumatic) and in such case the cervix is not visualized.
3. Stenosis of the vagina at the site of trauma (Fig. 3).

The next diagnostic step is to perform an endoscopic evaluation through the suprapubic tract to inspect the bladder, bladder neck, and proximal urethral stump. Urethral avulsion injury may typically be observed at three different levels:

1. Proximal urethra.
2. Mid-urethra.
3. Bladder neck-proximal urethra.

Furthermore, some patients also exhibit a) meatal stenosis, or b) concomitant urethrovaginal fistula and/or vaginal stenosis. Some patients who have suffered urethral injury or avulsion as a result of pelvic fracture present to the Emergency Room with concomitant pelvic lesions of varying severity leading to surgical repair of differing complexity [8]. These concomitant lesions include injuries of the vulva (bruising, hematoma, laceration), vaginal canal (simple or severe tears, complete circumferential avulsions eventually leading to complete fibrotic obliteration, fistulation), uterovaginal prolapse (due to severe disruption of the uterovaginal ligaments), and rectal injuries (eventually, requiring more than simple repair and a temporary colostomy) (Table 1). Venn et al. highlighted that some series are not strictly comparable among them [8]. In some of the studies, patients were treated primarily elsewhere, while in others they were referred to tertiary institutions

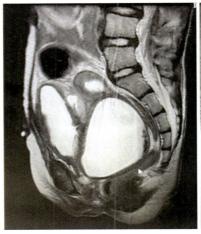
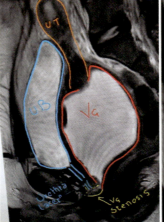
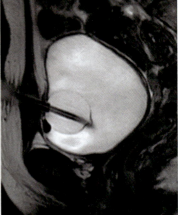

Fig. 1 Magnetic Ressonance Imaging

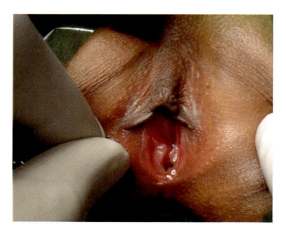

Fig. 2 Meatal injury

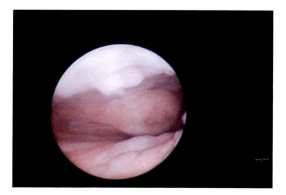

Fig. 3 Vaginoscopy showing cervix

after receiving conservative procedures. These included suprapubic catheter placement, urethral dilatations, urinary diversion (ileal conduit or bilateral cutaneous ureterostomies) of variable duration, and even anastomotic urethroplasty before referral for definitive treatment [4, 10, 12, 17–19].

Clinical presentation varies widely in a spectrum from simple longitudinal or transverse vaginal tear to "open book" injury with pubic diastasis and concomitant urethral, vaginal, and rectal injuries. Some of these patients receive initial treatment elsewhere and are referred later to tertiary, academic centers for definitive repair. Most of these patients present with urinary incontinence of different severity. In Patel's systematic review, 53% of the female patients with pelvic

Table 1 Types of urethral injury

Urethra in continuity/laceration/tear
Isolated urethral injury
Anterior and posterior longitudinal urethral lacerations and anterior vaginal tear
Wide, open urethra and genitourinary prolapse; small vaginal laceration
Midurethral stricture; no other injury
Urethral avulsion-distraction-rupture
Total urethral rupture; vaginal laceration
Total urethral rupture; partial vaginal laceration
Total urethral rupture; partial vaginal and rectal lacerations
Total urethral rupture; total vaginal laceration; 75% trans-sphincteric rectal rupture
Total urethral rupture; total vaginal laceration; complete supra-sphincteric rectal rupture

Adapted and modified from Ref. [8]

fracture urethral injury were managed in the acute setting. Of these, 20% underwent primary urethral alignment with a catheter and 80% underwent anastomotic urethroplasty. Forty-seven percent of the patients received a delayed repair [21].

Treatment

Anastomotic Urethroplasty for Female Pelvic Fracture Urethral Injury

In our Kulkarni Reconstructive Urology Center, in Pune, India, patients usually undergo surgery within the first 24 h following hospital admission [22]. Upon admission patients receive a single dose of preoperative antibiotic prophylaxis. Intraoperatively, we use the dorsal lithotomy position. Preoperative endoscopy is a critical tool of evaluation, and the urethra is best visualized with a 0-degree endoscope. The best instrument for this has proved to be the 7 Fr mini nephroscope or a 4.5 Fr ureteroscope, which is passed in a retrograde fashion from the meatus for evaluation of the distal urethra.

Urethrovaginal fistula should be suspected in every female patient with pelvic fracture urethral injury, which was present in most of our patients.

If possible, a guidewire is inserted transurethrally into the bladder with the external end brought out through the introitus. Vaginoscopy is then performed displaying a normal vagina and cervix in most instances (Fig. 3). Occasionally, a post-traumatic transverse vaginal septum preventing visualization of the cervix or stenosis of the vagina at the site of trauma is seen. The next step is to perform endoscopy through the suprapubic catheter tract to assess the bladder, the bladder neck, and the urethra proximal to the site of injury. Urethral avulsion at the bladder neck, proximal or middle thirds of the urethra can be seen. Some patients also exhibit meatal stenosis and/or concomitant urethrovaginal fistula and/or vaginal stenosis.

Surgical Approach

An abdominal approach is invariably used in young girls. In adult females, the vaginal approach may be possible and, therefore, is licit to attempt it. Patients are placed in the dorsal lithotomy position for this surgery.

Transection at Bladder Neck

The bladder can be transected and disrupted at the level of the bladder neck. When suprapubic endoscopy is performed a dimple can be seen, suggesting the position of bladder neck. Identification of the ureteric orifices and trigone also helps to locate the position of the transected bladder neck. Surgery is performed through a lower abdominal incision. The extraperitoneal, perivesical space is entered and the bladder is dropped down by releasing it from the anterior attachments. A posterior and superior pubectomy is then performed. All scar tissue should be excised. The urethral stump distal to the injury is carefully incised over a dilator inserted from the meatus. The safest way to open the bladder neck is to perform the incision under suprapubic endoscopic guidance with a 12 Fr mini nephroscope. The anastomosis between the bladder neck and urethra is performed with six 5-0 polydiaxone sutures. Initially, sutures on the posterior wall are placed and tied. Then a 14 Fr silicon catheter is passed across the vesicourethral anastomosis followed by placement of the anterior sutures. The omentum should be mobilized and transposed onto the anastomosis. The use of a drain should be optional.

Transection at Proximal Urethra Level

In cases that involve transection at the level of the proximal urethra, a small urethral stump remains attached to the bladder. The surgical steps were similar to the ones previously described for the bladder neck injury, except that the anastomosis is between the 2 urethral ends. This is more challenging than bladder neck repair because of the very narrow space to work in the female pelvis.

Transection at Mid-Urethral Level

This was the most common injury site seen in female pelvic fracture at our Center. This particular injury is almost always associated with a urethrovaginal fistula, which can be missed. The mid-urethra is transected allowing creation of a fistula between the distal urethra and the anterior vaginal wall. Intraoperative endoscopy with a 7Fr or 12Fr mini nephroscope, determined by the patient's age, is very critical in these patients. The endoscopic evaluation through the meatal orifice and distal urethral stump reveals the urethrovaginal fistula. A guidewire is inserted through the distal urethral stump, vaginal fistula, and back through the proximal urethral stump. The surgical steps are similar to but more difficult than the previously described procedure. A wider posterior and superior pubectomy is usually needed, (Fig. 4a–e) until healthy edges of both proximal and distal urethral stumps are clearly visualized. Once the distal urethra is opened, the guidewire is inserted and pulled through the abdominal incision. The vaginal fistula is then clearly apparent. The edges are freshened, and the fistula tract is closed with interrupted absorbable (polydiaxone) sutures. A stay suture is then taken and kept long. This omentum is mobilized and tucked between the urethral anastomosis and the anterior vaginal wall, to produce an intermediate layer. Occasionally, the vagina is also transected in the traumatic process involving the mid-urethra. The resultant scarring may cause the formation of a vaginal septum, leading to

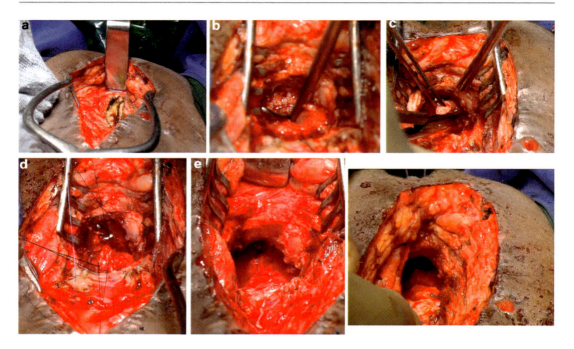

Fig. 4 (**a**) Abdominal approach, post pubectomy. (**b**) Dilator in distal urethra from meatus. (**c**) Scar excision. (**d**) Sutures in proximal urethra. (**e**) Anastomosis

vaginal compartmentalization and separation of the uterus and proximal vagina from the distal vagina. These patients may complain of amenorrhea and hematocolpos. Diagnosis is evident on ultrasound, which depicts these findings. Usually, vaginoscopy does not allow visualization of the cervix and confirms the presence of a septum. These anomalies can be treated either with laser incision of the septum or a vaginal pull-through technique.

Transection at Meatus

Infrequently, the injury can be found at the level of meatus, which is typically associated with a vaginal injury (Fig. 3). The meatus becomes hypospadiac and the vaginal injury heals with dense fibrotic tissue causing stenosis of the vaginal outlet. These patients urinate through the vagina, where the urine is collected. These patients complain of intermittent urinary incontinence.

The diagnosis is confirmed by vaginoscopy with a small caliber endoscope. Such patients require vaginotomy (similar to episiotomy). Vaginal examination (a difficult exam in children due to a narrow introitus, and thus difficult access) frequently reveals an almost bony scar on the posterior vaginal wall. Older patients may eventually require a vaginal pull-through procedure, with distal mobilization of the healthy edges of the vagina to be sutured to the introitus.

Results

In Kulkarni Reconstructive Urology Center, in Pune, 22 patients underwent treatment, including 10 prepubertal girls (median age 9 years) and 12 adult women (median age 25 years). Median time from injury to surgery was 10 months. Urethral injury was mainly in the proximal urethra in five cases (22.7%, four girls and one adult woman), in the mid-urethra in ten (45.5%, four prepubertal girls and six adult women), in the distal urethra in six cases (27.3%, two prepubertal girls and four adult women), while one case presented with total urethral loss. Eight of the ten patients presenting with mid-urethral injury, a transabdominal approach was utilized, and in six (two girls and four adult women) a urethrovaginal fistula repair was performed. All six patients with distal pelvic fracture urethral distraction defects were treated transvaginally. Twenty percent of the prepubertal girls (2/10) in our series with distal injury had vaginal introital stenosis and needed episiotomy. Two patients presented with a transverse vaginal septum, most likely due to trauma. A vaginal pull-through procedure was necessary. One patient with total urethral loss required a bladder wall flap. A complex urethral reconstruction with a Martius flap with overlying labial skin was necessary to reconstruct the vaginal wall. Overall, 77.3% (17/22) patients maintained nocturnal and diurnal urinary continence. Of those with proximal urethral injury, 60% (3/5) were continent at night and day. Median postoperative Qmax was 18 ml/min. At a median follow-up of 36 months, only one patient with proximal urethral avulsion required a revisional surgery but was continent thereafter.

Discussion

The experience with management of urethral injuries associated with pelvic fracture in females has evolved slowly over the last few decades, and only scarce reports are available in the literture. The true incidence of female urethral injuries is uncertain. However, overall female pelvic fractures are less common in females than in males with a ratio of 1:5 [8]. The lower incidence of urethral injuries could be attributed to the female urethra being protected by the bony pelvis. This lower incidence can be explained by the flexibility provided by the vagina as well as inherent elasticity of the female urethra in adults. Perry et al. reported that patients presented with extravasation and persistent incontinence, a probable reflection that these patients were overlooked initially [5]. In these instances, a longitudinal urethral laceration is a possible etiology, which is usually a less serious injury and associated hemorrhagic vaginal injuries are similarly less common [8]. In these cases, urethral catheterization is usually not difficult and urinary drainage is easily achieved. On the contrary, more serious injuries involving total urethral transverse laceration or avulsion are associated with other pelvic visceral injuries rendering urethral catheterization impossible.

Podesta et al. reported a concurrent vaginal laceration in 75–87% of cases [23]. Singh et al. reported a case of urethral distraction defect causing complete urethrovaginal avulsion [24]. This also explains why in our series we found more urethrovaginal fistulae in young girls as compared to adult counterparts. Blandy et al. reported a series of five females with ruptured urethra. One patient had a concomitant rectal injury, and four had bladder and urethral injuries. No further details were given [25]. Mundy et al. reported their experience of 12 females with urethral injuries [8]. Patient age ranged from 7 to 51 years. Nine patients had concomitant vaginal injuries. Four patients had rectal injuries, and five patients had urethral continuity preserved due to a longitudinal urethral injury. Two of these twelve patients presented on follow-up with sphincter weakness urinary incontinence. The cause of incontinence could be related to direct urethral damage or damage to innervation, or both. However, the authors suggested a mixed etiology for the incontinence [8].

In our experience, the majority of patients were continent after the urethroplasty. Five patients reported nocturnal incontinence. It is our belief that the fear of incontinence should not deter the urologist from performing anastomotic urethroplasty in female urethral injuries following pelvic fracture. An artificial urinary sphincter can be a therapeutic option, although this was not necessary in our series. Moreover, the evidence supporting its role in the treatment of urinary incontinence following pelvic fracture urethral injury in females is almost inexistent.

An algorithm is proposed to assist the reconstructive urologist in the evaluation and surgical treatment of these patients (Figs. 5 and 6). We suggest categorizing patients into two groups according to age: young/prepubertal girls, and adult females. In young girls, a urethrovaginal fistula should always be suspected in the context of urethral injury. Anastomotic urethroplasty is the recommended procedure via abdominal approach. The urethra can be accessed through posterior and superior pubectomy keeping the rim of the pubic bone intact. The urinary incontinence rate is very low in these patients. A tailored approach is recommended for these patients to either lengthen the urethra if short or a full reconstruction in case of total urethral loss. In such instances, harvesting vaginal or bladder flaps for urethral reconstruction is an option. A bladder pubovaginal stenosis should be suspected in distal urethral injuries. Such patients can present with amenorrhea and hematocolpos in the adolescent age. Scar excision, good tension-free anastomosis, and omental interposition are critical steps in anastomotic urethroplasty.

Total Urethral Loss in Female Pelvic Fracture Urethral Injury

Urethral loss can occur as a result of traumatic injury and less frequently due to iatrogenic injury. The latter etiology is predominant in the industrialized world and typically results from anterior vaginal or urethral surgery. Traumatic urethral loss can result from road traffic accident, obstetric injury, and civil and war violent trauma, including rape and other types of sexual assault. Urethral loss following pelvic fracture urethral injury can

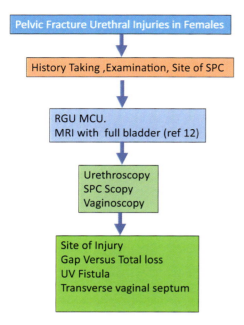

Fig. 5 Investigation algorithm for management of female pelvic fracture urethral injury

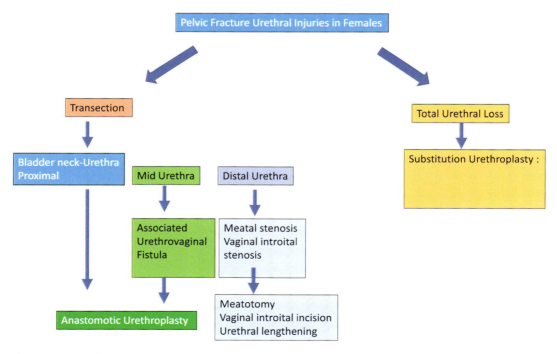

Fig. 6 Algorithm for management of female pelvic fracture urethral injury

be classified as: a) primary, where initial injury is responsible for the urethral loss, and b) secondary, if it results from iatrogenic injury associated with the management of avulsion injuries. The actual incidence of urethral loss following pelvic fracture urethral injury in females is also unknown. It can only be speculated from the type of surgeries reported for this condition in the published literature. Neourethral reconstructions are more commonly performed for congenital defects as well as following obstetric or iatrogenic causes. In a series of 74 cases, Flisser and Blaivas reported that only three received a vaginal flap for traumatic urethral loss [26]. In a systematic review by Patel et al., a total of 158 women with traumatic urethral injuries were identified [20]. Of these, 63% (99/158) were pediatric patients and 37% (59/158) were adults. Of these injuries, 53% (83/158) were managed immediately in the acute setting. A delayed repair was performed in 47% (75/158) patients, 4% (3/75) of them due to a delay in diagnosis resulting in delayed repair. In 21% (16/75) of the patients, a delayed repair was electively performed. The cause of the delayed repair was a delay in presentation in 75% (56/75) of the patients. Of these 75 patients who had a delayed repair, 40% (30/75) were adult women and 60% (45/74) were prepubertal girls. All delayed repairs required either an abdominal or a combined abdominovaginal approach. The main reasons for these approaches were the presence of dense scarred tissue compromising surgical access significantly and/or a need to reconstruct a severely damaged bladder neck. In this systematic review, the most common delayed repair procedure used in 43% (32/75) of the patients was a retropubic or transpubic anastomotic urethroplasty. Of these 75 patients who underwent a delayed repair, 28% (21/75) had an anterior bladder wall flap and 6.6% (5/75) underwent definitive continent urinary diversion via a Mitrofanoff or Mainz-type procedure. From this, it can be assumed that the prevalence of traumatic urethral loss would range from 4% to 35%. Complications after delayed surgical reconstruction included urethral stricture (3%), fistula formation (4%), vaginal stenosis (4%), and urinary incontinence (31%) [20]. The delayed repair was associated with the highest rates of post-treatment urinary incontinence, vaginal stenosis, and need of urinary diversion among the three most common types of repair (Table 2).

Before the surgical procedure, some pertinent questions should be addressed. How is the vaginal health? Is the vaginal introitus adequate? Is the bladder neck intact or damaged? Is the bladder capacity adequate? What are the patients' expectations? Is the patient willing to do CISC? Will the patient accept a Mitrofanoff-type diversion? Will urinary incontinence be acceptable? What are the patient's expectations regarding sexual life?

The goals of surgical reconstruction are to create a continent urethra of appropriate length that allows volitional, painless, and unobstructed passage of urine. The neourethra should also have sufficient length to prevent voiding into the vagina. Blaivas et al. believe that these goals can almost always be achieved with a single procedure [27]. The same authors state that the three approaches to post-traumatic female urethral reconstruction are anterior bladder flaps, posterior bladder flaps, and vaginal wall flaps. They recommend vaginal flaps as the best option. In cases where urethrovaginal fistulae are present, surgical

Table 2 Outcomes after surgical repair of pelvic fracture urethral injury in females

Repair type (N)	Stricture (%)	Fistula (%)	Incontinence (%)	Vaginal stenosis (%)	Urinary diversion (%)
Primary Realignment (17/158; 11%)	9/15 (60%)	2/15 (12%)	0/15 (0%)	0/15 (0%)	0/15 (0%)
Primary Anastamotic Repair (66/158; 42%)	2/66 (3%)	4/66 (6%)	6/66 (9%)	0/66 (0%)	2/66 (3%)
Delayed Repair (75/158; 47%)	2/75 (3%)	3/75 (4%)	23/75 (31%)	3/75 (4%)	5/75 (7%)

Adapted and modified from Ref. [20]

options include primary closure, peninsula flaps, bilateral labial pedicle flaps, and labial island flaps. Due to the shorter urethral length, there is a potentially greater risk of incontinence and neurosensory dysfunction following female surgical urethral reconstruction, in general.

To repair distal urethral loss, we favor the Jackknife prone position, and buccal mucosal graft should be harvested before patient surgical positioning. If the injury is proximal with unhealthy distal urethra or a complete loss of urethra, a number of options exist:

1. Bladder flap (Tanagho and modifications) [28–34]
2. Young Dees bladder neck reconstruction [35, 36]
3. Tubularized pedicle labia minora flap [37, 38]
4. Lateral vaginal flap [39]
5. Tubularized buccal mucosa graft with buttock flap [40]
6. Appendix [41]
7. Intestinal segment [42–45]
8. Ileovesicostomy [46]
9. Mitrofanoff with bladder neck closure [47]
10. Ileal conduit/continent diversion [48]
11. Singapore flap [49]
12. Suprapubic catheter

General principles of repair include adequate exposure of the operative site, a tension-free, multilayered closure, adequate blood supply of the flap, a concomitant anti-incontinence procedure including a pubovaginal sling, appropriate use of tissue interposition to fill the operative space and for vascularity, adequate bladder drainage, meticulous hemostasis, and detailed attention to catheter care to prevent damage to the repair.

Patients with an intact bladder neck but near complete urethral loss may undergo reconstruction by the vaginal route [35]. However, vaginal access for urethral repair is difficult especially in Type 2 fracture associated with narrow vaginal hiatus, vaginal stenosis, scarring especially in children, and also after failure of a primary repair [20]. For these indications, either abdominal or combined abdominal and vaginal approaches are preferable. A bladder flap tube is the ideal tissue for urethral substitution in females. It is well vascularized, and hence healing is good with less fibrosis or fistulation. The mucosa is suitable for handling urine and the detrusor tonus is expected to contribute to urinary continence. A sufficiently long tube can be created to bridge any length of female urethral defect, the bladder neck can be suspended to restore adequate vesicourethral angle, and a supra levator position of the newly formed bladder neck can be achieved allowing better access for repair when associated with vesicovaginal fistula.

Prior to the reconstructive procedure, urodynamic examination is essential to diagnose an atonic bladder wall as this is not an appropriate material and especially if associated with a hyperactive neurogenic bladder. An anterior bladder wall flap, either as a classical Tanagho type, a modified flipped anterior wall flap (vertical or oblique), or a T-shaped flap, can be fashioned for use [28, 31, 33]. The rationale of the procedure is to incorporate the ventral condensation of circular fibers that extend above the internal meatus for about 2.54 cm (1 inch). The tube formed from this material has enough tonus to provide an exclusive effect and sphincteric function and is adequate to replace damaged sphincter segment. Tanagho stressed the quality of the muscles in the tube rather than the length [28].

Procedure

The patient is positioned in the low lithotomy position. After patient prepping and draping, the bladder is partially filled through a sterile suprapubic catheter. A suprapubic midline incision (alternatively, a Pfannenstiel incision can also be used) is made, the peritoneum is mobilized for a limited area on the anterior bladder surface, and sharp dissection is carried out to release the bladder and bladder neck from the pubic symphysis also by excising the extensive and dense scarred tissue using care to preserve the adventitia on the bladder. With a finger in the vagina, the sharp and blunt dissection is continued to create sufficient space up to the vestibular area. This step can be assisted by simultaneous dissection from the vaginal side. The Tanagho flap is formed by marking the bladder wall area with the bladder half distended for about 6 × 4 cm and disconnecting it at the bladder neck. Alternatively, disconnecting the flap proximally produces a reverse Tanagho or a flipped anterior wall flap [31]. The flap can be oriented obliquely if the site of the suprapubic catheter is in the way or if there is a linear scar. Some authors have used a reverse Boari flap for this kind of reconstruction [29]. In the presence of a concomitant vesicovaginal fistula, the bladder must be mobilized from the vagina, which should be followed by closure of the vagina and bladder in opposite directions. Next, the flap is tubularized in two layers over a catheter (10 Fr in girls and 14 Fr in adults). The advantage of the flipped flap is the anterior location of the suture line unlike the posterior suture line in the Tanagho flap. For a similar reason, Hemal et al. preferred an oblique flap to avoid a vertical suture line abutting the anterior vaginal wall thus reducing the chance of fistula formation [30]. Unlike the vertical or oblique flap, in the bladder flipped flap the bladder neck remains caudal in a more anatomical location instead of a higher location in the former. Before bringing out a circular omentum flap for interposition or Martius fat pad is placed, the tube is exteriorized and sutured to the vagina to create a neomeatus. Lv et al. described a T-shaped flap, with one arm of the flap forming the posterior wall and the other forming the anterior wall of the tube with a lateral suture line [33]. Elkins et al. performed the Tanagho-type procedure through a vaginal approach in all the 20 cases of extensive urethral damage due to obstructed labor [50]. This may not be possible in pelvic fracture urethral injury.

Bladder flaps are more commonly used for urethral substitution in cases of extensive urethral loss or proximal urethral injuries [30, 37]. Bladder flaps are typically well vascularized thus promoting good wound healing and aiding in urinary continence. Bladder flaps can be mobilized in two different types. Vertical flaps are longer but more prone to fistulation. On the other hand, oblique bladder flaps may be shorter but have better blood supply. Bladder flaps are more adequate for severe urethral loss associated with trauma. Following bladder flap neourethral reconstruction, up to 80% of these patients report partial or total continence and void normally [37]. However, other authors reported urinary incontinence at 3-month follow-up [30]. If urinary incontinence occurs, it can be addressed accordingly, including a pubovaginal sling, at a later time. Some surgeons prefer to include an anti-incontinence procedure at the same time with the use of fascial slings as these are easy to harvest and use the graft, thus avoiding a second procedure. Synthetic slings are contraindicated in patients following urethral reconstruction in the settings of hypovascularized tissues such as in severe traumatic injury with concurrent urethrovaginal fistula, or following partial or total urethral loss.

Huang et al. reported their experience with management of traumatic urethral injury in a cohort of 44 girls, 40 of whom presented with urethrovaginal fistula [35]. Transpubic reconstruction of the urethra using a modified Young-Dees-Leadbetter procedure with simultaneous repair of the urethrovaginal fistula was performed in 35 patients. Twenty-three percent (8/35) patients required more than one procedure (twice in five and three times in three). The authors concluded that the transpubic approach remains the method of choice to treat total urethral distraction and obliterative urethral stenosis, especially with concomitant urethrovaginal fistula. However, this technique has not been reported widely.

After bladder wall flap, a pedicled tubularized labia minora flap is also a popular surgical technique. Radwan et al. used these two techniques in their 16 female patients who required urethral reconstruction [37]. Six patients underwent a proximally based anterior bladder tube (Tanagho flap) and ten received a labia minora pedicled tube. All ten patients with a labia minora flap had a transobturator mid-urethral sling placed at the time of surgery. They concluded that both bladder tube and labia minora pedicled tube with a simultaneous mid-urethral sling operation have a good success rate with only slight complications and are equally effective in the management of total urethral loss in females. Xu et al. [38] have also reported on the use and efficacy of the pedicle tubularized labial urethroplasty for urethral repair following traumatic urethral injuries associated with urethrovaginal fistulae. A rectangular or oval incision is made in an adjacent healthy, hairless portion of the labia minora as close to the site of the urethra as possible. The size of the incision should be large enough to roll into a tube over 16 Fr catheter. The incision is deepened around the labia and a pedicled flap is raised on an anterior or posterior blood supply. The flap is passed beneath the vaginal wall and rotated so that the mucosal surface forms the inner wall of the reconstructed urethra. In case of extensive vaginal scarring a linear incision at the site of new urethra is made sufficient to elevate flaps for covering the graft. The critical step is to ensure adequate exposure and mobilization of the remaining scarless proximal urethra or bladder neck for the anastomosis of the tubularized flap.

The vaginal wall flap was popularized by Flisser and Blaivas, mostly in obstetric injury and other conditions [26]. In their series of 74 cases, only 3 were of traumatic etiology. The following factors prevented the use of this technique: Type 2 pelvic fracture, vaginal scarring, vaginal stenosis, compromised blood supply, and young girls. If the vaginal wall tissue is adequate, then a rectangular incision of required length and of width sufficient to be rolled over a 16Fr catheter is made. The flap is tubularized by suturing in the midline without tension. In some instances, a lateral vaginal flap will be required. The vaginal wall can be closed primarily, or if there is insufficient tissue for primary closure, it is usually possible to elevate another adjacent broad-based vaginal or labia minora rotational flap to cover the wound. Some surgeons have used gracilis myocutaneous and rectus pedicle flaps to facilitate closure, although Blaivas et al. found it unnecessary.

In 2001, Park and Hendren described their experience with the use of tubularized buccal mucosal graft with a buttock flap for urethral reconstruction in seven girls aged 3–13 years. The underlying pathological condition was a severely scarred urethra or urethral loss following previous major surgeries for congenital malformations, such as cloacal exstrophy, cloacal malformation, and other iatrogenic urethral injuries. None of these patients had suffered traumatic loss of urethra as a result of pelvic fracture [40].

They concluded that in select prepubertal girls with difficult urethral reconstructive problems a tubularized buccal mucosal graft may be effectively used when local tissue is unhealthy, fibrotic, and unsuitable for creating a supple new urethra.

Appendix, ileal segment, and colon have been used as alternative sources for neourethral formation [41–43]. The use of an ileal segment through a Yang-Monti technique with rectus muscle flap in a 5-year-old girl was reported by Kannaiyan and Sen in 2009 [44]. The little girl presented with post-traumatic urinary incontinence due to rupture of the bladder neck into the vagina. The short female urethra is often totally lost in pelvic distraction injury and needs to be replaced. Several options have been reported [30, 35, 41, 43]. In some complex settings where neourethral reconstruction is not possible, then one may have to resort to continent diversion with or without closure of the bladder neck. Bladder neck closure can be effectively achieved through a vaginal approach. However, when a Mitrofanoff procedure or a noncontinent diversion (ileovesicostomy) is performed, a layered bladder neck closure can be performed transabdominally. Urinary continence, need for clean intermittent self-catheterization, and sexual health following vaginal injury are important issues related to urethral loss. Vaginal anatomical and functional restoration, whenever possible and with help from plastic surgeons, will improve general outcomes and quality of life.

Any neourethral reconstruction should aim to restore normal voiding following the same principles as in men. If urinary incontinence occurs, it should be dealt with appropriately at a later stage. Surprisingly, continence is highly satisfactory after bladder flap procedures. The urinary continence in females is a complex mechanism and is expected to be severely damaged or nonexistent after an insult that results in total loss of the urethra. However, the literature on the outcomes of these reconstructive procedures state otherwise. To simplify, a tube of adequate length (its relevance has been questioned by Tanagho), an intact bladder neck (continence mechanism apparently located in mid-urethra), mucosa coaptation (difficult to assess in tissues like labia minora and oral mucosal graft), vaginal buttress, intra-abdominal portion, and intact neural mechanisms are key factors for global success and optimal functional outcomes. In some cases, urinary continence could be achieved by additional maneuvers such as bladder neck tightening, bladder neck suspension, hitching the vagina to the pubis, and use of autologous fascial slings at the time of reconstruction. A transobturator sling was used in all the cases of tubularized pedicled labia minora flap but the continence rate was similar or worse than Tanagho bladder flap without concomitant anti-incontinence procedure [37]. Blaivas advocates an anti-incontinence procedure at the same time of reconstruction as he reports urinary incontinence rates as high as 50–84% if not addressed simultaneously [51]. It is assumed that a secondary procedure is required to correct continence optimize success rates.

Conclusion

Female pelvic fracture urethral injuries are uncommon and may be underdiagnosed especially if a meticulous vaginal examination is routinely performed in the presence of blood at the vaginal introitus as well as careful endoscopic and/or imaging studies in females with voiding problems and associated vulvar hematoma or edema in the context of acute trauma. These injuries occur in females less often than in males. The most common type and location of pelvic fracture urethral injury is avulsion of the mid-urethra, realizing that an associated vaginal injury is likely. The presence of a concomitant urethrovaginal fistula should always be suspected. Due to its anatomic location and physical characteristics, the female urethra seems relatively resistant to injury, and in general, a more severe injury is needed to cause more significant damage as compared to male urethra. Traumatic urethral injury associated with pelvic fracture in prepubertal girls can result in technically demanding management scenarios. More severe pelvic fracture is usually associated with significant urethral avulsion and greater urethral loss requiring more complex repair. Partial urethral injury or urethral transection without considerable displacement is better managed by primary repair of the transected urethra, which can reduce morbidity. Primary repair may not be possible in patients with major injury. These patients should be managed with deferred appropriate reconstruction after preliminary suprapubic cystostomy. Complete urethral loss may be treated with a bladder or labial flap tubed neourethra. In specific cases, concomitant treatment of urinary incontinence can be effectively advocated with good outcomes. Apparently, the transpubic approach remains the method of choice for repairing complete urethral disruption and severe urethral stricture, especially when associated with urethrovaginal fistula. Thus, reconstruction of the post-traumatic urethral injury in females is challenging, and a careful evaluation of patients afflicted with this type of urethral injury is highly critical. Unfortunately, due to its relatively low incidence, long-term outcome data are almost inexistent for contemporary techniques of female urethral reconstruction, making the optimum management of female urethral distraction defects to be founded on low-quality literature. According to scarce literature available, primary anastomotic repair of a female urethral distraction defect via a vaginal approach as soon as the patient is hemodynamically stable appears to be an excellent solution. Furthermore, the available literature also advises that most pelvic fracture urethral injuries are best repaired with delayed anastomotic urethroplasty, mostly through the abdominal approach, which can lead to excellent outcomes. High success rates have also been reported with use of bladder flaps, vaginal flaps, and buccal mucosal graft for urethral reconstruction. These surgeries require specialized expertise.

For cases of complete urethral loss where delayed anastomotic urethroplasty is not feasible and vaginal and labial tissue is inadequate to raise a flap, the flipped anterior bladder wall tube may be a suitable therapeutic choice. If this option is not possible either, then some form of urinary diversion should be considered as a last resort.

References

1. Simpson-Smith A. Traumatic rupture of the urethra: eight personal cases with a review of 381 recorded ruptures. Br J Surg. 1936;24:309–32.
2. Antoci JP, SchiC MR Jr. Bladder and urethral injuries in patients with pelvic fractures. J Urol. 1982;128:25–6.
3. Bredael JJ, Kramer SA, Cleeve LK, Webster GD. Traumatic rupture of the female urethra. J Urol. 1979;122:560–1.
4. Patil U, Nesbitt R, Meyer R. Genitourinary tract injuries due to fracture of the pelvis in females: Sequelae and their management. Br J Urol. 1982;54:32–85.
5. Perry MO, Husmann DA. Urethral injuries in female subjects following pelvic fractures. J Urol. 1992;147:139–43.
6. Barach E, Martin G, Tomlanovich M, Nowak R, Littleton R. Blunt pelvic trauma with urethral injury in the female: a case report and review of the literature. J Emerg Med. 1984;2:101–5.
7. Carter CT, Schafer N. Incidence of urethral disruption in females with traumatic pelvic fractures. Am J Emergency Med. 1993;11:218–20.
8. Venn SN, Greenwell TJ, Mundy AR. Pelvic fracture injuries of the female urethra. BJU Int. 1999;83:626–30.
9. Kulkarni SB, Surana S, Desai DJ, Orabi H, Iyer S, Kulkarni J, Dumawat A, Joshi PM. Management of complex and redo cases of pelvic fracture urethral injuries. Asian J Urol. 2018;5(2):107–17.
10. Thambi Dorai CR, Boucaut HAP, Dewan PA. Urethral injuries in girls with pelvic trauma. Eur Urol. 1993;24:371–4.
11. Williams DI. Rupture of the female urethra in childhood. Eur Urol. 1975;1:129–33.
12. Casselman RC, Schillinger JF. Fractured pelvis with avulsion of the female urethra. J Urol. 1977;117:385–6.
13. Parkhurst JD, Coker JE, Haverstadt B. Traumatic avulsion of the lower urinary tract in the female child. J Urol. 1981;126:265–7.
14. Ahmed S, Neel KF. Urethral injury in girls with fractured pelvis following blunt abdominal trauma. Br J Urol. 1996;78:450–3.
15. Chatelain C, Giuli R, Farge C, Kuss R. Traumatic rupture of the female urethra associated with a fracture of the pelvis involving the pubic symphysis block. J Urol Nephrol (Paris). 1970;76:108–13.
16. Pokorny M, Pontes JE, Pierce JM Jr. Urological injuries associated with pelvic trauma. J Urol. 1979;121:455–7.
17. Goldman HB, Idom CG Jr, Dmochwoski RR. Traumatic injuries of the female external genitalia and their association with urological injuries. J Urol. 1998;159:956–9.
18. Joshi PM, Kulkarni SB. Management of pelvic fracture urethral injuries in the developing world. World J Urol. 2020;38(12):3027–34.
19. Kulkarni SB, Joshi PM, Hunter C, Surana S, Shahrour W, Alhajeri F. Complex posterior urethral injury. Arab J Urol. 2015;13(1):43–52.
20. Patel DN, Fok CS, Webster GD, Anger JT. Female urethral injuries associated with pelvic fracture: a systematic review of the literature. BJU Int. 2017;120(6):766–73.
21. Joshi PM, Desai DJ, Shah D, Joshi DP, Kulkarni SB. Magnetic resonance imaging procedure for pelvic fracture urethral injuries and recto urethral fistulas: a simplified protocol. Turk J Urol. 2021;47(1):35–42.
22. Joshi PM, Bandini M, Yepes C, Bhadranavar S, Sharma V, Bafna S, Kulkarni SB. Pelvic fracture urethral injury in females. Soc Int Urol J. 2022;3(2):77–86.
23. Podestá ML, Jordan GH. Pelvic fracture urethral injuries in girls. J Urol. 2001;165(5):1660–5.
24. Singh RK, Kaushal D, Khattar N, Nayyar R, Manasa T, Sood R. Pediatric pelvic fracture urethral distraction defect causing complete urethrovaginal avulsion. Indian J Urol. 2018;34(1):76–8.
25. Blandy JP. Urethral stricture. Post Med J. 1980;56:383–418.
26. Flisser AL, Blaivas JG. Outcome of urethral reconstructive surgery in a series of 74 women. J Urol. 2003;169:2246–9.
27. Blaivas JG, Purohit RS. Post-traumatic female urethral reconstruction. Curr Urol Rep. 2008;9(5):397–4.
28. Tanagho EA. Bladder neck reconstruction for total urinary incontinence: 10 years of experience. J Urol. 1981;125(3):321–6.
29. Ackermann D, Zingg EJ. Harnröhrenrekonstruktion bei der Frau mittels Blasenplastik [Reconstruction of the urethra in women using a bladder flap]. Urologe A. 1984;23(1):46–9. German. PMID: 6539017.
30. Hemal AK, Dorairajan LN, Gupta NP. Posttraumatic complete and partial loss of urethra with pelvic fracture in girls: an appraisal of management. J Urol. 2000;163(1):282–7.
31. Ahmed S. Construction of female neourethra using a flipped anterior bladder wall tube. J Pediatr Surg. 1995;30:1728–31.
32. Nayyar R, Jain S, Sharma K, Pethe S, Kumar P. A novel anterior bladder tube for traumatic bladder neck contracture in females: initial results. Urology. 2020;139:201–6.
33. Lv R, Jin C, Shu H, et al. Bladder neck reconstruction in girls' pelvic fracture bladder neck avulsion and urethral rupture. BMC Urol. 2020;20:179. https://doi.org/10.1186/s12894-020-00741-z.
34. Woodard JR, Marshall VF. Reconstruction of the female urethra to reduce post traumatic incontinence. Surg Gynecol Obstet. 1961;113:687.
35. Huang CR, Sun N, Wei-ping, Xie HW, Hwang AH, Hardy BE. The management of old urethral injury in young girls: analysis of 44 cases. J Pediatr Surg. 2003;38(9):1329–32. https://doi.org/10.1016/s0022-3468(03)00390-7. PMID: 14523814.

36. Ahmed S, Kardar AH. Construction of a neourethra in girls: follow-up results. Paediatr Surg Int. 2000;16:584–5.
37. Radwan Abou Farha MO, Soliman MG, et al. Outcome of female urethral reconstruction: a 12-year experience. World J Urol. 2013;31:991–5.
38. Xu YM, Sa YL, Fu Q, et al. Transpubic access using pedicle tubularized labial urethroplasty for the treatment of female urethral strictures associated with urethrovaginal fistulas secondary to pelvic fracture. Eur Urol. 2009;56:193–200.
39. Kelemen Z, Romics I, Pajor L. Substitution of the distal female urethra with a vaginal flap and pedicled skin island. BJU Int. 2002;89:459–61.
40. Park JM, Hendren WH. Construction of female urethra using buccal mucosa graft. J Urol. 2001;166(2):640–3. PMID: 11458109.
41. Sheldon CA, Gilbert A. Use of the appendix for urethral reconstruction in children with congenital anomalies of the bladder. Surgery. 1992;112:805–11.
42. Lavanya K, Sen S. Urethral substitution with ileum in traumatic bladder neck-vagina fistula. J Indian Assoc Pediatr Surg. 2009;14(2):76–7.
43. Xu YM, Qiao Y, Sa YL, Zhang J, Zhang HZ, Zhang XR, Wu DL, Chen R. One-stage urethral reconstruction using colonic mucosa graft: an experimental and clinical study. World J Gastroenterol. 2003;9:381–4.
44. Kannaiyan L, Sen S. Urethral substitution with ileum in traumatic bladder neck-vagina fistula. J Indian Assoc Pediatr Surg [serial online]. 2009. [cited 2023 Jan 2];14:76–7. Available from: https://www.jiaps.com/text.asp?2009/14/2/76/55159
45. Zimmern PE, Studer UE, Hadley HR, Raz S. Urethral replacement using ileum with an intussuscepted ileal valve for continence. J Urol. 1985;134(2):414–7.
46. Monti PR, Lara RC, Dutra MA, de Carvalho JR. New techniques for construction of efferent conduits based on the Mitrofanoff principle. Urology. 1997;49(1):112–5. https://doi.org/10.1016/S0090-4295(96)00503-1.
47. Khoury AE, Agarwal SK, Bägli D, Merguerian P, McLorie GA. Concomitant modified bladder neck closure and Mitrofanoff urinary diversion. J Urol. 1999;162(5):1746–8.
48. Mahran MR, Ghoneim MA. The application of the modified rectal bladder in management of the compromized urethral damage. Scand J Urol Nephrol. 1994;28(1):49–53. https://doi.org/10.3109/00365599409180470. PMID: 8009193.
49. Zorn KC, Bzrezinski A, St-Denis B, Corcos J. Female neo- urethral reconstruction with a modified neurovascular pudendal thigh flap (Singapore flap): initial experience. Can J Urol. 2007;14:3449–54.
50. Elkins, et al. Tanagho-like procedure in 20 West African woman with extensive damage due to obstructed labour. Obstet Gynecol. 1992;79(3):455–60.
51. Blaivas JG. Treatment of female incontinence secondary to urethral damage or loss. Urol Clin North Am. 1991;18:355–63.

Surgical Repair of Urethral Diverticula

49

S. Saad, N. Osman, O. A. Alsulaiman, and C. R. Chapple

Contents

Introduction	857
Etiopathogenesis	858
Diagnosis	858
Clinical Presentation	858
Evaluation	859
Classification	860
Management	860
Surgical	861
Outcomes	865
Conclusion	865
References	866

Abstract

Female diverticula represent a significant clinical problem when they occur. It is thought that they result from blockage of the drainage duct of a paraurethral gland. Urethral diverticula always communicate directly with the urethra. In this chapter we describe the use of the prone position which we believe facilitates accurate surgical excision of a urethral diverticulum.

Keywords

Female urethra · Diverticula · Surgery · Prone position

Introduction

Female urethral diverticula (UD) are focal fluid-filled sac-like structures in the periurethral tissue invariably communicating with the urethra and expanding the overlying urethral sphincteric tissues over them. Although the true incidence of female UD is unknown, they are estimated to occur in 0.6–6% of females [1, 2] and up to 40% females with lower urinary tract symptoms

---

The operative pictures unless stated otherwise remain the copyright of C. R. Chapple

S. Saad · N. Osman · O. A. Alsulaiman ·
C. R. Chapple (✉)
Department of Urology, Sheffield Teaching Hospitals NHS Foundation Trust, Sheffield, UK
e-mail: sanadsaad@gmail.com; nadir.osman@nhs.net; oasulaiman@kfshrc.edu.sa; c.r.chapple@sheffield.ac.uk; c.r.chapple@shef.ac.uk

© Springer Nature Switzerland AG 2023
F. E. Martins et al. (eds.), *Female Genitourinary and Pelvic Floor Reconstruction*,
https://doi.org/10.1007/978-3-031-19598-3_50

(LUTS) [3]. A UD, once diagnosed, can be surgically challenging [1]. UD can be completely asymptomatic or present with dyspareunia, incontinence, discharge, urinary retention, or infection. UD are rare in males where they arise because of trauma or partial duplication of the urethra. This chapter will deal exclusively with female UD.

Etiopathogenesis

Although there are a few reports of congenital UD described in female infants [4, 5], the majority of UD in females are diagnosed in adulthood [1]. The most widely accepted theory of pathogenesis was first popularized by Routh in 1890 and later expanded upon by Young and Wahle in 1996 (Fig. 1). The periurethral glands are tubuloalveolar glands located posterolaterally along the whole length of the urethra within the submucosal layer. These glands secrete mucin which can act as a urethral sealant to aid continence [6]. They are most prominent in the distal two-thirds of the urethra [1]. Consequently, the distribution of UD mirrors the anatomical location of periurethral glands and are usually found in the middle to distal third of urethra at 3 or 9 o'clock positions [7]. UD are composed of a single cyst-like structure connected to the urethra by a neck or ostium. They can lie in any configuration often ventral to the urethra [8] or extend partially around the urethra like a "saddlebag" or dorsally or circumferentially surround the entire urethra [9] as seen in Fig. 2.

The prevalent theory on etiology is that UD arise because of recurrent infections of a periurethral gland with subsequent abscess formation. As these glands drain into the urethra during excision of a UD, it has to be considered that the urethra will always be opened. It is also important to appreciate that UD stretch the whole wall of the adjacent urethra including the intrinsic smooth muscle over them which has implications for the surgical approach which is used. Marsupialization of a UD or failure to take account of surgical anatomy will inevitably result in the development of a urethral fistula.

Diagnosis

Clinical Presentation

Patients usually present in the third to seventh decade of life with variable symptoms [1]. As such, UD are prone to misdiagnosis which can lead to delays in diagnosis with one study estimating an average time to diagnosis following development of symptoms of 9 months [10]. The classically described "three D's" – dysuria, dribbling, and dyspareunia – are frequently seen. Other common symptoms are storage lower urinary tract symptoms (LUTS) (namely frequency, urgency, and post-void dribbling/incontinence) as well as dyspareunia, infection (UTI), and pain [1]. At least a third of patients present with recurrent UTIs, probably due to urinary stasis in the UD. Other symptoms include an anterior vaginal wall mass, urethral discharge, voiding LUTS, urinary retention, or hematuria. The latter may point towards a diverticular stone or malignancy, both of which are rare [6]. It is

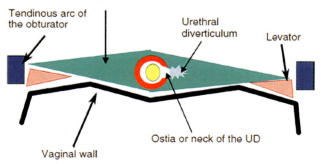

Fig. 1 UD as conceptualized by Young and Wahle forming between the layers of urethropelvic ligament. (Reproduced from Ref. [1] with permission from Elsevier)

Fig. 2 Different variations of UD. (Reproduced from Ref. [1] with permission from Elsevier)

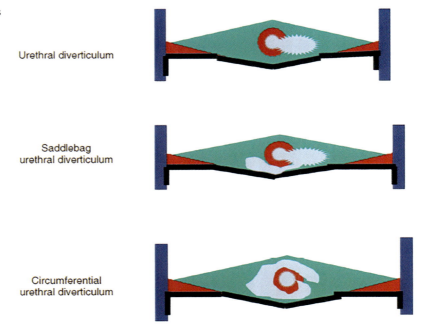

important to note that 10–20% of UD are picked up incidentally on imaging or examination [11].

An anterior vaginal wall mass is the most common finding on clinical examination. This may be more tender during an acute infection, and compression may express a purulent urethral discharge per urethra. There may be coexisting stress urinary incontinence (SUI) associated with pelvic organ prolapse (POP) and/or urethral hypermobility at this stage to assist in future prognosis [12].

While an anterior vaginal wall mass is the commonest finding on examination, smaller diverticula and those located laterally or anteriorly may not be palpable.

Evaluation

Urine Studies

Further evaluation includes urinalysis +/− microscopy and culture to assess for urinary infection or hematuria. If symptoms are principally storage and/or if malignancy is suspected, urine cytology should be checked. Malignant change is, however, very rare in urethral diverticula occurring in <1%.

Cystourethroscopy

This can be carried out to attempt to visualize the urethral defect. It is also important to evaluate the bladder for any other causes in patients with LUTS. The ostium of a urethral diverticulum is usually located posterolaterally at 4 and 8 o'clock positions [1] but identifying them on endoscopy is highly variable (15–89%) [13–15]. Helpful maneuvers to improve visualization are by milking the diverticulum during examination which may express fluid, as well as occluding the proximal urethra and moving the scope distally with continuous irrigation both to allow UD distension and improve the endoscopic view [1, 6].

Magnetic Resonance Imaging (MRI)

MRI is the gold standard in imaging of UD [6]. High-resolution, detailed, multi-planar images of UD help in not only diagnosing UD but also aids surgical planning. UD have decreased signal intensity as compared to surrounding tissues on T1 weighted images and increased intensity on T2 weighted images [1]. It is essential to request that the MRI to be performed after the patient voids so that the UD fills up with urine otherwise UD may be missed or mischaracterized [6]. Invasive endoluminal coils may be placed rectally or vaginally for greater resolution due to improved signal-to-noise ratio [16].

Voiding Cystourethrogram (VCUG)

VCUG is a widely available imaging technique that has a reported sensitivity of 44–95% [14, 17] and a diagnostic accuracy of 65% [6]. It is dependent on the patient's ability to void with enough pressure to distend the diverticulum during micturition. A VCUG is considered as nondiagnostic if it does not demonstrate a UD but has no post-void images [1]. This may occur if the ostium is narrow, the diverticulum is partially filled or contains debris, or the patient is unable to generate a good flow either due to pain or embarrassment [1, 6]. Consequently, VCUG is not used widely anymore as it is invasive, time-consuming, and technically challenging [18].

VCUG is also essential to demonstrate and characterize stress incontinence in those patients experiencing it preoperatively, and filling cystometry will allow identification of bladder dysfunction such as detrusor overactivity.

Ultrasonography

Although multiple techniques have been described (transabdominal, translabial, transvaginal, and transurethral), the transvaginal approach provides good information about the location and size of UD. The benefits of this test are its wide availability and ease of use; however, the accuracy and interpretation is operator dependent. Also, smaller size UD may be inadvertently compressed and therefore missed [19].

Double Balloon Positive Pressure Urethrography (PPU)

This technique, which was popular during the mid-twentieth century, utilizes a special catheter (Trattner catheter) that has two balloons separated by several centimeters. [1]. This is inserted into the urethra with one balloon positioned at the external urethral meatus and the other at the bladder neck to seal and isolate the urethra upon inflation. Infusion of contrast at slight pressure distends the urethra and forces contrast into the UD so the cavity can be visualized. Although this technique provides great images and is not dependent on the patient voiding successfully, it is not used in contemporary practice as the Trattner catheter is not widely available, and the advent of transvaginal ultrasonography and MRI has rendered the test obsolete [6].

Classification

Two classification systems are available for UD. The simpler of the two was proposed by Leng and McGuire [20] that divides UD into two categories: those with a preserved periurethral fascial layer (UD) and those without (pseudo-diverticulum). While it has potential surgical implications in our experience, we have not found this to be useful. The second system, proposed by Leach et al. [21], is a staging system for UD based on location, number, size, site of urethral communication, anatomy, and continence of the patient. This is termed the L/N/S/C3 classification system.

While both systems provide forms of classification, in our experience with MRI imaging, we do not find that either provides substantive benefit in the preoperative assessment of patients.

Management

Conservative

UD can be managed conservatively. There is a paucity in the literature on the natural history of UD if left untreated. There is no established timeline on the progression of symptoms, complexity, or size. Conservative management is reserved for those patients who are asymptomatic, medically unfit, or do not desire surgical management. However, patient counselling is vital in patients who choose not to undergo

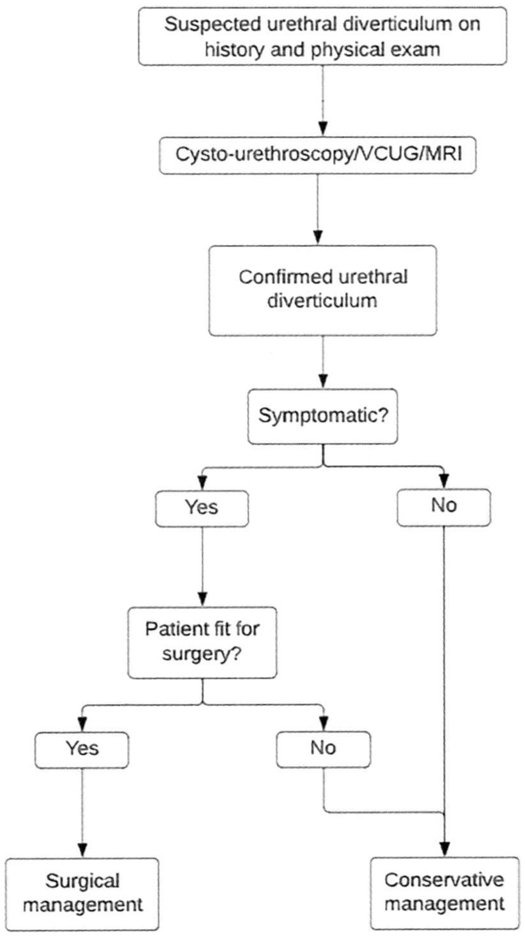

Surgical

Symptomatic patients who are fit for surgery should be offered surgical excision of a UD.

Since Hey's description in 1805 of transvaginal incision of UD and packing the cavity with lint [7], many surgical techniques have been described to treat UD. These include marsupialization, fulguration, obliteration with injection of cellulose or polytetrafluoroethylene, endoscopic deroofing, excision, and transurethral incision [1, 6, 33]. While a systematic review of surgical techniques for management of UD in 1947 patients could not determine differences in surgical outcomes and complications between various surgical techniques [34], the question has to be asked as to how robust this conclusion is, as contemporary experience would suggest that the most appropriate surgical approach is complete excision of a UD.

For occasional patients who have a very distal diverticulum and who don't wish to undergo major reconstruction, marsupialization of the diverticulum into the vagina has been described as an option [1, 35]. This is achieved via a deep ventral incision into the urethra, thereby incorporating the anterior vaginal wall into the diverticulum. This approach has been described by Spenge and Duckett (1969) and has the benefits of reduced operating time, blood loss, and recurrence rate [36, 37]. However, caution must be exercised not to aggressively extend the incision ventrally which may cause damage to the proximal or distal sphincteric mechanisms leading to SUI [1]. Another significant complication of this procedure in sexually active women is dyspareunia, which may result from creation of a pseudo-septum due to marsupialization of the urethra with respect to the anterior vaginal wall [1]. In rare cases where the UD is highly symptomatic, e.g., acute infection not responding to antibiotics, and a complete excision cannot be performed, e.g., pregnancy, a diverticulotomy can be performed via a transvaginal incision into the UD cavity to create a urethrovaginal fistula. While this can decompress the UD until such a time when definitive excision and reconstruction can safely be performed [35]. We would not recommend this course of

Fig. 3 An algorithm for management of urethral diverticula. *VCUG* voiding cystourethrography, *MRI* magnetic resonance imaging (based on EAU Guidelines on non-neurogenic female LUTS [43])

primary operative management, as there are multiple reports in literature of carcinomas arising in UD [22–31]. Some of these carcinomas may be asymptomatic and not identified on imaging [32]. Conservative management includes low-dose prophylactic antibiotics and digital compression of the anterior vaginal wall to produce post-void emptying of the UD to prevent urinary stasis and infection (Fig. 3). Patients should undergo long-term follow-up [1].

Fig. 4 Incision to lay the diverticulum open. (Reproduced from Ref. [35] with permission from Elsevier)

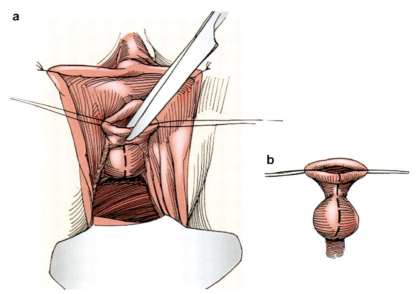

action because of the inevitable consequences in terms of sphincteric damage and the subsequent more complex reconstruction (Fig. 4).

Clearly, the gold standard procedure with results >90% is transvaginal excision of UD with urethral reconstruction [12, 33, 39].

Preoperative Preparation

Preoperatively, as surgery cannot proceed in the presence of an acute UTI, patient's urine should be rendered sterile by administration of culture-sensitive antibiotics, especially in patients with recurrent UTIs. Patients with atrophic vaginitis should be treated preoperatively with the regular application of topical estrogen therapy for several weeks prior to the surgery to improve the quality of tissues at the time of surgery. Patients can also be encouraged to "milk" the diverticulum after voiding to prevent urinary stasis and UTIs, although this may not be possible with patients with pain due to UD or a noncommunicating UD [1].

In order to obtain the best results with urethral diverticulectomy which is technically complex surgery, it is best performed in experienced hands.

To provide optimal exposure at the time of surgery, we would recommend the considerable advantage of carrying out this surgery with the patient placed in the prone position [42].

Preoperative patient counselling is vital to manage expectations over postoperatively outcomes.

Operative Technique

While tissue planes are hard to identify especially in patients with recurrent infections causing tissue fibrosis.

The principles of transvaginal urethral diverticulectomy are those of any reconstructive urological procedure. These are:

- Mobilizing a well-vascularized anterior vaginal wall flap(s).
- Preserving the periurethral fascia and the underlying urethral sphincteric tissues.
- Identifying and excising the UD down to its opening into the urethra (ostium).
- Complete removal of entire UD wall or sac (mucosa) usually piecemeal to preserve sphincteric tissue thereby preserving continence as far as possible.
- Watertight tension-free urethral closure using figure of eight sutures.
- Multilayered closure with absorbable sutures using suture lines that do not overlap.
- Obliteration of dead space during wound closure.

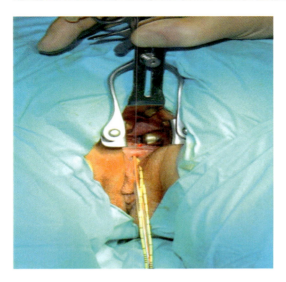

Fig. 5 Access to vagina and urethra of patient in prone position with catheters exiting the external urethral meatus

In our center, we prefer the prone surgical position due to good access especially in patients with more complex and proximal diverticula with full padding of all pressure areas (Fig. 5). Initially the patient is placed in the supine position. A suprapubic catheter is inserted, if desired ureteric catheters are passed (it is impossible to insert these in the prone position). A 16F urethral catheter is introduced. The posterior vaginal wall is retracted with a Parkes anal retractor (as shown in Fig. 6) to gain adequate exposure. Infiltration with a weak adrenaline solution is performed beneath the vaginal mucosa. After marking a U flap on the anterior vaginal wall with the base of the U at the distal urethral meatus and limbs extending towards the bladder neck, an incision is made along these lines (Fig. 7). This incision provides good exposure laterally in line with the mid-vagina and can be extended proximally if needed. By carefully dissecting within the space between the vaginal

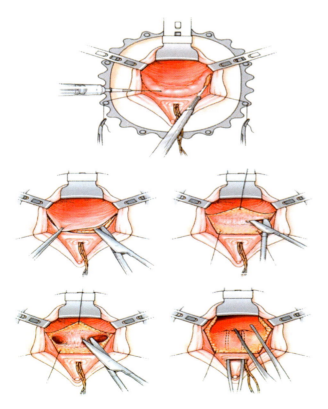
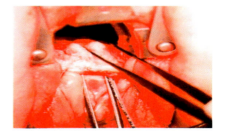

Fig. 6 Surgical technique showing patient in prone position with Parkes retractor in place. A U-shaped vaginal flap is raised with stay sutures to provide good access to the urethral diverticulum

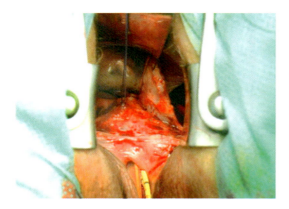

Fig. 7 Raised U-shaped vaginal flap

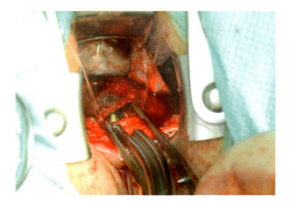

Fig. 8 Urethra open post-diverticulectomy with ureteric and urethral catheters seen in the urethra. Stay sutures in lateral walls of vagina to help with urethral repair and vaginal closure

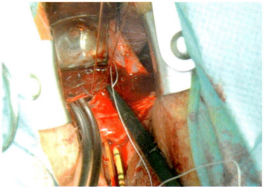

Fig. 9 Figure of eight sutures used for urethral and vaginal closure

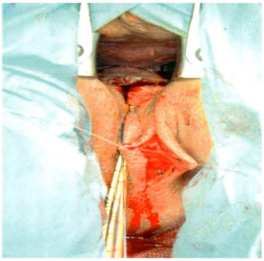

Fig. 10 Left labial incision to harvest a Martius fat pad for grafting

wall and periurethral fascia, a well-vascularized anterior vaginal wall flap is raised.

The periurethral fascia is incised transversely and the proximal and distal layers are carefully developed with a combination of sharp and blunt dissection to avoid inadvertent entry into the UD. Also, this tissue should be preserved as it can be used as another layer of closure. The UD is opened to identify the lumen with a fine suction device and its outline is dissected down to its origin with careful sharp dissection. In most cases, the UD needs to be opened to facilitate dissection, but with smaller lesions, it can be left intact. The mucosal surface of the UD must be removed completely to prevent recurrence [14, 38].

Once the UD is completely excised, the Foley catheter comes into view (Fig. 8). The urethral defect should be closed with 4-0 absorbable suture in a watertight tension-free closure including full-thickness of the urethral wall using figure of eight sutures (Fig. 9). The periurethral flaps are approximated transversely with 3-0 absorbable suture taking care to close all dead space. A Martius flap can be used to cover the urethral closure (Figs. 10 and 11). In our experience, this is only necessary in approximately 15% of cases to help prevent fistulae from forming, where the vaginal tissue and submucosal layers are deficient or where there is a significant dead space.

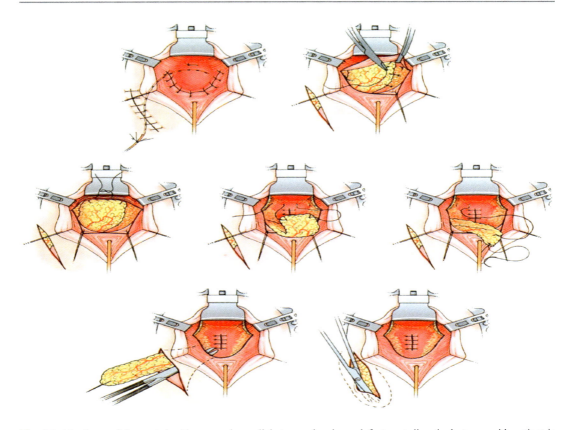

Fig. 11 Martius graft harvested with a vascular pedicle to repair a large defect post-diverticulectomy with patient in prone position

Postoperatively, a vaginal pack is placed which is removed within 24 h. Antispasmodics can be used to treat bladder spasms. We discharge the patient with a urethral and suprapubic catheter which is left in situ for 3 weeks.

Outcomes

Outcomes of this procedure are good with reported cure rates between 84% and 98% [33]. The reoperation rate is 2–13% after primary repair during a mean follow-up of 12–50 months [12, 39–41]. We have reported our outcomes using the modified prone jack-knife position which provides excellent exposure and ergonomics [42].

Early complications include UTI (0–39%), de novo urinary retention (0–9%), and de novo SUI (3.8–33%) [12, 33, 39, 41], whereas delayed complications include urethral stricture (0–5.2%) and fistula (0.9–8.3%) [1].

Conclusion

UD is an uncommon though important cause of LUTS in females that is often overlooked as a potential differential diagnosis. The current gold standard in diagnosis is a post-void MRI. Management is based on the patient's symptomatology and preference. The recommended surgical approach with highest reported cure rates is transvaginal excision and reconstruction. Patient counselling is vital to manage post-op expectations as surgery can cause significant complications such as incontinence, fistula formation, and UD may also recur. We recommend the routine use of the jack-knife procedure. For the rare cases with a dorsal diverticulum, then a supra-urethral surgical approach is recommended.

References

1. Cox L, Rovner ES. Bladder and female urethral diverticula. In: Partin AW, Peters CA, Kavoussi LR, Dmochowski RR, Wein AJ, editors. Campbell-Walsh-Wein urology. Amsterdam: Elsevier; 2020. p. 2964–92.
2. Nitti VW. Urethral diverticulectomy. In: Vaginal surgery for the urologist. Amsterdam: Elsevier; 2012. p. 115–26.
3. Stewart M, Bretland PM, Stidolph NE. Urethral diverticula in the adult female. Br J Urol. 1981;53(4):353–9.
4. Glassman TA, Weinerth JL, Glenn JF. Neonatal female urethral diverticulum. Urology. 1975;5(2):249–51.
5. Marshall S. Urethral diverticula in young girls. Urology. 1981;17(3):243–5.
6. Osman NI, Chapple CR. Urethral diverticula. In: Oxford textbook of urological surgery. Oxford, UK: Oxford University Press; 2017. p. 295–9.
7. Rovner ES. Urethral diverticula: a review and an update. Neurourol Urodyn. 2007;26(7):972–7.
8. Vakili B. Anterior urethral diverticulum in the female: diagnosis and surgical approach. Obstet Gynecol. 2003;102(5):1179–83.
9. Rovner ES, Wein AJ. Diagnosis and reconstruction of the dorsal or circumferential urethral diverticulum. J Urol. 2003;170(1):82–6. Discussion 86
10. Rufford J, Cardozo L. Urethral diverticula: a diagnostic dilemma. BJU Int. 2004;94(7):1044–7.
11. Baradaran N, et al. Female urethral diverticula in the contemporary era: is the classic triad of the "3Ds" still relevant? Urology. 2016;94:53–6.
12. Reeves FA, Inman RD, Chapple CR. Management of symptomatic urethral diverticula in women: a single-centre experience. Eur Urol. 2014;66(1):164–72.
13. Davis BL, Robinson DG. Diverticula of the female urethra: assay of 120 cases. J Urol. 1970;104(6):850–3.
14. Ganabathi K, et al. Experience with the management of urethral diverticulum in 63 women. J Urol. 1994;152 (5 Part 1):1445–52.
15. Leach GE, Bavendam TG. Female urethral diverticula. Urology. 1987;30(5):407–15.
16. Daneshgari F, Zimmern PE, Jacomides L. Magnetic resonance imaging detection of symptomatic non-communicating intraurethral wall diverticula in women. J Urol. 1999;161(4):1259–62.
17. Jacoby K, Rowbotham RK. Double balloon positive pressure urethrography is a more sensitive test than voiding cystourethrography for diagnosing urethral diverticulum in women. J Urol. 1999;162(6):2066–9.
18. Lee JW, Fynes MM. Female urethral diverticula. Best Pract Res Clin Obstet Gynaecol. 2005;19(6):875–93.
19. Keefe B, et al. Diverticula of the female urethra: diagnosis by endovaginal and transperineal sonography. AJR Am J Roentgenol. 1991;156(6):1195–7.
20. Leng WW, McGuire EJ. Management of female urethral diverticula: a new classification. J Urol. 1998;160 (4):1297–300.
21. Leach GE, Sirls LT, Ganabathi K, Zimmern PE. L N S C3: a proposed classification system for female urethral diverticula. Neurourol Urodyn. 1993;12(6):523–31. https://doi.org/10.1002/nau.1930120602.
22. Gonzalez MO, Harrison ML, Boileau MA. Carcinoma in diverticulum of female urethra. Urology. 1985;26 (4):328–32.
23. Hickey N, Murphy J, Herschorn S. Carcinoma in a urethral diverticulum: magnetic resonance imaging and sonographic appearance. Urology. 2000;55(4): 588–9.
24. Marshall S, Hirsch K. Carcinoma within urethral diverticula. Urology. 1977;10(2):161–3.
25. Patanaphan V, et al. Adenocarcinoma arising in female urethral diverticulum. Urology. 1983;22(3):259–64.
26. Rajan N, et al. Carcinoma in female urethral diverticulum: case reports and review of management. J Urol. 1993;150(6):1911–4.
27. Prudente de Toledo W, et al. Carcinoma in diverticulum of female urethra. Urol Int. 1978;33(6):393–8.
28. Seballos RM, Rich RR. Clear cell adenocarcinoma arising from a urethral diverticulum. J Urol. 1995;153 (6):1914–5.
29. Tesluk H. Primary adenocarcinoma of female urethra associated with diverticula. Urology. 1981;17(2):197–9.
30. Thomas RB, Maguire B. Adenocarcinoma in a female urethral diverticulum. Aust N Z J Surg. 1991;61(11): 869–71.
31. Tines SC, Bigongiari LR, Weigel JW. Carcinoma in diverticulum of the female urethra. AJR Am J Roentgenol. 1982;138(3):582–5.
32. Chung DE, et al. Urethral diverticula in women: discrepancies between magnetic resonance imaging and surgical findings. J Urol. 2010;183(6):2265–9.
33. Greiman AK, Rolef J, Rovner ES. Urethral diverticulum: a systematic review. Arab J Urol. 2019;17(1):49–57.
34. Bodner-Adler B, Halpern K, Hanzal E. Surgical management of urethral diverticula in women: a systematic review. Int Urogynecol J. 2016;27(7):993–1001.
35. Freilich, D.A. and Rovner, E.S. (2019) "Female Urethral Diverticulum," in Hinman's Atlas of Urologic Surgery. Amsterdam: Elsevier, pp. 647–654.
36. Roehrborn CG. Long term follow-up study of the marsupialization technique for urethral diverticula in women. Surg Gynecol Obstet. 1988;167(3): 191–6.
37. Spenge HM, Duckett JW. Diverticulum of the female urethra: clinical aspects and presentation of a simple operative technique for cure. J Urol. 1970;104 (3):432–7.

38. Fortunato P, Schettini M, Gallucci M. Diagnosis and therapy of the female urethral diverticula. Int Urogynecol J Pelvic Floor Dysfunct. 2001;12(1):51–7.
39. Crescenze IM, Goldman HB. Female urethral diverticulum: current diagnosis and management. Curr Urol Rep. 2015;16(10):71.
40. Nickles SW, et al. Simple vs complex urethral diverticulum: presentation and outcomes. Urology. 2014;84(6):1516–9.
41. Stav K, et al. Urinary symptoms before and after female urethral diverticulectomy – can we predict de novo stress urinary incontinence? J Urol. 2008;180(5):2088–90.
42. Osman NI, et al. The modified prone Jack-knife position for the excision of female urethral diverticula. Eur Urol. 2021;79(2):290–7.
43. Harding CK, et al. EAU guidelines on non-neurogenic female LUTS. 2022. Retrieved 5 Feb 2023, from https://uroweb.org/guidelines/non-neurogenic-female-luts/chapter/introduction

Part VI

Ureteral Reconstruction

Surgical Reconstruction of Ureteral Defects: Strictures, External Trauma, Iatrogenic, and Radiation Induced

Gillian Stearns and Jaspreet S Sandhu

Contents

Introduction	872
Etiology	872
Nephrolithiasis	872
Radiation	872
Trauma	873
Malignancy	873
Iatrogenic	873
Diagnosis	874
Timing of Repair	874
Preoperative Stenting	874
Treatment	875
Endoscopic	875
Ureteroureterostomy	876
Ureteroneocystostomy	877
Psoas Hitch	877
Boari Flap	878
Transureteroureterostomy	879
Ileal Ureter	880
Robotic and Laparoscopic Approaches	881
Robotic Ureteroureterostomy	881
Ureteroneocystostomy	882

G. Stearns
Carolinas Medical Center, Charlotte, NC, USA
e-mail: gillian.stearns@atriumhealth.org

J. S. Sandhu (✉)
Memorial Sloan Kettering Cancer Center, New York, NY, USA
e-mail: sandhuj@mskcc.org

© Springer Nature Switzerland AG 2023
F. E. Martins et al. (eds.), *Female Genitourinary and Pelvic Floor Reconstruction*,
https://doi.org/10.1007/978-3-031-19598-3_51

Horizons 882
Conclusion 883
References 883

Abstract

Ureteral injury and stricture present a challenge for the urologist, both in terms of identification and repair. Signs of injury and stricture may be quite subtle or develop months after the initial insult. Multiple options are available to the urologist in terms of treatment from endoscopic repair to ureteral reconstruction depending on the location, timing, length, and etiology. It is imperative for the urologist to be facile with the multiple options available as the patient's anatomy or disease may require change in plan during the operation in order to achieve a tension-free anastomosis. In some settings, the ureter may be unable to be reconstructed and options including bowel interposition, autotransplantation, or nephrectomy may need to be considered. This chapter reviews etiology of strictures as well as options for surgical management and possible emerging technologies for repair.

Keywords

Reconstruction · Trauma · Radiation · Nephrolithiasis

Introduction

Ureteral defects, either as a result of trauma, ureteral stones, malignancy, or surgical intervention are a significant source of morbidity for the patient. Although these can be initially managed with percutaneous nephrostomy or ureteral stents, repair is usually needed to help preserve renal function as well as patient health. Left untreated patients can suffer pain, infection, urinoma, renal failure, or, at worst, loss of a renal unit. A variety of etiologies exist, both benign and malignant. Symptoms of a ureteral stricture can be insidious and a high index of suspicion must be held in order to evaluate for ureteral injury. Once the injury is identified, a variety of options are available for the treatment of the defect ranging from stent placement to bowel interposition. A tension-free anastomosis is the hallmark of surgical repair and various techniques can be used to augment repair to help facilitate this.

Etiology

Nephrolithiasis

Impacted stones are a potential source for ureteral stricture. Roberts et al. discovered that an impacted stone for more than 2 months duration is associated with a 24% risk of ureteral stricture [1]. Iatrogenic ureteral injury most commonly occurs during stone extraction in urologic cases and some series reported ureteroscopy as the leading case of ureteral injury [2]. With the decrease in size of endoscopic equipment, increase in flexible ureteroscopy and access sheaths, the rate of ureteral injury has decreased. More recent studies show a rate of ureteral stricture following ureteroscopy at 0.6% [3]. Possible factors leading to ureteral damage include irradiated field, surgeon inexperience, longer surgery times, stone size, and presence of congenital abnormalities [4, 5].

Radiation

Patients who undergo retroperitoneal or pelvic radiation are at higher risk for development of ureteral stricture. Stricture formation secondary to radiation is caused by microvascular injury and stromal fibrosis, leading to fibrosis [6]. It is imperative that tumor recurrence be ruled out as the most common cause of hydronephrosis following treatment of pelvic malignancy is tumor recurrence rather than stricture. Hydronephrosis secondary to radiation-induced stricture tends to develop later compared to tumor recurrence, with one study showing tumor recurrence at a median of 16 months compared to 45 months for a radiation-induced stricture [7]. Overall risk of developing ureteral stricture following radiation for cervical cancer has been shown to be 1.7–2.1% [8].

Trauma

Isolated ureteral injuries are rare. Of all genitourinary injuries, 1–2.5% is ureteral and account for 4% of all penetrating and less than 1% of blunt trauma. Most ureteral trauma occurs from penetrating as opposed to blunt mechanism [9]. Ureteral injuries tend to be subtle and a high index of suspicion is required to avoid a delay in diagnosis. This is further complicated as most of these patients also have concurrent injuries and approximately one-third mortality rate. Greater than 90% of patients with ureteral injury also have an abdominal or visceral injury [9].

The mechanism of ureteral injury in penetrating trauma is twofold. They both directly transect tissue but also disrupt the adventitial blood supply. In ex vivo studies, damage has been found at least 2 cm away from the site of injury [10].

Malignancy

Malignancy is a source of ureteral stricture that should be ruled out before embarking on any form of reconstruction. While the most common malignant etiology of the ureter is upper tract urothelial cancer, other tumors such as breast, prostate, ovarian, colon, and cervical cancer have also led to stricture [11]. Obstruction secondary to malignancy can occur in a variety of fashions. Tumor can directly infiltrate the ureteral lumen, blocking the flow of urine. There can also be extrinsic compression of the ureter from tumor or an adjacent organ, such as colon, ovary, or cervix. Thirdly, edema can induce fibrosis and inflammation leading to ureteral stricture [11].

Iatrogenic

Ureteral injury can occur in urologic, gynecologic, vascular, and colorectal surgeries, as the ureter is in proximity to anatomic structures that are common sites of gynecologic and general surgery, such as gonadal and uterine vessels, the cervix, iliac arteries, inferior mesenteric, and sigmoid vessels as well as colon and rectum [12]. Most ureteral injuries occur due to thermal damage [9].

Gynecologic injuries have accounted for 52–82% of iatrogenic ureteral injuries; however, recent studies show that ureteral injury occurs in approximately 0.3% of gynecologic cases [13, 14]. There is some evidence in the gynecologic literature that a laparoscopic approach may increase the likelihood of ureteral injury. Tanaka et al. reported an increase 2.6 to 35 times the rate of ureteral injury in abdominal hysterectomy, for an overall rate of 0.2–6% [15]. Vaginal hysterectomy is associated with the lowest incidence of ureteral injury, at 0.2 per 1000 cases, although some of this may be related to selection bias [13, 16]. The most common site for injury is near the uterosacral ligaments as visualization can be difficult [9, 13].

Colon and rectal cases account for 9% of ureteral injuries. Abdominal-perineal resection (APR) and low anterior resection (LAR) are the most common cases in which a ureteral injury occurs. The rate of injury is approximately 0.3–5% [13]. Other studies have shown rates of 0.18% [17].

Vascular injuries near the ureters may lead to increased inflammation or devascularization, which can allow for ureteral stricture. This is a process that may be developed over months and may be unrecognized initially. This occurs in approximately 1–2% of procedures [18]. Risk factors associated with ureteral injury during intra-abdominal vascular surgeries include a previously operated field, placement of a graft anterior to the ureter, and large, dilated aneurysms [9].

Ureteral obstruction after urinary diversion (i.e., for cystectomy with ileal conduit for bladder cancer) is usually due to subsequent ureteroenteric strictures [19]. These patients are treated the same as distal ureteral injuries.

Diagnosis

In the setting of iatrogenic injury, ideally the defect is noted still in the operating room. Sadly, approximately 50–70% of ureteral injuries are not identified until after the operation [20]. This is especially true with minimally invasive procedures, so a high index of suspicion must be maintained [21]. Most common presenting symptoms include abdominal pain, port site pain, fever, and leukocytosis [9, 21]. Depending on the nature of the injury, flank pain may or may not be identified. A urinoma may form and present as a flank mass.

The majority of ureteral defects are visualized on computed tomography (CT scans) for varying reasons. CT Urogram is ideal for anatomy as well as visualization of any possible urinary extravasation that usually accompanies ureteral injury. This allows an estimate of the size and length of the stricture, which will play a role in options for management. Ureteroscopy may be required with or without retrograde/anterograde pyelography to further delineate the defect itself. Stent placement can also be attempted at the time of cystoscopy. Renal function should also be assessed, as kidneys with poor function may not improve with a reconstructive repair. If renal impairment is suspected (e.g., atrophy on CT scan), a nuclear renal scan should be performed to adequately determine split renal function.

Timing of Repair

Ideally the ureter is repaired at the time of injury recognition. However, only about 35% are identified at the time of injury [13]. If the ureteral injury cannot be repaired within 2 weeks of the injury, a waiting period of 6 weeks to 3 months is recommended. This is thought to decrease inflammation, edema, fibrosis, and adhesions. Authors have showed identical results with immediate repair [12, 22]. Ahn et al. looked at immediate repair and found that delayed repair did not improve the outcomes of the procedure. Those that underwent repair reported no cases of chronic flank pain, recurrent pyelonephritis, persistent severe hydronephrosis, or compromised renal function. No further intervention was needed in either the late or immediate repair group with a mean follow-up of 32.75 months [23].

However, other surgeons advocate for a period of ureteral rest. A recent article by Lee et al. showed that, in robotic repairs of proximal and mid-ureteral stricture, patients who underwent ureteral rest, described as 4 weeks, managed only with percutaneous nephrostomy tube, did better during their definitive repair. They were less likely to require buccal mucosa grafting. 90.7% of their repairs with ureteral rest were successful at 12 +months follow-up, compared to 77.5% of those patients who did not have ureteral rest [24].

Preoperative Stenting

Some surgical specialties, in particular gynecology and colorectal surgery, have used preoperative ureteral catheterization. It has been shown in other studies that resection of large pelvic masses, prior radiation, malignancy, inflammatory disease, or operating in a previously operated field increase the rate of ureteral injury [25]. The use of the catheters themselves does not appear to avoid ureteral injury, especially in the setting of bleeding, but has helped in the identification of ureteral injury

[26]. In colorectal surgery, a study looked at both open and laparoscopic colectomies. While the rate of ureteral injury was low overall (14/5729), placement of ureteral stents did not appear to help with identifying ureteral injuries [25]. At our institution, we use preoperative stents in cases where the ureter is deviated due to prior surgery or large bulky tumors. We also use them in some cases where significant fibrosis is expected such as those patients with bulky tumors who have undergone neoadjuvant chemoradiotherapy (e.g., large colorectal tumors).

A recent review of the National Surgical Quality Improvement Program (NSQIP) showed a lower rate of ureteral injury post colectomy. However, univariate analysis showed a higher rate of ileus, wound infection, urinary tract infection, and 30-day readmission in patients who had stent placement [27].

Ureteral stents are being used preemptively in some institutions at the time of high-dose vaginal brachytherapy for cervical cancer. This may allow modification of the ureteric dose and improve stricture free rates. Desmanes et al., in a study of 289 patients with cervical cancer, reported a stricture rate of 11% in 255 unstented patients versus a stricture rate of 0% in 34 stented patients [28]. Placement of the stents themselves is not without complications. Anuria has been reported in between 1% and 5% of cases [9]. The rate of ureteral injury during the stent placement itself is approximately 1% [29]. Stent placement itself is not always successful. Therefore, the risks and benefits of ureteral stent placement should be weighed prior to prophylactic usage.

Treatment

Endoscopic

Endoscopic management is a good option for patients in an acute setting or those in poor health. It is a less ideal option for patients with a stricture of >2 cm as it is unlikely these strictures will improve without definitive reconstruction [30].

If the injury is recognized immediately, attempting ureteral stent placement is a reasonable option and may be feasible. If this is not possible, percutaneous nephrostomy tube placement can be done to keep the upper tract drained until definitive management can be planned.

Ureteral dilation is an option for the management of ureteral strictures, which became more popular as endourologic technique and tools have advanced. This may be accompanied by either retrograde or anterograde balloon dilation. In these situations, a pyelogram is performed and a guidewire is introduced. A balloon dilator is advanced over the wire. This dilator is approximately 4 cm long and 5–8 mm in diameter. Proper position is ensured with radio-opaque markers. As the balloon is inflated, a waist will appear at the site of the stricture. This waist will ultimately disappear with continued dilation. The pressure is held for 10 min after which time the balloon is removed and a ureteral stent is placed. This stent is left in place for 2–4 weeks.

Balloon dilation has been found to be best with short, iatrogenic strictures. Success rates for these procedures has varied widely over time from 18% to 83% [31, 32]. A more recent literature review showed a success rate of 60% ± 10% at 3 months and 54% ± 14% at 6–12 months postoperatively [33].

In addition to balloon dilation, some centers will also perform an endopyelotomy with Holmium laser, cold knife, or cutting electrode. This involves making a full thickness incision along the length of the stricture until periureteral fat is seen and including 2–3 mm of normal ureteral tissue. Due to the proximity of the great vessels, care must be taken to avoid vascular injury. In the proximal ureter, this is performed laterally to avoid vascular injury. At the area where the ureter crosses the iliacs, this is performed anteriorly, and medially in the distal ureter [31, 34]. Holmium laser remains the method of choice given the ability to easily manipulate this through a small ureteroscope, the urologist's familiarity with the Holmium laser, as well as the availability of the laser. Objective success with the Holmium laser was seen in a cohort by Gnessin et al. in 26 out of 33 patients [31]. Cold knife endopyelotomy was thought to be attractive given the lack of heat source, thereby minimizing damage to adjacent tissues, with success rates listed between 62% and 80%; however, the knife itself can be difficult to pass through a non-dilated ureter, and therefore tends to be limited to distal ureteral strictures only [31, 34]. Until recently there was a cutting balloon option called Acucise, but it is no longer on the market.

Outcomes

Success rate in these procedures is difficult to standardize as stricture etiology, length of stenting, and length of stricture differ. Most failures were noted within 1 year of intervention [31, 32]. If stricture recurs, repeat endopyelotomy or dilation is not recommended due to low success rates and formal reconstruction is recommended. Radiographic follow-up with diuretic renography is recommended for at least 2 years post procedure [32].

For patients who underwent stent placement, usually further procedures are required. In one study of 25 ureters who had attempted recanalization and stent placement, 18 of 25 were able to be stented, but only 6 had a patent ureter at 13 months, whereas the others required repeat dilation [35].

Ureteroureterostomy

Short defects in the upper two-thirds of the ureter above the iliac bifurcation are appropriate choices for ureteroureterostomy. Ureteroureterostomy is also appropriate for intraoperative consults or in trauma to the ureter. These repairs should be tension free to avoid likelihood of re-stricture, as tension on an anastomosis often leads to stricture. Unfortunately, the surgeon will not know the degree of ureteral mobility until the time of surgery so other options must be considered preoperatively [30].

The ureter, if this is being repaired as a separate surgery, can be approached through a flank, anterolateral, or midline incision. Incision location may be determined by the level of the defect. The ureter can be identified either extra- or transperitoneally. If the ureter is difficult to identify, it can be found reliably as it crosses the iliac artery bifurcation. Once the ureter is found, it should be freed up and mobilized, either bluntly or sharply, taking care to preserve as much surrounding tissue as possible to avoid disruption of the adventitia, which may disrupt ureteral blood supply. If the ureter has been transected iatrogenically or divided secondary to penetrating trauma, both ends of the ureter must be identified. In the setting of ureteral stricture, the diseased segment is excised after ureteral mobilization. The anastomosis must be created with healthy, well-vascularized tissue. Once the stricture has been removed, stay sutures of a 4-0 or 5-0 are placed at each end of the ureter. If the ureteral length is insufficient, the kidney itself may be mobilized and a nephropexy performed.

The ends of the ureter should be cut obliquely to allow for a wide anastomosis. The ureteral ends may also be spatulated 180° apart to help facilitate the repair. In patients with injury secondary to electrocautery or missile injuries, extensive debridement should be performed as tissue devitalization may continue after the injury. Once the ends are prepared, sutures of 4-0 or 5-0 absorbable suture are used through the apex of the spatulated ureter and out through the middle of the non-spatulated side of the opposite ureteral end. The knots should be tied outside the lumen of the ureter. The two sutures should be placed 180° apart and held to help facilitate the repair. The anastomosis can be completed in either a running or interrupted fashion on one side and then rotated to perform the anastomosis on the other side. Placement of a double-J stent should be done prior to the completion of the anastomosis. Once the repair is complete, omentum can be wrapped around the ureter to help facilitate healing, particularly in patients with history of radiation, concomitant bowel or pancreatic injuries, or vascular grafts. The stent usually remains in place 2–4 weeks postoperatively [36].

Ureteroneocystostomy

For defects in the distal third of the ureter, ureteroneocystostomy is preferred. This may be performed in isolation or with the addition of a psoas hitch or Boari flap to help ensure a tension-free anastomosis.

It is usually best to approach the ureter from above the affected portion and progress distally. The ureter is then dissected as far as possible distally into the healthy ureteral portion to maximize length. Care should be taken to avoid disruption of the ureteral adventitia and ureteral blood supply during ureteral dissection. If the ureter has been injured iatrogenically, especially during attempts to ligate internal iliac vessels, the ureteral blood supply may be more tenuous than expected [13].

Anastomosis can be either refluxing or non-refluxing, although most use a refluxing method after a higher incidence of stricture was found leading to decreased renal function. The neocystostomy should be performed on the anterior or posterior portions of the bladder rather than the lateral sides to avoid kinking with bladder filling (Fig. 1).

Psoas Hitch

If additional length is needed and the ureter will not reach sufficiently, a psoas hitch can be performed. This procedure was first described by Zimmerman et al. in 1960 [37]. The psoas hitch may provide up to 5 cm of length in addition to a ureteroneocystostomy and allow mobilization of the bladder above the level of the iliac bifurcation, but a psoas hitch alone may not be sufficient if the defect extends above the level of the pelvic brim [36]. The bladder must also have sufficient mobility, so a small, contracted bladder is a relative contraindication [30].

The procedure can be approached either through a lower midline of Pfannenstiel approach. In order to help facilitate bladder mobility, the peritoneum should be dissected off the bladder dome and the space between the rectum and bladder developed. The superior vesical pedicles can be ligated contralaterally or bilaterally. Contralateral mobilization of vasculature should be minimized, if possible should be avoided in cases where the ipsilateral internal iliac artery has previously been ligated (e.g., in the setting of prior resection of large ipsilateral pelvic tumors). The bladder is then opened at its widest point transversely. The bladder should be distended prior to selecting cystotomy site, because too small of a

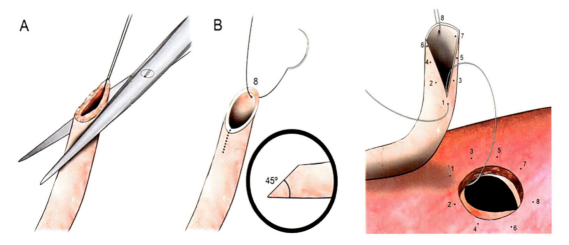

Fig. 1 This illustrates how to spatulate the ureter as well as how to perform an interrupted anastomosis, ensuring that all knots are located on the outside of the ureter so as not to disrupt the repair or lead to stone formation. (Illustration courtesy of Simon Kimm, MD)

cystotomy will limit bladder mobility and therefore the length of the defect that can be covered. The bladder should be opened slightly more than half the circumference of the bladder. The bladder is then brought to the psoas muscle at a level superior and lateral to the iliac bifurcation. This can be accomplished by placing two fingers inside the bladder. A stay stitch can be placed through the ureter to determine if the anastomosis would be tension free. If further ureteral length is required, proximal mobilization of the ureter or opening the contralateral endopelvic fascia may help. The bladder is then fixed to the psoas minor tendon or psoas major muscle with three to six 2-0 absorbable sutures. Care must be taken to avoid entrapment of the genitofemoral nerve, which has been noted post-procedurally, especially if sutures are placed too deeply into the muscle.

Once the sutures are placed but prior to tying these down, the site of the ureteroneocystostomy should be selected. Ideally the ureter is anastomosed at an immobile portion of the bladder to avoid intermittent obstruction with bladder filling. The ureter is pulled into the bladder using a stay suture and can be trimmed once obvious that adequate ureteral length is present. A refluxing anastomosis is appropriate in most adults. The ureter is spatulated anteriorly and is anastomosed to the bladder using interrupted 4-0 or 5-0 absorbable sutures. A ureteral stent is placed prior to completion of the anastomosis. A Foley catheter is usually kept to gravity drainage to allow for healing of the cystotomy for at least 7–10 days. Cystogram may be performed prior to catheter removal [36] (Fig. 2).

Boari Flap

The Boari flap was first described by Boari in 1894 in a canine model and first used in a patient in 1936 to close a significant ureteral defect [38]. It allows the bridging of up to 15 cm of ureteral defects provided adequate bladder capacity exists. Occasional reports have described the flap being able to reach the renal pelvis. The initial approach, bladder mobilization, and ureteral dissection are identical to the approach for the psoas hitch described above.

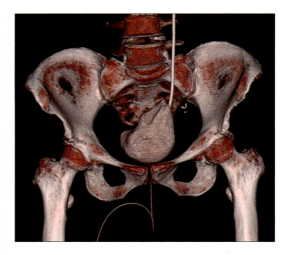

Fig. 2 This CT Urogram reconfiguration was performed post psoas hitch and illustrates the appearance of the bladder and ureter post-reconstruction. The bladder has been elevated almost to the level of the pelvic inlet

The Boari flap is used in addition to a psoas hitch to help decrease the length of the Boari flap needed. After bladder mobilization and psoas hitch, the site for the base of the flap is identified. Again, this should be on a fixed portion of the bladder. The base of the flap should be approximately 3–5 cm wide. If a longer flap is necessary, the base should be wider in order to ensure adequate blood supply. The length of the flap is measured. A stay suture is placed in each end of the flap apex and then the flap is developed using electrocautery. The flap is then brought to the ureter, which is then anastomosed apex either directly or in a tunneled fashion. A stent is placed across the defect. The bladder is then closed and the flap rolled into a tube over the stent using a running 3-0 absorbable suture on the mucosa and interrupted 2-0 absorbable stitch on the muscular and adventitia. A drain is placed and cystogram is performed prior to removal of ureteral and urethral catheters [36].

Outcomes

Wenske et al. looked at the functional outcomes of patients who underwent open ureteroneocystostomy for both benign and malignant obstruction. Resolution of hydronephrosis was noted in 81% of patients with a median follow-up of 48.7 months. Only 39% of these patients had a malignant etiology, most commonly transitional cell carcinoma. In this study, malignancy was not found to be an adverse indicator of continued poor renal function [39]. Van den Heijkant showed that while there was a higher immediate complication rate in patients who underwent ureteroneocystostomy with psoas hitch, most did not require surgical reintervention and were only transient in nature. Also noted was no change in oncologic outcome [40]. This was also echoed in the gynecologic literature. In a study of 46 women who underwent ureteroneocystostomy with or without psoas hitch, a higher rate of complications was noted in patients that had received prior radiation, but overall the outcomes allowed for a successful reconstruction with negative surgical margins [41]. In patients with malignant obstruction, ureteroneocystostomy was found to be a durable and effective option for management of stricture. As noted in the prior manuscript [41], patients who underwent radiation, in particular salvage or palliative radiation, were at a higher risk of failure [42].

In iatrogenic injuries, similar results have been found. One study of iatrogenic general surgical and gynecologic injury showed no adverse events with a median follow-up of 33 months [43].

Transureteroureterostomy

If ureteral length is insufficient to reach the bladder, a transureteroureterostomy may be performed. To perform a transureteroureterostomy, a transperitoneal midline approach is used to gain access to both ureters. The bowel is reflected and packed superiorly. The ureters are usually visualized as they pass over the iliac vessels. The retroperitoneum can be accessed in one of two ways: two separate incisions over each individual ureter as they cross the iliacs, or a single curved incision can be made beginning over the left distal ureter across the midline along the small bowel mesentery up the right line of Toldt. This second option allows for more extensive bowel mobilization.

Mobilization of the ureters should be kept to a minimum to avoid disruption of the adventitial blood supply. If further mobilization is needed the ipsilateral gonadal vessel can be ligated. After dividing the affected ureter as distally as possible, a tagging suture is placed on the distal aspect of the divided ureter to allow the ureter to pass through a retroperitoneal tunnel. Attention should be turned to the affected ureter as it passes through to avoid any kinking or twisting of the ureter, and ensuring that no tension is placed on the ureter. The tunnel should be made superiorly to the inferior mesenteric vessels as placement below this may lead to ureteral kinking [30, 36].

A vertical ureterotomy is made at least 1.5 cm in length on the anteromedial portion of the healthy ureter. Stay sutures may be used distal to the level of the anastomosis on the unaffected ureter to allow for touch-free ureteral manipulation. The affected ureter is spatulated unless it is sufficiently dilated. The anastomosis is performed using 4-0 or 5-0 sutures in either a running or interrupted fashion. Prior to completion of the anastomosis, a ureteral stent is typically placed and may help with the anterior wall anastomosis.

The patient should undergo renal ultrasound and/or diuretic renal scan to assess function and drainage of the kidney approximately 2 months postoperatively. Immediate postoperative complications include urinoma, pyelonephritis, prolonged anastomotic drainage, and recurrent stricture. Risk of these complications is elevated by excessive ureteral mobilization or prior radiation [36]. Later complications include small bowel obstruction, stone disease leading to obstruction of the common ureteral segment, late ureteral obstruction secondary to tumor recurrence, or compression of the affected ureter by the inferior mesenteric vessels.

The only absolute contraindication to transureteroureterostomy is insufficient ureteral length, both on the affected as well as the recipient side. Approximately one-half of the original ureteral length is required for a transureteroureterostomy to be feasible [43]. Relative contraindications include disease processes, which affect the contralateral renal unit such as a history of nephrolithiasis, retroperitoneal fibrosis, urothelial malignancy, chronic pyelonephritis, and a history of abdominopelvic radiation [30, 43].

Outcomes

Pisters et al. looked at the safety and feasibility of transureteroureterostomy in patients undergoing multiple organ resection. Patients showed stable renal function with a median follow-up of 15 months. Three out of twelve patients had a cancer recurrence leading to recurrent hydronephrosis and need for reintervention [44]. Another study showed that transureteroureterostomy is technically feasible; however, it does carry a higher risk of complications, occurring in approximately 24% of patients. The most common complication noted was urine leak. Ten percent of patients required reintervention for obstruction with a mean follow-up of 6 years [45].

Ileal Ureter

In instances where the bladder is insufficient for Boari flap or the defect is unable to be corrected with other reconstructive approaches, ileal interposition remains an option for management.

Prior to the procedure, a mechanical or antibiotic bowel prep may be used. A midline or flank incision can be used to access the affected ureter. If a flank incision is used, the incision should begin between the 11th and 12th ribs, continue toward the midline, and end as a paramedian incision. The peritoneum is entered and the small bowel packed away from the operative field. The ipsilateral colon is reflected superior-medially and the affected ureter is identified. The affected portion of the ureter is dissected to the level of healthy tissue, potentially up to the renal pelvis. The peritoneum should be mobilized away from the dome and lateral bladder. The length of ileum should be selected for ureteral replacement.

The ileal segment should be selected from the preterminal ileum. The dissection should be deep enough from the proximal end to reach the renal pelvis and the distal end to reach the bladder. The bowel is divided and the remaining bowel is restored to continuity in the same fashion as is done for an ileal conduit. The mesenteric defect is closed to prevent internal hernia formation. The mesentery of the ascending colon is incised and the ileal segment was passed into the retroperitoneum. The ileal segment is rotated to place the distal end near the bladder and the proximal end near the proximal edge of the defect. The mesenteric defect is again closed, taking care not to compress or kink the mesenteric vessels.

The proximal opening of the ileal segment is closed, usually with a running 3-0 Vicryl. Prior to completion of the anastomosis, a double-J stent is placed and the ileoureteral anastomosis of the spatulated ureter is performed in a single layer, either in an interrupted or running fashion in an end-to-side anastomosis (i.e., "Bricker"). 4-0 or 5-0 Vicryl is typically used for the anastomotic stitch. If the entire ureter is unable to be used, the renal pelvis will be opened widely and an end-to-end anastomosis is used. If the renal pelvis is small, the ileum may require tapering. To do this, the proximal opening of the ileum is partially closed on the anti-mesenteric side. The pyeloileal anastomosis is also performed in one layer with either running or interrupted sutures.

The ileocystostomy is performed beginning on the posterior bladder wall approximately 1–2 cm above and lateral to the native ureteral orifice. This helps to avoid kinking and possible obstruction during bladder filling. The bladder is opened anteriorly along the midline and a section of bladder is removed in the area of intended anastomosis. The anastomosis is performed in two layers with a running mucosal apposition suture and interrupted seromuscular-detrusor suture.

Early complications from surgery may include obstruction secondary to mucus plug, edema, or a kink. Other early complications may include urinoma formation or urinary extravasation. If preoperative renal function is normal, metabolic anomalies are uncommon [46].

In a patient who develops a progressively dilated ileal segment with worsening metabolic abnormalities, bladder outlet obstruction should be ruled out. Some case reports have identified malignancy developing in the intestinal segments [46]. Some experts recommend endoscopic surveillance beginning 3 years after surgery.

Contraindications to ileal interposition include a baseline creatinine of greater than 2 mg/dL, as the ileum will absorb urine and in those patients with baseline renal failure ultimately developed hyperchloremic metabolic acidosis [47]. Other contraindications include bladder outlet obstruction, inflammatory bowel disease, or radiation enteritis [30]. Urodynamics can be considered prior to surgery to evaluate for possible obstruction. If necessary, bladder outlet obstruction procedures should be performed prior to reconstruction [46]. Some patients may need to self-catheterize if they are unable to empty their bladder completely after an ileal ureter interposition.

Outcomes

A large series of patients who underwent ileal ureter showed 75% of patients had a stable creatinine at 36 months. Common adverse effects included fistula and anastomotic stricture. No patients complained of excess mucus production [48]. Another recent study showed patients did well immediately postoperatively with postoperative complications including urine leak, wound infection, and low grade fever, but these were limited to Clavien-Dindo Grade 1 and 2. One patient died 15 months postoperatively of fulminant hepatitis. The remaining patients had a median follow-up of 68 months and one patient reported a paraumbilical hernia. Otherwise, 10/36 patients reported one incidence of urinary tract infection. 4/36 had deterioration of renal function as determined by decreasing eGFR and decreased renographic clearance. Three of these patients had baseline moderate to severe chronic kidney disease and the fourth had prolonged urinary leakage in the early postoperative period [49].

Robotic and Laparoscopic Approaches

As urologists have become more facile and comfortable with minimally invasive techniques, minimally invasive ureteral repairs are being utilized with increasing frequency. The first ureteral repairs were described in 1993 with laparoscopy in pediatric patients with vesicoureteral reflux [50]. Since the first published case by Youannes et al. in 2001, ureteroneocystostomy for stricture disease has been occurring robotically with increasing frequency [51]. Benefits include decreased blood loss, improved cosmesis, and decreased length of hospital stay [52].

Ureteral identification can be challenging in a minimally invasive setting without the tactile feedback present in open cases. This can be compounded in situations with inflammation where surgical planes may be distorted. Assessment of preoperative imaging and clamping of the Foley catheter with or without administration of a diuretic may help with ureteral distension and increased peristalsis; it may help to identify the ureter more easily. Indocyanine green has also been used to identify the extent of a stricture.

In a malignant setting, large ureteral masses are usually easily identifiable. In the setting of a smaller ureteral mass, maneuvers such as concurrent ureteroscopy may be helpful to the surgeon to isolate the affected area and minimize the resection of healthy tissue to help facilitate repair [52].

Robotic Ureteroureterostomy

Robotic ureteroureterostomy is performed with the patient in a 60° flank position without any flexion of the table to minimize anastomotic tension. The ipsilateral arm is secured to the patient's side to prevent robotic arm interference. Ports are placed along the lateral border of the rectus muscle in a straight line configuration. A 12 mm camera port is placed at the level of the 11th rib and 2–8 mm ports are placed, one at the level of the anterior superior iliac spine and one two finger breadths below the costal margin. If necessary, an additional port can be placed near the xiphoid to help facilitate liver retraction and one or two assistant ports can be placed between the three primary ports. The robot is docked perpendicular to the patient.

After the colon is reflected and Gerota's fascia is entered, the ureter and gonadal vein are identified. The ureter is carefully dissected and once the stricture isolated, it is transected. The scar is resected to healthy, bleeding margins. The distal ureter is spatulated laterally and proximal ureter is spatulated medially, opposite to the site of the segmental blood supply. The anastomosis is performed using a 4-0 polyglactin suture in an interrupted fashion. Two polyglactin sutures may be placed in the periureteral tissues to help decrease tension. After the anastomosis of the posterior wall is performed, a double-J stent is placed with the aid of a guidewire. The remainder of the anastomosis is completed over the stent. Gerota's fascia is then closed over the repair. This prevents bowel adhesion and contains any possible urine leaks into the retroperitoneum [52].

Outcomes

Several cases of robotic ureteroureterostomy have been reported, both in adult and pediatric literature. Among adult patients, successful repair has been reported in post-ureteroscopy ureteral stricture and post-segmental resection for upper tract urothelial carcinoma [53, 54]. In a comparison of laparoscopic to robotic ureteroureterostomy, Sun et al. found equivalent outcomes between those undergoing robotic and those undergoing laparoscopic reconstruction. The robotic group reported decreased length of stay and mean operative time [55].

Ureteroneocystostomy

Ureteroneocystostomy is performed transperitoneally. Patient positioning and port placement are similar to the ureteroureterostomy described above, but may vary slightly between surgeons. The posterior peritoneum is incised over the iliac vessels and the ureter is isolated. A vessel loop is passed around the ureter to help with ureteral manipulation. The bladder itself is not mobilized initially in order to allow for improved traction during ureteral dissection [52]. Once the ureter is appropriately dissected, the ureter is transected proximally to the diseased segment. A clip can be placed on the ureter if resection is being performed secondary to malignancy to prevent cancerous cells from seeding the peritoneal cavity.

The bladder is then mobilized by dividing the urachus and opening the space of Retzius. The bladder can be filled with 200–300 ml to help facilitate dissection. To ensure a tension-free anastomosis, several maneuvers can be used. The bladder can be mobilized from the anterior abdominal wall with incision of the peritoneum lateral to the medial umbilical ligaments. The urachus can be divided. The contralateral superior vesicle vascular pedicle can be ligated in order to help mobilize the bladder further. As in open repair, a psoas hitch or Boari flap can be utilized to help with bridging the defect. The area around the ureteral stump is scored and ultimately dissected out if this is being performed for an oncologic etiology. If it appears a tension-free anastomosis cannot be completed with ureteroneocystostomy alone, a psoas hitch or Boari flap can be performed. Reimplantation is performed on the posterior wall of the bladder lateral to the dome. A stent is placed in a retrograde fashion. The mucosa of the bladder and ureter are anastomosed. This is usually performed in at least two layers to allow for watertight closure. Patients are usually left with the stent and Foley catheter postoperatively to keep the bladder decompressed to facilitate healing.

Outcomes

A study by Lee et al. of 3 patients showed the feasibility of performing robotic ureteroneocystostomy in the adult population. No stricture recurrence was noted at a median of 2 years postoperatively [56]. These findings were also found in studies by Patil et al. and Wason et al. [57, 58]. In a comparison between open, laparoscopic and robotic ureteroneocystostomy, Elsamra et al. analyzed over 100 open, laparoscopic and robotic cases and the outcomes were found to be the same across the three groups, but the minimally invasive options had lower blood loss and a decreased hospital stay [59].

Horizons

With the success of buccal mucosa being used in the treatment of urethral strictures, it has also begun to be used in the treatment of ureteral defects beginning with the first repair documented in 1999 by Naude [60]. The advantages that allow it to be easily used in urethral repair carry over to the use of ureteral repair including thick epithelium and highly vascular lamina propria [52]. Zhao et al. reported a 90% success rate using buccal mucosa in a multi-institutional study [61].

Conclusion

While ureteral injury and stricture can be a source of significant distress and morbidity for the patient, multiple modalities exist to help temporize and treat the defect, hopefully serving to protect the renal unit and maximize renal function in both the short- and long-term setting.

References

1. Roberts W, Caddedu J, Micali S, et al. Ureteral stricture formation after removal of impacted stone. J Urol. 1998;159:723.
2. Roberts DB, Pearl M. Complications of ureteroscopy. Urol Clin North Am. 2004;31:157.
3. El-Abd A, Suliman M, Farha M, et al. The development of ureteric strictures after ureteroscopic treatment for ureteric calculi: a long-term study at two academic centers. Arab J Urol. 2014;12:168.
4. Huffman JL. Ureteroscopic injuries to the upper urinary tract. Urol Clin North Am. 1989;16:249.
5. Bas O, Tuygun C, Dede O, et al. Factors affecting complication rates of retrograde flexible ureteroscopy: analysis of 1571 procedures-a single center experience. World J Urol. 2017;35:819.
6. Tran H, Arsovska O, Paterson R, et al. Evaluation of risk factors and treatment options in patients with ureteral stricture disease at a single institution. Can Urol Assoc J. 2015;9:E921.
7. McIntyre J, Eifel P, Levenback C, et al. Ureteral stricture as a late complication of radiotherapy for stage IB carcinoma of the uterine cervix. Cancer. 1995;75:836.
8. Fokdal L, Tanderup K, Potter R, et al. Risk factors for ureteral stricture after radiochemotherapy including image guided adaptive brachytherapy in cervical cancer: results from the EMBRACE studies. Int J Radiat Oncol Biol Phys. 2019;103:887.
9. Brandes S, Eswara J. Upper urinary tract trauma. In: Wein AJ, Kavoussi LR, Campbell MF, Walsh PC, editors. Campbell-Walsh urology. Philadelphia: Elsevier; 2020.
10. Amato J, Billy L, Gruber R, et al. Vascular injuries. An experimental study of high and low velocity missile wounds. Arch Surg. 1970;101:167.
11. Vasudevan V, Johnson E, Wong K, et al. Contemporary management of ureteral strictures. J Clin Urol. 2019;12:20.
12. Gild P, Kluth L, Vetterlein M, et al. Adult iatrogenic ureteral injury and stricture – incidence and treatment strategies. Asian J Urol. 2018;5:101.
13. Burks F, Santucci R. Management of iatrogenic ureteral injury. Ther Adv Urol. 2014;6:115.
14. Wong J, Bortoletto P, Tolentino J, et al. Urinary tract injury in gynecologic laparoscopy for benign indication: a systematic review. Obstet Gynecol. 2018;131:100.
15. Tanaka Y, Asada H, Kuji N, et al. Ureteral catheter placement for prevention of ureteral injury during laparoscopic hysterectomy. J Obstet Gynaecol Res. 2008;34:67.
16. Elliott S, McAninch J. Ureteral injuries: external and iatrogenic. Urol Clin North Am. 2006;33:55.
17. Eswara J, Raup V, Potretzke AM, et al. Outcomes of iatrogenic genitourinary injuries during colorectal surgery. Urology. 2015;86:1228.
18. Brandes S, McAninch J. Reconstructive surgery for trauma of the upper urinary tract. Urol Clin North Am. 1999;26:183.
19. Amin K, Vertosick E, Stearns G, et al. Predictors of benign uretero-enteric anastomotic strictures after radical cystectomy and urinary diversion. Urology. 2020;144:225.
20. Ostrzenski A, Radolinski B, Ostrzenka K. A review of laparoscopic ureteral injury in pelvic surgery. Obstet Gyneol Surv. 2003;58:794.
21. Parpala-Sparman T, Paananen I, Santala M, et al. Increasing number of ureteric injuries after the introduction of laparoscopic surgery. Scand J Urol Nephrol. 2008;42:422.
22. Ambani S, Skupin P, Małaeb B, et al. Does early ureteroneocystostomy after iatrogenic ureteral injury jeopardize outcome? Urology. 2020;136:245.
23. Ahn M, Loughlin L. Psoas Hitch reimplantation in adults – analysis of a modified technique and timing of repair. Urology. 2001;58:184.
24. Lee Z, Lee M, Lee R, et al. Ureteral rest is associated with improved outcomes in patients undergoing robotic ureteral reconstruction of proximal and middle ureteral strictures. Urology. 2021;152:160.
25. Palaniappa N, Telem D, Ranasinghe N, et al. Incidence of iatrogenic ureteral injury after laparoscopic colectomy. Arch Surg. 2012;147:267.
26. Chou M, Wang C, Lien R. Prophylactic ureteral catheterization in gynecologic surgery: a 12-year randomized trial in a community hospital. Int Urogynecol J. 2009;20:689.
27. Coakley K, Kasten K, Sims S, et al. Prophylactic ureteral catheters for colectomy: a national surgical quality improvement program-based analysis. Dis Colon Rectum. 2018;61:84.
28. Desmanes D, Banerjee R, Cahan B, et al. Ureteral stent insertion for gynecologic interstitial high-dose-rate brachytherapy. Brachytherapy. 2015;14:245.
29. Bothwell W, Bleicher R, Dent T. Prophylactic ureteral catheterization in colon surgery. A systematic review. Dis Colon Rectum. 1994;37:330.

30. Nakada S, Best S. Management of upper urinary tract obstruction. In: Wein AJ, Kavoussi LR, Campbell MF, Walsh PC, editors. Campbell-Walsh urology. Philadelphia: Elsevier; 2020.
31. Gnessin E, Yossepowitch O, Holland R, et al. Holmium laser endoureterotomy for benign ureteral stricture: a single center experience. J Urol. 2009;182:2775.
32. Wolf J, Elashry O, Clayman R. Long-term results of endoureterotomy for benign ureteral and ureteroenteric strictures. J Urol. 1997;158:759.
33. Lu C, Zhang W, Peng Y, et al. Endoscopic balloon dilatation in the treatment of benign ureteral strictures: a meta-analysis and systematic review. J Endourol. 2019;33:255.
34. Meretyk S, Albala D, Cayman R, et al. Endoureterotomy for treatment of ureteral strictures. J Urol. 1992;147:1502.
35. Koukouras D, Petsas T, Liatsikos E, et al. Percutanous minimally invasive management of iatrogenic ureteral injuries. J Endourol. 2010;24:1921.
36. Glenn G. Ureteral stricture. In: Glenn J, Keane T, Brendler C, et al., editors. Glenn's urologic surgery. Philadelphia: Lippincott Williams & Wilkins; 2004.
37. Zimmerman I, Precourt W, Thompson C. Direct uretero-cysto-neostomy with the short ureter in the cure of ureterovaginal fistula. J Urol. 1960;83:115.
38. Graziano M, Thompson P. The story of the Boari flap. J Urol. 2008;179:309.
39. Wenske S, Olsson C, Benson M. Outcomes of distal ureteral reconstruction through reimplantation with Psoas Hitch, Boari flap, or ureteroneocystostomy for benign or malignant ureteral obstruction or injury. Urology. 2013;82:231.
40. Van den Heijkant F, Vermeer T, Vrijhof E, et al. Psoas hitch ureteral reimplantation after surgery for locally advanced and locally recurrent colorectal cancer: complications and oncological outcome. Eur J Surg Oncol. 2017;43:1869.
41. Federico A, Gallotta V, Foscha N, et al. Surgical outcomes of segmental ureteral resection with ureteroneocystostomy after major gynecologic surgery. Eur J Surg Oncol. 2020;46:1366.
42. Paick J, Hong S, Park M, et al. Management of postoperatively detected iatrogenic lower ureteral injury: should ureteroureterostomy really be abandoned? Urology. 2006;67:237.
43. Crissell M, Rushton H. Transureteroureterostomy. In: Glenn J, Keane T, Brendler C, et al., editors. Glenn's urologic surgery. Philadelphia: Lippincott Williams & Wilkins; 2004.
44. Pisters P, Pettaway C, Liu P, et al. Is transureteroureterostomy performed during multi-organ resection for non-urothelial malignancy safe and effective? J Surg Oncol. 2012;106:62.
45. Iwaszko M, Krambeck A, Chów G, et al. Transureteroureterostomy revisited: long-term surgical outcomes. J Urol. 2010;183:1055.
46. Grimm MO, Ackerman A. Ureteral reconstruction. In: Glenn J, Keane T, Brendler C, et al., editors. Glenn's urologic surgery. Philadelphia: Lippincott Williams & Wilkins; 2004.
47. Austen M, Kalble T. Secondary forms of malignancy in different forms of urinary diversion using isolated gut. J Urol. 2004;172:831.
48. Armatys S, Mellon M, Beck S. Use of ileum as ureteral replacement in urological reconstruction. J Urol. 2009;181:177.
49. Ali-el-Dein B, El Hafnawy A, D'Elia G, et al. Long-term outcome of Yang-Monti Ileal ureter: a technique suitable for mild, moderate loss of kidney function and solitary kidney. Urology. 2021;152:153.
50. Atala A, Kavoussi L, Goldstein D, et al. Laparoscopic correction of vesicoureteral reflux. J Urol. 1993;150:748.
51. Yohannes P, Gershbaum D, Rotariu P. Management of ureteral stricture disease during laparoscopic ureteroneocystostomy. J Endourol. 2001.15:839.
52. Andrade H, Kaouk J, Zargar H, et al. Robotic ureteroureterostomy for treatment of a proximal ureteric stricture. Int Braz J Urol. 2016;42:1041.
53. Raheem A, Alatawi A, Kim D, et al. Feasibility of robot-assisted segmental ureterectomy and ureteroureterostomy in patient with high medical comorbidity. Int Braz J Urol. 2017;43:779.
54. Sun G, Yan L, Ouyang W, et al. Management for ureteral stenosis: a comparison of robotic-assisted laparoscopic ureteroureterostomy and conventional laparoscopic ureteroureterostomy. J Laparoendosc Adv Surg Tech A. 2019;29:1111.
55. Babbar P, Yerram N, Sun A, et al. Robot-assisted ureteral reconstruction – current status and future directions. Urol Ann. 2008;10:7.
56. Lee D, Schwab C, Harris A. Robotic-assisted ureteroureterostomy in the adult: initial clinical series. Urology. 2010;75:570.
57. Patil N, Mottrie A, Sundaram B, et al. Robotic-assisted laparoscopic ureteral reimplantation with psoas hitch. A multi-institutional, multinational evaluation. Urology. 2008;72:47.
58. Wason S, Lance R, Given R, et al. Robotic-assisted ureteral re-implantation: a case series. J Laparoendosc Adv Surg Tech A. 2015;25:503.
59. Elsamra S, Theckumparampil N, Garden B, et al. Open, laparoscopic, and robotic ureteroneocystostomy for benign and malignant ureteral lesions: a comparison of over 100 minimally invasive cases. J Endourol. 2014;28:1455.
60. Naude J. Buccal mucosa grafts in the treatment of ureteric lesions. BJU Int. 1999;83:751.
61. Zhao L, Weinberg A, Lee Z, et al. Robotic ureteral reconstruction using buccal mucosa grafts: a multi-institutional experience. Eur Urol. 2017;73:419.

Techniques of Ureteral Reimplantation

51

Andrew Lai, Rabun Jones, Grace Chen, and Diana Bowen

Contents

Introduction	886
Endoscopic Management	887
Open Ureteral Reimplant Techniques	887
Indications and Preoperative Considerations	887
General Approach	888
Open Ureteral Reimplant (Fig. 1)	888
Psoas Hitch (Fig. 2)	890
Boari Flap (Fig. 3)	891
Minimally Invasive Ureteral Reimplant	893
Special Consideration: Ureteroneocystostomy with Tapering (Fig. 5)	894
Postoperative Management	895
Complications	895
Anti-Refluxing Techniques	895
Indications and Preoperative Considerations	896
Intravesical Techniques	896
Patient Positioning	896
Initial Dissection	896
Mobilizing the Ureter	896
Cross-Trigonal (Cohen) Ureteral Reimplantation (Fig. 6)	897
Intraextravesical (Politano-Leadbetter) Technique	898
Ureteral Advancement (Glenn-Anderson) Technique	898
Other Techniques	898
Spatulated Nipple Technique	899
Closing the Bladder	899
Extravesical Ureteral Reimplantation	899

A. Lai · R. Jones · G. Chen
Department of Urology, University of Illinois at Chicago, Chicago, IL, USA

D. Bowen (✉)
Department of Urology, Northwestern University Feinberg School of Medicine, Chicago, IL, USA
e-mail: diana.bowen@nm.org

Patient Positioning and Dissecting Down to the Bladder 899
Open Lich-Gregoir Technique (Fig. 7) 899
Using a Laparoscopic or Robotic Approach for Extravesical Reimplantation (Fig. 8) ... 900
External Tunnel (Barry) Technique 901
Detrusorrhaphy (Hodgson-Firlit-Zaontz) Technique 902
Intraextravesical Technique (Paquin) 902
Postoperative Management 902
Complications 902
Obstruction 902
Persistent or Recurrent Vesicoureteral Reflux 903

Special Considerations 903
Reoperation 903
Duplication Anomalies 903
Transplant Kidney Ureteroneocystostomy 904
Reimplant into Bowel Segment 904

References 905

Abstract

Ureteral reimplantation (ureteroneo-cystostomy) is a reconstructive operation during which the distal ureter is reimplanted into the bladder. The most common indications for this surgery are ureteral obstruction, trauma, and vesicoureteral reflux. A basic understanding of ureteral reimplantation is crucial as the surgery is often performed on an urgent or emergent basis. The surgery may be performed via an open, laparoscopic, or robotic approach, and further characterized by an intra- or extravesical approach. A key additional feature is whether a refluxing or anti-refluxing anastomosis is performed. There is limited data on head-to-head comparisons among individual techniques and ultimately the choice is dependent on patient factors, surgeon experience, and the clinical scenario. Relatively few robust studies have been performed in the adult population, and much of the data are extrapolated from the pediatric literature.

Keywords

Ureteroneocystostomy · Ureteric reimplantation · Hydronephrosis · Ureteral injury · Ureteral stricture · Ureteral trauma · Inadvertent ureteral ligation · Ureteral reconstruction · Psoas hitch · Boari flap

Introduction

Ureteral reimplantation (or ureteroneocystostomy) is a broad term for a reconstructive operation that has multiple indications for it as well as a diverse array of techniques that fall under it. The process of removing and then reimplanting the ureter into the bladder includes several variations in technique, but the degree of difficulty and need for delicate tissue handling remains high regardless. A reconstructive surgeon's armamentarium must include a basic ureteral reimplantation foundation of knowledge as often times the surgery is performed on an urgent or emergent basis.

The major difference between the array of techniques lies in the etiology of the problem and characteristics of the patient – is it an obstructive phenomena or refluxing? Was there an intraoperative injury to the ureter during a pelvic surgery that cannot be managed conservatively? What is the age and health status of the patient? Obstruction and reflux can also coexist, most often in children, and so a careful preoperative history and radiologic investigation is imperative. Although obstruction or ureteral injury are more common reasons for reimplantation in adulthood, there are also cases of symptomatic reflux that present at this time, whether congenital or from a prior surgical intervention (such as a kidney transplant).

This chapter will cover the myriad of techniques for ureteral reimplantation and the clinical scenarios in which one would consider each option. Traditional open surgery for both refluxing and anti-refluxing anastomoses are the cornerstone of ureteral reimplantation, but minimally invasive techniques incorporating these fundamentals have evolved and now play an important role in the urologists' armamentarium. In addition, there are several special considerations that will be discussed at the end of the chapter.

Endoscopic Management

Although not the focus of this chapter, consideration should always be given to less invasive possibilities for management. Ureteral stent placement often precedes a ureteral reimplantation if obstruction of the ureter is diagnosed. In many cases of iatrogenic ureteral injury, especially in ureteroscopy, a ureteral stent can be placed and allow complete healing. However in more severe trauma or obstruction, this is a temporary management paradigm as it would require ureteral stent changes every few months to prevent infection and stone formation. This is most commonly employed in patients who are not fit for major reconstructive surgery, or with an ongoing pelvic disease process. Some distal ureteral strictures, however, can be managed with balloon dilation or incision of the UVJ. Balloon dilation of non-malignant strictures less than 2 cm has been shown effective in case series with success rates ranging from 57% to 89% over short-term follow-up [1, 2]. Endoureterotomy via cold knife incision, electrocautery, or laser excision for these types of strictures have also seen success rates from 60% to 86% [3]. Longer strictures (> 2 cm) have seen abysmal rates less than 40%. Overall, long-term success rates are unclear due to the paucity of high-quality evidence [4].

In cases of vesicoureteral reflux that leads to febrile urinary tract infection, endoscopic injection of bulking agents around the ureteral orifice has been performed for many years. Early injection materials were Polytetrafluorethylene (Polytef™) and Tegress™/Uryx™ (ethylene vinyl alcohol copolymer; however long-term results were poor and migration of the particles was seen [5, 6]. Dextranomer Hyaluronic acid (Deflux™), a cross-linked polysaccharide, has emerged as a viable option currently and has seen encouraging success rates as the technique has been disseminated. In the pediatric population, the double hydrodistention-implantation technique (Double HIT) using Deflux™ has been shown to be successful in the long term for reducing febrile urinary tract infections [7]. However the degree of reflux on preoperative evaluation is of utmost importance as success rates tend to decrease with increasing grade [8, 9]. Some literature suggest that clinically meaningful success rates remain high [10]. Importantly, the outcomes regarding endoscopic injection for reflux in adults is extrapolated from the pediatric experience as it has not been studied robustly in adults.

Open Ureteral Reimplant Techniques

Indications and Preoperative Considerations

Indications for ureteroneocystostomy vary and include ureteral trauma, ureteral stricture, malignancy, ureterovaginal fistula, and less commonly a congenital obstruction (megaureter). Ureteral strictures may occur due to radiation or complications from prior surgery, or following a kidney transplant from various factors (see section on "Kidney Transplant Ureteroneocystostomy"). In general, ureteral reimplantation can be accomplished as a refluxing technique – without a detrusor tunnel – as most adult patients will not be at high risk for ascending urinary tract infections. For ureteral reimplantation with the primary indication of febrile urinary tract infections, and vesicoureteral reflux, see section on "Anti-Refluxing Techniques."

When performed electively, obtaining and reviewing preoperative cross-sectional abdominal and pelvic imaging is essential. Computed tomography or magnetic resonance imaging with an excretory phase is preferable. Considerations of the etiology of the initial injury should be made, as the ureteral blood supply and history of pelvic radiation or surgery may increase the complexity of the case as well as inform the approach used. Often in cases of elective reimplant, the initial injury or obstruction has been acutely relieved with a nephrostomy tube or an indwelling ureteral stent. Depending on clinical circumstance, the surgeon may elect to remove the ureteral stent several weeks preoperatively to decrease inflammation. Some have advocated that removal of the foreign body decreases inflammation and, in the setting of strictures, allows the diseased segment of the ureter to fully mature. Removal of the indwelling stent should not come at the cost of renal injury secondary to re-obstruction. For planning purposes, retrograde and/or antegrade ureterograms should be obtained to assess the exact location and length of the ureteral defect, and to rule out concomitant ureteral problems. If the kidney has been chronically obstructed and appears to have poor renal parenchyma, a diuretic renal scan to understand the differential function (ideally with the nephrostomy tube open) can help determine if the kidney should be salvaged. In cases of pelvic radiation or preexisting bladder concerns, a cystogram with or without urodynamic testing may be obtained to ensure there is sufficient bladder capacity and safe detrusor pressures especially if a psoas hitch or boari flap are being considered.

Ureteral reimplantation may be necessary intraoperatively in cases of iatrogenic ureteral injury in pelvic surgery, or acute trauma. In these situations, when timely diagnosis and management is prudent, the surgeon should assess stability of the patient and whether the reimplant can be accomplished via the mode of the original surgery (i.e., laparoscopic or robotic) or if one should favor an open surgical approach, especially if other concurrent injuries are discovered or the pelvic anatomy is not favorable.

General Approach

Ureteral surgery requires delicate tissue handling to preserve the blood supply and ensure a healthy anastomosis. Ureteral reimplantation is typically performed by dismembering the ureter from the native ureterovesical junction of the bladder, or wherever the site of obstruction is located, and reattaching it in a different location, most often the dome of the bladder. Ureteral reimplant is an appropriate choice if there is a diseased segment of the mid-to-distal third of the ureter, either at the time of the initial insult or in a delayed manner. Although ureteroureterostomy is an appropriate choice for mid to proximal ureteral strictures, distal pathology is best handled with reimplantation into the bladder as the distal ureteral stump is at risk for devascularization. After resection of the diseased segment or transection of the ureter, ureteral mobilization is performed to ensure a tension-free anastomosis into the bladder. For injuries involving the distal 3–4 cm of the ureter, ureteral reimplantation can usually be accomplished alone. If this cannot be performed, a psoas hitch with or without an accompanying Boari-Ockerblad flap, is necessary to bridge the gap. Generally, a psoas hitch should suffice if the defect falls distal to the pelvic brim, as the psoas hitch technique can provide up to 5 additional centimeters of length when compared to primary ureteral anastomosis alone. The Boari flap can be used to overcome a defect between ureter and bladder of up to 10–15 cm in length [1]. Relative contraindications to these measures include known malignancy of the bladder, a small capacity or contracted bladder, irradiated bladder, and poor bladder function. In these cases, the bladder pathology should be addressed prior to definitive management of the ureter to ensure the risk of complications is minimized.

Open Ureteral Reimplant (Fig. 1)

The patient is positioned supine or if rigid cystourethroscopy is planned during the surgery, the patient is positioned in dorsal lithotomy. If retrograde pyelography was not performed preoperatively, it is done at the start of the case and at that time a small caliber open-ended catheter may be passed over a wire to help with identification of the ureter, assuming the obstruction is not complete, or can be left in the distal ureter up to the level of obstruction. Leave the bladder distended with the foley clamped to facilitate initial bladder dissection. If the reimplant is being performed due

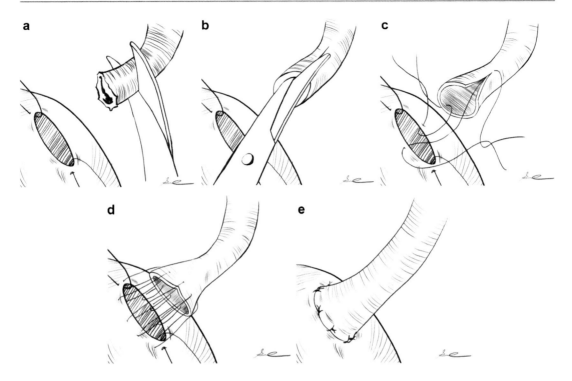

Fig. 1 Open ureteral reimplant. (**a**) Freshen the edge of the ureter. (**b**) Spatulate the ureter. (**c**) The first two sutures, held for traction. (**d**) Completing the approximation with interrupted sutures (indwelling ureteral stent not pictured). (**e**) Complete maturation of the anastomosis

to iatrogenic injury, the original laparotomy incision is utilized.

Either a Pfannensteil or a low midline incision below the umbilicus is made, and a foley catheter should be placed and accessible on the surgical field to allow for intraoperative distension of the bladder. Dissection is carried down through Campers and Scarpa's fascia to the anterior rectus sheath using blunt and electrocautery dissection. The anterior rectus sheath, composed of the aponeurosis of the external and internal oblique muscles, can then be dissected either transversely or longitudinally depending on the skin incision. Incise the transversalis fascia at its midline between the bellies of the rectus muscle. Enter the space of Retzius and develop this space bluntly, mobilizing the lateral bladder walls. Place a self-retaining retractor and retract the bladder gently to the opposite side of the injury for exposure.

Attention is then turned to the ureter. The dissection may be continued extraperitoneally to identify the ureter. Alternatively, and if a longer length of ureter needs to be mobilized, open the peritoneum. Determine if the colon needs to be medialized for visualization. Open the retroperitoneum at the level of the iliac vessels. Using anatomic landmarks of the psoas muscle and/or the gonadal vessels can assist in identifying the ureter. Once identified, gently free it from the surrounding structures by lifting up on the adventitia and coming around it with a fine right angle. Encircling the ureter with a vessel loop then assists with traction. Take caution in minimizing trauma to the vasculature surrounding the healthy ureter. The ureter should always be mobilized with a healthy amount of intact periureteral tissue. Dissect down to the ureterovesical junction and the area of injury. The distal ureteral stump is then suture ligated with a 2–0 or 3–0 absorbable suture or surgical clips, and the proximal ureter is freed. At this time, determine if the length of ureter if sufficient for reimplant alone and that the segment for reimplant appears healthy.

Ureteroneocystostomy can be performed via an extravesical technique without opening the bladder, or intravesically by making a sagittal incision in the bladder and choosing the location of the neo-orifice subsequent to this. If reimplanting extravesically, remove any perivesical fat in the future location of the neo-orifice to prepare for the new hiatus. Make a 1–2 cm incision through the serosa and detrusor muscle on the superolateral aspect of the bladder dome. Dissect down through the seromuscular layer, but do not yet incise the mucosa. Prepare the ureter by ensuring the edges appear healthy and then perform spatulation for approximately 1–2 cm using Potts scissors (Fig. 1). Make a small buttonhole in the bladder mucosa and drain the bladder contents. If performed without a detrusor tunnel, then place an apical 4–0 or 5–0 interrupted monofilament suture (e.g., PDS) from the detrusor muscle and mucosa of the bladder to the distal extent of the ureter as a full thickness bite. This is followed by a second suture from the spatulated crotch of the ureter to the bladder neo-orifice opposite the first. Holding up on these first two sutures for traction, continue placing interrupted monofilament sutures of detrusor muscle and mucosa to the ureter. Insert the indwelling double-J ureteral stent once half of the anastomosis has been completed. If a detrusor tunnel (anti-refluxing mechanism) is planned and the ureter can reach a site further than the dome under no tension, then the anastomosis of the ureter is to bladder mucosa only, following by a detrusor tunnel over it. This technique is described later. If intravesical, close the cystostomy in two layers of 3–0 running polyglactin suture. Confirm a watertight anastomosis by irrigating the bladder.

Psoas Hitch (Fig. 2)

When the distal third of the ureter is not suitable for direct reimplant due to injury or poor tissue quality, the bladder can be brought cephalad to meet the ureter by performing a psoas hitch. This technique involves mobilizing the dome of the bladder and anchoring it to the psoas muscle, and may be performed alone or as an adjunct to other complex reconstructive techniques (e.g., Boari flap –described below, transureteroureterostomy, or ileal ureter substitution).

To perform the psoas hitch, there are no additional considerations with regard to patient positioning, especially when performed concurrently with another pelvic surgery. After ligating the ureter and determining the length available, then mobilize the bladder enough to ensure that the dome of the bladder can reach the level of the iliac vessels. This may require ligation of the round ligament in females, and attention to the vas deferens in males. Approximate the distal ureteral stump and the bladder using holding sutures to ensure that the anastomosis will remain tension-free. Then, identify the genitofemoral nerve within the psoas muscle to avoid injury or entrapment from suture placement. Place several 2–0 interrupted polyglactin sutures from the psoas muscle to the detrusor muscle of the dome of the bladder, taking care to prevent mucosal perforation (Fig. 2). These are placed in a vertical orientation along the fibers of the psoas tendon, taking care to avoid the genitofemoral and the ilioinguinal nerves. Do not tie down these sutures until a tension-free ureterovesical anastomosis can be ensured. Place an indwelling ureteral stent of appropriate size. The ureter is then anastomosed to the superolateral aspect of the bladder dome. Although at this point a refluxing or anti-refluxing anastomosis can be performed (see individual procedure sections for technique), typically in this case where a psoas hitch has to be employed, there is not enough length to accomplish this safely.

If the bladder has been opened with an anterior cystostomy for an intravesical approach, the bladder dome can be elevated from within using one's finger. Some surgeons utilize this approach to a psoas hitch in order to gain tactile feedback on any tension left on the bladder.

Benefits of the psoas hitch over the Boari flap include technical simplicity, minimal or no need for dissection or ligation of vesical vascular supply, ease of future endoscopic surveillance and manipulation, and fewer voiding difficulties [11]. Psoas hitch may not be a suitable option for a small, contracted bladder, as it may not have the mobility needed to reach the psoas muscle.

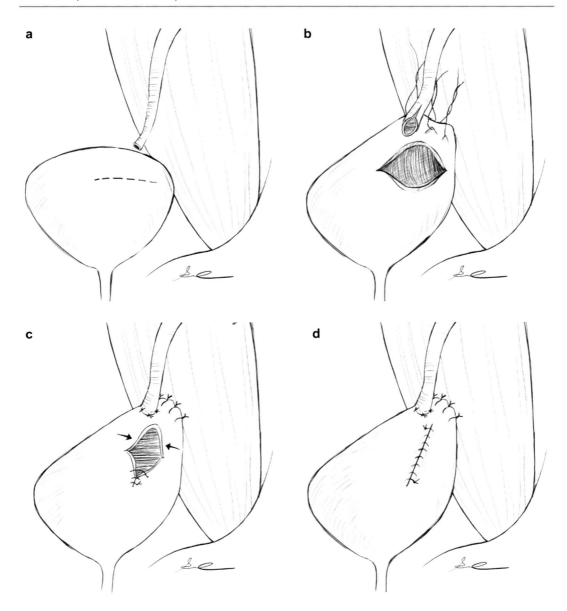

Fig. 2 Psoas hitch. (**a**) Anticipated cystotomy marked with proximal ureter prepared. (**b**) Interrupted sutures approximating the psoas muscle with the seromuscular layer of the bladder. (**c**) Ureteral stent placement after maturation of the ureteral neo-orifice (not pictured). (**d**) Closure of the cystotomy in two layers

Boari Flap (Fig. 3)

If more mobility is necessary despite ureteral and bladder mobilization, a Boari flap can be considered. When performed open it may be ideal to perform this as an extraperitoneal approach. This may not be possible however in cases of ureteral fibrosis or recent intra- or transperitoneal intervention. If there is significant fibrosis, a retroperitoneal approach can risk injuring the iliac vein, and an intraperitoneal approach may be required. If beginning in an extraperitoneal fashion, the peritoneum should be mobilized medially near the site of the defect, with care is taken to also medialize either the vas deferens or the round ligament and identify healthy ureter proximal to the defect.

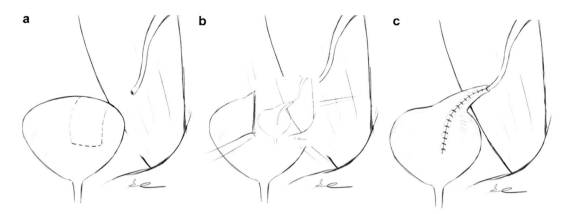

Fig. 3 Boari flap. (**a**) Planning the flap on the bladder. (**b**) Incision and tubularization of the flap with ureteral reimplantation. (**c**) Closure of the cystotomy

Peritoneum should then be divided and mobilized from the posterolateral bladder in order to begin preparing a flap; this peritoneal tissue can be used to cover the Boari flap anastomosis at the conclusion of the procedure, or omentum can be brought down. The ureter is prepared by excising the diseased portion, spatulating the healthy end, and placing a fine (4–0 polyglactin) stay suture at the distal aspect of healthy spatulated ureter. In order to fully mobilize the bladder toward the affected side, the contralateral side's superior vesical pedicle may be divided. If needed, in very rare cases, the inferior vesical pedicle may also be divided to allow for full mobility.

The bladder should then be instilled with 250–300 cc of sterile saline via the foley catheter, and a measuring tape can be used to evaluate the distance from the distal aspect of the healthy ureter to the posterior bladder wall, as well as to help plan the flap outline on the bladder. The width of the flap should be 4 cm at the base to minimize the risk of ischemia, and at least 3 cm at the apex to avoid excessive compression of the ureter. The length from the flap base to apex should cover the distance of the ureter-to-bladder defect, plus an additional 3–4 cm if a non-refluxing or tunneled anastomosis is needed (this is covered in detail in the following sections). The ratio of bladder flap length to base should adhere to the principle of 3:1 or smaller to prevent flap ischemia. Once the flap is planned and marked with a marking pen or cautery, the four corners of the flap are marked with 3–0 Vicryl stay sutures (Fig. 3). Cystotomy may be made with cutting current, beginning along the apex (distal) edge of the flap. A 5-French open-ended catheter or feeding tube may be placed in the contralateral ureter in order to protect against injury during closure of the flap.

At this time, the surgeon may elect to perform a psoas hitch in conjunction with the boari flap, which relieves tension from the ureterovesical anastomosis and can make it technically more straightforward. Using a finger through the existing cystotomy, the ipsilateral posterior bladder wall is elevated toward the psoas tendon and hitched in place with 2–0 polyglactin sutures. After performing a psoas hitch, the spatulated distal ureteral stump and superior edge of the bladder flap are anastomosed with multiple interrupted 4–0 or 5–0 absorbable sutures.

After completing the ureterovesical anastomosis but prior to approximating the tube portion of the Boari flap, a wire is placed gently into the new ureteral orifice and used to guide a double- J stent into the renal pelvis. The stent should be of adequate length so that the distal curl of the stent lies in the dependent portion of the bladder. The contralateral 5-Fr. feeding tube or ureteral catheter may be removed. The bladder tube is then closed in the standard two-layered fashion: running 4–0 polyglactin to close mucosa and interrupted or running 3–0 polyglactin to reapproximate muscularis and adventitia. The integrity of the closure can be assessed by instilling sterile saline into the bladder. The previously dissected peritoneum can be secured around the ureterovesical anastomosis for further coverage. Additionally, the superior edge of the Boari flap may be approximated to the adventitia of the distal ureter with 4–0 polyglactin suture.

Minimally Invasive Ureteral Reimplant

Ureteral reimplantation and the associated ancillary techniques of psoas hitch and Boari flap can also be performed via minimally invasive techniques. The exact approach is dictated by the situational context of the injury, timing of diagnosis, surgeon experience, and patient-specific factors. Given the delicate tissue handling and suturing required, robotic assistance when available is helpful above traditional laparoscopic capabilities. When performed robotically, the patient may be positioned supine or in dorsal lithotomy, with or without a bump placed under the affected side's hip. The patient must be secured to allow for steep Trendelenberg positioning to assist in moving the bowel contents away from the pelvis. Trocars include a 12 mm camera port at an infraumbilical or supraumbilical site, two 8 mm assistant robotic ports, each placed 8 cm lateral from the umbilicus, a fourth 8 mm robotic port placed on the pathologic side 3 cm above the iliac crest (optional), a 12 mm assistant port placed on the contralateral side 3 cm above the iliac crest, and if needed, an additional 5 mm assistant port triangulated between the camera port and the 8 mm robotic port (Fig. 4). The nondominant robot arm houses a bipolar Maryland forceps, the dominant arm contains the monopolar scissors or hook, and the fourth robotic arm (if used) may contain the Prograsp or Cadiere forceps (Intuitive Surgical Sunnyvale, Calif.).

Several intraoperative considerations should be appreciated when compared to an open approach. During ureteral identification and dissection, the use of a hook can be an atraumatic tool for handling

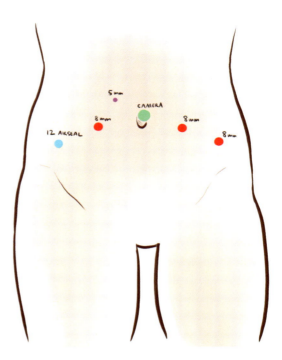

Fig. 4 Robot arm placement using da Vinci Xi system

of the ureter. Additionally, a vessel loop wrapped around the ureter can provide traction when approaching the ureterovesical junction. The use of monofilament suture is preferred, although absorbable V-lock sutures can be used if the ureteral anastomosis is planned to be made in running fashion and can facilitate holding tension.

In situations of suspected vascular compromise or complex anatomy, a tool within the robotic approach is the use of indocyanine green (ICG)-enhanced fluorescence, a technique that has gained popularity across surgical specialties and particularly in urologic surgery [12]. Intraureteral injection of ICG has been shown as an alternative to an indwelling ureteral stent to assist in the identification of the ureter, given that tactile feedback is very limited with the robotic approach. While this gives direct visual feedback of the location of the ureter, it does require preoperative planning. ICG may also be given intravenously to assess for ureteral viability. Currently, only small studies have evaluated its use, and none offer strong evidence over standard or lighted ureteral stents [13].

There has been recent literature describing a non-transecting robotic reimplant with side-to-side ureteral anastomosis that has shown promising results in small case series [14]. This technique avoids extensive posterior dissection of the ureterovesical junction and thus decreases risk of vascular compromise. Intravenous ICG is utilized to demonstrate good blood supply to the proximal ureter. A ureterotomy is made proximal to the diseased segment followed by the cystotomy. The anastomosis is then run with two monofilament sutures, with an indwelling ureteral stent placed after one side of the anastomosis is complete. This technique is usually paired with psoas hitch and/or Boari flap to relieve tension on the anastomosis. Because of the long anastomosis, lower rates of anastomotic stricture have been suggested.

Special Consideration: Ureteroneocystostomy with Tapering (Fig. 5)

Severely dilated ureters may present a challenge for reimplanation given the wide caliber. A persistent megaureter from childhood or a new process causing obstruction may cause the ureter to become tortuous and redundant. In these cases, tapering (tailoring) of the distal ureteral segment can facilitate urine propulsion and prevent reflux by allowing the ureter to be tunneled into the bladder. These cases can be done both open and robotic. If a stent is able to be placed prior to surgery, this is helpful. The megaureter is identified and dissected down to the UVJ. The ureter is transected at the point of obstruction; this site can be utilized for the neo-orifice in most cases as the ureter is redundant with sufficient length. The ureter is then straightened and a red

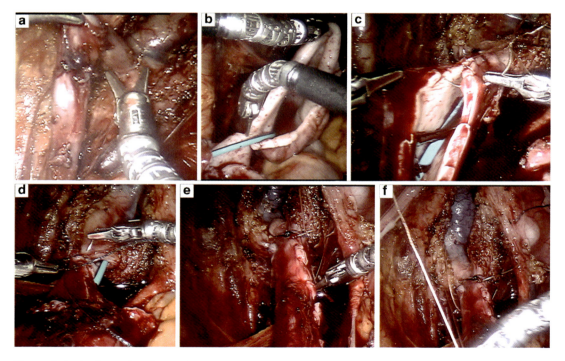

Fig. 5 Robotic dismembered tapered tunneled ureteral reimplant using V-lock. (**a**) Dissect the ureter to the UVJ or site of obstruction. (**b**) Assess the megaureter with stent in place, consider adding an additional 10 Fr catheter for sizing. Excise excess ureter. (**c**) Perform an interrupted anastomosis of the distal most ureter to narrow the lumen of the ureter for reimplantation. (**d**) Place the ureteral stent into the neo-orifice and perform the ureteral-bladder anastomosis – in this case a running V-lock was used to help keep tension and avoid the need for placement of additional ports. (**e**) Complete the ureteral tapering. (**f**) The detrusor tunnel has been prepared (blue mucosa) and the now-tapered distal ureter (see below) will next be secured within the detrusor tunnel

rubber catheter or 10 Fr tube can be placed adjacent to the ureteral stent to help estimate the degree of tailoring necessary. Excisional tapering is then performed by trimming the ureter for approximately 5–6 cm (Fig. 5). The incisions should gently flare back out proximally so there is not an abrupt transition of ureteral caliber. If there is concern for blood supply in this ureter, then the redundant ureteral wall can be folded in and plicated. However in most cases, excisional tapering is reasonable. The ureter is then reapproximated with interrupted sutures at the distal extent, to allow for further trimming if necessary. This is done with a 4–0 or 5–0 absorbable monofilament suture. The rest of the anastomosis may be run. The additional feeding tube or catheter is then removed. The ureteral stent is inserted into the bladder and the ureter is then anastomosed to the bladder mucosa of the natural orifice with either interrupted sutures or a running monofilament or V-lock. A detrusor tunnel is then made in standard fashion and the ureter placed into the tunnel. Caution should be emphasized to not obstruct the ureter given its width even despite the tapering. The stent is left in for several weeks and the catheter should be left for 3–5 days.

Postoperative Management

Following any type of ureteroneocystostomy, a closed suction drain is placed in the pelvis, away from the ureterovesical anastomosis. A foley catheter is left in place in addition to a double-J stent. The drain is typically removed prior to the patient's discharge home, however a drain fluid creatinine may be sent for analysis prior to removal. If the drain creatinine is elevated and there is concern for a urine leak, prolonged drainage with the foley catheter and pelvic drain should be undertaken. In the absence of a known leak, typically the foley catheter remains until a cystogram is performed to confirm integrity of the repair, which may be done 10–14 days postoperatively. If the repair is more difficult than typical, a Boari flap is utilized, the patient has comorbidities that suggest poor wound healing such as diabetes mellitus, or if the tissue is irradiated, the drains should be kept longer. If the cystogram is negative for anastomotic leak, the foley may be removed with subsequent removal of the ureteral stent between 4 and 8 weeks postoperatively.

Complications

Common complications of dismembered ureteral reimplant include hematuria, infection, and bladder spasms, however, the most common problem seen is urinary leak. Typically, these resolve with conservative management and prolonged urinary drainage or diversion. If a urinoma is suspected, radiographic imaging can be utilized and drainage of the urinoma may be indicated if the patient is symptomatic or if infection is suspected. Long-term complications include recurrent obstruction, de novo vesicoureteral reflux, and changes in bladder function. Follow-up imaging with renal bladder ultrasonography should be obtained in all patients to monitor for re-obstruction, with diuretic renography utilized if there is concern. If patients develop a pattern of febrile urinary tract infections, then voiding cystourethrogram can be obtained to rule out vesicoureteral reflux.

Anti-Refluxing Techniques

While the typical adult ureteral reimplantation occurs due to obstruction or injury and can safely be performed without a lengthy detrusor tunnel, the most common indication for an anti-refluxing ureteral reimplantation is definitive correction of vesicoureteral reflux (VUR). Other indications include conditions commonly found in the pediatric age group – obstructing megaureter, ureterocele, and ectopic ureter. If the surgery is performed to prevent infections, then a detrusor tunnel should be created to pin the ureter within it. Importantly, the previous surgical techniques described can all be done with the addition of a detrusor tunnel to mitigate post-operative VUR, however this does require more ureteral length.

Many techniques have been described in the last several decades specifically to correct VUR, and can be categorized generally by intravesical or extravesical approach.

Indications and Preoperative Considerations

Vesicoureteral reflux is diagnosed on voiding cystourethrogram (VCUG) where it is important to assess both the filling and voiding phases, as well as the capacity of the bladder and any urethral abnormalities that may be apparent. Patients with recurrent, febrile urinary tract infections or those with scarring of the kidneys are candidates for these procedures. Vesicoureteral reflux in adults is unlikely to resolve as it does in childhood. Careful thought must be given to the pros and cons of performing this surgery open or with robotic assistance, based on patient factors and body habitus, grade of reflux, and comfort of the surgeon.

Prior to performing a unilateral anti-refluxing reimplant for primary vesicoureteral reflux, assessment of contralateral ureteral reflux should be made. In the pediatric literature, new contralateral reflux after unilateral repair can be found in 6–18% [15]. Although risk of contralateral reflux exists, it is reasonable to only perform unilateral reimplant as the likelihood of significant clinical effects from contralateral VUR is very low. Just as in refluxing techniques, the bladder is important to understand and assess for any neuropathic changes. In a very small, contracted bladder, creating a tunnel that is long enough may prove challenging. In these cases, and if the reflux is low grade, endoscopic injection may be warranted.

Principles of ureteral reimplantation are to correct vesicoureteral reflux and prevent ureteral obstruction. To accomplish this, adherence to Paquin's 5:1 ratio of ureteral tunnel length to ureteral diameter has been recommended [16]. Recent modeling, however, has suggested that the ratio may be an overestimate of needed tunnel length [17].

Intravesical Techniques

There are many intravesical techniques that have been described to correct reflux. The most commonly performed are the Cohen, Politano-Leadbetter, and Lich-Gregoir, which are described below as well as highlighting several others. The initial approach is similar and described separately.

Patient Positioning

The patient should be placed in supine position with a soft pelvic bump underneath. If cystourethroscopy is planned prior, the patient should be placed in dorsal lithotomy position with option to reposition after foley catheter placement. The patient should be scrubbed with antimicrobial scrub from mid-thigh up to the umbilicus.

Initial Dissection

To gain access to the bladder, begin with a low transverse or Pfannenstiel incision along Langer's lines, approximately 1 cm above the pubic symphysis. Dissect down to the anterior rectus sheath and open the fascia in a transverse curvilinear fashion. Incise the transversalis fascia at its midline between the bellies of the rectus muscle, carry the dissection down to the pubis. Place a self-retaining retractor or ring retractor such as the Dennis-Browne retractor. Enter the space of Retzius and develop this space bluntly. Expose the bladder by removing any perivesical fat. Distend the bladder with a transurethral foley catheter for better visualization. Incise the bladder with a vertical incision distally until a few centimeters from the bladder neck and place a large stay suture to secure the apex. Open the bladder proximally enough to visualize the bladder floor but keep the dome intact to facilitate retraction. Secure the bladder with stay sutures or Allis clamps. Adjust the self-retaining retractor such that cranial retraction is achieved at the dome of the bladder with several moistened sponges.

Mobilizing the Ureter

Begin by intubating the ureter with a 5 fr feeding tube, and secure it to the bladder mucosa just adjacent at the ureteral orifice with a 4–0 polyglactin suture. Inject 1:100,000 lidocaine with epinephrine just under the mucosa around the orifice. Score the bladder mucosa circumferentially with bovie electrocautery around the ureteral orifice. Keeping tension on the feeding tube, mobilize the ureter circumferentially by insinuating a clamp or tenotomy scissors between the ureter and its bladder attachments. Once the initial bands have been lysed and correct plane is found, the end of the dissection can be done bluntly with a peanut to ensure the vas deferens and peritoneum are not pulled up into the field. The ureter is considered adequately mobilized when it can reach the skin level. Close the detrusor muscle defect with interrupted 3–0 vicryl suture, ensuring that the hiatus is not too tight. Closing the hiatus too tightly about the ureter can result in ureteral obstruction from kinking or ischemia that leads to stricture formation. In cases of significantly dilated tortuous ureters, the dissection can also be done extravesically to develop a straight length of the ureter.

Cross-Trigonal (Cohen) Ureteral Reimplantation (Fig. 6)

The cross-trigonal (Cohen) ureteral reimplantation technique, described in 1975, has historically been the most common approach to ureteral reimplantation for vesicoureteral reflux in the pediatric population. After adequate mobilization of the ureter, a submucosal tunnel is created across the trigone resulting in the new ureteral orifice localized just above the contralateral ureteral orifice. Using sharp dissection to establish the correct plane just under the bladder mucosa, create the submucosal tunnel from the hiatus of the ipsilateral ureter to the point planned to be the new ureteral orifice. This point should be just cephalad to the contralateral ureteral orifice and in keeping with the 5:1 rule. The mucosa over the neo-orifice site is incised and a vessel loop can be passed through the tunnel to hold traction upward and allow passage of a right angle clamp toward the old hiatus and ureter. Then the ureter is mobilized with feeding tube through the submucosal tunnel and mature the ureterovesical anastomosis. Close the floor of the posterior wall of the hiatus, followed by the mucosa overlying it.

To mature the ureterovesical anastomosis, first trim the ureteral edge and consider a slight spatulation. Place anchoring interrupted 4–0 polyglactin or chromic stitches at the 4- and 6-o'clock positions to approximate the detrusor muscle and mucosa to the transmural ureteral tissue. Then continue to reapproximate the ureter full thickness

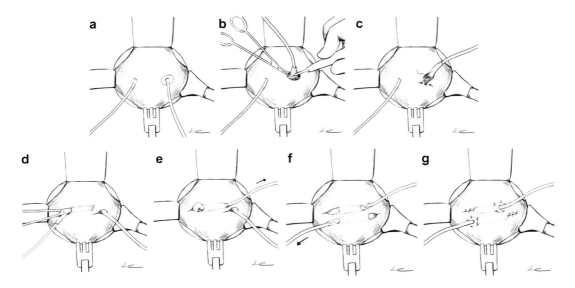

Fig. 6 Transtrigonal (Cohen) bilateral ureteral reimplantation. (**a**) Scoring the bladder mucosa circumferentially after intubating the ureters. (**b**) Mobilization of the ureter. (**c**) Closure of the detrusor defect. (**d**) Creation of the submucosal tunnel across the trigone. (**e**) Transferring the ureter through the tunnel. (**f**) Creation of the submucosal tunnel across the trigone. (**g**) Transferring the ureter through the tunnel

to the bladder urothelium with interrupted 5–0 polyglactin or chromic sutures [18].

If performing a bilateral cross-trigonal reimplant, mobilize and mature one side prior to creating the submucosal tunnel for the contralateral ureter (Fig. 6). The hiatus left by the ipsilateral ureteral orifice can be considered for the maturation site of the contralateral ureteral orifice, provided that the trajectory does not kink the ureter. Intubate both ureters at the end of the case and gently inject saline, then remove the feeding tubes to watch for efflux. This will ensure that no ureteral kinking or twisting has been created.

Intraextravesical (Politano-Leadbetter) Technique

The Politano-Leadbetter technique, first described in 1958, employs similar principles but keeps the ureter "anatomically aligned." It is considered more challenging to perform and does require additional extravesical dissection, which may increase complication rates. After adequate mobilization of the ureter, a transmural incision is made through the posterior wall of the bladder cranial to the existing orifice. Make the incision over the tip of a right-angle clamp that is tunneled from the original hiatus. Transfer the distal ureter to the full thickness neohiatus with the use of extravesical dissection and close the detrusor of the original hiatus. The ureter can then be trimmed and passed back submucosally to the mucosal hiatus. Spatulate the distal anterior ureter and anchor the ureter to the bladder mucosa with 4–0 chromic sutures. The anchoring stitches should approximate the transmural ureteral tissue and the detrusor muscle of the bladder about the orifice. Then reapproximate the spatulated ureteral urothelium to the bladder urothelium with full-thickness interrupted 5–0 chromic sutures. Intubate the ureter to ensure that no ureteral kinking or twisting has been created. The urothelium of the neohiatus should then be closed in running fashion.

Certain cases may require the extension of the submucosal tunnel, such as ureteral kinking. In this situation, a new orifice can be created more distally toward the bladder neck. The ureter can be tunneled further through a second tunnel submucosally. The new ureteral orifice can be created similarly to the described technique above, in which an incision is made over a right-angled clamp. The approximation of the ureter and ureterovesical anastomosis technique would be performed as above [19].

Of note, although it is not commonly performed aside from specific institutions, transvesical laparoscopic approach has been described and suggested to be feasible in small case series [20]. Using three 3 mm laparoscopic trocars and a 3 mm laparoscopic camera [21] has been suggested by the authors.

Ureteral Advancement (Glenn-Anderson) Technique

The Glenn-Anderson Technique is a technique that advances the ureteral orifice distally on the ipsilateral side (as opposed to the Cohen Technique). After adequate mobilization of the ureter, create a submucosal tunnel toward the bladder neck. Make the incision over a right-angled clamp, which will become the new urethral orifice. From the original hiatus, incise a portion of the posterior bladder wall cephalad and transfer the ureter cephalad. Then close the floor of the bladder with interrupted 2–0 sutures, taking care not to make the floor around the ureter too tightly. Then move the distal ureteral through the submucosal tunnel and mature the ureterovesical anastomosis as described above. Intubate the ureter to ensure that no ureteral kinking or twisting has been created.

Other Techniques

Sheath Approximation (Gil-Vernet) Technique

The Gil-Vernet Technique (Gil-Vernet Trigonoplasty) was described in the last several decades as an alternative to ureteral mobilization.

Due to the association of lateral ectopia and megatrigone with VUR, this procedure reduces the distance between the laterally displaced ureteral orifices and the bladder outlet. The principle of this technique embraces the theory that the muscle fibers intrinsic to the transmural ureter carry some sphincteric function to prevent VUR; not mobilizing the ureter thereby may help in preventing reflux.

After opening the anterior wall of the bladder, make a transverse incision that extends between both ureteral orifices, just cephalad to the orifices. This exposes the underlying trigonal muscle. A single nonabsorbable mattress suture is then taken at the base of each distal ureter, capturing the periureteral Waldeyer sheath and intrinsic ureteral muscle fibers. Tying down the mattress suture then advances both ureters together medially toward the midline [22].

There is a lack of studies that evaluate this technique, but no ureterovesical junction obstruction has also been reported in the literature [23].

Spatulated Nipple Technique

The Spatulated Nipple Technique is a good alternative for the obstructing megaureter indication, for which ureteral tapering may need to be performed. This procedure is also useful if the bladder capacity is inadequate to adhere to Paquin's ureteral tunneling ratio.

Ensure that 2 cm of the distal ureter has been mobilized and brought through the bladder. Anchor the base of the ureter to the neohiatus with 4–0 absorbable suture, much like the first step of ureteral orifice maturation. Then, spatulate the ureter and evert the distal lumen. Reapproximate the distal ureteral urothelium to the bladder urothelium with interrupted 5–0 chromic or polyglactin sutures. Then close the everted spatulated portion of the ureter with interrupted 5–0 chromic or polyglactin sutures. Intubate the ureter to ensure that no ureteral kinking or twisting has been created.

Few studies published results, but small case series with intermediate follow-up show high success rates [24].

Closing the Bladder

The bladder should be closed in two layers. The urothelial layer should be closed with running 3–0 absorbable suture. Then close the seromuscular layer with a running 2–0 or 3–0 absorbable suture.

Extravesical Ureteral Reimplantation

Both intravesical and extravesical reimplantation techniques have been shown to definitely and safely correct VUR, but the literature is mostly limited to the pediatric population. Those who advocate for an extravesical approach describe shorter mean operative times, avoidance of gross hematuria, reduced bladder spasms postoperatively, and shorter hospital length of stay [25–28]. Those who advocate for an intravesical approach cite increased risk of urinary retention (about 8%), especially after bilateral ureteral reimplant [29–32]. However this is typically transient, and a focus on optimizing bowel and bladder function prior to surgery further mitigates this risk.

Patient Positioning and Dissecting Down to the Bladder

The patient should be positioned similarly as described for the intravesical approach. The bladder should be approached similarly as also described in the intravesical ureteral reimplantation section above. The bladder should be distended, either by foley catheter insertion or initial cystoscopy. Isolate the distal ureter and wrap with a vessel loop atraumatically.

Open Lich-Gregoir Technique (Fig. 7)

The Lich-Gregoir technique has been described to reduce hospital stay and bladder spasms postoperatively [33]. Once the ureter has been dissected distally, the intramural portion of the ureter is freed from the detrusor muscle in the bladder down to the vesical subepithelium. Divide the

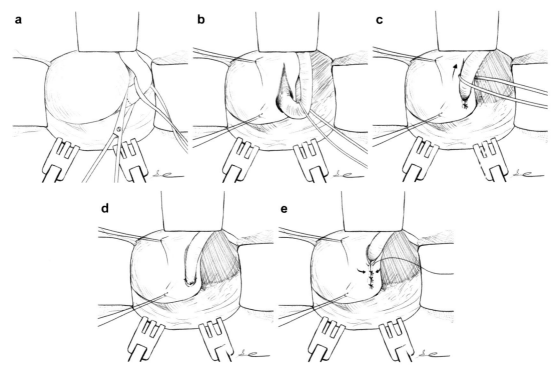

Fig. 7 Open (Lich-Gregoir) ureteral reimplantation. (**a**) Optional transection of the distal ureter. (**b**) Mobilization of the bladder medially with seromuscular incision. (**c**) Placement of the ureter in between the detrusor flaps. (**d**) Completion of ureterovesical anastomosis (if transection of ureter was performed). (**e**) Closure of detrusor flaps over the distal ureter

detrusor muscle into flaps with a 3 cm groove cut vertically to the UVJ. Place the ureter in this groove, and the detrusor muscle is closed overtop to cover.

A modification to this technique has been described, in which the detrusor myotomy is ended in an inverted Y distally to allow for easier reapproximation of the muscle [34].

Using a Laparoscopic or Robotic Approach for Extravesical Reimplantation (Fig. 8)

A growing number of urologists are utilizing the da Vinci robotic system as a minimally invasive option to perform ureteral reimplantation. Currently, there is no consensus on the role of robot-assisted laparoscopic ureteral reimplant in the management of VUR [35]. Concerns have been raised for high costs, longer operative times, and higher 90-day complication rates, particularly at sites with limited robotic experiences [36]. However, more contemporary series have published comparable success rates to other treatment modalities with low complication rates [37]. Considerations for a robotic approach versus open have been described above in the section for Psoas Hitch. In addition, older patients may benefit from a minimally invasive approach given the morbidity of the incisions for open ureteroneocystostomy.

When performed in a minimally invasive fashion, port placement includes an umbilical camera port and at least two robotic arm ports in the mid-clavicular line with or without an assistant port. The ureter is noted coursing along the retroperitoneum to the bladder and the peritoneum is opened over the site of the expected ureterovesical junction (Fig. 8). In a female, the incision is made anterior to the broad ligament and careful dissection around the ureterine vessels is undertaken. In a male, the vas deferens should be swept superiorly.

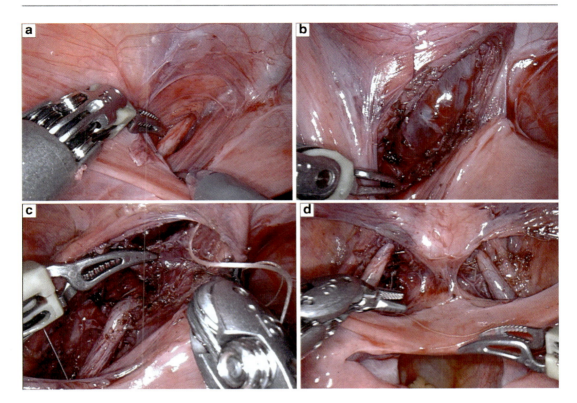

Fig. 8 Robotic approach for extravesical reimplantation. (**a**) Identify the UVJ by incision peritoneum and mobilize the distal ureter. This is done via an anterior approach through the broad ligament. (**b**) Creation of detrusor tunnel. Bladder mucosa is seen bulging out with bladder partially filled to facilitate dissection. (**c**) Perform detrusorrhaphy by pinning the ureter against the bladder mucosa with detrusor flaps. (**d**) Visualization of new ureteral hiatus and tunnels after bilateral extravesical reimplantation performed

The ureter is identified and mobilized sufficiently proximally, taking care to not devascularize it. A hitch stitch with a 2–0 prolene can be placed through the bladder, taking note of the natural tunnel the ureter will lie in. The bladder should be partially filled to facilitate dissection and also help assess the tunnel length. A detrusor tunnel is next created using electrocautery as well as blunt dissection to expose the bladder mucosa for several centimeters. If there is an inadvertent injury to the bladder mucosa, close this with a 5–0 chromic suture. A ureteral advancement stitch may be placed at the 6 o'clock position under the ureter to help prevent shortening of the tunnel by ureteral migration. The tunnel is then closed over the ureter in either a bottom-up approach or top-down approach, using 4–0 interrupted polyglactin suture. Insinuating a needle driver between the ureter and closed detrusor muscle is reassuring that the tunnel is not too tight.

External Tunnel (Barry) Technique

The Barry Technique has been described for its use in renal transplantation. Once at the bladder has been approached, the submucosal tunnel should be created between two 2-cm transverse incisions that are 3 cm apart. The incisions should pass through the detrusor muscle to the bladder mucosa. A traction suture should be placed superomedially to the planned re-anastomotic site. Open the submucosal tunnel space with a right-angle clamp to the full 2-cm incision width of each incision. Then sharply divide the bladder mucosa of the caudal incision. Spatulate the distal ureter, and pass it from the cephalad incision to the caudal incision. Reapproximate the ureteral urothelium to the bladder urothelium using 4–0 polyglactin sutures, starting with the apex, 3-, and 9-o'clock positions. Then place one 12-o'clock full thickness suture in horizontal mattress fashion beginning on the side of the bladder serosa. Close the caudal incision with 3–0 polyglactin suture in interrupted fashion [38].

Detrusorrhaphy (Hodgson-Firlit-Zaontz) Technique

Once the bladder has been approached, dissect the distal ureter away from the bladder with the help of a vessel loop around the ureter for traction, remaining outside of Waldeyer sheath. Dissect down using electrocautery to the submucosa of the bladder, following the course of the ureter. Plan to place two 4–0 polyglactin sutures through the seromusculayers of the bladder and ureter. About the 5-o'clock position of the bladder at the caudal end of the incision, pass the first suture from the outside seromuscular layers of the bladder in caudal-to-cranial fashion. Then pass the suture through the ureter in cranial-to-caudal fashion, producing a mattress-type suture. Repeat this with the second suture starting with the 7-o'clock position. Then close the detrusor incision over the ureter to create the submucosal tunnel using 3–0 polyglactin or chromic suture.

Ureteral advancement in addition to the described procedure has been described as a modification of the technique, with a high rate of VUR resolution (93%) [39].

Intraextravesical Technique (Paquin)

As with the procedures above, initially dissect the distal ureter down to the bladder serosa. Wrap a vessel loop around the ureter for traction. Ligate and divide the ureter just outside the bladder using electrocautery. Open the bladder in oblique fashion from the dome of the bladder down to the planned reinsertion site distally. Then create a submucosal tunnel from the incision site toward the reinsertion site. Reanastomose the ureteral urothelium to the bladder urothelium with 5–0 chromic or polyglactin suture. Close the bladder in two layers as described above.

Postoperative Management

In the pediatric population, most surgical techniques have been described without the placement of a ureteral stent. However, for adults, especially in the setting of a post-radiation, trauma, or otherwise hostile surgical field, a ureteral stent may be placed to help prevent urinary extravasation or acute obstruction from edema. If there is concern for poor tissue healing, stents can remain up to 6 weeks; in this situation, retrograde contrast imaging should be considered to evaluate for any urinary extravasation at the anastomosis.

Foley catheters deserve similar consideration. In a trauma or post-radiation setting, an indwelling foley catheter should be placed intraoperatively and remain for about 7–10 days with postoperative retrograde contrast imaging prior to removal. In an otherwise healthy surgical field, foley catheters should remain for approximately 3–5 days with retrograde contrast imaging at the discretion of the surgeon.

Complications

Postoperatively, one must look for obstruction and persistent or recurrent VUR. Other urologic complications include risk of urinary tract infections, urinary retention when bilateral reimplant is performed, oliguria/anuria, acute kidney failure, hematuria, urinary extravasation, and ureteral stent malfunction or migration. Other non-urologic complications include nausea/vomiting, ileus, constipation, blood loss anemia, abdominal pain, bowel injury, and sepsis [36].

Obstruction

Postoperative obstruction is typically diagnosed as hydronephrosis or hydroureteronephrosis on renal bladder ultrasound or other imaging. Patients may present with symptoms such as nausea, emesis, flank pain, and abdominal pain. Other signs include abnormal renal function seen on metabolic panels (especially if bilateral ureters were reimplanted) or infection (UTI, pyelonephritis, sepsis). Obstruction can be confirmed by renal diuresis scan. Mild hydronephrosis is common postoperatively, and is likely the result of postoperative edema, bladder spasms, stool retention/constipation, or ureter kinking or twisting. Mild hydronephrosis can be managed conservatively with follow-up renal ultrasonography several weeks postoperatively. High-grade hydronephrosis, especially in the setting of sepsis, should be managed by drainage of the obstruction; this can be accomplished by percutaneous nephrostomy tube or indwelling ureteral stent placement. Eventual endoscopic intervention or reoperation can be considered outside of the infectious period.

Persistent obstruction after several weeks is likely due to ureteral kinking, twisting, ischemia, or scarring. Kinking occurs when the neohiatus is created too tightly or the location of the neohiatus is too high or lateral on the bladder. As a result, the drainage of the ureter improves with bladder emptying. Ischemia is a result of over-aggressive dissection of ureter intraoperatively or ureteral kinking or twisting, resulting in stricture formation. Extravesical scarring can be seen in the context of urinary extravasation. All of these complications should be managed with immediate drainage of the obstruction (indwelling stent versus percutaneous nephrostomy tube). While some can be managed with endoscopic dilation or incision, reoperation is commonly required.

Persistent or Recurrent Vesicoureteral Reflux

Persistent or recurrent vesicoureteral reflux can be seen on postoperative voiding cystourethrogram or other contrast-imaging technique. Patients may present similarly to those with obstruction. This is typically a product of technical failure, in which inadequate ureteral tunneling or tapering has been achieved. As with obstruction, low-grade reflux is often transient and can be managed conservatively without further intervention. Follow-up renal and bladder ultrasonography (with pre- and post-void images) should be performed, although no imaging interval has been widely agreed upon. High-grade reflux can be offered endoscopic management (see discussion of Deflux above) or reoperation.

Special Considerations

Reoperation

Reoperative ureteral reimplantation poses a greater challenge as these take place in scarred operative fields, the ureter may lack robust blood supply, or the reasons for primary failure (i.e., bladder level) are still present. Studies in the pediatric population suggest that failure of initial ureteral reimplants fall in the 6–20% for recurrence of obstruction, and 2–5% for symptomatic reflux [26, 40, 41]. When this occurs, reoperative surgery generally necessitates open or robotic revision of the reimplant as it was not originally made with any detrusor tunnel. This is different than a kidney transplant recipient where tunneling is generally performed but may be deficient. In these cases, there is some literature to suggest that bulking agent injection may be a consideration [42, 43].

Duplication Anomalies

In cases of duplication anomalies andureteroceles associated with reflux or obstruction, ureteral reimplant may be indicated. A common sheath reimplant is performed for duplicated ureters. It is important to keep the two ureters attached by their common blood supply or risk devascularization. Cystoscopy and retrograde pyelogram may be helpful at the beginning of the case to establish the anatomy. They are reimplanted together by the standard techniques described above, ensuring the tunnel is wide and long enough. Placement of different colored holding sutures into the anterior lip of each ureter may help with orientation. If both ureters are located in the bladder without any other anomalies, then extravesical (robotic or open) as well as intravesical reimplantation are options. If there is a complicating intravesical factor, such as a ureterocele or diverticulum, then opening the bladder is important. A small ureterocele can be excised and the detrusor defect closed before reimplantation, however a large ureterocele is best marsupialized as the bladder defect is quite large and risks injury to important structures posterior to the bladder, or potentially the bladder neck. The ureters may be brought just past the contralateral orifice to obtain an adequate tunnel. It is important to relax the muscular hiatus if necessary where the ureters turn toward the contralateral wall to ensure there is no kinking. Before closing the hiatus, advance a feeding tube into both ureters and gently inject 5–10 cc of saline then remove the tubes to watch for efflux. Ureteral stents are generally only necessary if there is tapering of the ureter involved. A catheter should be left in place for 3–5 days if significant bladder wall dissection was done in the case of ureterocele. Counseling for large ureteroceles should include a small chance of stress incontinence postoperatively.

Transplant Kidney Ureteroneocystostomy

Reflux after transplant kidney can lead to significant infections given the immunocompromised status of the patient, placing the allograft at risk. Any patients with a complex congenital or reconstructed urinary tract, such as posterior urethral valves and those with an enterocystoplasty, may be at higher risk for reflux and complications as well. Preoperative testing should include a voiding cystourethrogram if the patient begins having urinary tract infections, and careful review of cross-sectional imaging to understand the transplant anatomy. Ureteral stricture should be ruled out. A preoperative urine culture is necessary and any bacteria should be treated ahead of surgery. At the time of surgery, performing cystoscopy with open-ended stent insertion into the transplant orifice is helpful prior to repositioning supine while keeping the catheters sterile. The prior transplant incision can be utilized, favoring the medial half for access to the bladder. The bladder is distended to allow palpation and identification, and the ureter is identified with use of the stent and a vessel loop placed around it. Place holding sutures and a self-retaining retractor for exposure and tension. The ureter is then dissected from the serosa and detrusor muscle of the bladder until the urothelium is visualized. The detrusor muscle is then opened in line with the ureteral path to create a tunnel approximately 4–5 cm long. As long as there is no concern for anastomotic stricture, the ureter does not need to be dismembered. The ureter is then placed into the tunnel against the bladder urothelium, and the detrusor muscle is closed with interrupted 4–0 absorbable sutures. A double-J ureteral stent can be placed and removed endoscopically several weeks later. A foley catheter is left for several days and antibiotics are continued for at least 24 h before transitioning back to suppressive doses.

Reimplant into Bowel Segment

Patients with a history complex bladder reconstruction are also of note. Spinal dysraphism and bladder exstrophy are examples of pertinent conditions. As these patients enter adulthood, their initial surgeries may be decades old. Obtaining all operative reports before embarking on a revision surgery in a patient such as this is paramount. Reimplantation into an interposed bowel segment may be necessary due to the changed anatomy, often on the anterior aspect of the neobladder. Placement of catheters into the bladder via any urinary stomas preexisting is important for initial dissection and identification of important structures. A ureteral stent is helpful and may need to be placed antegrade by interventional radiology prior to the surgery. If there is a suitable landing spot for the ureter to be reimplanted on the anterior native bladder wall then this can be done in typical tunneled fashion described earlier in the chapter. If the most suitable location is the bowel segment of an enterocystoplasty, this is reasonable as long as the bowel segment was not recently operated on and thus has a sturdy blood supply. Score parallel lines in the bowel serosa with electrocautery to develop a tunnel but the serosa is not lifted off, instead two parallel troughs are made. Mark the anterior side of the ureter with a 3–0 polyglactin long stay suture to keep the correct orientation. Spatulate on the opposite side. Open the neo-orifice and insert the distal end of the stent. Place 4–0 or 5–0 absorbable sutures through the posterior and anterior ureteral apices and tied to the bowel with full thickness bites; leave these long in order to expose for the remainder of the ureteroneocystostomy. Close the bowel tunnel over the ureter with interrupted 3–0 suture.

References

1. Byun S-S, Kim JH, Oh S-J, Kim HH. Simple retrograde balloon dilation for treatment of ureteral strictures: etiology-based analysis. Yonsei Med J. 2003;44(2):273–8.
2. Richter F, Irwin RJ, Watson RA, Lang EK. Endourologic management of benign ureteral strictures with and without compromised vascular supply. Urology. 2000;55(5):652–7.
3. Hafez KS, Wolf JS. Update on minimally invasive management of ureteral strictures. J Endourol. 2003;17(7):453–64.
4. Lucas JW, Ghiraldi E, Ellis J, Friedlander JI. Endoscopic management of ureteral strictures: an update. Curr Urol Rep. 2018;19(4):24.
5. Hurtado E, McCrery R, Appell R. The safety and efficacy of ethylene vinyl alcohol copolymer as an intra-urethral bulking agent in women with intrinsic urethral deficiency. Int Urogynecol J Pelvic Floor Dysfunct. 2007;18(8):869–73.
6. Kirchin V, Page T, Keegan PE, Atiemo KO, Cody JD, McClinton S, et al. Urethral injection therapy for urinary incontinence in women. Cochrane Database Syst Rev. 2017;25(7):CD003881.
7. Kalisvaart JF, Scherz HC, Cuda S, Kaye JD, Kirsch AJ. Intermediate to long-term follow-up indicates low risk of recurrence after double HIT endoscopic treatment for primary vesico-ureteral reflux. J Pediatr Urol. 2012;8(4):359–65.
8. Leung L, Chan IHY, Chung PHY, Lan LCL, Tam PKH, Wong KKY. Endoscopic injection for primary vesicoureteric reflux: predictors of resolution and long term efficacy. J Pediatr Surg. 2017;52(12):2066–9.
9. Rao KL, Menon P, Samujh R, Mahajan JK, Bawa M, Malik MA, et al. Endoscopic management of vesicoureteral reflux and long-term follow-up. Indian Pediatr. 2018;55(12):1046–9.
10. Kaye JD, Srinivasan AK, Delaney C, Cerwinka WH, Elmore JM, Scherz HC, et al. Clinical and radiographic results of endoscopic injection for vesicoureteral reflux: defining measures of success. J Pediatr Urol. 2012;8(3):297–303.
11. Kim D. Atlas of laparoscopic and robotic urologic surgery: Laparoscopic/Robotic Boari Flap Ureteral Reimplantation. Elsevier; 2017. p. 204–16.
12. Kaplan-Marans E, Fulla J, Tomer N, Bilal K, Palese M. Indocyanine Green (ICG) in urologic surgery. Urology. 2019;132:10–7.
13. Kanabur P, Chai C, Taylor J. Use of Indocyanine green for intraoperative ureteral identification in nonurologic surgery. JAMA Surg. 2020;155(6):520–1.
14. Slawin J, Patel NH, Lee Z, Dy GW, Kim D, Asghar A, et al. Ureteral reimplantation via robotic nontransecting side-to-side anastomosis for distal ureteral stricture. J Endourol. 2020;34(8):836–9.
15. Defoor WR. New contralateral vesicoureteral reflux-is it double trouble? J Urol. 2014;191(2):291–2.
16. Paquin AJ. Ureterovesical anastomosis: the description and evaluation of a technique. J Urol. 1959;82:573–83.
17. Kalayeh K, Brian Fowlkes J, Schultz WW, Sack BS. The 5:1 rule overestimates the needed tunnel length during ureteral reimplantation. Neurourol Urodyn. 2021;40(1):85–94.
18. Cohen SJ. The Cohen reimplantation technique. Birth Defects Orig Artic Ser. 1977;13(5):391–5.
19. Politano VA, Leadbetter WF. An operative technique for the correction of vesicoureteral reflux. J Urol. 1958;79(6):932–41.
20. Gill IS, Ponsky LE, Desai M, Kay R, Ross JH. Laparoscopic cross-trigonal Cohen ureteroneocystostomy: novel technique. J Urol. 2001;166(5):1811–4.
21. Baek M, Han DH. Transvesicoscopic Politano-Leadbetter ureteral reimplantation in children with vesicoureteral reflux: a novel surgical technique. Investig Clin Urol. 2019;60(5):405–11.
22. Gil-Vernet JM. A new technique for surgical correction of vesicoureteral reflux. J Urol. 1984;131(3):456–8.
23. Simforoosh N, Radfar MH. Current status of Gil-Vernet trigonoplasty technique. Adv Urol. 2008;2008:536428.
24. Tatlişen A, Ekmekçioğlu O. Direct nipple ureteroneocystostomy in adults with primary obstructed megaureter. J Urol. 2005;173(3):877–80.
25. Sriram K, Babu R. Extravesical (modified Gregoir Lich) versus intravesical (Cohen's) ureteric reimplantation for vesicoureteral reflux in children: a single center experience. Indian J Urol. 2016;32(4):306–9.
26. Silay MS, Turan T, Kayalı Y, Başıbüyük İ, Gunaydin B, Caskurlu T, et al. Comparison of intravesical (Cohen) and extravesical (Lich-Gregoir) ureteroneocystostomy in the treatment of unilateral primary vesicoureteric reflux in children. J Pediatr Urol. 2018;14(1):65.e1–4.
27. Schwentner C, Oswald J, Lunacek A, Deibl M, Koerner I, Bartsch G, et al. Lich-Gregoir reimplantation causes less discomfort than Politano-Leadbetter technique: results of a prospective, randomized, pain scale-oriented study in a pediatric population. Eur Urol. 2006;49(2):388–95.

28. McMann LP, Joyner BD. Outcomes of extravesical versus intravesical ureteral reimplantation. ScientificWorldJournal. 2004;4:195–7.
29. Fung LC, McLorie GA, Jain U, Khoury AE, Churchill BM. Voiding efficiency after ureteral reimplantation: a comparison of extravesical and intravesical techniques. J Urol. 1995;153(6):1972–5.
30. Barrieras D, Lapointe S, Reddy PP, Williot P, McLorie GA, Bägli D, et al. Urinary retention after bilateral extravesical ureteral reimplantation: does dissection distal to the ureteral orifice have a role? J Urol. 1999;162(3 Pt 2):1197–200.
31. Koyle MA, Butt H, Lorenzo A, Mingin GC, Elder JS, Smith GHH. Prolonged urinary retention can and does occur after any type of ureteral reimplantantion. Pediatr Surg Int. 2017;33(5):623–6.
32. Esposito C, Varlet F, Riquelme MA, Fourcade L, Valla JS, Ballouhey Q, et al. Postoperative bladder dysfunction and outcomes after minimally invasive extravesical ureteric reimplantation in children using a laparoscopic and a robot-assisted approach: results of a multicentre international survey. BJU Int. 2019;124(5):820–7.
33. Heidenreich A, Ozgur E, Becker T, Haupt G. Surgical management of vesicoureteral reflux in pediatric patients. World J Urol. 2004;22(2):96–106.
34. Lapointe SP, Barrieras D, Leblanc B, Williot P. Modified Lich-Gregoir ureteral reimplantation: experience of a Canadian center. J Urol. 1998;159(5):1662–4.
35. Baek M, Koh CJ. Lessons learned over a decade of pediatric robotic ureteral reimplantation. Invest Clin Urol. 2017;58(1):3–11.
36. Kurtz MP, Leow JJ, Varda BK, Logvinenko T, Yu RN, Nelson CP, et al. Robotic versus open pediatric ureteral reimplantation: costs and complications from a nationwide sample. J Pediatr Urol. 2016;12(6):408.e1–6.
37. Boysen WR, Akhavan A, Ko J, Ellison JS, Lendvay TS, Huang J, et al. Prospective multicenter study on robot-assisted laparoscopic extravesical ureteral reimplantation (RALUR-EV): outcomes and complications. J Pediatr Urol. 2018;14(3):262.e1–6.
38. Barry JM. Unstented extravesical ureteroneocystostomy in kidney transplantation. J Urol. 1983;129(5):918–9.
39. Zaontz MR, Maizels M, Sugar EC, Firlit CF. Detrusorrhaphy: extravesical ureteral advancement to correct vesicoureteral reflux in children. J Urol. 1987;138(4 Pt 2):947–9.
40. Mesrobian HG, Kramer SA, Kelalis PP. Reoperative ureteroneocystostomy: review of 69 patients. J Urol. 1985;133(3):388–90.
41. Guney D, Tiryaki TH. The prevalence of redo-ureteroneocystostomy and associated risk factors in pediatric vesicoureteral reflux patients treated with ureteroneocystostomy. Urol J. 2019;16(1):72–7.
42. Jung C, DeMarco RT, Lowrance WT, Pope JC, Adams MC, Dietrich MS, et al. Subureteral injection of dextranomer/hyaluronic acid copolymer for persistent vesicoureteral reflux following ureteroneocystostomy. J Urol. 2007;177(1):312–5.
43. Carrillo Arroyo I, Fuentes Carreterc S, Gómez Fraile A, Morante Valverde R, Tordable Ojeda C, Cabezalí BD. Technical challenges of endoscopic treatment for vesicoureteral reflux after Cohen reimplantation. Actas Urol Esp. 2019;43(7):384–8.

Part VII

Pelvic Pain, Irritative Voiding Disorders, and Female Sexual Dysfunction

Pathophysiology and Clinical Evaluation of Chronic Pelvic Pain

52

Elise J. B. De and Jan Alberto Paredes Mogica

Contents

Introduction: Why Treat Chronic Pelvic Pain?	910
Causes of Chronic Pelvic Pain	910
Initial Assessment of Chronic Pelvic Pain	912
Special Populations	914
Laboratory and Imaging Studies	915
Differential Diagnosis by Organ System	915
Gynecological System	915
Male Genitalia	916
Urological	917
Musculoskeletal	918
Gastrointestinal	920
Vascular	921
Neurological	922
Multifocal Pain and Other Conditions	926
Treatment	926
Conclusion	927
Guidelines and Resources for Providers and Patients	928
Cross-References	928
References	928

Abstract

Chronic pelvic pain is a prevalent problem among the female and male population worldwide. This disorder is commonly multifactorial and although diagnosis and management can prove difficult for even the most experienced clinician, it is often straightforward and satisfying to treat. In more complex cases, a

E. J. B. De (✉)
Massachusetts General Hospital, Boston, MA, USA
e-mail: ede@mgh.harvard.edu

J. A. Paredes Mogica
Anahuac University, Mexico City, Mexico

© Springer Nature Switzerland AG 2023
F. E. Martins et al. (eds.), *Female Genitourinary and Pelvic Floor Reconstruction*,
https://doi.org/10.1007/978-3-031-19598-3_53

multidisciplinary team is best equipped to manage, as pelvic pain can result from any pelvic organ or system. Initial signs and symptoms that will aid in the diagnosis of a specific etiology and treatment can be tailored to underlying diagnosis, if found. In cases with no established diagnosis, symptoms can still be managed effectively based on information from the workup. Psychological referral can be especially important in these cases, but must be introduced as a holistic component care, clearly validating that the pain is physiologic. Mind-based approaches can not only address the loss associated with chronic pain but known techniques can reduce pain severity and impact. This chapter presents etiologies for chronic pelvic pain in a pragmatic, useable manner, including the signs and symptoms pointing to each organ system and causes of systemic pain, as well as treatment strategies to help patients cope with this disorder when idiopathic.

Keywords

Chronic pelvic pain · Endometriosis · Central sensitization · Painful bladder syndrome · Interstitial cystitis · Overactive bladder

Introduction: Why Treat Chronic Pelvic Pain?

The purpose of this chapter is to provide the genitourinary and reconstructive surgeon tools for success in chronic pelvic pain. Pain can often easily be addressed along with the surgical and functional conditions of our specialties – especially through engaging our multidisciplinary colleagues – producing better outcomes from both the patient and provider perspective.

The American College of Obstetricians and Gynecologists (ACOG) define chronic pelvic pain (CPP) as pain in the pelvic area (i.e., the lower part of the torso between the abdomen and legs, including the pelvic bones and reproductive organs) that lasts for 6 months or longer [1]. Its prevalence has been estimated to be about 10% in the general population, and between 5.7% and 26.6% in women [2, 3]. It is vital to remember that CPP is not a pathology exclusive to women – as it has been reported to be present in 2–16% of men [4]. Because of the high prevalence of CPP, regardless of clinical focus within pelvic floor disorders, it is important for pelvic specialists to become familiarized with strategies to diagnose and treat associated pain. This chapter provides the basic tools needed to achieve this goal, improving satisfaction for both patient and provider in the long run.

Causes of Chronic Pelvic Pain

Just as many organ systems in the pelvis can cause acute pelvic pain, the etiology of CPP is multifactorial [5]. Identifying a cause can be problematic at the time of initial assessment, and it is commonplace for a patient to remain without a diagnosis to guide management. Social and psychological confounders (e.g., anxiety and depression) interplay with symptoms, further complicating diagnosis and treatment [6].

A coordinated multidisciplinary approach is the most effective strategy to improve CPP [7]. If organ-specific symptoms are present, the underlying cause should be sought by the appropriate specialist according to the European Association for Urology Guidelines on Chronic Pelvic Pain (Fig. 1). Even if no cause is found, symptoms can often be managed effectively. Coping strategies used in the management of other chronic pain disorders have shown success in CPP patients.

Some authors have identified pelvic venous disorders and endometriosis as the most common causes of chronic pelvic pain in women [7, 8]. Other sources cite irritable bowel syndrome (IBS), psychological conditions, ovarian cysts, interstitial cystitis, and pelvic inflammatory disease (PID) as the most common etiologies associated with CPP [9, 10]. Most patients remain without a specific diagnosis. A study conducted in the UK (n = 483) reported that only approximately 50% of patients with CPP received a final diagnosis [9]. This

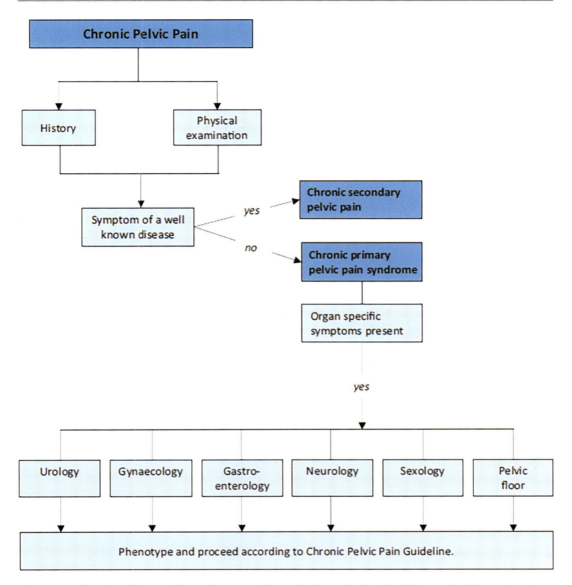

Fig. 1 Algorithm describing the diagnostic approach for chronic pelvic pain. (Reproduced from the European Association of Urology. D. Engeler (Chair), A.P. Baranowski, B. Berghmans, J. Borovicka, A.M. Cottrell, P. Dinis-Oliveira, S. Elneil, J. Hughes, E.J. Messelink (Vice-chair), A.C. de C Williams Guidelines Associates: B. Parsons, S. Goonewardene, P. Abreu-Mendes, V. Zumstein. EAU Guidelines on Chronic Pelvic Pain 2020. ISBN 978-94-92671-07-3. Available at: https://uroweb.org/guideline/chronic-pelvic-pain/#1_2)

number may reflect either the inherent complexity of CPP or a bias in medicine to stop investigating once the limits of one's specialty are reached – but it remains that these patients are left without an intellectual framework to understand their pain (Table 1).

An important division in the workup of CPP is whether pain is localized to the pelvis or systemic, for example, the patient who presents with CPP as well as other pain syndromes. Central sensitization plays an important role in perpetuating chronic pain. Pathologic changes occur within the central nervous system (CNS) and the hypothalamic–pituitary–adrenal axis that result in an exaggerated response to both

Table 1 Provides a list of possible CPP etiologies according to the organ system involved

Organ system	Possible diagnosis
Genitourinary	Endometriosis, adenomyosis, uterine fibroids, ovarian pathologies, pelvic inflammatory disease or adhesions, ectopic pregnancy, vulvar atrophy, dermatologic condition, or neuropathy, urethral diverticulum, skene's gland, prostatitis, prostatic utricle, epididymitis, Peyronie's disease, testicular pathologies, sexually transmitted disease, bladder outlet obstruction, interstitial cystitis, bladder or distal ureter stone, detrusor overactivity, urinary tract infection, cancer
Musculoskeletal	Myopathy; gait problems; osteitis; injury to bones, ligaments, or tendons; rheumatologic disease
Gastrointestinal	Irritable bowel syndrome, levator ani syndrome, proctalgia fugax, constipation, fissures, hemorrhoids, tumor, adhesions, chronic appendicitis, hernia, inflammatory bowel disease
Neurological	Upper and lower motor neuron syndromes, peripheral neuropathies (entrapment or small fiber), central sensitization
Vascular	Pelvic venous congestion, vasculitis

painful and non-painful stimuli. These changes give way to the development of allodynia (painful response to innocuous stimuli) and hyperalgesia (increased sensitivity to painful stimuli) [11].

Yet more work is needed to elucidate the mechanisms for chronification. Small fiber polyneuropathy has been identified in 64% of patients with complex (refractory or multisystem) chronic pelvic pain [12]. Current understanding of the pathophysiology of SFPN points to dysfunction of the small c-fibers, a-delta fibers, and postganglionic sympathetics in the peripheral nervous system. Traditionally, small fibers have been known to be responsible for the transduction of pain signals from the periphery. It is important to understand they are also a means for autonomic control and modulation of the immune response via the release of inflammatory mediators such as substance P and calcitonin-gene-related peptide (CGRP) [13–16]. This may help explain the presence of comorbidities such as fibromyalgia, IBS, migraine, interstitial cystitis (IC), and other conditions in patients with CPP. There is likely a dynamic relationship between the peripheral and central nervous system in chronification.

The following section discusses initial assessment along with important strategies needed to adequately manage CPP, whether a straightforward case or complex (refractory or multisystem) chronic pelvic pain.

Initial Assessment of Chronic Pelvic Pain

Validation

Validation of pain and assurance of resources – even by referral – has therapeutic benefit in and of itself, a knowledge that is second nature to most pelvic specialists reading this chapter.

Medical History

A good clinical history is vital in the assessment of CPP, but tools to protect the clinician's time are essential. Allowing the patient to "tell the story" for 5–10 min freely at the first visit provides important clues, such as pain, which resolves at night (pelvic venous congestion), starts after abdominal surgery (pelvic nerve entrapment) or foot surgery (pelvic floor muscle tension myalgia), or pain that arises unilaterally with relatively acute onset (partially obstructing distal ureteric stone). Characteristics of pain – time of onset, duration, intensity, radiation, quality, and aggravating factors – are standard pieces of information needed. Special care should be taken to include the obstetric, gynecologic, gastrointestinal, genitourinary, nervous, and skeletal systems. Organized, written information in advance of the interview can significantly improve the provider's capacity to process what can otherwise be overwhelming amounts of information. In the interest of completeness, data quality, and time efficiency, it is beneficial to provide patients with screening forms and validated tools to describe symptoms, as well as an inventory to keep track of prior assessments.

Questionnaires such as the Pelvic Pain Assessment Form by the International Pelvic Pain Society can provide valuable insight into the patient's presentation [17]. Helpful patient reported outcome measures include but are not limited to the Genitourinary Pain Index [18], the International Consultation on Incontinence Questionnaire Female Lower Urinary Tract Symptoms Modules (ICIQ-FLUTS) [19], the American Urological Association Symptom Score [20], the Pelvic Floor Distress Inventory [21], and the IMPACT Bowel Function Assessment Tool [22]. Webpage resources or books such as *Facing Pelvic Pain* (www.facingpelvicpain.org), can help patients engage and understand their diagnoses, which in turn can improve ease of management. On www.facingpelvicpain.org, patients learn about causes of pelvic pain, pelvic floor physical therapy, urodynamics and cystoscopy, and cognitive behavioral therapy in short videos. Patients can download the book and learn, in lay terms, about the causes and treatments of pelvic pain. The free downloadable "Treatment Map" for pelvic pain provides a space for the patient to write the story of the pain, alerts the provider to systemic pain issues, provides an inventory of anything that has been tried and response organized by therapeutic type, organizes a list of diagnostic studies already complete, details the list of current care providers, and ends with the next steps. This is of the utmost importance as the next step in management may vary considerably depending on the outcome of prior interventions (for example, difficulty voiding on anticholinergics may lead one to suspect bladder neck obstruction and thereafter to try an alpha blocker). Previous surgeries can provide clues to an underlying mechanism for CPP, especially if the onset of pain is related in time to the surgical intervention, which could raise suspicion for nerve entrapment. Surgeries of the spine and the genitourinary, gastrointestinal, and reproductive systems are all relevant when performing the initial workup of CPP [11, 16]. The authors find all of the above essential in the efficient approach to complex patients.

Physical Examination

The physical exam should be comprehensive, extending beyond the pelvic area. The musculoskeletal system, along with the abdominal wall and viscera, should be thoroughly examined as they are common contributors to pelvic pain [23]. Hernias can be identified by having the patient lift their head and shoulder half an inch off the table, engaging the abdominal muscles. Tenderness on the sacroiliac joints, pubic symphysis, and lower back are strong indicators of a musculoskeletal etiology. The FABER (flexion, abduction, external rotation) test can indicate an SI joint problem if pain is reproduced during these movements and the Carnett test (in which pain is reproduced when tensing abdominal wall muscles) can help rule out visceral origins of pelvic pain [24].

Neurological sources of pain can be demonstrable on exam. Simple dermatomes, reflexes, and gait should suffice for the reconstructive surgeon. Either during the exam or in the history form, the patient can map their pain for comparison to dermatome charts (Fig. 2). Reflexes, strength, observation of muscle atrophy, and ability to heel and toe walk will test the large nerve fibers. Clinical exam findings of decreased pinprick and thermal sensation and hyperalgesia, often most notable on the distal extremities, raise suspicion for a small fiber neuropathy. Affected areas can present with concomitant skin changes such as dry or shiny skin [25]. For patients in whom cutaneous allodynia is suspected, a cotton swab can be used to map a cutaneous distribution of pain [24].

For the pelvic exam itself, it is important to let the patient know the purpose of the examination and its importance in aiding the physician to establish a diagnosis. The six tenets of trauma-informed care can be found on the Centers for Disease Control website and apply to patients of all gender, education, and socioeconomic status [26]. The main concepts are safety, respect, and

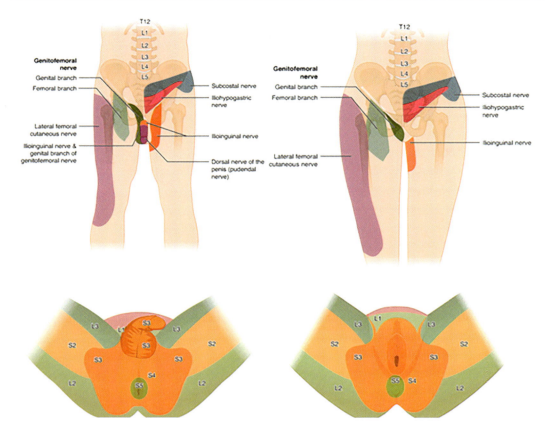

Fig. 2 The cutaneous innervation of the pelvic region in a man and woman, and the corresponding dermatomes. (Adapted by permission from [Springer Nature]: [Springer Nature] [Spinal Cord Stimulation: Pelvic Pain] by [Chen G.H., Hunter C.W.] [Copyright] (2018))

preserving locus of control. The authors' approach is to state the exam will be gentle but can stop at any time, and to ask if there are any considerations that will make the exam more comfortable. If there is apprehension, the examiner can offer waiting until the next visit to allow time to prepare. Breathing techniques can be used in the setting of patients developing anxiety during examination [24], or other strategies such as distracting with music.

During the pelvic exam, the provider should be on the lookout for signs of infection, vaginal or urethral discharge, inflammation, masses, cysts, pelvic organ prolapse or tenderness (e.g., prostate, urethra, cervix). The pelvic floor musculature should be examined for pelvic floor muscle tension myalgia and increased tone versus neurogenic hypertonicity, and for strength [24]. Specialized exam of problem areas can be helpful, for example, extracting a clipped hair fragment from under the clitoral prepuce or identifying a Peyronie's induration in the penile shaft.

Special Populations

Special consideration should be taken when addressing underage patients, victims of abuse or sexual coercion, and patients with disability. These patients might present with an array of problems unique to their background. The difficulty that might arise during communication may complicate diagnosis and treatment. Furthermore, poor communication can result in poor adherence to treatment. A multidisciplinary team should be involved in care. Gynecologists, urologists, physical therapists, psychologists, and pediatricians (in the case of underage patients) all play an important role in managing the varying complexities of chronic pelvic pain. Trauma informed care – preserving the patient's locus of control and providing a safe space – is essential to treatment.

Laboratory and Imaging Studies

Although a diagnosis can often be made with the medical history and physical exam alone, laboratory and imaging studies can be indicated at the time of initial workup. Studies should be ordered based on diagnostic suspicion, for example, urinalysis, sedimentation, and culture if a urinary tract infection (UTI) is suspected, a post void residual urine assessment in the case of urinary symptoms or suprapubic pain, and sexually transmitted infection (STI) screening for any possibility of sexual exposure. For any women of childbearing potential, a pregnancy test should be ordered [27].

Imaging studies such as ultrasonography can be useful in evaluating pelvic or visceral disease. It is often the first imaging study of choice when evaluating pelvic masses [28]. Studies such as computerized tomography (CT) scan or magnetic resonance imaging (MRI) could be considered if other tests prove to be equivocal, if hematuria is present, or if a specific diagnosis such as ureteric stone, osteitis pubis, or urethral diverticulum (MRI) is suspected. A diagnostic laparoscopic procedure could be performed in the setting of pain of unknown origin. There are no specific guidelines on when to perform cross-sectional imaging for pelvic pain, but if not already on file at the time of presentation, it should always be kept in the back of the physician's mind and performed at some point if pain does not resolve. Of importance is the consideration of an oncologic process as the source for chronic pelvic pain. Traction and invasion of adjacent structures, stimulation of nociceptors, ischemia, and muscle spasms are all mechanisms by which an oncologic process might manifest as pain within the pelvis.

The most common cancers implicated are those of the genitourinary and gastrointestinal system, but virtually any cancer can result in CPP if a pelvic structure becomes directly or indirectly involved [29]. Suspicion should arise in CPP in which no apparent etiology is found and in cases refractory to management. Imaging and/or endoscopy should be offered relatively early in the process. Lastly, spine imaging should be entertained in the setting of abnormal reflexes, heel/toe walking or gait, localized or radiating back pain not responding to physical therapy, or abnormal urodynamic testing seeking, for example, herniated disc, tumor, Tarlov cyst, or tethered spinal cord.

Differential Diagnosis by Organ System

A brief overview of the potential mechanism and pathophysiology by organ system is outlined.

Gynecological System

As discussed before, endometriosis is one of the most common pathologies associated with CPP. The prevalence of endometriosis has been estimated to affect 10% of reproductive age women, with a median delay in diagnosis of 7 years, a statistic that we as pelvic surgeons can impact positively [30]. Endometriosis is the presence of endometrial-like cells outside of the endometrial cavity. These are typically in the abdominal and pelvic cavities but have been found in the chest, vagina, bladder, abdominal wall, and beyond. The ectopic endometrial tissue gives rise to the cyclic characteristic of pain starting with menarche or after cessation of contraceptives. Signs and symptoms include painful menstruation (often with associated nausea and vomiting), painful sexual intercourse (dyspareunia), painful bowel movements, bloating, constipation or diarrhea, and palpable deposits of ectopic tissue at the posterior cul-de-sac upon examination. Ultrasonography and MRI can be used to diagnose endometriosis, but laparoscopy with direct visualization of the ectopic tissue is the gold standard [31, 32].

Adenomyosis (endometrial glands growing into the muscular layers of the uterus) and uterine fibroids are other disorders that are especially prevalent in women, and both can give rise to CPP. In both cases, heavy bleeding can be present during menstruation and surgery is usually considered to be the definitive cure for both.

Ovarian pathologies can also manifest as chronic pain in the pelvis – tumors as well as cysts are important diagnoses to consider. Pain can be exacerbated with movement, intercourse, and exercise. Ultrasound imaging is usually the test of choice for confirming diagnosis.

Other disorders that can result in CPP include pelvic inflammatory disease, chronic endometritis (diagnosed by biopsy), pelvic venous disorders (e.g., ovarian vein valve dysfunction, nutcracker syndrome, May-Thurner syndrome, discussed below), vaginal atrophy, and pelvic organ prolapse [33, 34].

Male Genitalia

It is important to remember that while CPP is more common in women, men can also be affected, and may encounter greater obstacles to care. Chronic Prostatitis/Chronic Pelvic Pain Syndrome (CP/CPPS) is perhaps the most discussed disorder associated with CPP in men. Prostatitis has been estimated to be present in 4.5–9% of men. Symptoms include pain in the perineum, suprapubic region, testes, or glans that can be worsened by urination or ejaculation. Voiding symptoms may be present [35–37]. Careful history taking and investigation of the prostate (e.g., expressed prostatic excretion culture) and pelvic musculature are warranted. The following instructions from Family Practice Notebook [38] are easy to follow:

Technique for Expressed Prostatic Secretion:

1. Patient with full Bladder and desires to void
2. Retract foreskin and cleanse penis
    a. Uncircumsized men maintain foreskin retraction
3. Collect midstream urine for pre-massage urine culture
4. Patient stops voiding
5. Examiner massages prostate from periphery to midline
    a. Not recommended in Acute Prostatitis
6. Collect a few drops of secretion from Urethra into post-massage urine culture cup
7. Collect 10 ml of urine for post-massage urine culture
8. Refrigerate urine samples
    a. Send both samples for urine microscopy of sediment
    b. Send both samples for urine culture

Interpretation:

1. Findings suggestive of Prostatitis
    a. Urine leukocytes >10 WBC/hpf in post-massage sample
    b. Post-massage urine culture positive
        i. Pre-massage urine culture sterile
        ii. Pre-massage <1 log colony/ml under post-massage
2. Findings suggestive of cystitis
    a. Significant bacteriuria in pre-massage sample

However, if initial intervention (antibiotic trial, anti-inflammatories) is not successful, further investigation should be performed. Further investigation of prostate causes should include assessment for prostatic or bladder neck obstruction. The latter is often overlooked but should be suspected in young men and those with small fiber neuropathy.

Pelvic floor tension myalgia can occur in men, and the puborectalis, iliococcygeus, and obturator internus muscles are easily examined at the time of digital rectal exam. Pelvic floor physical therapists certified in treatment of pelvic floor disorders can be found on locators such as the American Physical Therapy Association (https://aptapelvichealth.org/ptlocator/). Potentiators such as bicycle seats and poor vehicle or office ergonomics should be addressed. If there is any suspicion of pelvic floor muscle dysfunction this should be addressed concurrent with other initial measures and prior to more invasive approaches, such as those for chronic scrotal content pain below.

Chronic scrotal content pain (orchalgia) affects about 100,000 men in the United States each year. The differential diagnosis includes epididymitis, testicular torsion, tumors, obstruction, varicocele, epididymal cysts, hydrocele, iatrogenic injury following vasectomy or hernia repair, and referred pain from a variety of sources, including ureteral stone, indirect inguinal hernia, aortic or common iliac artery aneurysms, lower back disorders, interstitial cystitis, and nerve entrapment due to perineural fibrosis [39].

Surgical options include spermatic cord blocks, varicocelectomy, epididymectomy, targeted and standard microsurgical denervation of the spermatic cord (77–100% success rates), ultrasound-guided peri-spermatic cord and ilioinguinal cryoablation (59–75% success rates), botulinum toxin injection (56–72% success rates), targeted ilioinguinal and iliohypogastric peripheral nerve stimulation (72% success rate), radical orchiectomy (20–75% success rate), targeted robotic-assisted intra-abdominal denervation (71% success rate), and vasectomy reversal (69–100% success rates) [40].

Disorders involving ejaculatory ducts (e.g., cystic lesions such as a prostatic utricle), and penis (peyronie's, sexually transmitted infections) can cause localized chronic pelvic pain men.

Small fiber neuropathy should be considered in men with non-resolving pain, especially if other systemic pain or autonomic dysfunction is present.

Urological

The ureters, bladder, and urethra can contribute to the development of CPP. Several disorders that affect the bladder manifest as pain, pressure, or discomfort in the lower abdominal area. The diagnosis of Interstitial Cystitis /Bladder Pain Syndrome (IC/BPS) as delineated by the Society of Urodynamics, Female Pelvic Medicine, and Urogenital Reconstruction is "an unpleasant sensation (pain, pressure, discomfort) perceived to be related to the urinary bladder, associated with lower urinary tract symptoms of more than six weeks duration, in the absence of infection or other identifiable causes" [41]. The American Urological Association (AUA) chose this definition in the IC/BPS guideline, given the 6 weeks, to allow early intervention [42]. A key point in the definition is "in the absence of other identifiable causes" – therefore other etiologies such as pelvic floor muscle dysfunction, atypical infections (e.g., ureaplasma/mycoplasma), bladder neck obstruction, retention, distal ureteric stone, and urethral diverticulum should be considered [31, 43]. IC/BPS typically manifests with flare-ups and remissions.

The AUA Guideline on IC/BPS includes a helpful one-page algorithm with tiered recommendations (Fig. 3). The authors of this chapter almost always offer pelvic floor physical therapy (listed in second-line treatments) as part of the treatment approach.

Urethritis usually manifests with painful voiding (i.e., dysuria) and can radiate to adjacent structures such as the sacrum or the groin. A urinary tract infection (UTI) can give rise to urethritis but workup for a sexually transmitted infection should also be performed, especially if urine parameters are within normal limits [44]. Mycoplasma Genitalium and Ureaplasma can cause urethritis and can be transmitted sexually. They do not grow in standard culture media for UTI and are best identified by specific polymerase chain reaction techniques. It is reasonable to assess for these organisms in the setting of dysuria as soon as standard approach to UTI fails. Vulvar atrophy is a common cause of urethral pain, as the nerve endings are stabilized in the presence of estrogen. Bladder neck obstruction, stone, stricture, diverticulum, Skene's duct cyst, herpes, lichen sclerosis, nerve entrapment, and small fiber neuropathy should also be considered [45]. Topical irritants such as soaps, filamentous toilet paper, bleached or abrasive undergarments or pads, spermacides, friction, and wipes can lead to urethral pain in women.

Disorders affecting ureters are usually more acute and rarely manifest themselves as chronic pain but the authors have seen over five cases in CPP. Nonetheless, obstruction can manifest as pain in the lower back area that radiates to the groin or the suprapubic region. The healthcare

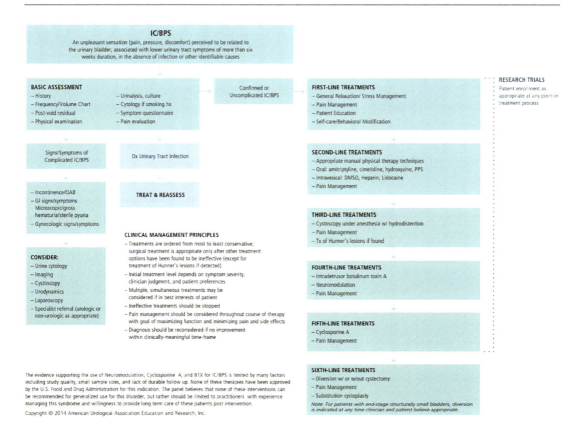

Fig. 3 Interstitial cystitis/bladder pain syndrome algorithm. (Reproduced from: Hanno PM, Erickson D, Moldwin R, et al.: Diagnosis and treatment of interstitial cystitis/bladder pain syndrome: AUA guideline amendment. J Urol 2015; 193: 1545)

provider should maintain a high level of suspicion in this setting if the pain is unilateral or was of relatively acute onset.

Musculoskeletal

The musculoskeletal system is an essential consideration in CPP. Pelvic floor tension myalgia/pelvic floor myofascial pain syndrome plays an important role in the pathophysiology of pelvic pain, both as a cause and a reaction. It has been estimated that up to 87% of women with CPP have increased tone of the pelvic musculature (the terms hypertonicity and dystonia refer specifically to neurologically based disorders of tone) [46–49]. LUTS are often present along with bowel symptoms, and sexual dysfunction. Upon physical examination of the piriformis, levator ani (puborectalis, pubococcygeus, and iliococcygeus), obturator, and coccygeus muscles, one appreciates a hard muscle that does not relax easily with pressure and verbal cues and does not elongate with stretch or pressure (Fig. 4) [49]. A practical reference is that normal firmness is equal to the resting compressibility of the thenar eminence, decreased is less, and increased would be equivalent to the compressibility of the thenar eminence when the thumb is opposed to the first (moderate) or fifth (severe) digits (Fig. 5) [50]. Pain, previously referred to as "trigger points," can be appreciated in addition to tone, and diagnosis can be made on vaginal or rectal exam without the need of imaging studies.

The pelvis plays a pivotal role in the transfer of weight to the lower extremities. It is to be expected that any disorder that affects

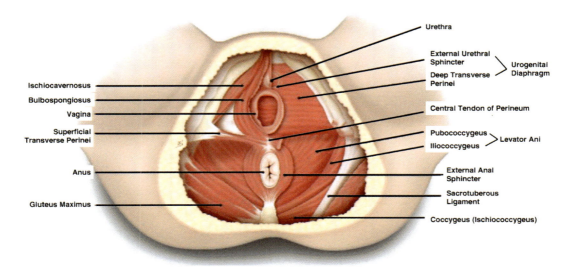

Fig. 4 Superficial (left) and deep (right) female pelvic floor musculature. (Image created by Ilaria Bondi. Reprinted by permission from [Springer Nature]: [Springer Nature] [Management of Fecal Incontinence: Current Treatment Approaches and Future Perspectives] by [Massimo Mongardini Manuel Giofrè] [Copyright] (2016))

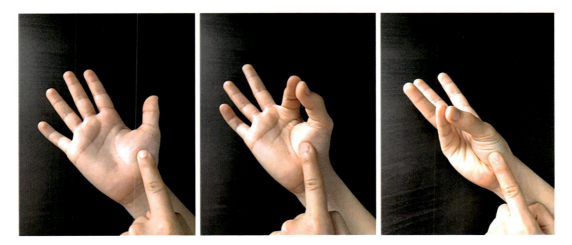

Fig. 5 The Pelvic Floor Muscle Overactivity (firmness) Manual Examination is a 4-point scale of hypertonicity based on comparison of the pelvic floor muscles to the thenar eminence. (**a**) Normal, (**b**) moderate, and (**c**) severe high tone

musculoskeletal structures (e.g., muscles, bones, tendons, and ligaments) in the pelvis can result in pelvic pain. Osteoporosis, fractures, scoliosis, foot injuries, and pubic symphysis diastasis are just examples of disorders that can result in pelvic pain. Young female athletes can present with osteitis pubis – or even osteomyelitis – likely due to microtrauma; painful isometric adductor contraction can be identified on exam with the patient supine, hips flexed, and the examiner's fist between the knees. Sacroiliac joint pain is identified with the FABER (flexion, abduction, external rotation) test, Fig. 6. Iliopsoas pain is interesting because it can mimic renal colic in addition to

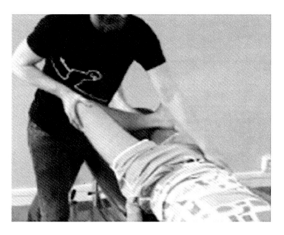

Fig. 6 FABER test: the examined leg is placed with the foot just proximal to the contralateral knee joint, the hip is moved into a combined flexion, abduction, and external rotation position, and the examiner places a hand on the contralateral side of the pelvis to minimize pelvic rotation. (Adapted section from original image: Pålsson, A., Kostogiannis, I. & Ageberg, E. Combining results from hip impingement and range of motion tests can increase diagnostic accuracy in patients with FAI syndrome. *Knee Surg Sports Traumatol Arthrosc* **28**, 3382–3392 (2020). https://doi.org/10.1007/s00167-020-06005-5. Creative Commons License: http://creativecommons.org/licenses/by/4.0/)

causing pelvic pain. With the patient supine and one leg bent, the examiner produces passive movement of the bent leg, palpating the psoas medial to the sartorius, under the ilioinguinal ligament, and up to its insertion on the spine. Particularly in thin patients, palpation will reproduce the pain.

Gastrointestinal

The innervation of gastrointestinal (GI) structures makes it possible for GI pain to be felt in the pelvis. Irritable bowel syndrome (IBS) is the diagnosis most associated with CPP. It is important to remember that IBS is considered a functional disorder – a diagnosis of exclusion, with no evidence of structural or biochemical abnormalities such as inflammatory bowel disease, celiac disease, severe constipation, ovarian cancer, or colon cancer. Diagnosis is currently set by the Rome IV criteria [51]. Symptoms are usually that of pain in the abdomen or pelvis that is relieved with defecation. It is typically accompanied by changes in stool frequency or consistency. It can be seen in association with other syndromes such as endometriosis and interstitial cystitis [51, 52].

Inflammatory bowel disease (IBD) is the term used to describe two inflammatory disorders: ulcerative colitis and Crohn's disease. Crohn's disease affects both the small and large intestine, and the inflammation can involve the full thickness of the bowel. Ulcerative colitis affects the innermost lining of just the large intestine, including the rectum. The clinical course is characterized by flares and remissions. Extraintestinal manifestations are common in IBD. Diagnosis is made by medical history, physical examination, and endoscopy with biopsy of the intestinal mucosa [53].

People with constipation-related pelvic pain may not be aware they are constipated. Constipation is more commonly caused by slow colon transit, pelvic floor issues, or a combination. Causes also include disorders of the colon (such as anal fissure, stricture, rectal inflammation, or colon cancer) or neurologic disorders (*Parkinson's disease* and spinal cord injuries).

Other gastrointestinal disorders that can give rise to CPP include abdominal or inguinal hernias, hemorrhoids, and rectal prolapse.

Functional anorectal pain disorders are defined by the Rome IV criteria as "Levator Ani Syndrome" (the equivalent of pelvic floor tension myalgia), unspecified functional anorectal pain, and "proctalgia fugax" [54]. Proctalgia fugax is characterized by episodes of sharp or stabbing fleeting pain that recur over weeks, are localized to the rectum, and last from seconds to 30 min with no pain between episodes. There are numerous precipitants including sexual activity, stress, constipation, defecation, and menstruation, although the condition can occur without a trigger. Treatment includes observation, inhaled salbutamol, and topical (surface) agents to relax the anal sphincter muscle for symptomatic relief during the event, such as diltiazem and glycerol nitrate.

Vascular

Vascular disorders in CPP can be classified as those arising from the arteries and those arising from the venous vasculature.

By far, the most common vascular disorders resulting in pelvic pain are those arising from the venous circulation of the pelvis. Some sources cite that up to 31% of all women presenting with chronic pelvic pain have some level of impairment in the pelvic venous circulation [8, 55]. The proposed mechanism in these cases is the development of venous hypertension within the renal, gonadal, iliac, or lower extremity veins. Pain is described as dull and is often relieved in the supine position (as venous pressure improves). Pelvic Congestion Syndrome presents with symptoms of pelvic pressure, aching, heaviness, throbbing that is worse with standing and at the end of the day and relieved with lying down. Up to one-third of women with pelvic venous congestion have vulvar-vaginal varicose veins, and up to 90% will have lower extremity varicose veins [56]. Adnexal point tenderness on examination with a history of post-coital ache – 94% sensitive and 77% specific for PCS [57]. The nutcracker syndrome (i.e., compression of the left renal vein by the mesenteric artery) and May-Thurner syndrome (i.e., compression of the left common iliac vein by the left external iliac artery) are two venous syndromes that can be associated with CPP, Figs. 7 and 8. Initial imaging includes venous duplex ultrasound, or more definitively, *computed tomography* (CT) *scan venogram*, or *magnetic resonance (MR) scan venogram*, which are excellent at evaluating venous anatomy, pelvic varicose veins, compression, obstruction, and dilated segments of gonadal (ovarian or testicular) veins.

Arterial causes of pelvic pain are much less common but should be considered. Arterial vasculitis, namely, giant cell arteritis, is associated with the development of polymyalgia rheumatica, which is associated with pain in the pelvic girdle [58]. The buildup of atherosclerotic plaques within the iliac arteries or even the abdominal aorta can impact perfusion to the pelvic area. Rarely, this can result in bladder symptoms and

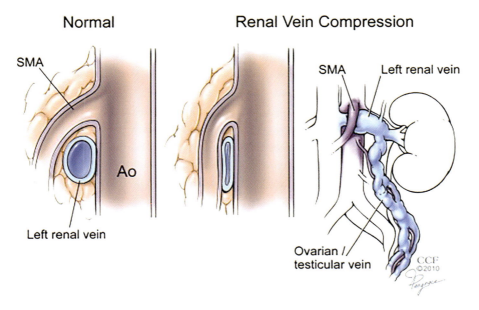

Fig. 7 Illustration of Nutcracker Syndrome. (Reprinted from The Nutcracker Syndrome, Annals of Vascular Surgery, Volume 25, Issue 8, 2011. Sridhar Venkatachalam, Kelly Bumpus, Samir R. Kapadia, Bruce Gray, Sean Lyden, Mehdi H. Shishehbor. Pages 1154–1164, ISSN 0890-5096, https://doi.org/10.1016/j.avsg.2011.01.002. With permission from Elsevier)

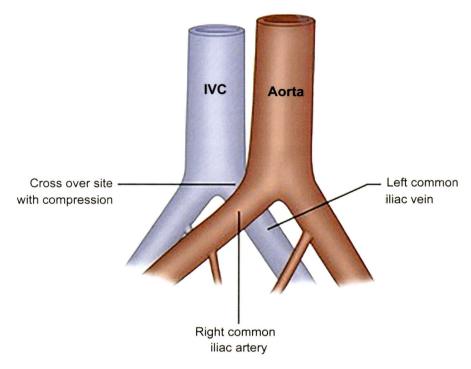

Fig. 8 Nonthrombotic iliac vein lesion. (Reprinted by permission from [Springer Nature]: [Springer Nature] [Nonthrombotic Iliac Vein Lesion (May-Thurner Syndrome)] by [Riju Ramachandran Menon] [Copyright] (2014))

sexual dysfunction. Aneurysm is a rare but serious etiology.

Neurological

Damage to the neurological structures supplying the pelvis can result in both acute and chronic pain. The innervation of the pelvic structures is supplied by the *hypogastric, lumbar, and sacral plexuses,* Fig. 9. The most common focal nerve injury associated with pelvic pain is pudendal neuralgia. In this disorder, the pudendal nerve is affected, either by direct compression (childbirth, biking, muscles, mesh) or damaged in conditions such as diabetes mellitus or viral infection. Pain in this condition is typically worse when sitting down, especially on hard surfaces, and is distributed along the rectum, genitalia, and the lower urinary tract. The Nantes criteria are used to diagnose this condition clinically and include: (1) pain in the anatomical territory of the pudendal nerve, (2) worsened by sitting, (3) the patient is not woken at night by the pain, (4) no objective sensory loss on clinical examination, and (5) positive anesthetic pudendal nerve block [59]. Sexual and sphincter dysfunction are also manifestations of pudendal neuralgia [59, 60]. Differential diagnosis for this pathology includes sacral radiculopathy (Tarlov cysts, sacral chordoma, arachnoititis, herpes) [61]. Back pain can radiate to the pelvis and/or lower extremities [60], and multiple discrete nerves originating outside the pelvis can lead to pelvic symptoms if injured (e.g., ilioinguinal nerve (L1), Obturator nerve (L2-L4), genitofemoral nerve [L1-L2]). In addition to history and physical exam, dermatomal maps and tables can be extremely helpful (Fig. 10) (Table 2). MRI can help delineate spinal lesions and targeted diagnostic nerve injections can clarify pain due to specific peripheral nerves.

Central nervous system causes of CPP have not always been diagnosed prior to presentation to the reconstructive surgeon.

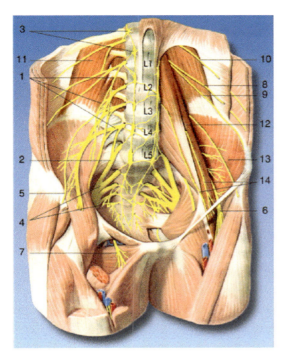

Fig. 9 Anatomy: lumbar plexus, sacral plexus, and coccygeal plexus. (1) Lumbar plexus, (2) lumbosacral trunk, (3) sympathetic trunk, (4) sacral plexus, (5) lateral femoral cutaneous nerve, (6) femoral nerve, (7) obturator nerve, (8) iliohypogastric nerve, (9) ilioinguinal nerve, (10) subcostal nerve, (11) quadratus lumborum muscle, (12) psoas major muscle, (13) iliacus muscle, (14) genitofemoral nerve. (Reprinted with permission from Danilo Jankovic (from Regional Nerve Blocks in Anesthesia and Pain Therapy, Traditional and Ultrasound-Guided Techniques; 4th ed. (2015), edited by Danilo Jankovic and Philip Peng, published by Springer))

Herniated disc can involve compression and irritation of the spinal cord or a radiculopathy of a spinal nerve root. The patient will report back pain, shooting pain, numbness that follows a specific dermatomal pattern (for example, a T10 through L1 disc herniation can *radiate* into the skin of the groin or abdomen), or sciatic symptoms. Persistent genital arousal disorder has also been attributed to the spine. Exam can reveal abnormal gait, pain with provocative maneuvers (such as pain with low back flexion or positive straight leg test that radiates pain with spine range of motion), and possible increased or decreased reflexes.

Tarlov Cysts are fluid-filled nerve root cysts found most often at the sacral level of the spine; small cysts can be a normal variant and are present in 5–10% of people. Symptoms vary but can present with pain over the buttocks and sacrum, pain with sitting, standing, or walking, or with bowel, bladder, or sexual dysfunction. Exam may reveal loss of or increased sensitivity to touch over the sacrum and buttock; patients might present with lower extremity weakness.

Spina bifida occulta (SBO) is a type of closed spinal dysraphism and it is not uncommon to find it in adults. *SBO* was the most common finding in a sample of young people imaged for low back pain in China [62]. Patients may report lower extremity symptoms, including weakness, as well as urinary, sexual, or bowel symptoms, pelvic pain, and impaired sensation of the genitals, bladder, or bowels. Sometimes, symptoms begin during growth spurts because of associated *tethered spinal cord*. Physical exam may demonstrate lower extremity atrophy and weakness, and the skin over the spine might present with an abnormal tuft of hair, dimple, or birthmark.

Tethered spinal cord is associated with spina bifida and is caused by tissue attachments that limit the movement of the spinal cord within the spinal column during growth, causing an abnormal stretching of the spinal cord. Patients may report back pain, shooting pain, weakness, or numbness in the legs, lower extremity spasms, and bowel or bladder dysfunction (over or underactive, as upper spinal levels can be affected). Physical exam may demonstrate lower extremity weakness, abnormally low or high reflexes, and diminished lower extremity sensation.

A recent retrospective report from the university of Iowa describes 24 newly diagnosed adult (aged 20–77) patients [63]. Non-dermatomal low-back or perineal pain occurred in 19, bladder dysfunction in 21, and motor, sensory, and reflex abnormalities in 21 patients. Of the 20 patients who elected surgery, 16 of 19 patients reporting low-back or perineal pain, 17 of 20 reporting motor and sensory complaints, and 12 of 20 patients normalized and 3 of 20 improved their bladder function postoperatively.

Cauda equina syndrome is caused by central spine nerve compression, such as stenosis in the lumbar region from a large herniated disc or tumor.

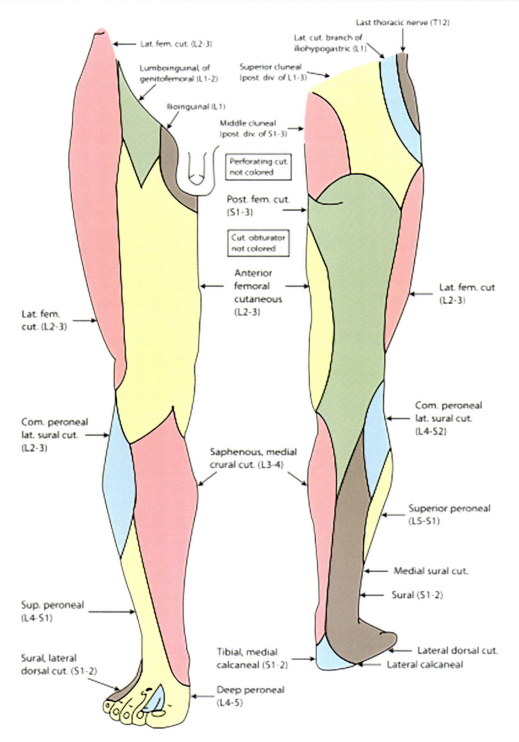

Fig. 10 Dermatomes of the pelvis and lower extremity. (Source: Henry Gray. Cutaneous nerves of the right lower extremity. Front and posterior views. Anatomy of the Human Body. 1918. Lea and Febiger. Available at: https://commons.wikimedia.org/wiki/File:Gray826and331.svg)

Table 2 Peripheral nerves of the pelvis and typical associated pain patterns. (Reproduced from Table 9-1 in Facing Pelvic Pain: *A Guide for Patients and Their Families.* De, EJB and Stern, TA, Eds. Massachusetts General Hospital Psychiatry Academy, Boston MA. Copyright 2021. ISBN-13: 978-1-951166-22-9. Available at: www.facingpelvicpain.org)

Peripheral Nerve	Area or Pattern of Pain
Ilioinguinal nerve	Pain, numbness and/or allodynia[a] on the groin and/or lateral waist with or without radiation to vulva, penis, or scrotum.
Iliohypogastric nerve	Pain, numbness, or allodynia in the lower abdominal wall or pubic region, sometimes hip and lateral thigh.
Genitofemoral nerve	Pain, numbness and/or allodynia on the groin, urethra, clitoris, anterior vulva in females; in males, symptoms are felt on the groin/crotch, scrotum, and base of the penis.
Obturator nerve	Pain, numbness and/or allodynia on the inner thigh. Also, can cause some hip instability.
Anterior abdominal cutaneous nerves.	Pin-point abdominal pain, often lateral to the rectus sheath (Applegate, 2002).
Pudendal nerve (rectal, perineal, vaginal, scrotal/penile branches)	Pain, numbness and/or allodynia on the *anus*, vulva/scrotum, penis, and perineum. Usually associated urinary and bowel urgency and frequency, pain on passing urine or stool. Genital arousal disorders, erectile dysfunction, and/or lack of vaginal lubrication may be present.
	May be described as knife-like pain or like a foreign-body sensation in the rectum, vagina, or perineum as well as an inability to sit; pain is often relieved by lying down, The Nantes Criteria is used as a diagnostic tool for pudendal nerve pain, also known as *pudendal neuralgia* (Labat Riant and Robert, 2008).
Lateral femoral cutaneous nerve	Pain and numbness of the lateral thigh is seen more frequently in those with obesity, wearing tight pants or belts, or with impingement secondary to prolonged hip flexion.
Sciatic nerve	Pain and numbness or allodynia on the buttocks, going down the back of the thigh, calf, and leg, to the sole of the foot. Sciatic *nerve entrapments* can cause difficulties walking and a foot drop.
S1 nerve root	Pain and numbness on the *external* aspect of the posterior thigh, calf, and leg and the exterior aspect of the foot. S1 nerve root entrapments can cause gait disturbances and loss of ankle stability.
S2 nerve root	Pain and numbness on the internal half of the posterior thigh, calf, and leg; internal surface of the foot; the vulva and clitoris (female); and penis and scrotum (male). Usually associated with urinary urgency and frequency. Genital arousal disorders, erectile dysfunction, and/or lack of vaginal lubrication might be present.
S3/4 nerve root (usually entrapped together because of proximity)	Pain and numbness on the buttock, anus, perineum, vulva, and clitoris (female), and penis and scrotum (male). Usually associated urinary and bowel urgency and frequency, pain on passing urine or stool. Often associated with vaginal and/or rectal foreign-body sensation.
Posterior femoral cutaneous nerve and *inferior cluneal nerves*	Inferior gluteal (buttocks) pain.

[a]Allodynia is when a stimulus that is usually sensed as gentle/subtle is perceived as a painful/unpleasant sensation; for example, underwear touching the skin or the touch of a cotton swab can be perceived as scratching, burning, or shocking

Symptoms might include lower extremity weakness and/or pain, decreased sensation in the legs and/or the lower pelvic/perineal region *("saddle anesthesia")*, new-onset difficulty urinating or urinary or bowel incontinence. If the above symptoms are acute, they require emergency evaluation. On exam one may note diminished perineal sensation, lower-extremity weakness, or reduced or absent reflexes in the legs.

Sacral tumor can involve benign or malignant growths impacting function of the sacral nerve roots. Patients might present with symptoms similar

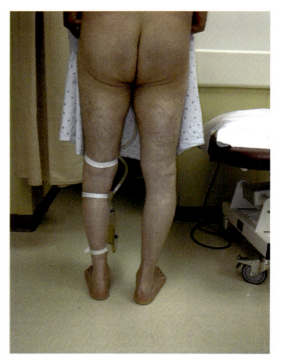

Fig. 11 Protracted history of benign sacral tumor impacting urinary, bowel, and sexual function and producing severe pelvic pain. Findings at the first visit of gluteal atrophy, left> right calf atrophy, and elevated post void residual prompted spinal MRI. Archive Elise De, MD, reproduced with permission of patient

to Tarlov cysts and herniated discs, such as back pain, lower extremity pain, lower extremity weakness, numbness or tingling, rectal dysfunction, urinary retention or incontinence, or erectile dysfunction. In the case of tumor, there may also be tenderness over the sacrum or a palpable mass. In chronic cases (Fig. 11) muscle atrophy might be noted.

Multifocal Pain and Other Conditions

There exist several conditions that can manifest as CPP in addition to extra pelvic symptoms. If a patient presents with multifocal pain or autonomic dysfunction, the workup shifts significantly.

Small fiber polyneuropathy has, as mentioned above, been identified in 64% of patients with complex (refractory or multisystem) chronic pelvic pain [12]. It involves dysfunction of the small c-fibers, a-delta fibers, and postganglionic sympathetics in the periphery, impacting transduction of pain signals from the periphery as well as autonomic function [12]. The Treatment Map at www.facingpelvicpain.org provides screening for the typical systemic symptoms (migraine, IBS, IC, gastroesophageal reflux, temporomandibular joint pain, foot pain, loss of hair on the extremities, tinnitus and other auditory malfunction, and other symptoms) prompting the provider to refer to an autonomic neurologist.

Multiple sclerosis, amyotrophic lateral sclerosis (ALS), Parkinson's disease, and Alzheimer's disease are all systemic neurological disorders that can manifest with the appearance of widespread pain. This occurs due to changes in the structural and biochemical level, resulting in disordered communication among neural pathways within the CNS [64, 65].

Rheumatological disorders can lead to CPP. As discussed before, polymyalgia rheumatica is the most common rheumatological disorder associated with CPP. Other disease processes such as rheumatoid arthritis, systemic lupus erythematosus, or ankylosing spondylitis can cause pelvic pain if the joints and structures of the pelvis become affected [66].

Central Sensitization: it should be emphasized that patients suffering from chronic pain disorders might have undergone central sensitization. This happens when repeated pain signals originate in the peripheral nervous system, resulting in increased neuronal excitability in second- and third-order neurons in the CNS. This increased excitability leads to typically non-painful stimuli being perceived as painful in patients with chronic pain disorders. Cognitive behavioral therapy, relaxation and mindfulness techniques, and exercise have been shown to have benefit in managing these patients [67–71].

Treatment

The treatment for chronic pelvic pain should be undertaken with a multidisciplinary approach in mind. The presence of CPP might be disabling to some people, so opioid-sparing symptom relief should be provided where possible and brisk referral to pain management where not. If a specific mechanism is found to be the source of chronic pain, then addressing the underlying etiology should be of primary focus. However, as discussed before, no underlying etiology is identified in a considerable percentage of patients suffering from CPP. In this case, the objective of management shifts to improvement of the patient's quality of life. This section will provide a brief overview of treatment in patients with CPP. For a comprehensive approach in the management of each individual disorder associated with CPP, refer to the European Guidelines on Chronic Pelvic Pain [71].

A conservative approach with physical therapy (where relevant on physical exam) and medication should be attempted before considering invasive procedures. Usually, medication should be directed at the underlying mechanism of pain. If no mechanism is elucidated, then medication should be directed at symptom relief [24].

Acetaminophen and nonsteroidal anti-inflammatory drugs (NSAIDs) are usually the first therapy attempted in patients with pain. Their adverse effect profile is manageable, and some patients are typically able to find some relief. In women, the use of oral contraceptives and progestogen can be effective in the management of cyclic menstrual pelvic pain. Endometriosis and related disorders should be considered.

For pelvic pain of suspected neuropathic origin, several medications can be used for its management, as catalogued in the Treatment Map. Pregabalin, gabapentin, tricyclic antidepressants, and serotonin-noradrenaline reuptake inhibitors are some options readily available for the treatment of CPP of neuropathic pain. Anesthetic and steroid injections could be considered for use in patients in whom focal radiculopathies can be identified. Chronic opioid use remains controversial and although it is sometimes employed for refractory CPP, it is best to initiate patients on opioids in consultation with a pain management specialist [24, 68–71].

Surgical procedures should rarely be performed in patients in whom no underlying mechanism for pain has been elucidated. Specific disorders such as bladder outlet obstruction, distal ureteric stone, endometriosis, tethered spinal cord, and nerve entrapment can benefit from surgical intervention. These interventions are not included in this chapter.

As is the case for other chronic pain disorders, the psychological and behavioral aspects of the disorder can and should be adequately managed. Psychological interventions play a crucial role in the management of CPP and should be attempted whenever possible. Cognitive Behavioral Therapy (focus on challenging negative behaviors and thoughts) has shown promise in the management of CPP. Mindfulness therapy, which focuses on the awareness of thoughts and sensations, is also a potentially effective approach to chronic pain [16, 68–71]. Comorbid conditions such as depression should also be addressed. It is important to introduce treating the brain as an important component of pain management – as pain is a cognitive process – but to assure the patient that the provider does not think the pain is "in the head."

Finally, other treatment modalities such as acupuncture and TENS units, and sophisticated techniques for neuromodulation, could provide some benefit in patients where other treatments have proved to be ineffective.

Conclusion

Chronic pelvic pain is a complex disorder that can result from alterations in virtually any organ system in the body. A significant fraction of patients suffering from chronic pelvic pain will not receive adequate diagnosis, and subsequently, will not receive adequate treatment. While this chapter provides clinicians with tools to diagnose and treat the chronic pelvic pain patient, a multidisciplinary team is essential to correctly manage this population. With the correct management, most of these patients will be able to achieve adequate control of this disorder, significantly improving their quality of life.

Guidelines and Resources for Providers and Patients

There are several resources that both healthcare providers and patients can use to better inform themselves about chronic pelvic pain. The following is a list naming some of these high yield resources.

- **Facing Pelvic Pain**: *A Guide for Patients and Their Family Members* (De E, Stern TA (eds). Due for publication September 2020; Massachusetts General Hospital Psychiatry Academy (via Amazon). Available at: www.facingpelvicpain.org
- **European Guidelines on Chronic Pelvic Pain**: Available at: http://uroweb.org/wp-content/uploads/EAU-Guidelines-Chronic-Pelvic-Pain-2015.pdf.
- **Interstitial Cystitis Network** Available at: https://www.ic-network.com/
- **World federation of Incontinent Patients** – Available at: https://wfip.org/
- **ICS Institute** – School of Pelvic Pain Available at: https://www.ics.org/institute/pelvicpain
- **AUA Guideline on IC/BPS** – Available at: https://www.auanet.org/guidelines/interstitial-cystitis-(ic/bps)-guideline
- **The Practical Management of Pain, 6th edition**. Editors: Benzon, HT, Turk D, Rathmell J, Wu C, Argoff C, Hurley R, and Nicol A. Elsevier, 2021.

Cross-References

▸ Bladder Dysfunction and Pelvic Pain: The Role of Sacral, Tibial, and Pudendal Neuromodulation
▸ Clinical Evaluation of the Female Lower Urinary Tract and Pelvic Floor
▸ Management of Vaginal Posterior Compartment Prolapse: Is There Ever a Case for Graft/Mesh?

References

1. American College of Obstetricians and Gynecologists. Chronic Pelvic Pain. 2011. Available at: https://www.acog.org/womens-health/faqs/chronic-pelvic-pain#:~:text=Chronic%20pelvic%20pain%20is%20pain,it%20may%20occur%20during%20menstruation. Last updated 2020. Accessed 6 June 2021.
2. Ahangari A. Prevalence of chronic pelvic pain among women: an updated review. Pain Physician. 2014;17(2):E141–7. PMID: 24658485.
3. Mathias SD, Kuppermann M, Liberman RF, Lipschutz RC, Steege JF. Chronic pelvic pain: prevalence, health-related quality of life, and economic correlates. Obstet Gynecol. 1996;87(3):321–7. https://doi.org/10.1016/0029-7844(95)00458-0. PMID: 8598943.
4. Smith CP. Male chronic pelvic pain: an update. Indian J Urol. 2016;32(1):34–9. https://doi.org/10.4103/0970-1591.173105.
5. Honorio B. Essentials of pain medicine. 4th ed. Elsevier; The Netherlands, Europe, 2018. p. 262.
6. Bryant C, Cockburn R, Plante A-F, Chia A. The psychological profile of women presenting to a multi-disciplinary clinic for chronic pelvic pain: high levels of psychological dysfunction and implications for practice. J Pain Res. 2016;9:1049–56.
7. EAU Guidelines. Edn. Presented at the EAU Annual Congress, Milan; 2021. ISBN 978-94-92671-13-4.
8. Meissner MH, Gloviczki P. Atlas of endovascular venous surgery (Second Edition) Chapter 21 – Pelvic venous disorders. 2019, p. 567–599. https://doi.org/10.1016/B978-0-323-51139-1.00021-8.
9. Zondervan KT, Yudkin PL, Vessey MP. Chronic pelvic pain in the community – symptoms, investigations, and diagnoses. Am J Obstet Gynecol. 2001;184(6):1149–55.
10. Grace VM, Zondervan KR. Chronic pelvic pain in New Zealand: prevalence, pain severity, diagnoses and use of the health services. Aust NZ J Public Health. 2004;28(4):369–75.
11. Chronic Pelvic Pain: ACOG practice bulletin, Number 218. Obstet Gynecol. 2020;135(3):e98–e109. https://doi.org/10.1097/AOG.0000000000003716. PMID: 32080051.
12. Chen A, De E, Argoff C. Small fiber polyneuropathy is prevalent in patients experiencing complex chronic pelvic pain. Pain Med. 2018;20(3):521–7. https://doi.org/10.1093/pm/pny001. PMID 29447372.
13. Albrecht PJ, Hou Q, Argoff CE, et al. Excessive peptidergic sensory innervation of cutaneous arteriole-venule shunts (AVS) in the palmar glabrous skin of fibromyalgia patients: implications for widespread deep tissue pain and fatigue. Pain Med. 2013;14(6):895–915.
14. Giannoccaro MP, Donadio V, Incensi A, Avoni P, Liguori R. Small nerve fiber involvement in patients referred for fibromyalgia. Muscle Nerve. 2014;49(5):757–9.
15. Caro XJ, Winter EF. The role and importance of small fiber neuropathy in fibromyalgia pain. Curr Pain Headache Rep. 2015;19(12):55.
16. De E, Stern TA. Facing pelvic pain: *a guide for patients and their family members*. Due for publication September 2020; Massachusetts General Hospital Psychiatry Academy (via Amazon).
17. International Pelvic Pain Society. Pelvic Pain Assessment Form. Documents and forms: history and physical. 2008. Available at: https://www.pelvicpain.org/IPPS/Professional/Documents-Forms/IPPS/Content/

Professional/Documents_and_Forms.aspx. Retrieved 23 September 2019. (Level III).
18. Clemens JQ, Calhoun EA, Litwin MS, et al. Validation of a modified National Institutes of Health chronic prostatitis symptom index to assess genitourinary pain in both men and women. Urology. 2009;74(5): 983–987.e9873. https://doi.org/10.1016/j.urology. 2009.06.078.
19. Brookes ST, Donovan JL, Wright M, Jackson S, Abrams P. A scored form of the Bristol Female Lower Urinary Tract Symptoms questionnaire: data from a randomized controlled trial of surgery for women with stress incontinence. Am J Obstet Gynecol. 2004;191:73–82.
20. Barry MJ, Fowler FJ Jr, O'Leary MP, Bruskewitz RC, Holtgrewe HL, Mebust WK, Cockett AT. The American Urological Association symptom index for benign prostatic hyperplasia. The Measurement Committee of the American Urological Association. J Urol. 1992;148(5):1549–57. https://doi.org/10.1016/s0022-5347(17)36966-5. discussion 1564. PMID: 1279218.
21. Barber MD, Walters MD, Bump RC. Short forms of two condition-specific quality-of-life questionnaires for women with pelvic floor disorders (PFDI-20 adn PFIQ-7). Am J Obstet Gynecol. 2005;193:103–13.
22. Bordeianou LG, Anger J, Boutros M, et al. Measuring pelvic floor disorder symptoms using patient-reported instruments: proceedings of the consensus meeting of the pelvic floor consortium of the American Society of Colon and Rectal Surgeons, the International Continence Society, the American Urogynecologic Society, and the Society of Urodynamics, Female Pelvic Medicine and Urogenital Reconstruction. Tech Coloproctol. 2020;24: 5–22. https://doi.org/10.1007/s10151-019-02125-4.
23. Yosef A, Allaire C, Williams C, Ahmed AG, Al-Hussaini T, Abdellah MS, et al. Multifactorial contributors to the severity of chronic pelvic pain in women. Am J Obstet Gynecol. 2016;215(760):e1–14. (Level II-3)
24. Speer LM, Mushkbar S, Erbele T. Chronic pelvic pain in women. Am Fam Physician. 2016;93(5):380–7. PMID: 26926975.
25. Hovaguimian A, Gibbons CH. Diagnosis and treatment of pain in small-fiber neuropathy. Curr Pain Headache Rep. 2011;15(3):193–200. https://doi.org/10.1007/s11916-011-0181-7.
26. Centers for Disease Control and Prevention. Infographic: 6 guiding principles to a trauma-informed approach. September 17, 2020. Available at: https://www.cdc.gov/cpr/infographics/6_principles_trauma_info.htm
27. Carrubba AR, et al. How to perform the physical examination in the female chronic pelvic pain patient: the pre-exam evaluation. J Minimally Invasive Gynecol. 25(7):S161–2.
28. Johns Hopkins Medicine. Pelvic ultrasound. [Internet] 2021 [cited 7 July 2021]. Available from: https://www.hopkinsmedicine.org/health/treatment-tests-and-therapies/pelvic-ultrasound#:~:text=A%20pelvic% 20ultrasound%20is%20a,vagina%2C%20fallopian% 20tubes%20and%20ovaries.
29. Rigor BM. Pelvic cancer pain. J Surg Oncol. 2000;75(4):280–300. https://doi.org/10.1002/1096-9098(200012)75:4<280::aid-jso13>3.0.co;2-q.
30. ACOG Practice Bulletin July 2010 Farquhar, C. endometriosis: clinical review. BMJ. 2007;334: 249–253.
31. Bishop LA. Management of chronic pelvic pain. Clin Obstet Gynecol. 2017;60(3):524–30. https://doi.org/10.1097/GRF.0000000000000299.
32. Kuhn A. Chronischer Beckenschmerz [Chronic pelvic pain]. Ther Umsch. 2019;73(9):573–5. https://doi.org/10.1024/0040-5930/a001039.
33. O'Brien MT, Gillespie DL. Diagnosis and treatment of the pelvic congestion syndrome. J Vasc Surg Venous Lymphatic Disord. 2015;3:96–106.
34. Erben Y, Gloviczki P, Kalra M, et al. Treatment of nutcracker syndrome with open and endovascular interventions. J Vasc Surg Venous Lymphatic Disord. 2015;3:389–96.
35. Krieger JN, Nyberg L Jr, Nickel JC. NIH consensus definition and classification of prostatitis. JAMA. 1999;282:236.
36. Litwin MS, McNaughton-Collins M, Fowler FJ, et al. The National Institutes of Health chronic prostatitis symptom index: development and validation of a new outcome measure. J Urol. 1999;162:369.
37. Polackwich AS, Shoskes DA. Chronic prostatitis/chronic pelvic pain syndrome: a review of evaluation and therapy. Prostate Cancer Prostatic Dis. 2016;19(2): 132–8. https://doi.org/10.1038/pcan.2016.8. Epub 2016 Mar 8. PMID: 26951713.
38. Moses S. Expressed prostatic secretion. Family Practice Notebook 2007. Available online at: https://fpnotebook.com/uro/Lab/ExprsdPrstcScrtn.htm
39. Sigalos JT, Pastuszak AW. Chronic orchialgia: epidemiology, diagnosis and evaluation. Transl Androl Urol. 2017;6(Suppl 1):S37–43.
40. Parekattil SJ, Ergun O, Gudeloglu A. Management of chronic Orchialgia: challenges and solutions – the current standard of care. Res Rep Urol. 2020;12:199–210. https://doi.org/10.2147/RRU.S198785. PMID: 32754451; PMCID: PMC7351977.
41. Hanno P, Dmochowski R. Status of international consensus on interstitial cystitis/bladder pain syndrome/painful bladder syndrome: 2008 snapshot. Neurourol Urodyn. 2009;28:274.
42. Hanno PM, Erickson D, Moldwin R, Faraday MM. Diagnosis and treatment of interstitial cystitis/bladder pain syndrome: AUA guideline amendment. J Urol. 2015;193:1545–53. https://doi.org/10.1016/j.juro.2015.01.086. ® © 2015 by American Urological Association Education and Research, Inc.
43. Metts JF. Interstitial cystitis: urgency and frequency syndrome. Am Fam Physician. 2001;64(7):1199–206. PMID: 11601802.
44. Young A, Toncar A, Wray AA. Urethritis. [Updated 2020 Dec 14]. In: StatPearls [Internet]. Treasure Island:

45. Ulmer WD, Gilbert JL, De EJB. Urethritis in women – considerations beyond urinary tract infection. Curr Bladder Dysfunct Rep. 2014;9:181–7. https://doi.org/10.1007/s11884-014-0246-7.

46. Bedaiwy MA, Patterson B, Mahajan S. Prevalence of myofascial chronic pelvic pain and the effectiveness of pelvic floor physical therapy. J Reprod Med. 2013;58(11–12):504–10.

47. Rogalski MJ, Kellogg-Spadt S, Hoffmann AR, Fariello JY, Whitmore KE. Retrospective chart review of vaginal diazepam suppository use in high-tone pelvic floor dysfunction. Int Urogynecol J Pelvic Floor Dysfunct. 2010;21(7):895–9.

48. Faubion SS, Shuster LT, Bharucha AE. Recognition and management of nonrelaxing pelvic floor dysfunction. Mayo Clin Proc. 2012;87(2):187–93. https://doi.org/10.1016/j.mayocp.2011.09.004.

49. Frawley H, Shelly B, Morin M, Bernard S, Bø K, Digesu GA, Dickinson T, Goonewardene S, McClurg D, Rahnama'i MS, Schizas A, Slieker-Ten Hove M, Takahashi S, Voelkl Guevara J. An International Continence Society (ICS) report on the terminology for pelvic floor muscle assessment. Neurourol Urodyn. 2021;40(5):1217–60. https://doi.org/10.1002/nau.24658. Epub 2021 Apr 12. PMID: 33844342.

50. Spettel S, Frawley HC, Blais DR, De EJB. Biofeedback treatment for overactive bladder. Curr Bladder Dysfunct Rep. 2012;7:7–13.

51. Ford AC, Lacy BE, Talley NJ. Irritable Bowel syndrome. N Engl J Med. 2017;376(26):2566–78. https://doi.org/10.1056/nejmra1607547.

52. Schmulson MJ, Drossman DA. What is new in Rome IV. J Neurogastroenterol Motil. 2017;23(2):151–63. https://doi.org/10.5056/jnm16214.

53. Sairenji T, Collins KL, Evans DV. An update on inflammatory Bowel disease. Prim Care. 2017;44(4):673–92. https://doi.org/10.1016/j.pop.2017.07.010. Epub 2017 Oct 5. PMID: 29132528.

54. Simren M, Palsson OS, Whitehead WE. Update on Rome IV criteria for colorectal disorders: implications for clinical practice. Curr Gastroenterol Rep. 2017;19(4):15. https://doi.org/10.1007/s11894-017-0554-0. PMID: 28374308; PMCID: PMC5378729.

55. Durham JD, Machan L. Pelvic congestion syndrome. Semin Intervent Radiol. 2013;30(4):372–80. https://doi.org/10.1055/s-0033-1359731.

56. Meissner MH, Gibson K. Clinical outcome after treatment of pelvic congestion syndrome: sense and nonsense. Phlebology. 2015;30(1 Suppl):73–80.

57. Beard RW, Highman JH, Pearce S, Reginald PW. Diagnosis of pelvic pain varicosities in women with chronic pelvic pain. Lancet. 1984;2:946–69.

58. Gonzalez-Gay MA, Barros S, Lopez-Diaz MJ, Garcia-Porrua C, Sanchez-Andrade A. Giant cell arteritis: disease patterns of clinical presentation in a series of 240 patients. Llorca J Med (Baltimore). 2005;84(5):269–76.

59. Labat JJ, Riant T, Robert R, Amarenco G, Lefaucheur JP, Rigaud J. Diagnostic criteria for pudendal neuralgia by pudendal nerve entrapment (Nantes criteria). Neurourol Urodyn. 2008;27(4):306–10. https://doi.org/10.1002/nau.20505.

60. Alexander CE, Varacallo M. Lumbosacral radiculopathy. [Updated 2021 May 4]. In: StatPearls [Internet]. Treasure Island: StatPearls Publishing; 2021. Available from: https://www.ncbi.nlm.nih.gov/books/NBK430837/

61. Modirian E, Pirouzi P, Soroush MR, Karbalaei-Esmaeili S, Shojaei H. Physical medicine and rehabilitation, HamidReza Zamani, General Surgeon, chronic pain after spinal cord injury: results of a long-term study. Pain Med. 2010;11(7):1037–43.

62. Li W, Xiong Z, Dong C, Song J, Zhang L, Zhou J, Wang Y, Yi P, Yang F, Tang X, Tan M. Distribution and imaging characteristics of spina bifida occulta in young people with low back pain: a retrospective cross-sectional study. J Orthop Surg Res. 2021;16(1):151. https://doi.org/10.1186/s13018-021-02285-w. PMID: 33618758; PMCID: PMC7898417.

63. Menezes AH, Seaman SC, Iii MAH, Hitchon PW, Takacs EB. Tethered spinal cord syndrome in adults in the MRI era: recognition, pathology, and long-term objective outcomes. J Neurosurg Spine. 2021:1–13. https://doi.org/10.3171/2020.9.SPINE201453. Epub ahead of print. PMID: 33740756.

64. Kumar B, Kalita J, Kumar G, Misra UK. Central post-stroke pain: a review of pathophysiology and treatment. Anesth Analg. 2009;108:1645–57.

65. Bermejo PE, Oreja-Guevara C, Diez-Tejedor E. Pain in multiple sclerosis: prevalence, mechanisms, types and treatment. Rev Neurol. 2010;50:101–8.

66. Fukunishi S, Fukui T, Nishio S, Imamura F, Yoshiya S. Multiple pelvic insufficiency fractures in rheumatoid patients with mutilating changes. Orthop Rev (Pavia). 2009;1(2):e23. https://doi.org/10.4081/or.2009.e23.

67. Engeler D, Baranowski AP, Borovicka J, et al. European Association of Urology. Guidelines on chronic pelvic pain. 2021. Available at: https://uroweb.org/wp-content/uploads/EAU-Guidelines-on-Chronic-Pelvic-Pain-2020.pdf

68. Sator-Katzenschlager SM, Scharbert G, Kress HG, et al. Chronic pelvic pain treated with gabapentin and amitriptyline: a randomized controlled pilot study. Wien Klin Wochenschr. 2005;117(21–22):761–8.

69. Haugstad GK, Kirste U, Leganger S, Haakonsen E, Haugstad TS. Somatocognitive therapy in the management of chronic gynaecological pain. A review of the historical background and results of a current approach. Scand J Pain. 2011;2(3):124–9.

70. Pak DJ, Yong RJ, Kaye AD, Urman RD. Chronification of pain: mechanisms, current understanding, and clinical implications Curr Pain Headache Rep. 2018;22(2) https://doi.org/10.1007/s11916-018-0666-8.

71. Voscopoulos C, Lema M. When does acute pain become chronic? Br J Anaesth. 2010;105(Suppl 1):i69–85. https://doi.org/10.1093/bja/aeq323.

Bladder Pain Syndrome: Interstitial Cystitis

53

Francisco Cruz, Rui Pinto, and Pedro Abreu Mendes

Contents

Introduction	932
Terminology	932
Epidemiology	933
Etiology	934
Pathology	935
Diagnosis	936
History Including Emotional Problems and Bowel and Sexual Dysfunction	936
Physical Examination	940
Laboratory Tests and Urodynamics	940
Cystoscopy and Bladder Biopsy	941
Biomarkers	942
Phenotyping BPS/IC Patients	944
Management	944
Conservative Measures	945
Interventional Pharmacotherapy	945
Oral Pharmacotherapy	946
Intravesical Pharmacotherapy	948
Intramural Treatments	948
Surgical Treatments	949
Future Developments in Terms of Animal Studies	950
Cross-References	950
References	950

F. Cruz (✉) · R. Pinto · P. A. Mendes
Department of Urology, Faculty of Medicine of University of Porto, Hospital São João, I3S Institute for Investigation and Innovation in Health, Porto, Portugal
e-mail: cruzfjmr@med.up.pt

Abstract

Bladder pain syndrome/interstitial cystitis (BPS/IC) is a terminology that reflects how little is known about the disease, or diseases, that are characterized by pain, localized to the bladder or systemic, associated with urological

© Springer Nature Switzerland AG 2023
F. E. Martins et al. (eds.), *Female Genitourinary and Pelvic Floor Reconstruction*,
https://doi.org/10.1007/978-3-031-19598-3_54

and non-urological symptoms. Historically it was associated to an intense pain-bladder inflammation and to pathognomonic bladder ulcerations justifying the name IC. It is now clear that BPS/IC may progress without inflammatory changes in the bladder wall, justifying the term BPS. Etiology is unknown and no biomarkers have been identified to support the diagnosis. Thus, the exclusion of confoundable diseases remains a fundamental step in the diagnostic workup of BPS/IC. Cure for BPS/IC is not yet known.

Keywords

Chronic pelvic pain · Interstitial cystitis · Painful bladder syndrome · Overactive bladder

Introduction

Bladder pain syndrome/interstitial cystitis (BPS/IC) is one of the few still enigmatic diseases involving the urinary bladder. Several factors have decisively contributed to this unfortunate outlook. The terminology has evolved over the years, and different societies still adopt different wording when referring to the disease [1]. Historically defined as a severe intense inflammatory disease, it was first described by Skene in 1887 and afterward characterized by the presence of bladder ulcerations by Hunner in 1915; it is now evident that BPS/IC may progress with symptoms of pain, localized or systemic, associated with both urological and non-urological symptoms but without pathological changes in the bladder wall [2]. In addition, the etiology is unknown, despite the multiple hypotheses put forward. It is therefore unclear if BPS/IC is a single disease with different stages of evolution or different diseases, which share similar symptomatology. Eventually, biomarkers could contribute to filling the gap left by the lack of pathognomonic pathological findings or specific symptomatology. However, a reliable biomarker is still missing [3]. Curative treatment for BPS/IC is yet to be discovered. The pursuit of specific phenotypes, of homogeneous groups of patients with more uniform pathological and symptomatology and more responsive to certain management strategies, is under debate.

Terminology

Initial descriptions of BPS/IC put a strong emphasis on the pan-inflammation of the bladder wall and urothelial denudation (Skene, 1887) or the presence of ulcerative lesions in the bladder, Hunner's lesions that for years become pathognomonic of the disease. The National Institute of Diabetes and Digestive and Kidney Diseases (NIDDK) made the first structured move to define criteria for the diagnosis of the disease [4]. According to NIDDK, the diagnosis of BPS/IC required the presence of pain, associated or not with frequency and urgency to void and present for at least 9 months. The identification of Hunner's lesions was enough to establish the diagnosis, while the visualization of glomerulations during cystoscopy and a bladder capacity inferior to 350 ml would strongly favor the diagnosis in patients with the classic symptoms. The importance of symptoms in the definition of BPS/IC becomes clear when the International Continence Society (ICS) defined this condition as the complaint of suprapubic pain related to bladder filling, accompanied by other symptoms such as increased daytime and nighttime frequency, in the absence of proven urinary infection or other obvious pathology [5]. In 2008, the International Society for the Study of BPS (ESSIC) reworded the definition and defined it as a disease characterized by chronic pelvic pain, pressure, or discomfort perceived to be related to the urinary bladder, with at least one other urinary symptom such as urgency or urinary frequency [6]. Since these symptoms are not specific, confusable diseases must be excluded as the cause of the symptoms. According to ESSIC, the term IC should be used only when Hunner's lesions (HL) are identified, whereas BPS should be considered as a pain syndrome involving but not limited to the bladder. The separation between BPS and IC as two different entities, the former being a chronic pain syndrome and the latter an inflammatory disease of the bladder associated with a painful perception, has since then prevailed [7, 8]. The American Urological Association (AUA) adopted the "Multidisciplinary Approach to the Study of Chronic Pelvic Pain" (MAPP) proposal defining BPS as a disease characterized by an unpleasant sensation, variably described as pain, pressure, or discomfort, seemingly related to the urinary bladder and associated with other lower urinary tract symptoms, lasting for more than 6 weeks, in the absence of infection or other identifiable cause [9].

The European Association of Urology (EAU) guidelines on chronic pelvic pain of 2018 followed the International Association for the Study of Pain (IASP) concept of chronic pain as a disease [10, 11]. Accordingly, chronic pelvic pain was defined as chronic pain perceived by the patients and/or by the physicians as related to pelvic organs or structures. Pain, pressure, or discomfort associated with the urinary bladder was typically accompanied by at least one other lower urinary tract symptom, such as an increase in the daytime and/or nighttime urinary frequency. Pain characteristics for the diagnosis of BPS/IC were also found important for the disease characterization. Pain should be associated with the bladder, increase with bladder filling, and be relieved by voiding. However, pain could also be constant. Localization was typically suprapubic but could also radiate to other areas, and confoundable diseases needed to be ruled out.

The new 2022 EAU version of the guidelines introduced the concept of chronic primary pelvic pain syndrome, which now requires the exclusion of an infection or other obvious pathology that may account for pelvic pain [7]. Pain perception in chronic primary pelvic pain syndrome may be focused on one single organ, the bladder, and in that case, the term BPS can be used. However, when systemic symptoms or diseases are present such as chronic fatigue, fibromyalgia, or Sjogren syndrome, then clinicians should consider a systemic disturbance rather than a local problem. The minimal duration of the symptoms to sanction a firm diagnosis is not clearly stated in the EAU guidelines of 2022, but European physicians tend to require 6 months as the minimum length of symptomatology to accept the pain as chronic, before establishing a diagnosis of BPS/IC.

Epidemiology

The lack of a specific symptom complex and a definition universally accepted makes the epidemiological studies particularly difficult. Pelvic pain may affect up to 10% of the population [12], but this number included diseases confoundable with BPS/IC, which better needed exclusion. The lack of an accepted definition, the unknown etiology, the absence of a validated diagnostic marker, and the variable pathological changes further make epidemiological studies difficult. Furthermore, different cultural responses to pain may explain the different prevalence across the world [13]. Therefore, the numbers shown below should not be interpreted as true differences in BPS/IC prevalence in different areas around the world but rather as different responses to the survey tools applied. In most surveys, affected women were typically young or in middle age.

In Japan, the incidence may be as low as 1.2 per 100,000 population [14], while in South Korea BPS/IC-like symptoms were identified in more than 16,000/100,000 [15]. In the United States, a questionnaire-based study suggested a prevalence in women of 20,000 per 100,000 [10], while another survey using different questionnaires found an upper figure of only 2700 per 100,000 [16]. In Finland, Leppilahti et al. [17] using the O'Leary-Sant Symptom and Problem Index questionnaire considered the disease present if the score was 7 or higher and concluded a prevalence of 230/100,000. In Austria, the prevalence was 306/100,000 women using the O'Leary-Sant questionnaire with a cutoff score of 12 [18]. In Spain, the incidence of BPS/IC in women using health units was 5400/100,000 [19]. In the Netherlands, Bade et al. [20] concluded, based on pathological findings, that the prevalence was only 16 per 100,000 female patients.

A recent survey conducted in five European countries, France, Germany, Italy, Spain, and the United Kingdom, deserves a particular mention

[21]. Patients were enrolled if they had experienced pain in the past 12 months and identified the bladder as the source of an unpleasant sensation, pain, pressure, or discomfort in the past month. Furthermore, patients had to indicate that the condition was diagnosed by a physician. Individuals with a history of bladder cancer and those who experienced bladder pain without physician diagnosis were excluded. The prevalence of overall bladder-related pain was 1220/100,000, but the diagnosis of BPS/IC was 440/100,000. Many texts tend to accept a balance prevalence between 300 and 400/100,000 subjects.

Etiology

It is unfortunate that after so many years of intense research and despite the multiple hypotheses raised, the etiology remains unknown.

The classic concept of a defect in the urothelial barrier function remains attractive. Increased permeability of the urothelium may allow different molecular weight urine solutes to escape to the bladder wall. Potassium and hydrogen ions can sensitize nociceptors and cause the release of neuropeptides and other neurotransmitters that may contribute to a neurogenic component of inflammation [22, 23]. Bladder nociceptors may also branch into other pelvic organs, including the colon. Therefore, once excited they may cause cross-sensitization at the spinal cord level, which might contribute to the coincidence of urinary and colonic symptomatology in many BPS/IC [24]. Toll-like receptors (TLR), particularly TLR-4, have also been identified as key players in the course of central pain sensitization [25]. In addition, the network of suburothelial bladder nociceptors is denser in BPS/IC patients which might also contribute to the disproportionate intensity of pain referred by BPS/IC patients [26].

Urine solutes that penetrate the bladder wall may also activate inflammatory cells like mast cells, leading to the release of inflammatory mediators into the bladder wall. Neurotransmitters such as histamine, leukotrienes, serotonin, and cytokines, all of which, can excite and sensitize bladder nociceptors [27]. In the end, the inflammatory process can also contribute to bladder fibrosis and angiogenesis [28].

The urothelial barrier is constituted by a sulfate polysaccharide glycosaminoglycan layer covering the urothelium and by tight junctions that interconnect the umbrella cells. Tight junctions, gap junctions, and desmosomes also contribute to maintaining the urothelium impermeable to urine and its solutes. The reasons why the urothelium of BPS/IC patients is leaky are unclear. Electron microscopy identified defects in intercellular junctions [29]. A decreased expression of tight junctions has been recognized [30] eventually caused by epigenetic abnormalities leading to the expression of abnormal microRNAs involved in tight junction expression [31].

The urothelium of BPS/IC patients seems to have a slower proliferative rate than that of normal people. An antiproliferative factor (APF) responsible for downregulation of genes that stimulates cell proliferation and upregulates genes that inhibit cell growth was identified in the urine of BPS/IC patients [32, 33]. Eventually, this APF could slow down the repair of the urothelium caused by different insults, and if maintained during a prolonged period, the urothelium may become thinner and leakier. In this context, an infectious etiology for BPS/IC becomes attractive. However, the evidence supporting infection as the cause of BPS/IC is very weak. Some patients may improve with the antibiotic doxycycline [34]. Microbiota of BPS/IC patients and normal women may be different. A smaller diversity abundance was observed in BPS/IC women, with more than 90% of the IC sequence reads belonging to the genus *Lactobacillus* [35]. The prevalence of *Candida* and *Saccharomyces* species was greater in women having a flare-up [36]. Furthermore, in two cohorts of patients with ulcerative BPS/IC, BK polyomavirus (BKPyV) was identified in the urine of virtually all the cases [37, 38]. The role of BKPyV, one of the five polyomaviruses, in causing urinary pathology is established in transplanted patients under immunosuppressive therapy. The polyomavirus BKV causes serious hemorrhagic cystitis in the recipients.

The role of toxic agents in the urine has also been put forward in the premise that they may function as cytotoxic agents to the bladder urothelium. Major urinary cationic metabolites are present in higher amounts in BPS/IC patients. Patients have higher levels of modified nucleosides, amino acids, and tryptophan in the urine. The cytotoxicity of cationic metabolites to isolated urothelial cells was significantly higher in BPS/IC patients than in controls [39]. Abnormal glycosylation of Tamm-Horsfall protein in BPS/IC patients may reduce the capacity of the protein to neutralize the toxic cations [40].

The intense T- and B-lymphocyte infiltrate is found in the bladder of ulcerative cases of BPS/IC or those with detectable antinuclear antibodies, as it occurs in Sjogren syndrome [41]. These findings are among those that have nurtured an autoimmune hypothesis for the disease. In Taiwan BPS/IC patients were associated with autoimmune diseases, especially Hashimoto's thyroiditis, ankylosing spondylitis, rheumatoid arthritis, and Sjogren's syndrome. Clinicians are recommended to be alert to the increased likelihood of this problem when investigating middle-aged women. The MAPP consortium found some evidence to suggest that rising pollen count in the air may trigger flares of BPS/IC [42].

The urothelium from BPS/IC patients [43] and felines with IC release more ATP [44] upon distention. The excess of ATP may then excite suburothelial sensory nerves expressing P3X3 receptors [45]. However, the reasons why more ATP is released by umbrella cells of IC patients and felines were never clarified.

Pathology

Pathology can be consistent with the diagnosis of BPS/IC, but there is no pathognomonic finding for this disease. The most important role of histopathology in the diagnosis of BPS is, therefore, the exclusion of confoundable diseases, in particular, carcinoma and carcinoma in situ and tuberculous cystitis [6, 46]. Old descriptions refer to a chronic, edematous involvement of the entire bladder wall with increased mast cell infiltration and chronic lymphocytic infiltrate and submucosal ulcerations [47]. However, a great variation in the histologic appearance of BPS/IC bladders and even variation among biopsies taken from the same patients over time may occur. Johansson and Fall, when looking into samples from ulcerative and non-ulcerative patients, in 1990, reported considerable pathological differences between patients with and without ulcers [48]. The ulcerative group had evidence of hemorrhage, granulation tissue, and intense inflammatory infiltrate, including mast cell and perineural inflammatory infiltrates. In contrast, the non-ulcerative patients had a relatively unaltered mucosa with a scant inflammatory response. The more common features were small, mucosal ruptures and suburothelial hemorrhages. Interestingly symptomatology did not differ between the two types of patients. These findings were confirmed almost 30 years later, by Akiyama et al. [49]. In BPS/IC patients with Hunner's lesions, pancystitis with B-cell abnormalities, and epithelial denudation predominated, associated with edema and fibrosis. Epithelial denudation in a sloughing manner was also found a distinct histological feature of the epithelium in Hunner's lesion patients. Intraepithelial lymphocytes were frequently seen. In contrast, BPS/IC patients without Hunner's lesions show minimal histological changes.

Whether a transition from non-ulcerative to ulcerative BPS/IC occurs, it is unknown, as repeated cystoscopies are not routinely performed. Further studies are necessary to clarify if we are dealing with two separate entities or just an evolution of the same disease, although in the light of actual knowledge the rationale is that there could be two different entities [50, 51].

Mast cells are more common in the bladder wall of patients with the ulcerative phenotype but may also be found in completely non-related bladder problems [52]. No mast cell-based phenotypes are accepted, and therefore the use of specific staining for identifying mast cells and determining their density in biopsy samples has shown little utility in clinical practice.

Diagnosis

The first step in the diagnosis of BPS/IC is the observation that the patients have the key symptoms accepted by the different societies and guidelines which are chronic pelvic pain, which may be described as pressure or discomfort, usually related to the urinary bladder associated with other urinary or painful complaints. Pain may be referred by 75% of the patients also outside the pelvic area, to the thighs, buttocks, the back, shoulders, and neck region [53, 54]. An intense urinary frequency may occult pain by preventing a reasonable bladder filling. In about one-fourth of the cases, pain may be referred to multiple areas at the same time although the pelvic region is generally maintained [53, 54]. Patients with a greater number of pain locations tend to have more intense pain and refer to sleep disturbance, depression, anxiety, psychological stress, and worse quality of life. The presence of Hunner's lesions does not visibly enhance pain intensity despite the empiric assumption going in the opposite view [55–57].

Diagnosis differs enormously among centers in Europe, North America or Asia, and Japan, something that does not constitute a surprise, as symptoms are not specific [8]. Moreover, a clear confusion may occur with more severe forms of overactive bladder (OAB) in which urgency may be taken as pain and frequency and nocturia as the urological symptoms accompanying PBS/IC. Nevertheless, a word of caution should be left here, since it may be difficult to distinguish the urge to pass urine due to the fear of pain from the urgency to pass urine to avoid incontinence [58]. Although a careful history may help to distinguish between pain and urgency, the pivotal symptoms of BPS/IC and OAB, respectively, the two conditions may occur simultaneously. Within a cohort of 144 women with BPS/IC, 69% had urinary incontinence associated with the strong desire to void, although pain scores were not modified by the presence of incontinence [59].

The symptoms of BPS/IC are fluctuant, with periods of symptom relapse or exacerbation intercalated with periods of little or no symptoms. There is no universal definition for flares. Flares can last less than 1 h or prolong for periods longer than 1 day and eventually persist for months [60]. Flares of all durations are associated with greater pain and severity of urological symptoms and cause an important disruption of patient activities. Furthermore, they increase the use of healthcare resources. Flares may be absent for years or repeat at very short intervals [61, 62]. In a recent MAPP study of a large BPS/IC patient cohort followed for 11 months, 24.2% reported no flares, 22.9% reported 1 flare, 28.3% reported 2–3 flares, and 24.6% reported ≥4 flares. During each flare, the average increase in pain intensity, using a 0 to 10 point VAS, was 2.6 [62].

Diagnosis is hampered by the lack of specific symptoms and pathological features. Reliable biomarkers do not exist yet, as explained before. Consequently, the exclusion of confoundable diseases is a fundamental step in the diagnostic workup of BPS/IC. Figure 1 shows a comprehensive list of diseases that may evolve with the same symptomatology of BPS/IC [6]. Identification or exclusion of such diseases is relevant for different reasons. The most obvious is that the failure to diagnose a confoundable disease will lead to the wrong diagnosis of BPS/IC. Also relevant, an unrecognized confoundable disease will not be treated. Thus, as van der Merwe and co-workers summarized [6], the confirmation of BPS/IC requires the confirmation of the presence of the classic symptoms and signs of the disease and the exclusion of the confusable diseases. History and physical examination, urine culture including tuberculosis investigation, cytology, and cystoscopy with bladder biopsy are probably enough to exclude most confounders. However, the reader should understand that the diagnostic path might vary markedly among centers in Europe, North America, or Asia.

History Including Emotional Problems and Bowel and Sexual Dysfunction

A thorough history should pay close attention to the location of pelvic and referred pain, the wording used by patients to describe it, the relations with bladder filling and voiding, and its fluctuations with time. The correlation of flare-ups with

Confusable disease	Excluded or diagnosed by[a]
Carcinoma and carcinoma in situ	Cystoscopy and biopsy
Infection with	
Common intestinal bacteria	Routine bacterial culture
Chlamydia trachomatis, Ureaplasma urealyticum	Special cultures
Mycoplasma hominis, Mycoplasma genitalium	
Corynebacterium urealyticum, Candida species	
Mycobacterium tuberculosis	Dipstick; if "sterile" pyuria culture for M. tuberculosis
Herpes simplex and human papilloma virus	Physical examination
Radiation	Medical history
Chemotherapy, including immunotherapy with cyclophosphamide	Medical history
Anti-inflammatory therapy with tiaprofenic acid	Medical history
Bladder-neck obstruction and neurogenic outlet obstruction	Uroflowmetry and ultrasound
Bladder stone	Imaging or cystoscopy
Lower ureteric stone	Medical history and/or hematuria: upper urinary tract imaging such CT or IVP
Urethral diverticulum	Medical history and physical examination
Urogenital prolapse	Medical history and physical examination
Endometriosis	Medical history and physical examination
Vaginal candidiasis	Medical history and physical examination
Cervical, uterine, and ovarian cancer	Physical examination
Incomplete bladder emptying (retention)	Postvoid residual urine volume measured by ultrasound scanning
Overactive bladder	Medical history and urodynamics
Prostate cancer	Physical examination and PSA
Benign prostatic obstruction	Uroflowmetry and pressure-flow studies
Chronic bacterial prostatitis	Medical history, physical examination, culture
Chronic non-bacterial prostatitis	Medical history, physical examination, culture
Pudendal nerve entrapment	Medical history, physical examination, nerve block may prove diagnosis
Pelvic floor muscle-related pain	Medical history, physical examination

CT = computed tomography; IVP = intravenous pyelogram; PSA = prostate-specific antigen.
[a] The diagnosis of a confusable disease does not necessarily exclude a diagnosis of BPS.

Fig. 1 List of BPS/IC confoundable diseases and the simplest methods to make a differential diagnosis [6]

emotional, stressful events, urinary tract infections (UTI), or other situations should be explored. Special attention must be given to previous pelvic operations, previous UTIs, bladder history, and previous urological diseases and treatments including pelvic radiation therapy. Associated allergic, inflammatory, and autoimmune diseases should be listed including allergies, rheumatoid arthritis, Crohn's disease, ulcerative colitis, and Sjögren's syndrome [63]. The latter is frequently associated with Hunner's lesions.

During the initial investigation, a 3–7-day voiding diary is extremely useful to estimate the day and nighttime voiding, the relation of pain with bladder activity, and the voided volume to estimate bladder capacity. In the follow-up, the bladder diary may be relevant to calculate the frequency and duration of flare-ups and duration of remissions and watch functional bladder capacity. A visual analogue scale (VAS) for pain, combined with the bladder diary, can estimate pain and at each visit can score the average, mildest, and worst pain, usually in the last 15-day period.

Multiple questionnaires were created to investigate the type of symptoms present, the bother they cause in daily activities, and the relationship with precipitating events. The O'Leary-Sant IC Symptom Index (OSSI) and Problem Index (OSPI) score (Fig. 2) are commonly used as a basic symptom score combined with a numeric quality of life (QoL) score [64]. The Pelvic Pain and Urgency/Frequency (PUF) questionnaire captures a wide variety of the symptoms including pain in the vagina, labia, lower abdomen, or urethra (Fig. 3). However validity is questionable as the prevalence of BPS/IC estimated by PUF is largely overestimated [65].

The Genitourinary Pain Index (GUPI) questionnaire (Fig. 4) was a modification of the National Institutes of Health-Chronic Prostatitis Symptom Index. GUPI differentiates women with the disease from those with incontinence or no diagnosis. GUPI scores correlated with OSPI

Interstitial Cystitis Symptom Index:

Q1. *During the past month*, how often have you felt the strong need to urinate with little or no warning?

0. ____ not at all
1. ____ less than 1 time in 5
2. ____ less than half the time
3. ____ about half the time
4. ____ more than half the time
5. ____ almost always

Q2. *During the past month*, have you had to urinate less than 2 hours after you finished urinating?

0. ____ not at all
1. ____ less than 1 time in 5
2. ____ less than half the time
3. ____ about half the time
4. ____ more than half the time
5. ____ almost always

Q3. *During the past month*, how often did you most typically get up at night to urinate?

0. ____ none
1. ____ once
2. ____ 2 times
3. ____ 3 times
4. ____ 4 times
5. ____ 5 or more times

Q4. *During the past month*, have you experienced pain or burning in your bladder?

0. ____ not at all
2. ____ a few times
3. ____ almost always
4. ____ fairly often
5. ____ usually

Add the numerical values of the checked entries; total score: _____

Interstitial Cystitis Problem Index:

During the past month, how much has each of the following been a problem for you?

Q1. Frequent urination during the day

0. ____ no problem
1. ____ very small problem
2. ____ small problem
3. ____ medium problem
4. ____ big problem

Q2. Getting up at night to urinate

0. ____ no problem
1. ____ very small problem
2. ____ small problem
3. ____ medium problem
4. ____ big problem

Q3. Need to urinate with little warning

0. ____ no problem
1. ____ very small problem
2. ____ small problem
3. ____ medium problem
4. ____ big problem

Q4. Burning pain, discomfort, or pressure in your bladder

0. ____ no problem
1. ____ very small problem
2. ____ small problem
3. ____ medium problem
4. ____ big problem

Add the numerical values of the checked entries; total score: _____

Fig. 2 The O'Leary-Sant IC Symptom Index and Problem Index score [64]

and OSSI scores, and GUPI is highly responsive to clinical changes. A reduction of 7 points indicates a treatment responder [66].

The UPOINT system was created to phenotype BPS/IC patients according to the predominant symptoms [67]. UPOINT is a mnemonic for a 6-point clinical classification system that categorizes the phenotype of patients into six clinically identifiable domains, urinary, psychosocial, organ-specific (including gynecology, gastrointestinal, sexual), infection, neurological/systemic, and muscular tenderness (Fig. 4) [65]. Increased symptom duration leads to a greater number of domains affected by the disease including those outside of the bladder, which may help clinicians to predict the global impact of symptoms on a patient's daily life. UPOINT is more useful in patients with chronic pelvic pain than in patients with BPS/IC since by definition all patients have urinary and bladder-specific complaints. This observation leads to the creation of the INPUT phenotyping system which stands for infection, neurologic/systemic, psychosocial impact, presence of ulcers, and tenderness of muscles [68]. Since many patients have more than one positive domain, whether UPOINT or INPUT systems are applied, it may facilitate the introduction of multimodal therapy ab initio specific for the affected domains, like pelvic floor physical therapy combined with intravesical therapy or Hunner's lesion fulguration, rather than a step-by-step approach.

Most questionnaires investigate pain and urinary symptoms together, both concurring to a total score. Although it is undeniable that pain, frequency, and nocturia may cause significant bother, only pain seems associated with symptoms of depression. These findings from the MAPP consortium suggest that pain and urinary

1. In the last week, have you experienced any pain or discomfort in the following areas?

a. Entrance to vagina   ☐₁ Yes ☐₀ No
b. Vagina   ☐₁ Yes ☐₀ No
c. Urethra   ☐₁ Yes ☐₀ No
d. Below your waist, in your pubic or bladder area   ☐₁ Yes ☐₀ No

⎫ Pain location

2. In the last week, have you experienced:

a. Pain or burning during urination?   ☐₁ Yes ☐₀ No
b. Pain or discomfort during or after sexual intercourse?   ☐₁ Yes ☐₀ No
c. Pain or discomfort as your bladder fills?   ☐₁ Yes ☐₀ No
d. Pain or discomfort relieved by voiding?   ☐₁ Yes ☐₀ No

⎫ Relationship with urination and intercourse

3. How often have you had pain or discomfort in any of these areas over the last week?

☐₀ Never   ☐₁ Rarely   ☐₂ Sometimes   ☐₃ Often   ☐₄ Usually   ☐₅ Always

4. Which number best describes your AVERAGE pain or discomfort on the days you had it, over the last week?

☐ 0   ☐ 1   ☐ 2   ☐ 3   ☐ 4   ☐ 5   ☐ 6   ☐ 7   ☐ 8   ☐ 9   ☐ 10
No Pain   Pain as bad as you can imagine

⎫ Frequency and intensity of pain

5. How often have you had a sensation of not emptying your bladder completely after you finished urinating, over the last week?

☐₀ Not at all   ☐₁ Less than 1 time in 5   ☐₂ Less than half the time   ☐₃ About half the time   ☐₄ More than half the time   ☐₅ Almost always

6. How often have you had to urinate again less than two hours after you finished urinating, over the last week?

☐₀ Not at all   ☐₁ Less than 1 time in 5   ☐₂ Less than half the time   ☐₃ About half the time   ☐₄ More than half the time   ☐₅ Almost always

⎫ Lower urinary tract symptoms

7. How much have your symptoms kept you from doing the kinds of things you would usually do, over the last week?

☐₀ None   ☐₁ Only a little   ☐₂ Some   ☐₃ A lot

8. How much did you think about your symptoms, over the last week?

☐₀ None   ☐₁ Only a little   ☐₂ Some   ☐₃ A lot

9. If you were to spend the rest of your life with your symptoms just the way they have been during the last week, how would you feel about that?

☐₀ Delighted
☐₁ Pleased
☐₂ Mostly satisfied
☐₃ Mixed (about equally satisfied and dissatisfied)
☐₄ Mostly dissatisfied
☐₅ Unhappy
☐₆ Terrible

⎫ Impact on daily tasks and Quality of life

Fig. 3 The Pelvic Pain and Urgency/Frequency (PUF) questionnaire [65]

Urology	Urinary flow, micturition diary, cystoscopy, ultrasound, uroflowmetry.
Psychology	Anxiety about pain, depression and loss of function, history of negative sexual experiences.
Organ specific	Ask for gynaecological, gastro-intestinal, ano-rectal, sexological complaints. Gynaecological examination, rectal examination.
Infection	Semen culture and urine culture, vaginal swab, stool culture.
Neurological	Ask for neurological complaints (sensory loss, dysaesthesia). Neurological testing during physical examination: sensory problems, sacral reflexes and muscular function.
Tender muscle	Palpation of the pelvic floor muscles, the abdominal muscles and the gluteal muscles.
Sexological	Erectile function, ejaculatory function, post-orgasmic pain.

Fig. 4 UPOINT classification [70]. (Drawing from Engeler et al., EAU guidelines 2022)

symptoms should be assessed separately and that the GUPI questionnaire is adequate for that purpose [69].

Episodes of stress and intense emotional burden may aggravate pain. Pain in the genital area like vulvodynia and dyspareunia may lead to sexual intercourse avoidance behavior. Patients in whom there is an association between IC/BPS and irritable bowel syndrome frequently report bowel pain and modifications in bowel habitudes. Bowel dysfunctions should be accessed since due to the phenomenon of pelvic crossed sensitization, disease flares can be caused by primary bowel dysfunction [71].

Diet should be investigated as symptoms may be aggravated by some food and drinking habitudes. Registering this information may be relevant to designing conservative management.

Physical Examination

A common physical examination should include palpation of the lower abdomen for bladder fullness and tenderness. A careful vaginal examination with pain mapping of the vulvar region and vaginal palpation for tenderness of the bladder, urethra, *levator*, and adductor muscles of the pelvic floor should be carried out gently. Tenderness might be graded from mild to severe. All the areas of pain referred by the patient should be evaluated.

A good rule of thumb is to discuss meticulously the procedures that will take place beforehand and avoid as much as possible painful procedures like bimanual vaginal examination. Consent for examination and the presence of a nurse in the room are part of good clinical practice. Physicians should discuss with patients the unlikely possibility of symptom aggravation after certain examination maneuvers.

Laboratory Tests and Urodynamics

Urine dipstick and urine culture must be obtained from all patients, including culture for *Chlamydia* in all female patients. If sterile pyuria is present, then culture for tuberculosis is mandatory. In women with frequent flare-ups, urine should be investigated for fungi [36]. Urine cytology should be considered in all patients at risk of having a bladder tumor or if hematuria is detected, both macro and micro. Vaginal and endocervical swabs for investigation of vaginal *ureaplasma* and fungi may be useful taking into consideration the recent observations related to the risk of flare-up and urine microbiome [36].

Urodynamics has little role in the diagnosis of IC/BPS. There are no data to support the recommendation of obtaining a flowmetry, filling cystometry, pressure-flow study, and measure of post-void residual urine volume in women with BPS/IC. An exception can be made for patients with severe OAB symptoms, including urgency incontinence, who might benefit from the use of anticholinergics or beta-3 agonists to control OAB symptoms. In addition, a suspicion of small, terminal, noncompliant urinary bladder justifies a careful urodynamic evaluation. As stated before, urodynamics is an invasive procedure, and patients should be aware of an aggravation of complaints after the examination.

A recent study on a small cohort tested the use of bladder anesthesia with lidocaine installation to investigate the changes in bladder volume filling at which pain was felt [72]. Women were asked to report their pain using a VAS at maximal cystometric capacity. Then, the urodynamic examination was repeated after intravesical instillation of 20 ml of 2% lidocaine or normal saline. Although on average the lidocaine bladder instillation increased the volume for maximal cystometric capacity, the individual analysis revealed that in about one-third of the lidocaine-treated subjects the local anesthetic did not improve pain. Interestingly the nonresponders to local anesthesia of the bladder had a worse quality of life and were more likely to have central sensitization syndromes. Whether the test will become useful to decide on initial treatment, future studies will tell.

The potassium chloride test is excluded from routine use in recently updated guidelines [7]. The 0.4 M tests were already excluded from the diagnostic workup due to a lack of specificity [73].

The subsequent modification of the test using 0.3 M potassium chloride solutions lacked again specificity to differentiate BPS/IC patients from OAB patients with detrusor overactivity [74]. The potassium chloride test was further modified to evaluate cystometric capacity with a 0.2 M solution, which may improve acceptability among patients [75]. Despite the claims that it is not painful in clinical practice, it also did not become popular.

Cystoscopy and Bladder Biopsy

In Europe, despite the intense controversy around it, EAU guideline orientations released in 2022 recommend cystoscopy on the premise that bladder inspection will be useful for the diagnosis, for phenotyping patients, and for ruling out confoundable bladder diseases [7]. The most typical lesions are Hunner's lesions which may not assume the aspect of bladder ulceration but rather look like a scar, sometimes covered with fibrin or a clot, with blood vessels converging to it, and surrounded by a reddened, eventually swollen bladder mucosa. Frequently, as the bladder distends (the pressure should not overpass 80 cm H_2O for about 5 min), these areas rupture, and bleeding occurs from the urothelium fissure causing the characteristic waterfall bleeding. Some researchers find Hunner's lesion in 50% or more of their patients, while other physicians rarely report one [76]. Moreover, the way cystoscopy is performed, under sedation or local anesthesia, and the criteria used by individual clinicians to identify Hunner's lesion may influence the prevalence. Other possible cystoscopy findings are glomerulations, which are small petechiae or submucosal hemorrhages, seen after hydrodistention of the bladder. NIDDK included glomerulations as one among a list of positive factors for diagnostic purposes in trials. However, glomerulations swiftly started to be used as pivotal diagnostic criteria. The reader should realize that a systematic review did not find a consistent relationship between glomerulations and BPS/IC. Moreover, the review did not find an association link between the severity of symptoms and the number of glomerulations, which can be found in healthy asymptomatic subjects [77].

Bladder tissue samples should be obtained from the lateral wall and dome or from specific areas where abnormal morphology of the mucosa is detected. A cold cup instrument is preferable to obtain tissue samples, which should include a representation of the detrusor layer. The pathologist should report on the characteristics of the urothelium and the presence of inflammatory infiltrates and eventually grade it, describe the intensity of fibrosis in the mucosa and detrusor layer, and estimate the intensity of mast cell infiltration. At this moment, it is unclear if a precise measurement of the density of mast cells is relevant. Mast cell information requires a specific staining, in addition to the conventional hematoxylin and eosin. In addition, a statement about the absence of signs suggestive of carcinoma in situ and tuberculous cystitis is helpful in the report, particularly if the patient is at risk of having these diseases.

A histological distinction between BPS/IC with and without Hunner's lesions is becoming very robust. In BPS/IC patients with Hunner's lesions, pancystitis with B-cell abnormalities and epithelial denudation predominates (see Fig. 5). The bladder tissue usually shows a dense subepithelial infiltration by inflammatory cells, predominantly lymphocytes and plasma cells, which often form lymph follicles. Intraepithelial lymphocytes are frequently seen. The plasma cell/lymphocyte ratio is significantly higher than in nonspecific chronic cystitis. Edema and fibrosis may be present, most likely as a result of chronic inflammation. Epithelial denudation in a sloughing manner is a distinct histological feature of the epithelium in Hunner's lesion patients and is much more intense than in patients with nonspecific chronic cystitis (Fig. 5). In contrast, BPS/IC patients without Hunner's lesions show minimal histological changes (Fig. 5). These findings seem to support the view that BPS/IC with and without lesions are two distinct phenotypes of the same disease or even two distinct conditions sharing common symptomatology [49].

Based on the cystoscopy findings with bladder distention and the pathological findings, the

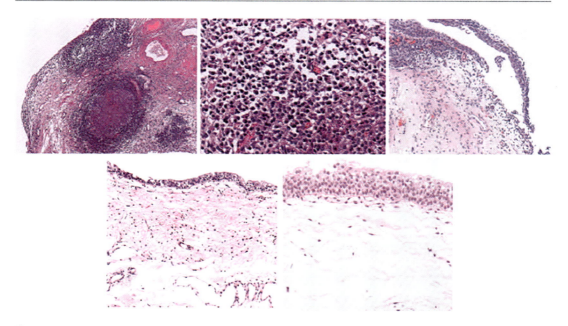

Fig. 5 Examples of histological findings in the bladder of patients with BPS/IC with Hunner's lesion (top) and without Hunner's lesion (bottom)

	Cystoscopy with hydrodistention			
	Not done	Normal	Glomerulations[a]	Hunner's lesion[b]
Biopsy				
Not done	XX	1X	2X	3X
Normal	XA	1A	2A	3A
Inconclusive	XB	1B	2B	3B
Positive[c]	XC	1C	2C	3C

[a] Cystoscopy: glomerulations grade 2–3.
[b] With or without glomerulations.
[c] Histology showing inflammatory infiltrates and/or detrusor mastocytosis and/or granulation tissue and/or intrafascicular fibrosis.

Fig. 6 Classification of BPS/IC based on biopsy and cystoscopic findings [6]

ESSIC association proposed a BPS/IC phenotyping method [6]. Bladder pain syndrome would be followed by a type of designation based on two symbols. The first symbol relates to cystoscopy with hydrodistention findings (1, 2, or 3, indicating an increasing grade of severity, normal, with glomerulations, or with Hunner's lesions, respectively) and the second to the histological characteristics of the biopsy (A, B, and C, indicating the severity of inflammatory findings). If largely used in clinical investigation, which is not yet the case, it would be possible to define cohorts with similar pathological and cystoscopy findings and study each cohort's natural history, prognosis, and response to different therapies. True IC would be the 3C group of patients (Fig. 6).

Biomarkers

A biomarker is an indicator of a biological process that can be used to confirm a diagnosis, detect remissions or relapses, and define the prognostic. An ideal biomarker should be susceptible to quick detection without the requirement of very sophisticated equipment usually not available in a normal clinical laboratory setting. The initial cost and the development of appropriate kits should not be viewed as drawback since technical progress can occur swiftly once a molecule of importance is identified.

The APF was the first biomarker to be investigated in IC/BPS. It was measured by complex methods using 3H thymidine incorporation by urothelial cells in the urine of IC patients, and it was identified as a low molecular weight peptide that inhibits the proliferation of bladder epithelial cells in vitro [78]. The increase of APF was accompanied by an increase in epidermal growth factor, IGF binding protein-3 and IL-6, and a decrease in heparin-binding epidermal growth factor-like growth factor and cyclic guanosine monophosphate. Of all these molecules, the APF had the least overlap in the BPS/IC and control groups. Other markers were not significantly different in the IC and control groups, including total glycosaminoglycans, epitectin, hyaluronic acid, IL-8, IL-1, and nitrates [79].

The gaseous free radical nitric oxide (NO) is an important biological mediator and cell signaling in smooth muscle relaxation, neurotransmission, and vasodilation. NO has an important role in the regulation of micturition, and marked differences between the subtypes concerning nitric oxide production, mirroring the differences in inflammatory bladder findings, were observed. All patients with Hunner's lesions had high levels of NO. None of the other BPS\IC patients had any significant increase in NO levels in the bladder. The NO increase was not related to symptoms but rather to the specific Hunner's lesion subgroup [80].

Nerve growth factor (NGF) has been explored as a potential biomarker under the premise that among other functions it is involved in neurogenic-mediated inflammatory pathways and sensitizes nociceptors, decreasing pain threshold and the volume to bladder voiding contractions [81]. Thus, the potential use of specific NGF blockers or antibodies could be a possibility in patients with high NGF expression. In the urine high NGF levels were detected in many patients with Hunner's lesion [82] although high levels of NGF mRNA were detected both in the ulcerative and non-ulcerative phenotypes [83]. Urinary levels may correlate with pain intensity [84].

Serum levels of NGF were increased in BPS/IC patients, which may contribute to explaining the systemic pain referred by many patients [85]. Although a recent metanalysis of 10 original studies involving 295 cases and 290 normal controls showed an increased level of urinary NGF in BPS/IC patients [86], one must not forget that the methods used to detect NGF in urine are not yet validated.

The 24-h urinary excretion of norepinephrine (NE) was increased in a small cohort of BPS/IC patients further supporting the role of stress in BPS/IC [87]. As in stress animal models, a similar increase was confirmed urinary NE levels could be used to select potential responders to alpha-1A antagonist medication [88].

Many interleukins and cytokines have been detected in the urine which may be seen as a consequence of the inflammatory process occurring in the bladder wall of BPS/IC patients [82, 89]. However none stood out as a candidate to separate BPS/IC from other urinary conditions or identify the ulcerative phenotype. Furuta et al. [90] measured 40 inflammatory urine biomarkers in BPS/IC patients with or without Hunner's lesions and OAB patients. Vascular endothelial growth factor (VEGF), interleukin-1α, IL-6, and chemokines including CCL2, CCL5, CXCL1, CXCL8, and CXCL10 were significantly increased in ulcerative and non-ulcerative BPS/IC phenotypes compared with OAB patients. A combination of biomarkers may increase the importance of biomarkers in BPS/IC. Increased urinary levels of CXCL10 and NGF may offer a more robust confirmation of the presence of Hunner's lesion phenotype [91].

Mass spectrometry global metabolite profiling of urine of BPS\IC women identified multiple metabolites capable of discriminating between BPS\IC and control subjects. Among them etiocholan-3α-ol-17-one sulfate (Etio-S), a sulfoconjugated 5-β reduced isomer of testosterone, distinguished female BPS/IC and control subjects with a sensitivity and specificity of 90%. Pelvic pain and the number of painful body sites correlate with Etio-S levels. The elevated levels of Etio-S persist for several months [92].

In the future, the urinary microbiome may also play a role as a biomarker. Microbiota diversity of BPS/IC patients is smaller than that of normal women, with more than 90% of the sequence reads belonging to the genus *Lactobacillus* [35]. A significantly greater prevalence of fungi (*Candida* and *Saccharomyces*) was detected in the midstream urine of women who reported a flare compared to those who did not [36]. Case patients were reflective of IC epidemiology with an age range from 26 to 88 years (median 58) and female predominance (41/50 F). There was a significant increase in the frequency of polyomavirus shedding between cases and controls ($p < 0.02$). Polyomavirus shedding, in particular BK viruria [36], was associated with vesical ulceration, a marker of disease severity, among interstitial cystitis cases after adjustment for age and sex. There was a significant association among cases between the presence of BK viruria and response to intravesical clorpactin therapy, which has anti-DNA virus activity and was more likely to improve symptoms in the presence of BK viruria. Two studies identified polyomavirus BKPyV shedding in the urine of most patients with ulcerative BPS/IC [32, 38]. Interestingly, BKPyV, one of the five polyomaviruses, is associated with serious hemorrhagic cystitis in transplanted patients under immunosuppressive therapy.

Quantitative PCR of stool DNA showed reduced levels of *E. sinensis*, *C. aerofaciens*, *F. prausnitzii*, *O. splanchnicus*, and *L. longoviformis* in the microbiota of BPS/IC patients [93]. As pelvic sensory neurons branch simultaneously to the bladder and the colon, one can hypothesize that those microorganisms have a protective role for colonic sensory terminals and that the reduced levels of these agents could be related to mechanisms of cross-sensitization that trigger or enhance bladder pain at a central level.

Phenotyping BPS/IC Patients

An etiopathogenesis is better identified and recognized in homogeneous than in heterogeneous groups. If one accepts this principle, it is logical to group BPS/IC patients with similar symptoms and signs to unravel the cause of a disease. Moreover, response to a particular treatment may be better in certain subgroups. In addition, patients with multi-organ symptoms may receive a combined treatment from the very beginning. The pathological classification of ESSIC based on the biopsy and cystoscopy findings was an important step ahead in this concept [94]. The introduction of the UPOINT and INPUT classification of symptoms goes in the same direction [67, 95]. The presence of symptoms originating in different organs will favor the introduction of a multimodal therapy from the very beginning of BPS/IC management.

Management

Whatever the form of management used, the key outcomes will always be an improvement in pain intensity, incidence, and severity of flare-ups and improvement of urinary symptoms like frequency and nocturia. Of notice the urinary symptoms, although usually seen as secondary outcomes in many clinical trials, may cause significant bother, eventually superior to that associated with pain as voiding at small volumes may prevent pain to reach intolerable levels. This form of evaluation is influenced by the subjective understanding and emotional situation of the patient. A painful situation of short duration unrelated to BPS/IC if concurring in time with a specific BPS/IC evaluation may increase the pelvic pain score. On the other hand, remissions may be seen in up to 50% of the cases, a rate that will cause an abnormal proportion of improvements after a specific treatment [96].

Functional problems in urology have always demonstrated a high rate of the placebo effect [97]. Several reasons have been forwarded. The condition may evolve into a natural improvement due to the natural history and regression to the mean of symptom scores used in the initial evaluation. Some chronic pain problems resolve or enter long periods of remission regardless of the treatment used. The physician's attention, patient and physician expectations about the treatment, and the reputation of the health unit influence the outcome of a treatment. Cost may affect positively or negatively the improvement perceived from a treatment. Interventional treatments and the overall awareness about the active drug can cause enormous placebo effects [98]. Improvement in lower urinary tract symptoms including frequency, urgency incontinence, or bladder pain is among the symptoms in which a larger placebo effect can be detected [99, 100]. Consequently, clinical trials using an inert comparator to estimate the placebo effect are essential before assuming that a certain agent is effective in BPS/IC management. Unfortunately, few BPS treatments have been subjected to placebo-controlled trials creating a high degree of uncertainty about the real efficacy of the treatment. However, even placebo-controlled trials may reveal serious flaws, coming from the potential experience of volunteers in previous trials and from the ethical concerns of assigning patients with severe pain to the placebo arm.

There is no cure for BPS/IC. Thus, the main goal of available treatments is to decrease the intensity of pain and lower urinary tract symptoms and increase the quality of life. With this in mind, the improvement of sexual life might play a relevant role in ameliorating the daily life of BPS/IC patients. Usually, a step-by-step approach is recommended. Nevertheless, the use of phenotyping systems can indicate at the initial visit more than one symptomatic organ system involved. In such cases, patients may benefit from receiving a multimodal therapy up front for the affected domains, like improving urinary frequency together with Hunner's lesion fulguration rather than a sequential approach.

Conservative Measures

Stress reduction, exercise, warm tub baths, and efforts by the BPS/IC patient to maintain a normal lifestyle all contribute to improving the overall quality of life. Behavioral therapy includes timed voiding, controlled fluid intake, pelvic floor muscle training, and bladder training, with a slow increase of voiding intervals. The objective is to avoid intense pain caused by excessive bladder filling, while slowly training the patients to accommodate higher urine volumes [101–103]. Soft tissue massage and other physical therapies associated or not with biofeedback may aid in muscle relaxation of the pelvic floor. The small size and non-randomization of most physiotherapeutic studies greatly limit the strength of the evidence [104]. Nevertheless, randomized clinical trials show that massage and teaching how to relax the pelvic muscle when the pain starts can be very rewarding [105]. Physical therapy with biofeedback combined with oral analgesic therapy is superior to pharmacotherapy alone [106]. Reducing mental stress may bring significant gains in terms of pain control in a vast majority of patients [107]. A curious study showed that pain caused by mental stress was observed only in patients with BPS [108].

Sexual counselling may help to overcome or at least reduce the limitations that pelvic pain and dyspareunia cause. Exploring alternatives to intercourse with vaginal penetration and discovering positions that do not cause pain are part of the strategies.

Many patients find that their symptoms are adversely affected by specific diets. Nevertheless, diets should be restricted on an individual basis. Triggering food may include caffeine, alcohol, artificial sweeteners, hot pepper, and beverages like cranberry juice. Although diet manipulation is one of the most frequently offered conservative treatments, there is little evidence to support a very strict diet, and attempts to increase urinary pH did not work in a small randomized trial [109].

Interventional Pharmacotherapy

Interventional pharmacotherapy is subdivided into two main arms according to the objective underlying its application (Fig. 7). Some of the interventions are directed to replenish the glycosaminoglycan (GAG) layer and decrease the urothelial permeability or to reduce inflammatory and autoimmune pathological mechanism in play. Other pharmacotherapies, in contrast, are simply directed to treat symptoms, namely, pain and

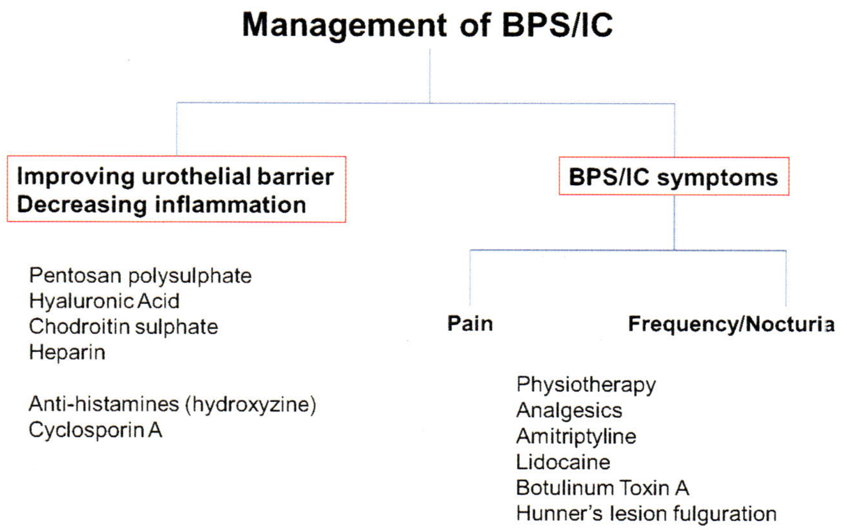

Management of BPS/IC

Improving urothelial barrier / Decreasing inflammation
- Pentosan polysulphate
- Hyaluronic Acid
- Chodroitin sulphate
- Heparin
- Anti-histamines (hydroxyzine)
- Cyclosporin A

BPS/IC symptoms

Pain / Frequency/Nocturia
- Physiotherapy
- Analgesics
- Amitriptyline
- Lidocaine
- Botulinum Toxin A
- Hunner's lesion fulguration

Fig. 7 Description of the most common pharmacological treatments used in the management of BPS/IC. The treatments are divided according to their main mechanism of action, potentially interfering in the pathophysiological mechanism on the left or being oriented to symptom control on the right

urinary symptoms. The common practice whatever the initial orientation is to introduce in the first place the agents that cause fewer side effects. The two strategies might be combined.

Oral Pharmacotherapy

Pentosan polysulfate sodium (PPS) is a heparin-like macromolecule that resembles urothelium GAG and remains the only oral therapy approved by the Food and Drug Administration (FDA). It is postulated that PPS reconstitutes the GAG layer and inhibits mast cell degranulation [110]. The recommended dose is usually 100 mg three times daily although higher doses are frequently used. However, not all studies showed the superiority of PPS over placebo. Positive [111–115] and negative trials [116, 117] have been reported. When observed, improvements increased with the duration of treatment, which in some patients may extend along 2 years, after which no further improvement or worsening should be expected [118]. A study suggested a higher efficacy in patients with Hunner's lesions [119]. Physicians should expect that half of the patients will stop the treatment within the first 3 months [118]. The frequency of adverse events is generally very low. However, recent concern about ocular side effects was raised. In a retrospective study in an eye center, PPS was the sole predictor of pigmentary maculopathy in one-third of the patients observed with that ophthalmologic condition [120]. Although a large commercial database did not confirm this association [121], an eye examination should be recommended for BPS/IC under long-term PPS treatment or who have recently noticed a decrease in visual accuracy

Cyclosporine is largely used in organ transplantation to prevent organ rejection. This immunosuppressive drug at an initial dose of 2.5–5 mg/kg daily and a maintenance dose of 1.5 to 3 mg/kg daily showed a good symptomatic improvement in pain and urological symptoms in 90% of the patients enrolled in a small cohort [122, 123]. Sairanen et al. [124] further found that cyclosporine A was far superior to PPS in reducing pain and frequency and in increasing bladder capacity. The necessity of a close vigilance of renal function and the risk associated with immunosuppression prevent its larger use. Cyclosporine is only recommended for refractory BPS/IC, especially that with Hunner's lesion [125]. A recent retrospective review of the outcome of 51 patients with the ulcerative phenotype reported a good general improvement in more than 80% of the cases [126].

Hydroxyzine is an antagonist of the histamine receptor type H1. These receptors are present in mast cells, and their blockade is expected to limit the release of pro-inflammatory neurotransmitters. In addition, hydroxyzine has weak anticholinergic and anxiolytic properties. At dosages of 25 to 50 mg daily, it reported a decrease of symptom severity in 40% of BPS/IC patients. In those with a history of allergies, the success rate can reach 55% [127]. However, placebo-controlled clinical trials conducted with hydroxyzine were negative [116, 128]. Cimetidine is another antagonist of histamine receptors, in this case, the H2 receptor subtype. It was tested in a small trial, but the results did not stimulate the progress into larger studies [129].

Tanezumab is a humanized anti-NGF monoclonal antibody that binds with high affinity and specificity to NGF, preventing it from interacting with receptors on nociceptive neurons. Hence, a good rationale for conducting a phase 2 trial existed. The modest efficacy (only 50% of patients having a 30% or greater reduction of pain score) and the serious adverse events including headache (20.6%), paresthesia (17.6%), and risk of bone necrosis at different joints [130] prevented further development of tanezumab. Other phase 2 placebo-controlled trials with a novel monoclonal antibody against NGF (EudraCT Number 2016-004138-12) took place afterward, but no positive reports were communicated [131].

Pain treatment is pivotal in the oral pharmacological management of BPS/IC patients. Many non-opioid analgesics including acetaminophen (paracetamol) and nonsteroidal anti-inflammatory drugs have a place in pain therapy. Patients with more severe symptoms can benefit from drugs used for chronic neuropathic pain syndromes like gabapentin [132] and pregabalin [129]. The introduction of these agents should be progressive. Opioids in very painful periods of the disease evolution can be of great utility, but the risk of drug addiction must be evaluated and discussed with the patients and relatives.

Amitriptyline, a tricyclic antidepressant, has anticholinergic and sedative properties by decreasing 5-hydroxytryptamine reuptake. It stabilizes mast cells and blocks the actions of histamine. Although largely recommended by guidelines [7], clinical trials could not demonstrate a clear superiority of amitriptyline over placebo. Only the sub-analysis of the study conducted by the Interstitial Cystitis Collaborative Research Network for doses above 50 mg/day showed efficacy, however with increased risk of side effects [133].

Several drugs have been investigated in small clinical trials without subsequent developments. In the list of drugs tested are immunosuppressive agents such as methotrexate, cyclosporine A, and azathioprine with severe side effects. Montelukast, a selective antagonist of the leukotriene D4 receptor used, is used in asthma management and prevents mast cell degranulation. After a small positive trial [134], no further studies were surprisingly carried out, particularly in those patients with intense mast cell infiltration in the bladder wall. Some reasoning can be given to conducting small exploratory studies with C-kit inhibitor, IL-10 (anti-inflammatory cytokine), TNF-alpha inhibitors, quercetin, or suplatast (helper T-cell inhibitor).

Daily low-dose sildenafil proved to be a well-tolerated and effective treatment in a small placebo-controlled clinical trial [135] and in an open study [136]. In a small 3-month trial, tadalafil 5 mg/day decreased pain intensity and urinary frequency and increased volume voided. No obvious differences between ulcerated and non-ulcerated patients were observed. Two patients stopped treatment due to persistent headache and/or tachycardia [136].

Other drugs investigated for BPS/IC include microRNA manipulation, APF antagonists, selective cannabinoid type-1 receptor agonists, and phosphodiesterase type-5 inhibitors. APF antagonists revert tight junction damage in laboratory models [137]. MicroRNA manipulation may mediate the downregulation of NK-1 receptors in BPS/IC [138]. Selective cannabinoid type-1 receptor agonists significantly decrease inflammatory activity in the urothelium [139]. A combination of TRPV1 and TRPV4 antagonists was effective in an animal model of bladder pain [140].

Intravesical Pharmacotherapy

Intravesical therapy is another important treatment option in BPS/IC management. It opens the possibility of applying drugs directly to the bladder, either using high doses or delivering substances that are not suitable for systemic use.

Dimethyl sulfoxide (DMSO) is the only intravesical therapy approved by the FDA for BPS/IC although it is not recommended in the last version of EAU guidelines [7]. DMSO is an organic solvent, a by-product of the paper pulp industry, which has analgesic and anti-inflammatory properties, muscle relaxant, and collagen dissolution effects. Ulcer-type BPS/IC patients may refer to symptomatic relief in frequency and pain after instillation although no improvement was observed in maximum bladder capacity [141]. After instillation, patients may exhale a typical garlic odor, particularly when they receive more than 50 ml of 50% DMSO per week. DMSO is often combined in intravesical cocktail solutions (lidocaine, heparin, and/or sodium bicarbonate) that are administered weekly or biweekly.

Alkalinized lidocaine, as a local anesthetic, has an immediate effect on the mean pain, which may last for up to 8 days after the instillation [142]. Unfortunately, the effect is usually short-lasting requiring frequent if not daily instillations. Attempts to produce a device that once put in the bladder would slowly release the lidocaine have failed. Electromotive drug administration for lidocaine may increase the penetration of the local anesthetic into the bladder wall. Accordingly, Rosamilia et al. [143] described a good response in 85% of the patients with the effect persisting for 6 months in 25%. Despite this excellent report, intravesical lidocaine use is restricted to periods of unbearable pain and resistant to other therapies.

Intravesical therapy may offer the possibility of reconstituting the GAG layer with higher doses of PPS or with a dose that is not suitable by oral route. In a recent study, simultaneous oral and intravesical PPS showed a significant advantage over placebo or oral PPS alone [144]. GAG layer restitution has also been attempted with chondroitin sulfate, hyaluronic acid, and heparin. Nevertheless, controlled clinical trials concluded that sodium chondroitin sulfate or hyaluronic acid was negative or showed a high recurrence rate during the first year. The exception might be the instillation of high molecular weight hyaluronic acid at a concentration of 0.08% [100, 145]. One trial examined the effect of the intravesical instillation of Bacillus Calmétte-Guerin (BCG), although the rationale for BCG instillation, which is used in bladder cancer prevention, remains unclear. Anyway, the study concluded that BCG instillation has no clinical effect on BPS/IC [127].

Sensory-type C fibers are responsible for pain transmission in BPS/IC. Thus, desensitizing the TRPV1 receptor and inactivating C fibers can be an alternative approach. Several short reports claimed a beneficial effect of resiniferatoxin (RTX) applied intravesically. Nevertheless, the only large placebo-controlled trial comparing RTX solutions in different concentrations against placebo was negative [146]. No further developments, including the production of alternative formulations of RTX, followed. The intravesical route was never used to investigate the synthetic TRPV1 antagonists synthetized by the industry.

Intramural Treatments

Botulinum toxin type A (BoNT/A) has the temporary ability to inhibit the release of neurotransmitters like substance P and calcitonin gene-related peptide from pain-related sensory neurons. In addition, BoNT/A decreases the trafficking of pain receptors which decreases their expression in the membrane of pain afferents, in particular in the peripheral endings. Also, BoNT/A reduces ATP release from the urothelium [147]. Moreover, BoNT/A decreases the urinary levels of NGF, which sensitizes bladder nociceptors and increases their responsiveness [84].

A small number of women treated with BoNT/A injections (onabotulinum toxin A 100 U and 200 U) throughout the whole bladder reported improvement in pain and urinary symptoms in a large proportion of patients for 3–5 months [148]. However many women reported severe voiding difficulties [149]. Taking into consideration that most bladder nociceptors course in the trigone, Pinto et al. [84] restricted the injections of onabotulinum toxin A 100 U to the trigone, in 10 sites (10 U/1 ml each). All patients reported subjective improvement at 1- and 3-month follow-up in pain, daytime and nighttime voiding frequency, O'Leary-Sant score, and QoL. Retreatment was equally effective in all cases, with a similar duration of the effect up to four consecutive treatments [150]. Clinically relevant increases of post-void residual urine did not occur [150]. Interestingly, the improvement in pain may be similar in patients with and without Hunner's lesions [57].

One randomized study compared onabotA 200 U or 100 U injected in 40 suburothelial sites followed by hydrodistention 2 weeks later against hydrodistention only. All women remained on PPS throughout the study [55]. Pain reduction and urodynamic improvement were observed at 3 months in the arms that received onabotA, without any relevant differences between the two doses. In placebo-controlled trials, trigonal-only injections of onabotA 100 U, but not saline, caused a marked reduction in pain intensity. The proportion of patients who achieved a 50% or greater reduction in the pain visual analogue scale was 60% for onabotA vs 22% for placebo. No cases of urinary retention occurred compared to BPS/IC women [151]. Metanalyses concluded that among the different treatment options for BPS/IC, BoNT/A bladder injections have the highest probability of decreasing bladder pain [152].

Hydrodistension under anesthesia in addition to being a diagnostic tool can be also used as a treatment for BPS/IC. Under anesthesia, the bladder is filled at a maximal pressure of 80 cm H2O and kept distended for 5 min. Long-term symptom-free periods may follow the procedure. Exactly why this procedure has therapeutic benefits for some patients is still unknown. A recent study examined patients with BPS/IC who were treated with hydrodistension and subsequent bladder training. Of the 361 patients recruited into this uncontrolled study, only 13.4% described urgency symptoms 8 weeks after hydrodistension, and more than 80% of patients showed improvement in their BPS/IC flares of pain associated with menstruation and sexual intercourse [153]. Nevertheless, long-term results are not encouraging [154], and the treatment is not recommended by the European guidelines [7].

Surgical Treatments

Since 1971 that transurethral resection or fulguration of Hunner's lesion has been used to relieve pain and urinary symptoms in patients presenting with the ulcerative BPS/IC phenotype [155–158]. The efficacy of transurethral resection and transurethral coagulation is similar, the average symptom-free time being around 12 months without recognizable different effects in pain and urological symptoms. Although generally low, the incidence of bladder injury may be higher after transurethral resection than after coagulation, 7.9% vs 3.4%, respectively [157]. Although long symptom-free periods, up to 3 years, have been reported in a significant proportion of patients [155], most patients will require repeat interventions at much shorter intervals. One center reported that after an initial fulguration 13% of patients will request another within 1 year, the rate increasing to 57% at 4 years [158]. Fulguration of Hunner's lesion with laser or electric current seems to provide similar outcomes [159].

Major surgical procedures are the last resource in the treatment of BPS/IC patients. The level of evidence regarding cystectomy and/or urinary diversion is weak and limited only to case series, the majority of results being mixed if not negative. Reports suggest that better results are expected in patients with the ulcerative phenotype or with low (less than 250–350 mL) bladder capacity under anesthesia. The fluctuating natural history of disease and inconsistent results of major surgeries should be extensively discussed with the patient. Referral to an experienced center with a multidisciplinary team approach is mandatory. Psychological evaluation and support are strongly recommended. In addition, the potential consequences of any major surgery on sexual life, intended pregnancies, and the possible voiding difficulties, which might require intermittent catheterization for urine removal, need a thorough discussion with the patients.

Three major surgical approaches are commonly reported: supratrigonal cystectomy with bladder augmentation, subtrigonal cystectomy with an orthotropic bowel bladder creation, and complete cystectomy with the formation of an ileal conduit. Supratrigonal cystectomy with subsequent bladder augmentation represents the most favored technique even though the conservation of the trigone may be the cause of failure to achieve a complete pain-free state [160–163]. However, the relapse of pain when the bladder trigone is left in place is not an inevitable event as seen in some surgical series [160].

Future Developments in Terms of Animal Studies

BPS/IC is a chronic pain condition for which better treatments are eagerly needed, but the introduction of new therapies with proven clinical benefits has been slow. A review of existing preclinical in vivo models for BPS/IC in rodents included the review of 1055 BPS/IC publications. Most models were by far bladder centric, followed by complex mechanisms and stress-induced models which together represented only 15% of the models used. The most frequently used models were instillation of irritants, autoimmune models, and water avoidance stress. Remarkably, although pelvic pain is a hallmark of BPS/IC and the endpoint for the development of novel therapies, only a small proportion of the studies examined endpoints associated with pain. Therefore, the models need to be refined to better reflect clinical reality. In such a process, standardized endpoints need to be defined [164].

Cross-References

▶ Behavioral Modification and Conservative Management of Overactive Bladder and Underactive Bladder Disorders
▶ Electrophysiologic Evaluation of the Pelvic Floor
▶ Neuroanatomy and Neurophysiology
▶ Overview of Diagnosis and Pharmacological Treatment of Overactive and Underactive Bladder Disorders

References

1. Malde S, Palmisani S, Al-Kaisy A, Sahai A. Guideline of guidelines: bladder pain syndrome. BJU Int. 2018;122(5):729–43.
2. Meijlink JM. Interstitial cystitis and the painful bladder: a brief history of nomenclature, definitions and criteria. Int J Urol [Internet]. 2014;21(S1):4–12. Available from: https://onlinelibrary.wiley.com/doi/10.1111/iju.12307.
3. Charrua A, Mendes P, Cruz C. Biomarkers for bladder pain syndrome/interstitial cystitis. Curr Bladder Dysfunct Rep [Internet]. 2021;16(1):12–8. Available from: http://link.springer.com/10.1007/s11884-020-00626-9.
4. Wein AJ, Hanno PM, Gillenwater JY. Interstitial cystitis: an introduction to the problem. In: Interstitial cystitis [Internet]. London: Springer London; 1990. p. 3–15. Available from: http://link.springer.com/10.1007/978-1-4471-3293-6_1.
5. Abrams P, Cardozo L, Fall M, Griffiths D, Rosier P, Ulmsten U, et al. The standardisation of terminology of lower urinary tract function: report from the standardisation sub-committee of the international continence society. Am J Obstet Gynecol. 2002;187(1):116–26.
6. van de Merwe JP, Nordling J, Bouchelouche P, Bouchelouche K, Cervigni M, Daha LK, et al. Diagnostic criteria, classification, and nomenclature for painful bladder syndrome/interstitial cystitis: an ESSIC proposal. Eur Urol [Internet] 2008;53(1):60–7. Available from: https://linkinghub.elsevier.com/retrieve/pii/S0302283807011657.
7. Engeler D, Baranowski AP, Berghmans B, Borovicka J, Cottrell AM, Dinis-Oliveira P, et al. EAU guidelines on chronic pelvic pain 2022. Eur Urol. 2022.
8. Malde S, Palmisani S, Al-Kaisy A, Sahai A. Guideline of guidelines: bladder pain syndrome. BJU Int [Internet]. 2018;122(5):729–43. Available from: https://onlinelibrary.wiley.com/doi/10.1111/bju.14399.

9. Landis JR, Williams DA, Lucia MS, Clauw DJ, Naliboff BD, Robinson NA, et al. The MAPP research network: design, patient characterization and operations. BMC Urol. 2014;14(1):1–17.
10. Engeler D (Chair), Baranowski AP, Berghmans B, Borovicka J, Cottrell AM, Dinis-Oliveira P, Elneil S, Hughes J, Messelink EJ (Vice-chair), AC de C Williams Guidelines Associates: Pacheco-Figueiredo L, Parsons B SG. EAU guidelines on chronic pelvic pain. Eur Urol [Internet]. 2018. Available from: https://linkinghub.elsevier.com/retrieve/pii/S0302283804003975.
11. Cohen M, Quintner J, van Rysewyk S. Reconsidering the International Association for the Study of Pain definition of pain. Pain Rep [Internet]. 2018;3(2):e634. Available from: https://journals.lww.com/01938936-201804000-00003.
12. Verhaak PFM, Kerssens JJ, Dekker J, Sorbi MJ, Bensing JM. Prevalence of chronic benign pain disorder among adults: a review of the literature. Pain. 1998;77(3):231–9.
13. Campbell CM, Edwards RR. Ethnic differences in pain and pain management. Pain Manag [Internet]. 2012;2(3):219–30. Available from: https://www.futuremedicine.com/doi/10.2217/pmt.12.7.
14. Ito T, Miki M, Yamada T. Interstitial cystitis in Japan. BJU Int. 2000;86(6):634–7.
15. Lee JW, Yoo KH, Choi H. Prevalence of bladder pain syndrome-like symptoms: a population-based Study in Korea. J Korean Med Sci [Internet]. 2021;36(46):1–8. Available from: https://jkms.org/DOIx.php?id=10.3346/jkms.2021.36.e293.
16. Clemens JQ, Link CL, Eggers PW, Kusek JW, Nyberg LM, McKinlay JB. Prevalence of painful bladder symptoms and effect on quality of life in black, hispanic and white men and women. J Urol [Internet]. 2007;177(4):1390–4. Available from: http://www.jurology.com/doi/10.1016/j.juro.2006.11.084.
17. Leppilahti M, Sairanen J, Tammela TLJ, Aaltomaa S, Lehtoranta K, Auvinen A. Prevalence of clinically confirmed interstitial cystitis in women: a population based study in Finland. J Urol. 2005;174(2):581–3.
18. Temml C, Wehrberger C, Riedl C, Ponholzer A, Marszalek M, Madersbacher S. Prevalence and correlates for interstitial cystitis symptoms in women participating in a health screening project. Eur Urol [Internet]. 2007;51(3):803–9. Available from: https://linkinghub.elsevier.com/retrieve/pii/S0302283806009845.
19. Morales-Solchaga G, Zubiaur-Libano C, Peri-Cusí L, Adot-Zurbano JM, Arlandis-Guzmán S, Franco-de Castro A, et al. Bladder pain syndrome: prevalence and routine clinical practice in women attending functional urology and urodynamics units in Spain. Actas Urol Esp (English Ed [Internet]). 2019;43(2):62–70. Available from: https://doi.org/10.1016/j.acuroe.2019.01.006.
20. Bade JJ, Rijcken B, Mensink HJ. Interstitial cystitis in The Netherlands: prevalence, diagnostic criteria and therapeutic preferences. J Urol. 1995;154(6):2035–7. https://doi.org/10.1016/s0022-5347(01)66684-9.
21. Hakimi Z, Houbiers J, Pedersini R, Vietri J. The burden of bladder pain in five European countries: a cross-sectional study. Urology [Internet]. 2017;99:84–91. Available from: https://doi.org/10.1016/j.urology.2016.08.038.
22. Parsons CL, Lilly JD, Stein P. Epithelial dysfunction in nonbacterial cystitis (interstitial cystitis). J Urol [Internet]. 1991;145(4):732–5. Available from: http://www.jurology.com/doi/10.1016/S0022-5347%2817%2938437-9.
23. Hurst RE, Van Meerveld BG, Wisniewski AB, VanGordon S, Lin HK, Kropp BP, et al. Increased bladder permeability in interstitial cystitis/painful bladder syndrome. Transl Androl Urol. 2015;4(5):563–71.
24. Malykhina AP. Neural mechanisms of pelvic organ cross-sensitization. Neuroscience. 2007;149(3):660–72.
25. Orr NL, Noga H, Williams C, Allaire C, Bedaiwy MA, Lisonkova S, et al. Deep dyspareunia in endometriosis: role of the bladder and pelvic floor. J Sex Med [Internet]. 2018;15(8):1158–66. Available from: https://doi.org/10.1016/j.jsxm.2018.06.007.
26. Mukerji G, Yiangou Y, Agarwal SK, Anand P. Transient receptor potential vanilloid receptor subtype 1 in painful bladder syndrome and its correlation with pain. J Urol. 2006;176(2):797–801.
27. de Groat WC, Yoshimura N. Afferent nerve regulation of bladder function in health and disease. In: Canning BJ, Spina D, editors. Sensory nerves, handbook of experimental pharmacology 194, [Internet]; 2009. p. 91–138. Available from: http://link.springer.com/10.1007/978-3-540-79090-7_4.
28. Kim A, Han J-Y, Ryu C-M, Yu HY, Lee S, Kim Y, et al. Histopathological characteristics of interstitial cystitis/bladder pain syndrome without Hunner lesion. Histopathology [Internet]. 2017;71(3):415–24. Available from: https://onlinelibrary.wiley.com/doi/10.1111/his.13235.
29. Lee YK, Jhang J-F, Jiang Y-H, Hsu Y-H, Ho H-C, Kuo H-C. Difference in electron microscopic findings among interstitial cystitis/bladder pain syndrome with distinct clinical and cystoscopic characteristics. Sci Rep [Internet]. 2021;11(1):17258. Available from: https://doi.org/10.1038/s41598-021-96810-w.
30. Zhang CO, Wang JY, Koch KR, Keay S. Regulation of tight junction proteins and bladder epithelial paracellular permeability by an antiproliferative factor from patients with interstitial cystitis. J Urol. 2005;174(6):2382–7.
31. Monastyrskaya K, Sánchez-Freire V, Hashemi Gheinani A, Klumpp DJ, Babiychuk EB, Draeger A, et al. MiR-199a-5p regulates urothelial permeability and may play a role in bladder pain syndrome. Am J Pathol [Internet]. 2013;182(2):431–48. Available from: https://doi.org/10.1016/j.ajpath.2012.10.020.

32. Winter BJ, O'Connell HE, Bowden S, Carey M, Eisen DP. A case control study reveals that polyomaviruria is significantly associated with interstitial cystitis and vesical ulceration. Hurst R, editor. PLoS One [Internet]. 2015;10(9):e0137310. Available from: https://doi.org/10.1016/j.juro.2015.09.075.
33. Keay S, Seillier-Moiseiwitsch F, Zhang C-O, Chai TC, Zhang J. Changes in human bladder epithelial cell gene expression associated with interstitial cystitis or antiproliferative factor treatment. Physiol Genom [Internet]. 2003;14(2):107–15. Available from: https://www.physiology.org/doi/10.1152/physiolgenomics.00055.2003.
34. Burkhard FC, Blick N, Hochreiter WW, Studer UE. Urinary urgency and frequency, and chronic urethral and/or pelvic pain in females. Can doxycycline help? J Urol. 2004;172(1):232–5.
35. Siddiqui H, Lagesen K, Nederbragt AJ, Jeansson SL, Jakobsen KS. Alterations of microbiota in urine from women with interstitial cystitis. BMC Microbiol [Internet]. 2012;12(1):205. Available from: http://bmcmicrobiol.biomedcentral.com/articles/10.1186/1471-2180-12-205.
36. Nickel JC, Stephens A, Landis JR, Mullins C, Van Bokhoven A, Lucia MS, et al. Assessment of the lower urinary tract microbiota during symptom flare in women with urologic chronic pelvic pain syndrome: a MAPP Network Study. J Urol [Internet]. 2016;195(2):356–62. Available from: https://doi.org/10.1016/j.juro.2015.09.075.
37. Van der Aa F, Beckley I, de Ridder D. Polyomavirus BK A potential new therapeutic target for painful bladder syndrome/interstitial cystitis? Med Hypotheses [Internet]. 2014;83(3):317–20. Available from: https://doi.org/10.1016/j.mehy.2014.06.004.
38. Van der Aa F, Beckley I, de Ridder D. Polyomavirus BK – a potential new therapeutic target for painful bladder syndrome/interstitial cystitis? Med Hypotheses [Internet]. 2014;83(3):317–20. Available from: https://linkinghub.elsevier.com/retrieve/pii/S0306987714002321.
39. Parsons CL, Shaw T, Berecz Z, Su Y, Zupkas P, Argade S. Role of urinary cations in the aetiology of bladder symptoms and interstitial cystitis. BJU Int. 2014;114(2):286–93.
40. Parsons CL, Proctor J, Teichman JS, Nickel JC, Davis E, Evans R, et al. A multi-site study confirms abnormal glycosylation in the Tamm-Horsfall protein of patients with interstitial cystitis. J Urol [Internet]. 2011;186(1):112–6. Available from: https://doi.org/10.1016/j.juro.2011.02.2699.
41. Leppilahti M, Tammela TLJ, Huhtala H, Kiilholma P, Leppilahti K, Auvinen A. Interstitial cystitis-like urinary symptoms among patients with Sjögren's syndrome: a population-based study in Finland. Am J Med. 2003;115(1):62–5.
42. Javed I, Yu T, Li J, Pakpahan R, Milbrandt M, Andriole GL, et al. Does Pollen trigger urological chronic pelvic pain syndrome flares? A case-crossover analysis in the multidisciplinary approach to the study of chronic pelvic pain research network. J Urol [Internet]. 2021;205(4):1133–8. Available from: http://www.jurology.com/doi/10.1097/JU.0000000000001482.
43. Sun Y, Chai TC. Augmented extracellular ATP signaling in bladder urothelial cells from patients with interstitial cystitis. Am J Physiol – Cell Physiol. 2006;290(1):27–35.
44. Birder LA, Barrick SR, Roppolo JR, Kanai AJ, De Groat WC, Kiss S, et al. Feline interstitial cystitis results in mechanical hypersensitivity and altered ATP release from bladder urothelium. Am J Physiol – Ren Physiol. 2003;285(3 54–3):423–9.
45. Cockayne DA, Hamilton SG, Zhu QM, Dunn PM, Zhong Y, Novakovic S, et al. Urinary bladder hyporeflexia and reduced pain-related behaviour in P2X3-deficient mice. Nature. 2000;407(6807):1011–5.
46. Engeler D (Chair), Baranowski AP, Berghmans B, Borovicka J, Cottrell AM, Dinis-Oliveira P, SE, Hughes J, Messelink EJ (Vice-chair), A.C. de C Williams Guidelines Associates: Parsons B, Goonewardene S, Abreu-Mendes P VZ. EAU guidelines on chronic pelvic pain. In: EAU guidelines edn presented at the EAU Annual Congress Milan 2021 [Internet]. 2021. p. 681–9. Available from: https://linkinghub.elsevier.com/retrieve/pii/S0302283804003975
47. Smith BH, Dehner LP. Chronic ulcerating interstitial cystitis (Hunner's ulcer). A study of 28 cases. Arch Pathol [Internet]. 1972;93(1):76–81. Available from: http://www.ncbi.nlm.nih.gov/pubmed/5007000.
48. Johansson SL, Fall M. Clinical features and spectrum of light microscopic changes in interstitial cystitis. J Urol [Internet]. 1990;143(6):1118–24. Available from: https://doi.org/10.1016/S0022-5347(17)40201-1.
49. Akiyama Y, Homma Y, Maeda D. Pathology and terminology of interstitial cystitis/bladder pain syndrome: a review. Histol Histopathol. 34(1):25–3.
50. Logadottir Y, Fall M, Kåbjörn-Gustafsson C, Peeker R. Clinical characteristics differ considerably between phenotypes of bladder pain syndrome/interstitial cystitis. Scand J Urol Nephrol [Internet]. 2012;46(5):365–70. Available from: https://www.tandfonline.com/doi/full/10.3109/00365599.2012.689008.
51. Fall M, Nordling J, Cervigni M, Dinis Oliveira P, Fariello J, Hanno P, et al. Hunner lesion disease differs in diagnosis, treatment and outcome from bladder pain syndrome: an ESSIC working group report. Scand J Urol [Internet]. 2020;54(2):91–8. Available from: https://doi.org/10.1080/21681805.2020.1730948.
52. Moore KH, Nickson P, Richmond DH, Sutherst JR, Manasse PR, Helliwell TR. Detrusor mast cells in refractory idiopathic instability. Br J Urol. 1993;72(2):17–21.
53. Tripp DA, Nickel JC, Wong J, Pontari M, Moldwin R, Mayer R, et al. Mapping of pain phenotypes in female

patients with bladder pain syndrome/interstitial cystitis and controls. Eur Urol. 2012;62(6):1188–94.
54. Lai HH, Jemielita T, Sutcliffe S, Bradley CS, Naliboff B, Williams DA, et al. Characterization of whole body pain in urological chronic pelvic pain syndrome at baseline: a MAPP Research Network Study. J Urol [Internet]. 2017;198(3):622–31. Available from: https://doi.org/10.1016/j.juro.2017.03.132.
55. Kuo HC, Chancellor MB. Comparison of intravesical botulinum toxin type A injections plus hydrodistention with hydrodistention alone for the treatment of refractory interstitial cystitis/painful bladder syndrome. BJU Int. 2009;104(5):657–61.
56. Killinger KA, Boura JA, Peters KM. Pain in interstitial cystitis/bladder pain syndrome: do characteristics differ in ulcerative and non-ulcerative subtypes? Int Urogynecol J [Internet]. 2013;24(8):1295–301. Available from: http://link.springer.com/10.1007/s00192-012-2003-9.
57. Pinto R, Lopes T, Costa D, Barros S, Silva J, Silva C, et al. Ulcerative and nonulcerative forms of bladder pain syndrome/interstitial cystitis do not differ in symptom intensity or response to onabotulinum toxin A. Urology [Internet]. 2014;83(5):1030–4. Available from: https://linkinghub.elsevier.com/retrieve/pii/S0090429514000636.
58. Clemens JQ, Bogart LM, Liu K, Pham C, Suttorp M, Berry SH. Perceptions of "urgency" in women with interstitial cystitis/bladder pain syndrome or overactive bladder. Neurourol Urodyn [Internet]. 2011;30(3):402–5. Available from: https://onlinelibrary.wiley.com/doi/10.1002/nau.20974.
59. Dubinskaya A, Tholemeier LN, Erickson T, De Hoedt AM, Barbour KE, Kim J, et al. Prevalence of overactive bladder symptoms among women with interstitial cystitis/bladder pain syndrome. Female Pelvic Med Reconstr Surg [Internet]. 2022;28(3):e115–9. Available from: https://journals.lww.com/10.1097/SPV.0000000000001166.
60. Sutcliffe S, Colditz GA, Goodman MS, Pakpahan R, Vetter J, Ness TJ, et al. Urological chronic pelvic pain syndrome symptom flares: characterisation of the full range of flares at two sites in the Multidisciplinary Approach to the Study of Chronic Pelvic Pain (MAPP) Research Network. BJU Int [Internet]. 2014;114(6):916–25. Available from: https://onlinelibrary.wiley.com/doi/10.1111/bju.12778.
61. Stanford E, McMurphy C. There is a low incidence of recurrent bacteriuria in painful bladder syndrome/interstitial cystitis patients followed longitudinally. Int Urogynecol J. 2007;18(5):551–4.
62. Sutcliffe S, Gallop R, Henry Lai HH, Andriole GL, Bradley CS, Chelimsky G, et al. A longitudinal analysis of urological chronic pelvic pain syndrome flares in the Multidisciplinary Approach to the Study of Chronic Pelvic Pain (MAPP) Research Network. BJU Int. 2019;124(3):522–31.
63. Keller JJ, Chen Y-K, Lin H-C. Comorbidities of bladder pain syndrome/interstitial cystitis: a population-based study. BJU Int. 2012;110(11 Pt C):E903–9.
64. O'Leary MP, Sant GR, Fowler FJ Jr, Whitmore KE, Spolarich-Kroll J. The interstitial cystitis symptom index and problem index. Urology. 1997;49(5A Suppl):58–63. https://doi.org/10.1016/s0090-4295(99)80333-1.
65. Parsons CL, Dell J, Stanford EJ, Bullen M, Kahn BS, Waxell T, et al. Increased prevalence of interstitial cystitis: previously unrecognized urologic and gynecologic cases identified using a new symptom questionnaire and intravesical potassium sensitivity. Urology [Internet]. 2002;60(4):573–8. Available from: https://linkinghub.elsevier.com/retrieve/pii/S0090429502018290.
66. Clemens JQ, Calhoun EA, Litwin MS, McNaughton-Collins M, Kusek JW, Crowley EM, et al. Validation of a modified National Institutes of Health chronic prostatitis symptom index to assess genitourinary pain in both men and women. Urology [Internet]. 2009;74(5):983–987.e3. Available from: https://linkinghub.elsevier.com/retrieve/pii/S0090429509022006.
67. Shoskes DA, Nickel JC, Rackley RR, Pontari MA. Clinical phenotyping in chronic prostatitis/chronic pelvic pain syndrome and interstitial cystitis: a management strategy for urologic chronic pelvic pain syndromes. Prostate Cancer Prostatic Dis [Internet]. 2009;12(2):177–83. Available from: https://www.nature.com/articles/pcan200842.
68. Crane A, Lloyd J, Shoskes DA. Improving the utility of clinical phenotyping in interstitial cystitis/painful bladder syndrome: from UPOINT to INPUT. Can J Urol [Internet]. 2018;25(2):9250–4. Available from: http://www.ncbi.nlm.nih.gov/pubmed/29680002.
69. Griffith JW, Stephens-Shields AJ, Hou X, Naliboff BD, Pontari M, Edwards TC, et al. Pain and urinary symptoms should not be combined into a single score: psychometric findings from the MAPP Research Network. J Urol [Internet]. 2016;195(4 Part 1):949–54. Available from: http://www.jurology.com/doi/10.1016/j.juro.2015.11.012.
70. Nickel JC, Shoskes D, Irvine-Bird K. Clinical phenotyping of women with interstitial cystitis/painful bladder syndrome—a key to classification and potentially improved management. J Urol [Internet]. 2009;182(1):155–60. Available from: https://doi.org/10.1016/j.juro.2009.02.122.
71. Akiyama Y, Luo Y, Hanno PM, Maeda D, Homma Y. Interstitial cystitis/bladder pain syndrome: the evolving landscape, animal models and future perspectives. Int J Urol Off J Japanese Urol Assoc. 2020;27(6):491–503.
72. Offiah I, McMahon SB, O'Reilly BA. Interstitial cystitis/bladder pain syndrome: diagnosis and management. Int Urogynecol J [Internet]. 2013;24(8):1243–56. Available from: http://link.springer.com/10.1007/s00192-013-2057-3.

73. Gordon Z, Parsons CL, Monga M. Intravesical ethanol test: an ineffective measure of bladder hyperpermeability. Urology. 2003;61(3):555–7.
74. Philip J, Willmott S, Irwin P. Interstitial cystitis versus detrusor overactivity: a comparative, randomized, controlled study of cystometry using saline and 0.3 M potassium chloride. J Urol. 2006;175(2):566–71.
75. Daha LK, Riedl CR, Lazar D, Simak R, Pflüger H. Effect of intravesical glycosaminoglycan substitution therapy on bladder pain syndrome/interstitial cystitis, bladder capacity and potassium sensitivity. Scand J Urol Nephrol. 2008;42(4):369–72.
76. Bade J, Ishizuka O, Yoshida M. Workshop 8: future research needs for the definition/diagnosis of interstitial cystitis. Int J Urol. 2003;10(Suppl):31–4.
77. Wennevik GE, Meijlink JM, Hanno P, Nordling J. The role of glomerulations in bladder pain syndrome: a review. J Urol [Internet]. 2016;195(1):19–25. Available from: https://doi.org/10.1016/j.juro.2015.06.112.
78. Keay S, Zhang CO, Trifillis AL, Hise MK, Hebel JR, Jacobs SC, et al. Decreased 3H-thymidine incorporation by human bladder epithelial cells following exposure to urine from interstitial cystitis patients. J Urol. 1996;156(6):2073–8.
79. Erickson DR, Kunselman AR, Bentley CM, Peters KM, Rovner ES, Demers LM, et al. Changes in urine markers and symptoms after bladder distention for interstitial cystitis. J Urol [Internet]. 2007;177(2):556–60. Available from: http://www.jurology.com/doi/10.1016/j.juro.2006.09.029.
80. Logadottir YR, Ehrén I, Fall M, Wiklund NP, Peeker R. Intravesical nitric oxide production discriminates between classic and nonulcer interstitial cystitis. J Urol. 2004;171(3):1148–51.
81. Dias B, Serrão P, Cruz F, Charrua A. Effect of water avoidance stress on serum and urinary NGF levels in rats: diagnostic and therapeutic implications for BPS/IC patients. Sci Rep [Internet]. 2019;9(1):14113. Available from: http://www.nature.com/articles/s41598-019-50576-4.
82. Tyagi P, Killinger K, Tyagi V, Nirmal J, Chancellor M, Peters KM. Urinary chemokines as noninvasive predictors of ulcerative interstitial cystitis. J Urol [Internet]. 2012;187(6):2243–8. Available from: https://doi.org/10.1016/j.juro.2012.01.034.
83. Homma Y, Nomiya A, Tagaya M, Oyama T, Takagaki K, Nishimatsu H, et al. Increased mRNA expression of genes involved in pronociceptive inflammatory reactions in bladder tissue of interstitial cystitis. J Urol [Internet]. 2013;190(5):1925–31. Available from: https://doi.org/10.1016/j.juro.2013.05.049.
84. Pinto R, Lopes T, Frias B, Silva A, Silva JA, Silva CM, et al. Trigonal injection of botulinum toxin A in patients with refractory bladder pain syndrome/interstitial cystitis. Eur Urol. 2010;58(3):360–5.
85. Liu HT, Kuo HC. Increased urine and serum nerve growth factor levels in interstitial cystitis suggest chronic inflammation is involved in the pathogenesis of disease. PLoS One. 2012;7(9):1–5.
86. Chen W, Ye D-Y, Han D-J, Fu G-Q, Zeng X, Lin W, et al. Elevated level of nerve growth factor in the bladder pain syndrome/interstitial cystitis: a meta-analysis. Springerplus [Internet]. 2016;5(1):1072. Available from: https://doi.org/10.1186/s40064-016-2719-y.
87. Charrua A, Pinto R, Taylor A, Canelas A, Ribeiro-da-Silva A, Cruz CD, et al. Can the adrenergic system be implicated in the pathophysiology of bladder pain syndrome/interstitial cystitis? A clinical and experimental study. Neurourol Urodyn [Internet]. 2015;34(5):489–96. Available from: http://doi.wiley.com/10.1002/nau.22542.
88. Matos R, Cordeiro JM, Coelho A, Ferreira S, Silva C, Igawa Y, et al. Bladder pain induced by prolonged peripheral alpha 1A adrenoceptor stimulation involves the enhancement of transient receptor potential vanilloid 1 activity and an increase of urothelial adenosine triphosphate release. Acta Physiol. 2016;218(4).
89. Jiang YH, Jhang JF, Kuo HC. Revisiting the role of potassium sensitivity testing and cystoscopic hydrodistention for the diagnosis of interstitial cystitis. PLoS One. 2016;11(3):1–9.
90. Furuta A, Yamamoto T, Suzuki Y, Gotoh M, Egawa S, Yoshimura N. Comparison of inflammatory urine markers in patients with interstitial cystitis and overactive bladder. Int Urogynecol J [Internet]. 2018;29(7):961–6. Available from: https://doi.org/10.1038/srep39227.
91. Niimi A, Igawa Y, Aizawa N, Honma T, Nomiya A, Akiyama Y, et al. Diagnostic value of urinary CXCL10 as a biomarker for predicting Hunner type interstitial cystitis. Neurourol Urodyn. 2018;37(3):1113–9.
92. Parker KS, Crowley JR, Stephens-Shields AJ, van Bokhoven A, Lucia MS, Lai HH, et al. Urinary metabolomics identifies a molecular correlate of interstitial cystitis/bladder pain syndrome in a Multidisciplinary Approach to the Study of Chronic Pelvic Pain (MAPP) Research Network Cohort. EBioMedicine [Internet]. 2016;7:167–74. Available from: https://doi.org/10.1016/j.ebiom.2016.03.040.
93. Braundmeier-Fleming A, Russell NT, Yang W, Nas MY, Yaggie RE, Berry M, et al. Stool-based biomarkers of interstitial cystitis/bladder pain syndrome. Sci Rep [Internet]. 2016;6(1):26083. Available from: https://doi.org/10.1038/srep26083.
94. Doggweiler R, Whitmore KE, Meijlink JM, Drake MJ, Frawley H, Nordling J, et al. A standard for terminology in chronic pelvic pain syndromes: a report from the chronic pelvic pain working group of the international continence society. Neurourol Urodyn [Internet]. 2017;36(4):984–1008. Available

95. Crane A, Lloyd J, Shoskes D. Improving the utility of clinical phenotyping in interstitial cystitis/painful bladder syndrome: from UPOINT to INPUT. J Urol [Internet]. 2017;197(4S):9250–4. Available from: https://doi.org/10.1016/j.juro.2017.02.928.
96. Hanno PM. Interstitial cystitis-epidemiology, diagnostic criteria, clinical markers. Rev Urol. 2002;4(Suppl 1):S3–8.
97. Benson H. The placebo effect. JAMA [Internet]. 1975;232(12):1225. Available from: http://jama.jamanetwork.com/article.aspx?doi=10.1001/jama.1975.03250120013012
98. Marberger M, Chartier-Kastler E, Egerdie B, Lee KS, Grosse J, Bugarin D, et al. A randomized double-blind placebo-controlled phase 2 dose-ranging study of onabotulinumtoxina in men with benign prostatic hyperplasia. Eur Urol. 2013;63(3):496–503.
99. Eredics K, Madersbacher S, Schauer I. A relevant midterm (12 months) placebo effect on lower urinary tract symptoms and maximum flow rate in male lower urinary tract symptom and benign prostatic hyperplasia – a meta-analysis. Urology [Internet]. 2017;106:160–6. Available from: https://doi.org/10.1016/j.urology.2017.05.011.
100. Barua JM, Arance I, Angulo JC, Riedl CR. A systematic review and meta-analysis on the efficacy of intravesical therapy for bladder pain syndrome/interstitial cystitis. Int Urogynecol J [Internet]. 2016;27(8):1137–47. Available from: https://doi.org/10.1007/s00192-015-2890-7.
101. Lowell Parsons C, Koprowski PF. Interstitial cystitis: successful management by increasing urinary voiding intervals. Urology [Internet]. 1991;37(3):207–12. Available from: https://linkinghub.elsevier.com/retrieve/pii/009042959180286G.
102. Chaiken DC, Blaivas JG, Blaivas ST. Behavioral therapy for the treatment of refractory interstitial cystitis. J Urol [Internet]. 1993;149(6):1445–8. Available from: http://www.jurology.com/doi/10.1016/S0022-5347%2817%2936411-X.
103. Jeong SJ, Lee SC, Jeong CW, Hong SK, Byun SS, Lee SE. Clinical and urodynamic differences among women with overactive bladder according to the presence of detrusor overactivity. Int Urogynecol J Pelvic Floor Dysfunct. 2013;24(2):255–61.
104. Loving S, Nordling J, Jaszczak P, Thomsen T. Does evidence support physiotherapy management of adult female chronic pelvic pain? A systematic review. Scand J Pain [Internet]. 2012;3(2):70–81. Available from: https://doi.org/10.1016/j.sjpain.2011.12.002.
105. Fitzgerald MP, Payne CK, Lukacz ES, Yang CC, Peters KM, Chai TC, et al. Randomized multicenter clinical trial of myofascial physical therapy in women with interstitial cystitis/painful bladder syndrome and pelvic floor tenderness. JURO [Internet]. 2012;187(6):2113–8. Available from: https://doi.org/10.1016/j.juro.2012.01.123.
106. Borrego-Jimenez P-S, Padilla-Fernandez B-Y, Valverde-Martinez S, Garcia-Sanchez M-H, Rodriguez-Martin M-O, Sanchez-Conde M-P, et al. Effects on health-related quality of life of biofeedback physiotherapy of the pelvic floor as an adjunctive treatment following surgical repair of cystocele. J Clin Med [Internet]. 2020;9(10):3310. Available from: https://www.mdpi.com/2077-0383/9/10/3310.
107. Koziol JA, Clark DC, Gittes RF, Tan EM. The natural history of interstitial cystitis: a survey of 374 patients. J Urol [Internet]. 1993;149(3):465–9. Available from: https://doi.org/10.1016/S0022-5347(17)36120-7.
108. Rothrock NE, Lutgendorf SK, Kreder KJ, Ratliff T, Zimmerman B. Stress and symptoms in patients with interstitial cystitis: a life stress model. Urology [Internet]. 2001;57(3):422–7. Available from: https://linkinghub.elsevier.com/retrieve/pii/S0090429500009882.
109. Nguan C, Franciosi LG, Buherfield NN, Macleod BA, Jens M, Fenster HN. A prospective, double-blind, randomized cross-over study evaluating changes in urinary pH for relieving the symptoms of interstitial cystitis. BJU Int. 2005;95(1):91–4.
110. Moutzouris DA, Falagas ME. Interstitial cystitis: an unsolved enigma. Clin J Am Soc Nephrol. 2009;4(11):1844–57.
111. Reiter M, Schwope R, Clarkson A. Sarcomatoid renal cell carcinoma: a case report and literature review. J Radiol Case Rep [Internet]. 2012;6(4):11–6. Available from: http://www.pubmedcentral.nih.gov/articlerender.fcgi?artid=3370693&tool=pmcentrez&rendertype=abstract.
112. Fritjofsson Å, Fall M, Juhlin R, Persson BE, Ruutu M. Treatment of ulcer and nonulcer interstitial cystitis with sodium pentosanpolysulfate: a multicenter trial. J Urol [Internet]. 1987;138(3):508–12. Available from: http://www.jurology.com/doi/10.1016/S0022-5347%2817%2943242-3.
113. Parsons CL, Schmidt JD, Pollen JJ. Successful treatment of interstitial cystitis with sodium pentosanpolysulfate. J Urol [Internet]. 1983;130(1):51–3. Available from: http://www.jurology.com/doi/10.1016/S0022-5347%2817%2950948-9.
114. Parsons CL, Benson G, Childs SJ, Hanno P, Sant GR, Webster G. A quantitatively controlled method to study prospectively interstitial cystitis and demonstrate the efficacy of pentosanpolysulfate. J Urol [Internet]. 1993;150(3):845–8. Available from: http://www.jurology.com/doi/10.1016/S0022-5347%2817%2935629-X
115. Mulholland SG, Sant GR, Hanno P, Staskin DR, Parsons L. Pentosan polysulfate sodium for therapy of interstitial cystitis. Urology [Internet]. 1990;35(6):552–8. Available from: https://linkinghub.elsevier.com/retrieve/pii/0090429590801165.
116. Sant GR, Propert KJ, Hanno PM, Burks D, Culkin D, Diokno AC, et al. A pilot clinical trial of oral pentosan

polysulfate and oral hydroxyzine in patients with interstitial cystitis. J Urol [Internet]. 2003;170(3): 810–5. Available from: http://www.jurology.com/doi/10.1097/01.ju.0000083020.06212.3d.
117. Holm-Bentzen M, Jacobsen F, Nerstrøm B, Lose G, Kristensen JK, Pedersen RH, et al. A prospective double-blind clinically controlled multicenter trial of sodium pentosanpolysulfate in the treatment of interstitial cystitis and related painful bladder disease. J Urol [Internet]. 1987;138(3):503–7. Available from: http://www.jurology.com/doi/10.1016/S0022-5347%2817%2943241-1.
118. Hanno PM. Analysis of long-term Elmiron therapy for interstitial cystitis. Urology [Internet]. 1997;49(5): 93–9. Available from: https://linkinghub.elsevier.com/retrieve/pii/S0090429597001799.
119. Fritjofsson Å, Fall M, Juhlin R, Persson BE, Ruutu M. Treatment of ulcer and nonulcer interstitial cystitis with sodium pentosanpolysulfate: a multicenter trial. J Urol [Internet]. 1987;138(3):508–12. Available from: https://doi.org/10.1016/S0022-5347(17)43242-3.
120. Hanif AM, Armenti ST, Taylor SC, Shah RA, Igelman AD, Jayasundera KT, et al. Phenotypic spectrum of pentosan polysulfate sodium-associated maculopathy: a multicenter study. JAMA Ophthalmol. 2019;137(11):1275–82.
121. Ludwig CA, Vail D, Callaway NF, Pasricha MV, Moshfeghi DM. Pentosan polysulfate sodium exposure and drug-induced maculopathy in commercially insured patients in the United States. Ophthalmology [Internet]. 2020;127(4):535–43. Available from:. https://doi.org/10.1016/j.ophtha.2019.10.036.
122. Sairanen J, Forsell T, Ruutu M. Long-term outcome of patients with interstitial cystitis treated with low dose cyclosporine A. J Urol. 2004;171(6 I):2138–41.
123. Forsell T, Ruutu M, Isoniemi H, Ahonen J, Alfthan O. Cyclosporine in severe interstitial cystitis. J Urol. 1996;155(5):1591–3.
124. Sairanen J, Tammela TLJ, Leppilahti M, Multanen M, Paananen I, Lehtoranta K, et al. Cyclosporine A and pentosan polysulfate sodium for the treatment of interstitial cystitis: a randomized comparative study. J Urol. 2005;174(6):2235–8.
125. Ogawa T, Ishizuka O, Ueda T, Tyagi P, Chancellor MB, Yoshimura N. Pharmacological management of interstitial cystitis/bladder pain syndrome and the role cyclosporine and other immunomodulating drugs play. Expert Rev Clin Pharmacol [Internet]. 2018;11(5):495–505. Available from: https://doi.org/10.1080/17512433.2018.1457435.
126. Vollstedt A, Tennyson L, Turner K, Hasenau D, Saon M, McCartney T, et al. Evidence for early cyclosporine treatment for Hunner lesion interstitial cystitis. Female Pelvic Med Reconstr Surg [Internet]. 2022;28(1):e1–5. Available from: https://journals.lww.com/fpmrs/Fulltext/2022/01000/Evidence_for_Early_Cyclosporine_Treatment_for.12.aspx.
127. Fall M, Oberpenning F, Peeker R. Treatment of bladder pain syndrome/interstitial cystitis 2008: can we make evidence-based decisions? Eur Urol [Internet]. 2008;54(1):65–78. Available from: https://linkinghub.elsevier.com/retrieve/pii/S0302283808003977.
128. Moldwin RM, Evans RJ, Stanford EJ, Rosenberg MT. Rational approaches to the treatment of patients with interstitial cystitis. Urology. 2007;69(4 Suppl).
129. Thilagarajah R, Witherow RO, Walker MM. Oral cimetidine gives effective symptom relief in painful bladder disease: a prospective, randomized, double-blind placebo-controlled trial. BJU Int [Internet]. 2001;87(3):207–12. Available from: http://doi.wiley.com/10.1046/j.1464-410x.2001.02031.x.
130. Evans RJ, Moldwin RM, Cossons N, Darekar A, Mills IW, Scholfield D. Proof of concept trial of Tanezumab for the treatment of symptoms associated with interstitial cystitis. J Urol [Internet]. 2011;185(5):1716–21. Available from: https://doi.org/10.1016/j.juro.2010.12.088.
131. Wang H, Russell LJ, Kelly KM, Wang S, Thipphawong J. Fulranumab in patients with interstitial cystitis/bladder pain syndrome: observations from a randomized, double-blind, placebo-controlled study. BMC Urol [Internet]. 2017;17(1):2. Available from: https://doi.org/10.1186/s12894-016-0193-z.
132. Sasaki K, Smith CP, Chuang YC, Lee JY, Kim JC, Chancellor MB. Oral gabapentin (neurontin) treatment of refractory genitourinary tract pain. Tech Urol. 2001;7(1):47–9.
133. Foster HEJ, Hanno PM, Nickel JC, Payne CK, Mayer RD, Burks DA, et al. Effect of amitriptyline on symptoms in treatment naïve patients with interstitial cystitis/painful bladder syndrome. J Urol. 2010;183(5):1853–8.
134. Bouchelouche K, Horn T, Nordling J, Larsen S, Hald T. The action of cysteinyl-leukotrienes on intracellular calcium mobilization in human detrusor myocytes. BJU Int. 2001;87(7):690–6.
135. Chen H, Wang F, Chen W, Ye XT, Zhou Q, Shao F, et al. Efficacy of daily low-dose sildenafil for treating interstitial cystitis: results of a randomized, double-blind, placebo-controlled trial – treatment of interstitial cystitis/painful bladder syndrome with low-dose sildenafil. Urology [Internet]. 2014;84(1):51–6. Available from: https://doi.org/10.1016/j.urology.2014.02.050.
136. Mendes PA, Dias N, Simaes J, Dinis P, Cruz F, Pinto R. Daily low dose of tadalafil improves pain and frequency in bladder pain syndrome/interstitial cystitis patients. Türk Üroloji Dergisi/Turkish J Urol [Internet]. 2022;48(1):82–7. Available from: https://turkishjournalofurology.com/en/daily-low-dose-of-tadalafil-improves-pain-and-frequency-in-bladder-pain-syndrome-interstitial-cystitis-patients-133783.
137. Keay S, Kaczmarek P, Zhang C-O, Koch K, Szekely Z, Barchi JJJ, et al. Normalization of proliferation and tight junction formation in bladder epithelial cells from patients with interstitial cystitis/painful bladder syndrome by d-proline and d-pipecolic acid derivatives of antiproliferative factor. Chem Biol Drug Des. 2011;77(6):421–30.

138. Freire VS, Burkhard FC, Kessler TM, Kuhn A, Draeger A, Monastyrskaya K. MicroRNAs may mediate the down-regulation of neurokinin-1 receptor in chronic bladder pain syndrome. Am J Pathol [Internet]. 2010;176(1):288–303. Available from:. https://doi.org/10.2353/ajpath.2010.090552.

139. Tambaro S, Casu MA, Mastinu A, Lazzari P. Evaluation of selective cannabinoid CB1 and CB2 receptor agonists in a mouse model of lipopolysaccharide-induced interstitial cystitis. Eur J Pharmacol [Internet]. 2014;729(1):67–74. Available from: https://doi.org/10.1016/j.ejphar.2014.02.013.

140. Charrua A, Cruz CD, Jansen D, Rozenberg B, Heesakkers J, Cruz F. Co-administration of transient receptor potential vanilloid 4 (TRPV4) and TRPV1 antagonists potentiate the effect of each drug in a rat model of cystitis. BJU Int. 2015;115(3):452–60.

141. Peeker R, Haghsheno MA, Holmäng S, Fall M. Intravesical bacillus Calmette-Guerin and dimethyl sulfoxide for treatment of classic and non-ulcer interstitial cystitis: a prospective, randomized double-blind study. J Urol. 2000;164(6):1912–6.

142. Nickel JC, Moldwin R, Lee S, Davis EL, Henry RA, Wyllie MG. Intravesical alkalinized lidocaine (PSD597) offers sustained relief from symptoms of interstitial cystitis and painful bladder syndrome. BJU Int. 2009;103(7):910–8.

143. Rosamilia A, Dwyer PL, Gibson J. Electromotive drug administration of lidocaine and dexamethasone followed by cystodistension in women with interstitial cystitis. Int Urogynecol J Pelvic Floor Dysfunct. 1997;8(3):142–5.

144. Davis EL, El Khoudary SR, Talbott EO, Davis J, Regan LJ. Safety and efficacy of the use of intravesical and oral pentosan polysulfate sodium for interstitial cystitis: a randomized double-blind clinical trial. J Urol. 2008;179(1):177–85.

145. Engelhardt PF, Morakis N, Daha LK, Esterbauer B, Riedl CR. Long-term results of intravesical hyaluronan therapy in bladder pain syndrome/interstitial cystitis. Int Urogynecol J. 2011;22(4):401–5.

146. Payne CK, Joyce GF, Wise M, Clemens JQ. Interstitial cystitis and painful bladder syndrome. J Urol. 2007;177(6):2042–9.

147. Cruz F. Targets for botulinum toxin in the lower urinary tract. Neurourol Urodyn [Internet]. 2014;33(1):31–8. Available from: https://doi.org/10.1002/nau.22445.

148. Smith CP, Nishiguchi J, O'Leary M, Yoshimura N, Chancellor MB. Single-institution experience in 110 patients with botulinum toxin A injection into bladder or urethra. Urology. 2005;65(1):37–41.

149. Giannantoni A, Porena M, Costantini E, Zucchi A, Mearini L, Mearini E. Botulinum A toxin intravesical injection in patients with painful bladder syndrome: 1-year followup. J Urol [Internet]. 2008;179(3):1031–4. Available from: http://www.jurology.com/doi/10.1016/j.juro.2007.10.032.

150. Pinto R, Lopes T, Silva J, Silva C, Dinis P, Cruz F. Persistent therapeutic effect of repeated injections of onabotulinum toxin A in refractory bladder pain syndrome/interstitial cystitis. J Urol [Internet]. 2013;189(2):548–53. Available from: https://doi.org/10.1016/j.juro.2012.09.027.

151. Pinto RA, Costa D, Morgado A, Pereira P, Charrua A, Silva J, et al. Intratrigonal onabotulinumtoxinA improves bladder symptoms and quality of life in patients with bladder pain syndrome/interstitial cystitis: a pilot, single center, randomized, double-blind, placebo controlled trial. J Urol [Internet]. 2018;199(4):998–1003. Available from: https://doi.org/10.1016/j.juro.2017.10.018.

152. Zhang W, Deng X, Liu C, Wang X. Intravesical treatment for interstitial cystitis/painful bladder syndrome: a network meta-analysis. Int Urogynecol J [Internet]. 2017;28(4):515–25. Available from: http://link.springer.com/10.1007/s00192-016-3079-4.

153. Hsieh C-H, Chang S-T, Hsieh C-J, Hsu C-S, Kuo T-C, Chang H-C, et al. Treatment of interstitial cystitis with hydrodistention and bladder training. Int Urogynecol J Pelvic Floor Dysfunct. 2008;19(10):1379–84.

154. Hanno P, Nordling J, Fall M. Bladder pain syndrome. Med Clin North Am. 2011;95(1):55–73.

155. Peeker R, Aldenborg F, Fall M. Complete transurethral resection of ulcers in classic interstitial cystitis. Int Urogynecol J Pelvic Floor Dysfunct. 2000;11(5):290–5.

156. Kerr WS. Interstitial cystitis: treatment by transurethral resection. J Urol. 1971;105(5):664–6.

157. Ko KJ, Cho WJ, Lee Y-S, Choi J, Byun HJ, Lee K-S. Comparison of the efficacy between transurethral coagulation and transurethral resection of Hunner lesion in interstitial cystitis/bladder pain syndrome patients: a prospective randomized controlled trial. Eur Urol. 2020;77(5):644–51.

158. Hillelsohn JH, Rais-Bahrami S, Friedlander JI, Okhunov Z, Kashan M, Rosen L, et al. Fulguration for hunner ulcers: long-term clinical outcomes. J Urol [Internet]. 2012;188(6):2238–41. Available from: https://doi.org/10.1016/j.juro.2012.08.013.

159. Rofeim O, Hom D, Freid RM, Moldwin RM. Use of the neodymium: YAG laser for interstitial cystitis: a prospective study. J Urol. 2001;166(1):134–6.

160. Linn JF, Hohenfellner M, Roth S, Dahms SE, Stein R, Hertle L, et al. Treatment of interstitial cystitis: comparison of subtrigonal and supratrigonal cystectomy combined with orthotopic bladder substitution. J Urol. 1998;159(3):774–8.

161. Kim HJ, Lee JS, Cho WJ, Lee HS, Lee HN, You HW, et al. Efficacy and safety of augmentation ileocystoplasty combined with supratrigonal cystectomy for the treatment of refractory bladder pain syndrome/interstitial cystitis with Hunner's lesion. Int J Urol [Internet]. 2014;21(S1):69–73. Available from: https://doi.org/10.1111/iju.12320.

162. Peeker R, Aldenborg F, Fall M. The treatment of interstitial cystitis with supratrigonal cystectomy and ileocystoplasty: difference in outcome between

classic and nonulcer disease. J Urol. 1998;159(5): 1479–82.
163. Elzawahri A, Bissada NK, Herchorn S, Aboul-Enein-H, Ghoneim M, Bissada MA, et al. Urinary conduit formation using a retubularized bowel from continent urinary diversion or intestinal augmentations: ii. Does it have a role in patients with interstitial cystitis? J Urol. 2004;171(4):1559–62.
164. Nunez-Badinez P, De Leo B, Laux-Biehlmann A, Hoffmann A, Zollner TM, Saunders PTK, et al. Preclinical models of endometriosis and interstitial cystitis/bladder pain syndrome: an Innovative Medicines Initiative-PainCare Initiative to improve their value for translational research in pelvic pain. Pain. 2021;162(9): 2349–65.

Female Sexual Dysfunction

Francisco E. Martins, Farzana Cassim, Oleksandr Yatsina, and Jan Adlam

Contents

Introduction	960
Definition	961
Consensus Classification Systems	962
Incidence, Prevalence, and Risk Factors	963
Female Pelvic Anatomy	965
The Vagina	965
The G-Spot	966
The Vulva	967
The Clitoris	968
Innervation	969
Vascular Supply	970
The Female Sexual Response Cycle	970
Physiology and Biochemistry of Female Sexual Response Cycle	974
Mechanisms of Sexual Arousal	974
Etiology and Pathophysiology of Female Sexual Dysfunction	975
Female Sexual Dysfunction in Specific Settings	977
FSD in the Post-Partum Period	977
FSD and Pelvic Organ Prolapse and/or Urinary Incontinence	978
FSD After Pelvic Surgeries	979

F. E. Martins (✉)
Department of Urology, University of Lisbon, School of Medicine, Hospital Santa Maria, Lisbon, Portugal

F. Cassim
Division of Urology, Stellenbosch University/Tygerberg Hospital, Cape Town, South Africa

O. Yatsina
Department of Urological Surgery, National Cancer Institute, Kyiv, Ukraine

J. Adlam
Department of Obstetrics and Gynaecoogy, Stellenbosch University/Tygerberg Hospital, Cape Town, South Africa

© Springer Nature Switzerland AG 2023
F. E. Martins et al. (eds.), *Female Genitourinary and Pelvic Floor Reconstruction*,
https://doi.org/10.1007/978-3-031-19598-3_55

Evaluation of Female Sexual Dysfunction 984
Treatment Options 985
Conclusion 987
References 987

Abstract

Female sexual dysfunction is a common medical problem with biological and psychosocial detrimental repercussions on a woman's quality of life. It is age-related, increasing in frequency as women age or enter menopause, progressive, and highly prevalent. It is also associated with socioeconomic impact. Female sexual dysfunction is defined as any disorder that decreases sexual desire, subjective arousal, vaginal lubrication, and increased difficulty in achieving orgasm. It may be associated with pain and discomfort with intercourse. The etiology is frequently multifactorial. It is a common complication of most oncologic pelvic surgeries, such as radical cystectomy and colorectal amputation, but also due to physical, mental, and social factors such as quality of relationship, depression, unemployment or other professional issues, life stressors, and woman's age and health status, especially cardiovascular diseases, which are also pathological conditions associated with aging and erectile dysfunction in males. Unlike the significant progress in research and treatment for male erectile dysfunction, specifically the development of pharmacological and other noninvasive therapeutic options, female patients have witnessed significantly less scientific and industry investment, and treatment is primarily restricted to psychological therapy. Nonetheless, treatment should be adjusted to the patient's needs and may potentially involve a multidisciplinary team approach including a psychotherapist/sexologist and a physician. Enormous work needs to be pursued to improve the care of women with female sexual dysfunction. This chapter will provide the most current and up-to-date knowledge on female sexual dysfunction, including basic science related to this medical problem, and reveal the latest therapeutic approaches available.

Keywords

Female sexual dysfunction · dyspareunia · sexual pain · desire disorder · arousal disorder · orgasmic disorder · treatment of female sexual dysfunction · evaluation of female sexual dysfunction · clitoris · vagina

Introduction

Human sexual function constitutes an integral part of life for species propagation and quality of life. Sexuality has captivated attention since ancient times shown by the number of art manifestations related to different aspects of sexuality, affection, love, emotional relationships, or gender differences. Sexual dysfunction can result in decreased quality of life with potential impact in procreation.

Scientific research in sexual dysfunction did not really initiate until the late 1920s with the pioneering studies on marital relationships by Hamilton and Davis independently in 1929 [1]. Davis surveyed the sex life of 2200 women from New York City [1]. Approximately two decades later, Kinsey published his magnificent work in two separate volumes on human male and female sexual behavior [2]. However, the awareness and management of female sexual dysfunction (FSD) has only made great progress since Master and Johnson's study in 1957 but published in 1966 and 1970 [3]. These publications were regarded as important landmarks in the research of female sexual dysfunction, describing the four-phased response of the female sexual cycle: (1) motivation, including desire or libido; (2) arousal or excitement; (3) orgasm; and (4) resolution.

Female sexual dysfunction is more complex and notably less clear than its male counterpart. It is currently known that female sexual dysfunction is age-related, progressive, and particularly prevalent, affecting 30–50% of women [4–7]. Until recently, FSD was thought to be psychogenic in nature. Nonetheless, this scenario has changed and FSD is now accepted as a multifactorial disease entity, which is associated with several medical and surgical diseases. Furthermore, epidemiologic studies in females have suggested the same pathogenic and risk factors behind male erectile dysfunction, such as aging, cardiovascular diseases, cigarette smoking, hypercholesterolemia, and pelvic surgeries for cervical, uterine cancer, and bladder malignancies, are associated with FSD [8]. Regardless of its cause, FSD can negatively affect a woman's quality of life.

Until recently, limited basic science and clinical research has focused on female sexual function. Consequently, our knowledge and perception of the anatomy and physiology of female sexuality, and the pathophysiology of FSD is scanty. Gradual progress has been made in this field based on our understanding of the pathophysiology of the male erectile response encouraged by recent advances in modern technology coupled with the latest interest in women's health issues.

This chapter discusses the definition, classification, pathophysiology, and therapeutic options of the female sexual dysfunction, as well as the recent advances in basic science and clinical research addressing this dysfunction.

Definition

In 1966, Masters and Johnson described four successive phases of the normal female sexual response cycle: excitement, plateau, orgasm, and resolution [6]. Kaplan, in 1979, altered this hypothesis by further subdividing the excitement phase into desire/libido and arousal, removing the plateau phase, thus giving rise to the three-dimensional model consisting of desire, arousal, and orgasm [9].

The *World Health Organization International Classification of Disorders-10* (ICD-10) defined sexual dysfunction as "the various ways in which an individual is unable to participate in a sexual relationship he or she would wish" [1]. In addition, the *Diagnostic and Statistical Manual of Mental Disorders* (DSM-IV), based on Kaplan's hypothesis, deals specifically with psychiatric disorders, defines female sexual dysfunction as "disturbances in sexual desire and in psychophysiological changes that characterize the sexual response cycle and cause marked distress and interpersonal difficulty" [10]. Both systems base their definitions and classifications firmly on the human sexual cycle sequence and timing, and on the conceptualization of sexual response as a "psychosomatic mechanism." Sexual arousal is a physiologic phase or state involving specific feelings and physiologic changes, usually associated with sexual activity related to the genitals [11]. In 2001, Basson proposed a five-phase model with a highlight on intimacy [12]. Desire and intimacy are key for woman's participation in sexual activity. A coordinated sequence of intimacy, sexual stimulation, emotional and sexual arousal, and desire occurs and culminates in psychologic and somatic pleasure and satisfaction.

In 1998, The Sexual Function Health Council of the American Foundation for Urologic Disease (AFUD) convened the first international interdisciplinary consensus conference panel with 19 experts in FSD. The former DSM-IV classification was expanded to include psychogenic and organic causes of the sexual response cycle, such as desire, arousal, orgasm, and sexual pain disorders [8]. This final system uses the major categories described in DSM-IV and ICD-10; however, the definitions have been modified to reflect current clinical and research patterns. An essential component of this new diagnostic and classification system is the addition of the new sexual pain disorder, a personal distress criterion, stressing the fact that a condition is considered a disorder only if it generates distress in the woman experiencing the condition [8].

Clear, consistent, uniform, and universally acceptable definitions of sexual complaint, sexual dysfunction, and sexual disorders are necessary for prevalence and etiology of FSD, as well as potential therapeutic interventions. As this stands currently, *sexual complaint* may be considered as the expression of discontent or discomfort associated with sexual activity. *Sexual disorder* relates to sexual dysfunction or problem that meets DSM-IV criteria for a sexual disorder, which includes malfunction and significant distress.

Consensus Classification Systems

In 1998, the AFUD Consensus Panel published a classification and definitions of female sexual dysfunction after evaluating and revising existing definitions and classifications of FSD [8]. Later in 2003, an update of this consensus was reported by the International Consensus Development Conference on Definitions and Classifications of Sexual Dysfunction [13]. Thus, the following definitions are currently recommended.

Hypoactive Sexual Desire Disorder (HSDD): Hypoactive Sexual Desire Disorder is the persistent or recurrent deficiency (or total absence) of sexual thoughts or fantasies and/or a lack of receptivity to or interest in sexual engagement leading to personal distress [8]. This first area of sexual dysfunction has been more highlighted and discussed in women and somewhat more neglected in epidemiologic analysis in men. It may result from psychogenic (emotional) causes, as well as physiologic factors, especially hormone deficiencies/disruptions such as menopause, medications, or surgical interventions, ending in decreased sexual desire [14, 15].

Sexual Aversion Disorder: This denotes the persistent or recurrent phobic repulsion to and avoidance of sexual activity with a sexual partner, leading to personal distress [8].

Sexual Arousal Disorder: This is a persistent or recurrent inability to attain or maintain sufficient erotic excitement, causing personal distress [8]. It can be divided into three types: (a) genital sexual arousal dysfunction, characterized by minimal vulvar swelling and vaginal lubrication; (b) subjective sexual arousal dysfunction, denoting absence or marked reduction of feeling of sexual arousal, excitement, and pleasure from any type of erotic stimuli; and (c) a combination of genital and subjective arousal dysfunction. These arousal disorders may include absent or reduced vaginal lubrication, decreased clitoral and labial engorgement and sensation, and absence of vaginal smooth muscle relaxation. They may occur because of psychogenic factors, or have a physiologic and medical basis, especially decreased vaginal and clitoral blood flow, previous pelvic trauma or pelvic surgery.

Orgasmic Disorder: This may be expressed in the difficulty, delay, or absence of attaining orgasm from any kind of sufficient erotic stimulation [8]. Ending in personal distress. It can be divided into primary (never achieved orgasm, eventual associated with emotional trauma or sexual abuse) or secondary to trauma, surgery, or hormonal deficiency. Anorgasmia has been reported in 24–37% of women seeking sex therapy for various reasons [16]. Serotonin reuptake inhibitors are among the pharmacological agents that can contribute to or exacerbate this condition Depending upon the dose and type of the drug, up to 50% of women have been shown to develop anorgasmia [16].

Sexual Pain Disorders: Dyspareunia: This is defined as recurrent or persistent genital pain linked to sexual activity, specifically vaginal intercourse [8]. Dyspareunia rates may range from 14% to 18% in the literature [9]. *Vaginismus* is the persistent or recurrent difficulty of the woman to allow vaginal penetration of a penis, a finger, and/or any object, despite of the woman's expressed desire to do so. This is expressed by involuntary spasms of the distal third of the vaginal musculature that prevent vaginal penetration and that cause personal distress. It may develop as a conditioned response to painful penetration, or due to psychogenic/emotional factors (Table 1) [1].

Disorders of the pelvic floor, sociopsychological factors and postmenopausal status may diminish vaginal lubrication and thus induce pain during sexual activity [17–19].

In terms of clinical applicability, these definitions should bear a degree of distress or bother from the sufferer, which would assist considerably

Table 1 Consensus classification system of female sexual disorders [4]

Sexual desire disorders
Hypoactive sexual desire disorder
Sexual aversion disorder
Sexual arousal disorder
Orgasmic disorder
Sexual pain disorders
Dyspareunia
Vaginismus
Other sexual pain disorders

data collection and interpretation, and possible future communication of that data. These definitions should also be further characterized in terms of duration (lifelong vs. acquired) and whether they are global or circumstantial. These definitions should have enough power to be used for comparative studies in terms of degree of dysfunction, and be internationally validated and accepted, such as the Female Sexual Function Index (FSFI) [20].

Incidence, Prevalence, and Risk Factors

Although FSD is acknowledged as a common health problem, its epidemiologic characteristics are ill-defined in evidence-based literature. Further well-conducted, longitudinal studies for FSD are immensely needed to obtain more accurate epidemiologic data. Unlike well-documented prevalence rates for male erectile dysfunction in the literature, its prevalence in FSD is surrounded by controversy, with reported rates ranging from 11% to 20% in some studies, 20–43% in other studies and even 91% in a further study using self-administered questionnaires [21–24]. This variation may be the result of distinct assessment methodologies, different age groups studied, difference in definitions used for the dysfunctions, the methods used for data selection and collection, duration, and degree of the dysfunction, and lastly the enormously general and unspecific definition of FSD in different study populations, making retrieval of population-based prevalence data more difficult and incurring in selection bias. Prevalence rates in clinical populations seeking help at gynecologic and uro-gynecologic clinics and general practitioners in London area have been estimated between 40% and 50% [25].

The results of a Committee on Sexual Dysfunctions in Men and Women convened in Paris in 2004, the panel reported that about 40–45% of adult women have at least one manifest sexual dysfunction [24]. Prevalence of low levels of sexual desire varied between 17% and 55%, this increasing with age, that is, 10% below 49 years of age, doubling to 22% for those aged 50–65, and then doubling again to 47% in women 66–74 years old [24]. The Committee also reported a general prevalence of manifest lubrication disorder in 8–15%, although other studies have revealed a higher rate of 21–28% in sexually active women [21, 25, 26]. Nonetheless, it is universally accepted that lubrication insufficiency becomes more prevalent with age > 50 years. Mercer et al. also found that 53.8% of women reported at least one sexual problem lasting ≥1 month over a 2-year period [26]. In another study with data derived from the US National Health and Social Health Survey, Laumann et al. reported that 43% of women were affected by sexual dysfunction [21].

There is a wide variation in reported rates for orgasmic dysfunction. In countries such as the United States, England, Sweden, and Australia, the average prevalence of manifest orgasmic dysfunction is 25% in women aged 18–74 years, although most of the studies did not report an age dependency. In some Nordic countries, using similar methodology, more than 80% of all sexually active women, regardless of age, reported some degree of orgasmic dysfunction [24]. The prevalence of vaginismus has been reported to be around 6% in two considerably diverse cultures such as Morocco and Sweden [24]. Although manifest dyspareunia has been reported to be as high as 18–20% in British and Australian surveys, it was as low as 2% in elderly British women [24].

Sexual dysfunction, regardless of sex, is often a multifactorial condition. There are several risk factors that are known to be common to men and women, including general health status, the presence of diabetes mellitus, the presence of hypertension and cardiovascular disease, simultaneous occurrence of genitourinary disease, psychiatric/psychologic disorders, including depression, anxiety, conflict within the relationship, fatigue, stress, lack of privacy, prior physical or sexual abuse, medications, and organic problems that result in uncomfortable or even painful sexual activity, such as endometriosis or atrophic vaginitis.

The presence of any serious medical condition is likely to alter sexual function due both to the condition itself and to the associated effect on psychological well-being. In a study of female sexuality, physical health was more solidly related to sexual problems than age alone in a study population cohort aged 57–85 years [27]. In the PRESIDE study, patient self-assessment of poor health was a significant correlate of distressing sexual problems, underlying the importance of assessing the prevalence of sexually related personal distress in accurately estimating the prevalence of sexual problems that may need clinical intervention. This prevalence of distressing sexual problems was highest in middle-aged women and was remarkably lower than the prevalence of sexual problems [28].

Evidence-based criteria should be established for evaluating risk factors for both male and female sexual dysfunctions. Nonetheless, despite all weaknesses found, diabetes mellitus and cigarette smoking should be considered independent risk factors for erectile dysfunction in men. However, cigarette smoking has not been found in descriptive analytical literature to be linked to female sexual dysfunction. Decreased lubrication has been suggested to be significantly linked to diabetes mellitus. Hypertension has also been associated with decreased lubrication, dyspareunia, vaginismus, and orgasmic dysfunction. Urinary incontinence has also been found to negatively impact all features of female sexual function, including sexual interest, desire, arousal, lubrication, and orgasm [24]. Psychiatric problems are also intimately associated with orgasmic dysfunction and dyspareunia [24]. Clearly, when specific types of sexual dysfunction were evaluated, distress-associated low desire rates followed an age-related pattern comparable to that for any sexual difficulty [29].

Menopausal status has a close correlation with age. The likelihood of the onset of sexual dysfunctions with menopause is apparently related to the specific type of sexual problem. It is well known that decreased lubrication leading to vaginal dryness and dyspareunia are commonly increased after menopause due to deficient estrogen levels in the vaginal tissue [30]. Additionally, a greater impact on sexual function may be induced by surgical compared to natural menopause [29]. In natural menopause, estrogen levels are low, but ovarian androgen production is preserved at premenopausal levels [31–33]. However, hormonal changes alone could not be directly linked to negative modifications in sexual activity, raising the possibility of an independent adverse mechanism on sexual physiology [29, 34].

Some studies have also linked cardiovascular diseases with sexual dysfunction, in both males and females [35]. In addition, Schwarz et al. found a high correlation between FSD and chronic compensated cardiac failure. In this report, 87% of middle-aged women with cardiac failure complained of some degree of sexual dysfunction, 80% of whom complained of decreased vaginal lubrication, resulting in a 76% rate of unsuccessful intercourse and 63% rate of anorgasmia, suggesting an altogether reduction in quality of life [36].

Unlike men, substantially less research on sexual dysfunction has been performed in diabetic women. However, recent studies have shown that sexual dysfunction was experienced more commonly in diabetic women, including decreased sex drive, reduced or absent arousal, vaginal dryness, difficulty in achieving and overall decreased sexual pleasure [37]. Notwithstanding these observations, the correlation between diabetes and FSD is debatable. Because a 73.3% incidence of psychosexual problems were detected in a study of diabetic women with FSD, and no direct association between sexual disorders and diabetic complications could be found, the authors of the study concluded that in diabetic women, sexual dysfunction had a predominantly psychogenic origin [38].

A global interpretation of these data related to cardiovascular diseases may drive the medical community to view FSD as an early marker/risk factor for cardiovascular diseases and therefore a life-threatening condition. Hence, it is critical that FSD must be better investigated and understood to improve women's quality of life and simultaneously prevent more serious, even fatal future consequences.

Female Pelvic Anatomy

Understanding female sexual anatomy is essential to understand female sexual function. The relevant anatomy is not only confined to the external genitalia, but also to the internal organs, pelvic floor, and the broader anatomy of the neurovascular structures involved. Synergistic actions between these structures allow sexual arousal, orgasm, and vaginal penetration.

The appearance of normal female external genitalia shows great variation. With today's ease of access and the pervasiveness of pornography, a false conception of normal vulvar anatomy is increasing and has led to reduced female confidence and body image. This is illustrated by the exponential rise in woman undergoing cosmetic genital procedures; the number of women undergoing labiaplasty in the United States went from 2142 in 2011 to 12,756 in 2018 [39].

Variation does not only exist among individuals, but the appearance and function of the genital tract changes with age, hormonal status, childbirth, and following pelvic or vulvar surgery.

The Vagina

The vagina is a fibromuscular tube that extends from the opening between the labia minora, known as the vestibule, to the uterus. The vagina is lined with non-keratinized stratified epithelium, which becomes estrogenized following puberty. With sexual arousal, vasocongestion will occur and these cells will produce a vaginal exudate that is responsible for vaginal lubrication [40]. In hypoestrogenic states, such as menopause, atrophy of smooth muscle, a reduction of vaginal-area blood flow, and loss of tissue elasticity will result in vaginal dryness and dyspareunia [41].

The angle between the vagina and the uterus is more than 90° to the uterine axis and this angle will vary depending on the content of the bladder and rectum. The total vaginal length varies with a mean of 9.8 cm ±1.3 cm. Patients who have undergone a total hysterectomy have a slightly shortened vaginal length with a mean of 8.9 ± 1.5 cm [42]. Many authors have investigated the association between vaginal length and sexual function, with particular concern that vaginal shortening following pelvic reconstructive surgery may lead to dyspareunia. A recent systematic review highlighted the lack of clarity in the literature regarding this question and could not demonstrate a statistically significant association. This was likely due the complexity and multifactorial nature of sexual function and dyspareunia. It is however still ideal to aim to maintain the most vaginal length, without compromising risks and benefits to the patient undergoing pelvic reconstructive surgery [43].

Vaginal support can be divided into three levels [44]:

- Level I: Cervix and upper third of the vagina attaches to the pelvic walls by the cardinal and uterosacral ligaments.
- Level II: Middle third of the vagina attaches laterally to the fascial structures (arcus tendinous fascia pelvis).
- Level III: Distal vagina fuses with the surrounding structures, namely, the levator ani muscles and the perineal body.

Pelvic organ prolapse occurs by a combined failure of the pelvic floor muscle and connective tissue. Woman with Pelvic organ prolapse often present with complaints of sexual dysfunction and are more likely to restrict sexual activity, report decreased libido, decreased sexual excitement, and difficulty achieving orgasm during intercourse.

Woman with urogenital prolapse are often treated with surgery. The data reporting on sexual function following reconstructive surgery is limited and conflicting, with some showing improvement and others showing deterioration [45]. Possible explanations for postoperative sexual dysfunction include:

- Narrowing and/or deviation of the vagina
- Reduced lubrication
- De novo urinary incontinence

Distally the vagina opens through the sagittal introitus just below the external urethral meatus. The introitus is capable of distention, especially during childbirth and to a lesser extent during sexual intercourse.

Just within the vaginal orifice, the hymen can be found. The shape of the hymen varies, and it may be annular, semilunar, cribriform, fringed, absent, or complete and imperforate. There is no known function for the hymen, however it has cultural significance in some societies, because of the belief that if unruptured it serves as proof of virginity. The hymen usually ruptures following the first sexual intercourse but may also rupture during nonsexual physical activity. Once ruptured, circumferential skin elevations are referred to as hymeneal remnants.

The arterial supply of the vagina originates from the anterior trunks of the internal iliac arteries by two vaginal arteries. These arteries also supply the vestibular bulbs, base of the bladder, and the adjacent part of the rectum. Collateral blood supply may be received from the uterine, internal pudendal, and middle rectal arteries.

Venous drainage of the vagina occurs by means of lateral plexuses that drain into two vaginal veins. Communications with uterine, vesical, and rectal plexuses occur, all of which ultimately drain into the internal iliac veins.

Lymphatic drainage of the vagina can be divided in three groups. The lymphatic vessels of the upper vagina follow the uterine artery and drain to the internal and external iliac nodes, vessels for the middle vagina follow the vaginal arteries and drain to the internal iliac nodes, and vessels draining the vagina below the hymen pass to the superficial inguinal nodes.

The innervation of the vagina is derived from the sacral nerve roots S2, S3, and S4. The upper vagina receives parasympathetic supply from the pelvic splanchnic nerves that is responsible for transudation. The lower vagina receives somatic supply from the pudendal nerve, which is responsible for contraction.

The G-Spot

The G-spot is named after the German gynecologist Ernst Graffenberg, who published a report in 1950 that described an area along the course of the urethral neck on the anterior vaginal wall as a distinct erotogenic zone. Over the past few decades this structure has received widespread attention; however this concept remains controversial without strong anatomic proof and continued debate if it truly exists [46].

Histologic evidence of the G-spot is conflicting. Some studies reported that the distal anterior vagina had a higher density of small nerve fibers [47, 48] while other studies reported regular distribution of nerves throughout the entire vagina and no site consistently demonstrating the highest nerve density [46, 49].

Furthermore, evidence regarding the presence of a specific anatomical organ is inconsistent. A case series by Ostrzenski in 2014 describes the presence of a tangled vein-like structure found lateral to the urethra in eight cadavers [50]. This study received criticism on its limitations, and in response Hoag et al. published a detailed and systematic report of 13 cadavers in which the erectile or spongy tissue described by Ostrzenski was not identified in the anterior vaginal wall along the urethra [51].

The presence of the G-spot has been explored with various imaging studies. One study compared urethrovaginal thickness on ultrasound in women who reported a history of vaginal orgasm to those who have never attained vaginal orgasm. In this study the woman who had experienced vaginal orgasm had a thickened urethrovaginal thickness, which may provide evidence of a G-spot; however this increased thickness may also be a consequence of stronger orgasmic contractions [52].

One observational study using magnetic resonance imaging (MRI) provided evidence for an in vivo morphological correlate to postmortem anatomical findings of a g-spot complex described by Ostrzenski [53]; however a more recent prospective observational study using imaging and histologic examination in live tissues could not find any evidence of a g-spot complex [54].

Some argue that the G-spot is represented by the Skene glands and their ducts. During stimulation these para-urethral glands secrete various amounts of fluid, biochemically similar to prostatic fluid. This has been described by some as female ejaculation.

The Vulva

The female external genitalia or the vulva extends inferiorly from the pubic arch. The vulva consists of non-erectile and erectile structures:

Non-erectile structures:

- Mons pubis
- Labia majora
- Vestibule of the vagina
- Greater vestibular glands

Erectile structures:

- Labia minora
- Clitoris
- Clitoral bulbs

The Mons Pubis

The mons pubis is a triangular hair-bearing area of skin and adipose tissue overlying the pubic symphysis and adjacent pubic bone. The base of the triangle is formed by the pubic hairline and the apex is formed by the glans clitoris inferiorly. Following puberty and continuing into adult life, the mons becomes more prominent with coarse hair and undergoes slight atrophy following menopause.

The Labia Majora

The labia majora are two paired longitudinal cutaneous folds that overlie adipose tissue. Each fold has an external pigmented surface covered with hair and an internal smooth, pink surface with large sebaceous follicles. Together they form the lateral boundaries of the vulva and extend inferiorly from the mons pubis to merge as the posterior fourchette, which overlies the perineal body. The average length of the labia majora from the most superior aspect of the clitoral hood to the posterior fourchette ranges between 7 cm and 12 cm and the distance between the posterior vulva and the anus rangers from 1,5 cm to 5,5 cm [55].

Intermixed in the adipose tissue of the labia majora is loose connective tissue, smooth muscle (resembling the scrotal dartos muscle), vessels, nerves, and a rich supply of sebaceous, apocrine, and eccrine sweat glands. In addition, the endings of the uterine round ligaments and a patent processus vaginalis may also reach the labia.

The underlying fascia of the labia is similar to that of the anterior abdominal wall, with a superficial fatty layer resembling Camper's fascia, and a deep membranous layer, Colles' fascia, which is continuous with Scarpa's fascia. Interestingly, infections and hematomas of the labia majora cannot spread to the thighs, but may spread to the anterior abdominal wall, this is due to Colles' fascia that lacks anterior attachments but has attachments inferiorly to the ischiopubic rami and posteriorly to the urogenital diaphragm.

Labia Minora

The labia minora are skin folds found adjacent to the vestibule, immediately medial to the labia majora. Theses pigmented, hairless skin folds lack adipose tissue, but contain a rich supply of nerve endings and sensory receptors. The anterior portions of each labium minus divide into superior and inferior folds. The superior folds unite in the midline over the glans of the clitoris to form the prepuce or clitoral hood and the inferior folds insert below the clitoris to form its frenulum. The posterior portion of each labium minus merge with the labia majora at the posterior fourchette. The labia minora is derived from the ectoderm and consists of keratinized epithelium while the vestibule and vagina are derived from the endoderm and consists of non-keratinized epithelium; this transition is demarcated by Hart's line.

The variation between dimensions of the labia minora is extremely large, with the average length measured from the frenulum of the clitoris to the posterior fourchette, ranging from 2 cm to 10 cm and the average width, extending from the hymen, ranging from 0,7 cm to 5 cm [55]. In some African populations the labia minora have been stretched up to 20 cm. The labia minora is often asymmetrical and sometimes a duplicated labial fold (labium tertium) may be present. Adhesions between the labia minora can also be seen in prepubertal girls and these may predispose them to urinary tract infections.

The dermis of the labia minora consists of thick connective tissue with elastic fibers and small blood vessels that form an erectile tissue similar to the penile corpus spongiosum. The labia minora are richly innervated over their entire surface, providing very sensitive sensory perception [56]. The labia minora may also contribute to sensory stimulation indirectly when traction or manipulation of the labia minora stimulates the clitoris due to their termination at the clitoral hood. It is therefore important to note that when labiaplasty is performed there is a risk to remove tissue that not only has many nerve endings contributing to sexual arousal, but that may result in further diminished sexual arousal due to the altered traction movement the labia minora has on the clitoris.

The Vestibule

The vestibule of the vagina contains the vaginal orifice, external urethral meatus, vestibular bulbs, openings of the two Bartholin's glands, and numerous, mucus, lesser vestibular glands. The vestibule is bordered laterally by the area between Hart's line and the hymen, anteriorly by the frenulum of the clitoris, and posteriorly by the posterior fourchette. The female corpus spongiosum or pars intermedia is found at the area between the frenulum of the clitoris and the external urethral meatus where the clitoral bulbs join anteriorly. The external urethral meatus is superior to the vaginal opening with the fossa navicularis below, found at the area between the hymen and the posterior fourchette. Two Skene glands that lie paraurethral at the posterior-lateral aspect of the urethral meatus line the urethra longitudinally to provide lubrication.

The Bartholin glands resemble the male bulbourethral glands. They flank the vaginal orifice and open into the posterior-lateral aspect of the vestibule at 5 and 7 o'clock. They are in contact and often overlapped by the posterior end of the vestibular bulb. The glands consist of tubule-acinar tissue, with secretory cells that secrete a clear or whitish mucus for lubrication during sexual arousal.

Some patients with dyspareunia may describe localized pain to the vestibule (vestibulodynia/vulvodynia), which may be provoked or unprovoked. However poorly understood and likely multifactorial, these patients have been shown to have a higher density of nerve endings in the vestibule, which could be contributory [57]. Some of these patients also have coexisting symptoms of painful bladder and urethral syndromes, which could be explained by the shared embryology of these tissue linings [58].

The Clitoris

The clitoris is widely accepted as the primary anatomical source of female sexual pleasure. The clitoris has external and internal components that are rooted in the labia minora, fat, and vasculature inferior to the pubic arch and symphysis. The clitoris can further be divided in to six components, namely:

- Glans
- Suspensory ligament
- Body (corpora)
- Root
- Paired crura
- Vestibular bulbs

The clitoris shares an intimate physiological and anatomical relationship with the urethra and distal vagina. Not only do these structures share innervation and vasculature, but due to their proximity they move in unity during sexual intercourse.

The External Clitoris

The external clitoris consists of the glans, prepuce, and frenulum. It is found at the superior portion of the vestibule and is covered by the anterior portions of the labia minora forming the prepuce and the frenulum. The average length varies from 1 cm to 2 cm and its diameter varies from 0,5 cm to 1 cm.

Superficial to the erectile tissue of the corpora cavernosa of the clitoral body the glans has a fibrovascular cap. This cap consists of specialized genital vascular tissue, which is the smallest segment of erectile tissue compared to other structures. The skin is thin, hairless, and directly overlies the dense vascular dermis. The glans receives somatic innervation for the dorsal nerve of the clitoris, a branch of the pudendal nerve. The nerve runs on the dorsum of the clitoral body at 11 and 1 'o'clock to end in abundant corpuscular receptors in the subepithelial tissues. The glans has the highest density of small nerves compared to any of the other clitoral components.

The Internal Clitoris

The body of the clitoris extends cephalad from the glans of the clitoris, it then folds back on itself and bifurcates at the pubic symphysis into the two crura. The crura attach to the ischiopubic rami laterally, laying over the urethra and lateral to the vaginal walls. The body and its crura contain the most erectile tissue, but has less innervation compared to other parts of the clitoris. The body of the clitoris is extremely vascular with sinus and smooth muscle trabeculae. It is surrounded by the tunica albuginea, a dense connective tissue sheath. The tunica albuginea has an incomplete midline septum that divides the body into two corpora. Branches of the dorsal nerves and vessels of the clitoris run over the outer surface of the body, while the deep clitoral arteries run within the erectile core of each corpora. The crura differs from the body as it is not completely surrounded by the tunica and lacks the surrounding and internal neurovascular structures described above.

The suspensory ligament of the clitoris is a thick fibrofatty, fan-shaped structure that arises from the fascia of the mons pubis to converge on the body of the clitoris and extending down into the medial labia majora. The ligament supports and restricts the body of the clitoris in such a way that the clitoris can rise upward on arousal but cannot accomplish pendular motion or straighten.

All the erectile tissues of the clitoris merge just beneath the skin of the vestibule in the root of the clitoris. The root is highly sensitive to direct stimulation.

The vestibular bulbs are two paired structures that lay beneath the labia majora. The two triangular structures are inferior to the body of the clitoris and between the urethra and crura. With sexual arousal the bulbs engorge, which provides stability to the vaginal walls and may possibly push the clitoral tissue toward the vaginal lumen aiding in perception of sensation and stimulation.

Innervation

The perineum receives its motor and sensory supply primarily from the pudendal nerve. The pudendal nerve stems from the ventral rami of the second, third, and fourth nerve roots, and runs deep to the piriformis muscle to enter the gluteal region through the greater sciatic foramen. It passes dorsal to the sacrospinous ligament, close to its attachment to the ischial spine to reenter the pelvis through the lesser sciatic foramen. The nerve enters the perineum through the pudendal canal on the lateral wall of the ischioanal fossa in the obturator fascia ventral to the sacrotuberous ligament. In the posterior part of the canal the nerve divides into three branches:

- Inferior rectal nerve
  - Sensory: Perianal skin
  - Motor: External anal sphincter
- Perineal nerve
  - Sensory: Medial labia majora, labia minora, and vestibule

- Motor: External urethral sphincter, bulbocavernosus, ischiocavernosus, and superficial transverse perineal muscles
- Dorsal nerve of the clitoris
  - Sensory: The clitoris

The vulva and perineum receive additional supply from the:

- Cutaneious branch of the ilioinguinal nerve
- Genital branch of the genitofemoral nerve
- Perinineal branch of the posterior femoral cutaneous nerve

Vascular Supply

The internal pudendal artery, a branch of the internal iliac artery is the main supply the perineum. The internal pudendal artery and vein follow the same course as the pudendal nerve. The internal pudendal artery's branches are:

- Inferior rectal artery, which supplies the anal canal
- Perineal artery, which supplies the superficial perineal muscles
- Posterior labial artery
- Artery to the bulb of the vestibule
- Dorsal and deep arteries of the clitoris
- Urethral artery

The vulva receives additional supply for the superficial and deep pudendal arteries that branch from the femoral artery. These supply the labia majora and form anastomoses with branches of the internal pudendal artery.

The Female Sexual Response Cycle

The female sexual response is complex, and models thereof have taken many forms over the years; in order to understand the response, the fundamental components of desire, arousal, and orgasm need to be reviewed.

In 1966, Masters and Johnson pioneered research on the sexual response [3]. They described four successive physiologic states the excitement, plateau, orgasmic, and resolution phases. This conceptualization only addressed the physical aspect of the sexual response cycle and failed to address the phase that initiated sexual activity, which led to Kaplan's interconnected three-phase model introducing sexual desire (Fig. 1) [49].

Ten years after the initial publication by Masters and Johnson, Robinson argued that the plateau phase was actually the final stage of the excitation phase. This led to a revised model, referred to as the modified linear model. In this model the sexual response commences with spontaneous sexual desire, followed by arousal, which

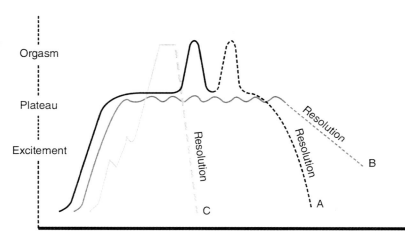

Fig. 1 Female sexual response cycle developed by Masters and Johnson [3]

may lead to orgasm and resolution, suggesting that female sexual response cycle proceeds one stage after the other in a direct linear fashion, mirroring the male sexual response cycle [59].

However, these linear models cannot consistently be applied to every patient's sexual response. For many patients these phases vary in sequence, overlap, repeat, or may be absent during some or all sexual encounters. Furthermore, subjective satisfaction with a sexual experience may not require achieving all response phases, including orgasm.

In response to these concerns, Basson conceptualized the human sexual response as a motivation/incentive-based cycle comprising of phases of physiologic response and subjective experience. In contrast Basson argued that the motivation for sexual activities was complex, and that the reasons to initiate sexual activity comprised of more than simply sexual desire. With the onset of sexual activity, a woman may become aroused, which could lead to a desire to continue the sexual activity, which in turn can then feedback to further increase arousal levels. Hence this pathway may be described as circular (Fig. 2) [59].

Desire

The former understanding of sexual desire or drive, based on the work of Masters, Johnson and Kaplan was considered to be the initiator of any sexual response. This was likened to the same physiologic urge to eat, sleep, or breathe. Desire has been linked to the hypothalamus and dopamine system. Increased activity of the dopamine system has been seen early in the sexual response and is believed to propagate to and activate other areas of the brain, including the limbic system [49].

As illustrated in Basson's circular model, desire does not always precede arousal, and may even be absent at the onset of sexual activity, only to be triggered during the actual sexual encounter. A study conducted in the United States with 3262 participants of multiple ethnicities found that 40% of these women reported infrequent or no sexual desire. However, most participants reported moderate to extreme satisfaction (86,3%) and moderate to extreme physical pleasure (89,6%) in their relationships. This provides evidence that sexual desire is not essential to the sexual response [60].

Arousal

Although not completely understood, it is generally accepted that sexual arousal in women consists of two components, genital arousal and subjective arousal. Genital arousal relates to the physiological genital changes in response to sexual stimuli. These changes include genital vasocongestion, clitoral engorgement, and vaginal lubrication. There are extragenital physiological changes associated with genital arousal and these include an increase in heart rate and blood pressure, hardening and erection of the nipples,

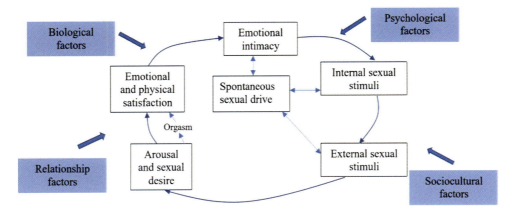

Fig. 2 Pathways of female sexual response [59]

sweating, skin flushing, and pupil dilatation. Subjective sexual arousal is the woman's experience of arousal also referred to as "cognitive sexual arousal," "mental sexual arousal," and feeling "turned on." It can be described as positive mental engagement and focus in response to sexual stimuli [61].

Sexual stimuli include erotic talking, sexual memories, and visual and physical stimulation. Physical stimulation may be nongenital as well as genital and non-penetrative as well as penetrative modalities.

Following sexual stimulation, the first observable sign of genital arousal is vaginal lubrication. Lubricating secretions are derived from a transudate that is formed by genital vasocongestion, and subsequent increased capillary pressure that forces fluid to the surface of the vaginal epithelium. Following the onset of vaginal lubrication, an increase in vasocongestion to the internal and external genitalia occurs. This leads to engorgement and swelling of the tissue of the vestibule and the venous plexus that surrounds the lower portion of the vagina. As the blood pools in these areas, the vaginal walls become dark purple. Muscle relaxation occurs allowing lengthening and dilatation of the vagina, protrusion of the clitoris, and engorgement of the vestibular bulbs. The clitoris retracts under the clitoral hood, and uterine elevation occurs, probably caused by the contraction of the parametrial muscle fibers that surround the vagina and uterus [61].

Subjective arousal is a report about an experience of sexual arousal. There is evidence suggesting that the anterior insular cortex provides the basis for all subjective feelings, contributing to emotional awareness and affecting subjective arousal downstream. For subjective arousal to occur a woman needs to be aware of erotic cues and have a positive appraisal of those cues. Following a sexual stimulus, the genital response is largely autonomic; however the subjective response depends on the level of attention given to the erotic stimulus and to other arousing cues, like her partner's excitement or her own genital sensations. The woman's appraisal of the sexual stimulus gives it emotional meaning and will influence both physiological and behavioral responses to the event. It is this appraisal of a sexual cue that will ultimately determine if subjective arousal will occur. Several psychological variables can distract women from erotic cues leading to an impaired ability to mentally engage in sexual activity, positively appraise a sexual stimulus, and experience subjective arousal. These include variables specific to the relationship and/or partner, beliefs and attitudes about sexuality, and a history of sexual abuse and/or negative sexual experiences [61].

The relationship between genital and subjective arousal might not always be concurrent. That is, mental appreciation for the sexual stimulus, as well the experience of nonsexual rewards, can occur with and without objective genital changes and/or an awareness of those changes. Moreover, the degree of connectivity between genital and subjective arousal seems to be unrelated to sexual arousal function and dysfunction in women. A meta-analysis looking at the agreement of self-reported and genital measures of sexual arousal in men and woman found that the correlation between genital and subjective arousal was highly variable in sexually healthy women [62]. This disconnection raises the question of what exactly sexual arousal in women is and whether physiological changes that occur in the absence of a subjective sexual experience should even be considered a sexual response.

A great degree of overlap between desire and arousal exists, and for many women and men, it is difficult to distinguish between desire and subjective arousal, reporting that sexual stimuli trigger both desire and subjective arousal simultaneously (Fig. 3) [63].

Orgasm

Masters and Johnson first described orgasm as "the few seconds during which the vasoconcentration and myotonia developed from sexual stimulation are released." However, this definition fails to express the multiple indicators that represent the objective and subjective complexities of an orgasm. A more contemporary working definition for the female orgasm has

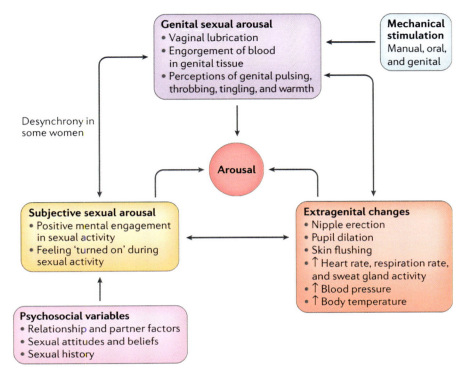

Fig. 3 Pathways of female sexual arousal and dysfunction [63]

been provided by Metson et al.: "an orgasm in the human female is a variable, transient peak sensation of intense pleasure creating an altered state of consciousness usually accompanied by involuntary rhythmic contractions of the pelvic striated circumvaginal musculature, often with concomitant uterine and anal contractions and myotonia that resolves the sexually induced vasocongestion (sometimes only partially), usually with an induction of well-being and contentment" [64].

Orgasms can arise from a wide range of even nongenital stimulations. For most heterosexual and same-sex couples, orgasms are induced by frictional, pressure, or vibrational stimulation of genital structures. These structures include the labia minora, clitoris, vagina, urethra, and in some the cervix. However, orgasms may occur completely independent of genital stimulation or coitus and have been seen to occur with skin, mouth, breast, nipple, and anal stimulation, with exercise, during epileptic attacks, and by drugs [65].

The spectrum of pleasure experienced ranges widely with some describing it as "just nice" to others experiencing an explosive condition that can even cause transient loss of consciousness. In contrast to men, woman can experience multiple orgasms. One study recorded the objective duration of an orgasm as 19.9 ± 12 s and subjective duration as 12.2 ± 9.8 s; in this study the objective duration did not correlate with subjective pleasure grading [66].

Pulsatile contraction for the pelvic floor muscles and rectum occur at and during orgasms and are associated with each wave of pleasure. These contractions are often accompanied with vocalizations, and a characteristic orgasmic face (open mouth, shut eyes, grimace). Uterine contractions also occur but some studies have shown these to already be present with arousal. Many have tried to explain the function(s) for these contractions; however all explanations have received criticism, these include:

- Ejecting paraurethral glandular secretions from the urethra; however this is not a feature seen in all women
- Emptying the vasocongested genital tissues, which is unlikely achieved in a single orgasm
- Ending sexual arousal; however women are serially multi-orgasmic
- Stimulating male arousal to induce ejaculation and capturing semen
- Creating pleasurable feelings; however voluntary contraction does not accomplish this

The neurochemical brain mechanisms of orgasm are extremely complex and beyond the scope of this chapter. However, a simplistic and useful working aid is that dopaminergic and adrenergic transmission is prosexual and orgasm-promoting while serotonergic is inhibitory of arousal and orgasm [65].

A notable gap in the frequency of orgasm during sex exists between heterosexual men and women. In fact, a recent study found that 75% heterosexual men always experienced an orgasm vs. only 33% of heterosexual woman when sexually intimate. Interestingly in the same study men reported that 41% of their heterosexual partners always experienced orgasm. This difference brings to light the occurrence of "faking" orgasms, which women will do for a variety of reasons including out of love for their partner, to protect their partner's self-esteem, intoxication, and to bring the sexual encounter to an end. Women in this study who experienced more frequent orgasms reported receiving more oral sex, having sex for longer durations, and being more satisfied with their relationships.

A rewarding experience and outcome, emotionally and physically, will enhance present and subsequent sexual motivation. Sexual satisfaction has received less study than sexual function/dysfunction but would appear to be a more relevant entity. There can be satisfaction despite dysfunction. Woman's satisfaction may or may not include orgasm(s) but usually requires freedom from pain and freedom from partner dysfunction, and a positive emotional conclusion.

Physiology and Biochemistry of Female Sexual Response Cycle

There are various factors that play a role in the physiology and biochemistry of female sexual arousal (FSA). It is impossible to explain female sexual function in terms of an uncomplicated physiological process [67]. The initial challenge arises when defining normal sexual function as previously discussed.

Mechanisms of Sexual Arousal

When broken down into a purely physical process, FSA comprises of neurological and physiological components. The autonomic nervous system, genital vasculature, and hormonal function must be optimal for FSA to occur. Studies of isolated tissues in organ baths have been done in order to determine the mechanisms of neurotransmitters and vasoactive substances. An integrated approach by means of studying signaling pathways in cells, and subsequent in vivo studies to confirm these processes has been used by various researchers [68].

On a peripheral level FSA is characterized by increased genital (vaginal and clitoral) blood flow. This in turn results in clitoral swelling and vaginal lubrication. Vaginal lubrication is thought to be a transudate from the vaginal vasculature. Vaginal length and diameter increase, and the vaginal wall becomes engorged, as do the labia and the cavernosal bodies in the clitoris.

Various in-depth animal studies in rats and rabbits were used to understand the impact of estrogen, estradiol, and androgens in sexual arousal. Trial subjects underwent bilateral oophorectomy Doppler flowmetry or laser oximetry was used to assess changes in genital blood flow. Peripheral hormone levels were also checked. Estrogen, estradiol, or testosterone were then supplemented (either individually or in combination) to determine their effect on the genital blood flow and lubrication status. It was found that estrogen and estradiol replacement improved genital blood flow to normal levels, whereas testosterone did not have the same effect.

The importance of nitric oxide (NO) in maintaining a healthy vaginal mucosa had also been well established. The lack of NO leads to decreased vaginal blood flow, and subsequent vaginal mucosal cell apoptosis. It is widely accepted that estrogen regulates vaginal NO synthase. This enzyme maintains normal levels of NO in vaginal tissue, and along with other factors, assists in preventing vaginal mucosal fibrosis. In the animal models used by Traish et al. among others, it has been noted that estrogen or estradiol supplementation reduces the activity of nitric oxide synthase (NOS), resulting in decreased levels of vaginal NO [68]. Supplementation with progesterone and testosterone, however, increased the activity of NOS.

The use of sildenafil in study animals who were both intact and having undergone bilateral oophorectomy was found to increase genital blood flow and lubrication [69]. The effect of sildenafil was significantly more pronounced in animals receiving estradiol. It can therefore be deduced that the NO-cGMP pathway has a role to play in FSA. Clinically, however, the use of sildenafil to treat FSD has had mixed outcomes and will be discussed in more detail later in this chapter.

Local neurotransmitters and regulatory nerve fibers are also important for FSA to occur. Hoyle et al., 1996 found that human vaginal tissue has nerve fibers containing NPY, VIP, NOS, CGRP, and substance P [70]. These may be involved in vaginal and clitoral engorgement, as well as vaginal lubrication. VIP has been found to cause vaginal wall relaxation, and its exact role is yet to be determined. The alpha-2 adrenergic system also plays a role in FSA. Preliminary organ bath studies on strips of vaginal and clitoral tissue showed contraction of these tissues, while alpha 1 and alpha 2 antagonists inhibited contractions to exogenous norepinephrine [68]. Further studies in these areas may provide more insight into the neurophysiological aspect of FSA, allowing improved understanding and therefore improved management of FSD.

Etiology and Pathophysiology of Female Sexual Dysfunction

The traditional dissociation of psychogenic and organic etiologies both in male and female sexual dysfunction is artificial, as both etiologic categories are intertwined. Psychologic pathologies can interfere with hormonal and neurologic physiologic mechanisms, as organic changes can induce psychologic alterations that interfere and exacerbate the preexistent dysfunction. However, for didactic purposes, etiologies will be categorized into primarily psychogenic and primarily organic or physical.

Psychological: The psychological causes of sexual dysfunction in women may include ***depression, anxiety,*** **and other** ***mood disorders*** that are correlated with low desire, arousal, and/or orgasm problems, and may cause a lack of interest in activities women enjoyed before, including sex. Low self-esteem, fear of being vulnerable or rejected, and feelings of hopelessness can also contribute to sexual dysfunction. Stress at home or work can significantly impact on sexual pleasure and satisfaction and may lower sex drive. ***Past physical trauma*** **or** ***sexual abuse*** **or any other negative experiences** may lead to low self-esteem, shame or guilt, increased anxiety, and a fear of intimacy, causing inhibition in expressing sexual feelings, which compromises sexual function. *Relationship issues* with the partner, such as unhappiness, boredom, or other strains may lead to sexual dysfunction. *Concerns about a negative consequence*, such as undesired pregnancy, sexually transmitted diseases, and partner's sexual dysfunction can also trigger a negative sexual response. *Specific circumstances*, such as intrapersonal factors leading to low sexual self-image due to infertility, premature menopause, and previous mastectomy or hysterectomy; relationship factors involving lack of trust, and decreased attraction toward a sex partner; sexual factors, for example, insufficiently erotic, private, and/or safe ambience; and cultural factors, especially restrictions on sexual activity imposed by a specific culture. Finally, *several distractions* associated with family, profession, financial constraints, or legal issues can also interfere with motivation, desire, and arousal.

Organic/Physical: Organic or physical causes may include vasculogenic, neurogenic, hormonal/endocrine, musculogenic, and genital lesions.

Vasculogenic. Cardiovascular risk factors, such as hypertension, diabetes mellitus, hyperlipidemia, and smoking are associated with vasculogenic erectile dysfunction in men. Although most studies have historically focused on men, atherosclerosis involving the aortoiliac and pelvic vasculature predisposes men and women to vascular insufficiency resulting in reduced hypogastric/pudendal arterial bed in women, causing clitoral and vaginal vascular insufficiency syndrome [71]. Decreased pelvic blood flow leads to vaginal wall and clitoral smooth muscle fibrosis [72]. Atherosclerosis of clitoral cavernosal arteries was shown to induce loss of corporal smooth muscle and replacement by fibrous connective tissue in human clitoris [72, 73]. Additional causes, such as pelvic irradiation, blunt trauma, and pelvic fractures can decrease vaginal and clitoral blood supply, thereby contributing to sexual dysfunction. It has also been postulated that chronic perineal pressure from bicycle riding can result in decreased vaginal and clitoral blood flow sexual dysfunction [7].

Causes of Vasculogenic FSD
- Atherosclerosis
- Vaginal Vascular Insufficiency Syndrome
- Pelvic injury to the iliohypogastric/pudendal vascular bed
- Pelvic fracture
- Blunt trauma
- Iatrogenic (Surgical injury)
- Chronic perineal pressure
- Cycling

Neurogenic. Neurologic disorders account for important causes of sexual dysfunction in both men and women. They include spinal cord injury (SCI) or diseases of the central or peripheral nervous system. The sacral reflex arc and upper motor neurons must be intact for a woman to experience orgasm and perceive sexual desire and arousal. The impact of SCI is precisely dependent upon the level and degree of the injury [74]. Complete upper motor neuron lesions affecting the sacral segments will produce a negative impact on psychogenic lubrication, whereas incomplete upper motor neuron lesions usually are associated with preservation of both psychogenic and reflex vaginal lubrication [73, 75]. Women with SCI have significantly more difficulty in achieving orgasm than normal controls [74]. More research will lead to better understanding of the neurophysiology of arousal and orgasm in SCI patients as well as in normal women.

Hormonal/endocrine. Estrogens, specifically estradiol, are critical in female sexual function. Estradiol is the main sex hormone in the female sexual physiology, which helps to maintain the integrity and stability of vaginal mucosal epithelium and is responsible for vaginal lubrication. Estradiol is a major player in the regulation of sexual physiology and nitric oxide production in the vagina and clitoris, including vasoprotective and vasodilator effects on the vaginal tissue. Estradiol improves vaginal sensation, vasocongestion, and secretions, enhancing arousal. Vaginal lubrication and sexual desire and frequency decrease after menopause, eventually contributing to vaginismus [76]. Estradiol deprivation leads to significant decrease in clitoral intracavernosal blood flow as well as vaginal and urethral blood flow [76, 77]. Important histological changes occur, such as diffuse clitoral fibrosis, thinned vaginal epithelium, diminished vaginal submucosal blood supply, ultimately impacting sexual function. Estrogen replacement therapy has shown improvement in vaginal lubrication and sexual desire in postmenopausal women [78].

Testosterone is the chief androgen in women, being produced predominantly by the adrenal glands and ovaries. Although circulating androstenedione is also an important androgen, testosterone, and its metabolite dihydrotestosterone, constitutes the most potent endogenous androgen in men and women. It is also the chief precursor of estrogens. Testosterone levels tend to fall with age. By the mid-40 s, circulating testosterone levels drop to roughly half of the levels of women in their 20 s. Nonetheless, no dramatic decrease is observed at the time of spontaneous menopause. A considerable decline, however, occurs after bilateral oophorectomy [79]. Low levels of testosterone correlate to reduced sexual desire, arousal, genital sensation, and orgasm. Testosterone influences sexual behavior through its direct action on the central nervous system. It has been demonstrated that testosterone might stimulate nitric oxide synthase activity, thereby promoting vascular smooth muscle relaxation [80]. Testosterone can also enhance libido in postmenopausal women due to oophorectomy. Unfortunately, androgen replacement therapy usually causes hirsutism, acne, and virilization.

Musculogenic. It is known that the pelvic floor muscles are actively involved in both male and female sexual function and response to sexual cycle. The levator ani and perineal membrane are the predominant muscles that participate in this function, especially, female genital arousal and orgasm. The bulbocavernosus and ischiocavernosus muscles form the perineal membrane, which contributes to and enhances sexual arousal and orgasm when it contracts voluntarily [78]. Additionally, these muscles are responsible for the rhythmic contractions during orgasm. The levator ani muscles also function as modulators of the motor responses during orgasm and vaginal receptiveness. Hypotonicity of the pelvic musculature may impact negatively on the sexual function cycle, causing vaginal numbness, coital anorgasmia, or urinary incontinence during intercourse or climaturia. Hypertonicity of the pelvic floor muscles can be a significant component of sexual pain disorders in both men and women. Moreover, pelvic pain disorders and pelvic organ prolapse are known to be correlated with sexual dysfunction [81].

Female Sexual Dysfunction in Specific Settings

Four specific scenarios will be discussed in greater detail as they constitute very common circumstances in the routine quality of life of women.

FSD in the Post-Partum Period

There is limited scientifically reliable literature on the deleterious impact of childbirth on sexual function. Nonetheless, lay press has published on women's concerns regarding the potential detrimental consequences of vaginal childbirth on their sexual function. These concerns fostered the concept of elective Caesarean section (C/S) to protect sexual function. A great number of healthcare providers recommend this option with up to 24% of obstetricians and 4.4% of midwives favoring elective C/S for themselves and their spouses [1, 82–85]. Curiously, urogynecologists showed even higher scores averaging 46% in favor of primary elective C/S [85].

The incidence of postpartum sexual dysfunction has been reported to range from 22% to 86% [86]. Surprisingly, only a few large, prospective articles have been published in the literature. Symptoms such as dyspareunia, loss of desire or reduced interest in sexual activity are highly prevalent in postpartum women, problems that can be compounded even further by emotional distress and increased family burden difficulties. The overall incidence of these problems ranges from 57% to 75% [87, 88]. A study by Glazener showed that 53% of women reported problems with sexual activity in the first 8 weeks after childbirth [89]. The author called attention to the importance of health education linked to sexual dysfunction in the antenatal period. Another study by Johanson et al. showed a higher rate of dyspareunia after assisted vaginal delivery (forceps or vacuum) compared to spontaneous vaginal delivery or C/S [90]. It is generally agreed within the literature that assisted vaginal delivery is associated with a higher risk of sexual dysfunction in the postpartum period. Yet, the literature on sexual dysfunction following C/S is notably deficient. The weaknesses detected in these studies are their retrospective nature, lack of a validated questionnaire, and no assessment of the various sexual function domains. However, in a recent and large study using a validated questionnaire, Buhling et al. reported persistence of dyspareunia for longer than 6 months in 3.4% of women after spontaneous, nontraumatic deliveries, and C/S, in 10% of women after episiotomy/leisure, and in 14% after surgical vaginal delivery [91]. Signorello et al. also reported that perineal trauma and traumatic or surgical vaginal delivery are associated with increased incidence and degree of dyspareunia [92].

Sexual interest usually recovers after childbirth; however, up to 57% of women still complain of diminished sexual interest at 3 months, and up to 37% at 6 months [93, 94].

Up to 57% of women complain of lubrication problems up to 6 months postpartum [93]. Prolong breast-feeding can result in vaginal atrophy due to hypoestrogenism, and this translates into deficient vaginal lubrication with subsequent dryness and dyspareunia. Deficient lubrication can be easily corrected with topical estrogens or nonhormonal lubricants.

Pregnancy may decrease the ability to achieve orgasm, with approximately 60% of pregnant women achieving orgasm through the second trimester [88]. However, the ability to achieve orgasm as well as other components of sexual function improves postpartum.

Physicians should include these high rates of persistent dyspareunia after surgical vaginal delivery in the antenatal counseling and informed consent discussion with patients. More research using standardized, validated sexual function questionnaires should be carried out to clarify and draw a scientifically sound conclusion on the relationship between the several components of sexual dysfunction and the different modes of delivery.

FSD and Pelvic Organ Prolapse and/or Urinary Incontinence

Pelvic organ prolapse and urinary incontinence are known to impact adversely female sexual function. Up to 45% of women with urinary incontinence avoid sexual intercourse for fear of urine leakage during intercourse. In a study involving 2153 women, Moran et al. noticed an overall 11% incidence of urinary incontinence during intercourse, with 69% reporting coital leakage on penetration, 20% on orgasm, and 11% had leakage on both penetration and orgasm [95]. The pathophysiology of this association in not clear but seems to be associated with the same factors causing stress urinary incontinence in the general population. Salonia et al. reported that 47% of women with incontinence had low sexual desire, and 46% of those with orgasmic difficulties had urge incontinence [19]. Yip et al. also reported that women with any type of urinary incontinence (stress or urge) noticed less sexual pleasure [96]. Other authors stressed the higher negative effect of a hyperactive bladder and younger age (< 60 years) on sexual activity compared to stress or mixed incontinence [97]. However, a worse result noticed by younger women might be biased as sexual activity declines with age.

The literature addressing the association between pelvic organ prolapse and sexual dysfunction is scanty and controversial. Handa et al. noticed that 52% of women with POP reported sexual problems. However, the difference was not significantly different from women without POP [98]. In another study comparing women with POP and or without UI with women without UI, Weber et al found no significant difference between the two cohorts in terms of sexual function phases [99]. However, in a study Barber et al. concluded that POP has a more detrimental effect on sexual function than UI, in contradiction to previous reports. Again, other authors found that UI/POP induced less frequent and less satisfactory sexual activity.

FSD After Pelvic Surgeries

The pelvic autonomic nerves are vital for the normal function of pelvic organs. The hypogastric plexus at the sacral promontory level originates in the sympathetic nerves, whereas the sacral roots of S2–S4 originate in the parasympathetic fibers (pelvic nerves). These two nerve systems form the major autonomic nerve supply to the pelvic organs.

Anti-Stress Urinary Incontinence Surgery

Burch colposuspension (and variants) was regarded as the "standard" surgical treatment for correcting stress urinary incontinence (SUI) prior to the advent of minimally invasive synthetic suburethral slings. There is deficient data in the literature regarding the impact of colposuspension on sexual function. In a study evaluating 55 women with SUI who reported coital incontinence prior to colposuspension, Moran et al. found that 65% had coital leakage with penetration, 16% with orgasm, and 18% with both. Eighty-one percent of the women were cured of coital incontinence after surgery [95].

There is no consensus regarding the effect of mid-urethral vaginal slings, tension-free vaginal tape (TVT), on female sexual function. The literature is contradictory with some studies claiming a decrease of postoperative dyspareunia [100, 101], while others show the opposite [102, 103]. Nonetheless, there is apparently consensus that TVT decreases coital incontinence rates by three- to sixfold [101, 103].

Regarding the transobturator mid-urethral slings, there seems to be a consensus that after surgery women report a decrease in coital incontinence and a significant improvement in sexual desire assessed by the FSFI validated questionnaire and a global positive impact on sexual function domains, including sexual satisfaction [104–106]. Women undergoing sling procedures for SUI should be informed that their sexual activity is likely to remain unchanged or even improve after the operation, but that dyspareunia may occur [106]. Interestingly, some authors noted not only improvement in sexual function in women after the transobturator mid-urethral sling placement, but also a significant improvement in the sexual activity of their partners [107]. The surgeon should be aware of the potential risk of injuring the dorsal nerve of the clitoris with the passage of the trocar [108].

Anterior Vaginal Repair

Globally, there has been a consensus that anterior vaginal wall repair is not only associated with an increase of postoperative dyspareunia and other sexual function aspects but may in fact improve previous sexual dysfunction in women [109]. Weber et al. compared three surgical procedures to treat cystocele and noted that the dyspareunia rate decreased from 30% before surgery to 22% after surgery [109]. In a retrospective analysis of 116 women undergoing anterior vaginal wall repair, Shen et al. reported that all types of transvaginal anterior wall surgery had a positive impact on the patients' health-related quality of life and female sexual function [110].

Posterior Vaginal Repair

Posterior colporrhaphy may be associated with dyspareunia with a significantly adverse effect on sexual activity. Levator ani surgical plication, also called levatorplasty, and an historical and practically abandoned method of rectocele repair, was commonly related to dyspareunia due to postoperative mid-vaginal narrowing [111]. In a study of 73 women, Komesu et al. compared the incidence of dyspareunia and overall improvement in sexual function using a validated questionnaire in 30 women who underwent posterior compartment repair to 30 who did not. There was a trend toward an increase in dyspareunia in the cohort that underwent posterior compartment repair and a decrease in the cohort that did not have posterior compartment surgery. However, an overall improvement in sexual function was noted in both cohorts [112]. Conversely, improvement of dyspareunia and its lower "de novo" incidence after surgery has also been reported with perineal body reconstruction and midline vaginal plication [113–115].

Apical Vaginal Prolapse

Dyspareunia and female sexual dysfunction may result from surgical repair of apical or vault vaginal prolapse. But because this repair frequently entails another simultaneous procedure, it is not easy to establish the true origin for the problem.

Transvaginal sacrospinous fixation procedure may result in dyspareunia through injury to the pudendal nerve, vaginal axis deviation, or vaginal narrowing. Holey et al. found that postoperative dyspareunia resulted most commonly from vaginal narrowing following excessive colpectomy during another simultaneous repair [116]. Several studies report rates of post-sacrospinous fixation dyspareunia to range from 8% to 16% [117–119]. Maher et al. compared sacrospinous fixation to iliococcygeal fixation, another method to suspend the vaginal vault in sexually active women [120]. They did not find any significant difference in the incidence of dyspareunia (10% vs. 14%) and buttock pain (14% vs. 19%). However, iliococcygeal fixation has been associated with vaginal shortening up to 3 cm and, therefore, bilateral iliococcygeal fixation should be discouraged in sexually active women with vaginal vault prolapse and short vaginal length due to potential severe dyspareunia following surgery. In a study of 33 women, Baessler and Schuessler noticed that preoperative dyspareunia disappeared in eight in nine patients who had abdominal sacrocolpopexy [121]. In contrast, Virtanen et al. observed that 44% of patients in their study developed dyspareunia 3 years following abdominal sacrocolpopexy [122]. Some studies comparing vaginal and abdominal approaches to vault prolapse repair showed inconsistent, even opposing, outcomes [120, 123].

Vaginal Repair Using Mesh

Use of mesh for stress urinary incontinence and vaginal prolapse repair has been highly controversial. Petros pioneered the intravaginal slingplasty using synthetic mesh in 2001 [124]. This was followed by numerous reports on the successful outcomes of the use of mesh, either synthetic or biological, in vaginal prolapse repairs, the main purpose being improved long-term results with low recurrence rates. However, there is a paucity of information related to the impact of mesh use on sexual health. Several studies including sexual function in their postoperative assessment reported favorable results [125]. In contrast, other studies reported a negative impact. Milani et al. noted an increase of dyspareunia anterior and posterior repairs of 20% and 0%, respectively [125–129].

Hysterectomy for Benign Conditions

The impact of hysterectomy on sexual function has been explored in numerous peer-reviewed research articles. Historically, the uterus was believed to have an important role in sexual activity, including orgasm, a sense of well-being and self-esteem, and femininity. These beliefs might interfere with female sexual function. A potential negative impact on sexual function, or even its loss, constitutes a major cause of anxiety for women planned for hysterectomy [130]. In fact, Bradford et al. showed that the physician has a critical role in mitigating this anxiety through education [131]. Nonetheless, despite the importance of this matter, the literature has not shown clarity and consistency, especially attributed to methodology discrepancies. Most reports suggest a favorable or unchanged sexual function outcome and quality of life, being predominantly influenced by the quality of partner relationship of preoperative dysmenorrhea [132].

In a nationwide Danish study, Lycke et al. showed that adjusted incidence rates of benign hysterectomy declined over time from 2000 to 2015 [133]. Nonetheless, simple hysterectomy for benign conditions remains the most frequently performed gynecologic operation globally, there have been limited prospective studies on postoperative sexual dysfunction. Most of the data derive from retrospective series, accounting for a major limitation. Most of these women are not evaluated for sexual function following hysterectomy. Dennerstein et al. reported a considerable decrease in their sex life after hysterectomy in 15–37% of the women in his historical series

[30, 134]. The reasons for this decrease in sexual activity included loss of desire, deficient vaginal lubrication, and preoperative dyspareunia and dysmenorrhea. In contrast, other studies reported improvement in sexual function following benign hysterectomy in 30–50% of patients [132, 135]. In a prospective study of sexual function after both abdominal and vaginal simple hysterectomy involving 1101 patients and using a validated questionnaire, Rhodes et al. noted that sexual function improved globally, including frequency of intercourse, strength of orgasm (but not frequency), desire, and vaginal lubrication [136]. Other studies have concluded that simple hysterectomy, whether performed abdominally, vaginally, or laparoscopically, has no adverse effect on sexual function in women [137, 138]. Several other studies assessing the effect of total hysterectomy on specific aspects of sexual function such as low desire, decreased arousal, and difficulty achieving orgasm, reported that most women either felt no change or felt improvement and benefits in sexual function [139, 140].

Kikku et al. compared total to subtotal abdominal hysterectomy and found that both methods significantly reduced dyspareunia after surgery, but with a significantly higher reduction in the subtotal group [141, 142]. However, recent randomized controlled trials did not support these conclusions [143, 144]. The previous belief that the cervix was essential to attain orgasm or that total hysterectomy induces damage to the local nerves causing sexual dysfunction is not corroborated by current literature.

In a randomized controlled trial assessing sexual pain and psychologic outcomes after laparoscopic-assisted vaginal total hysterectomy versus supracervical laparoscopic hysterectomy, Flory et al. noted that the parameters of sexual function improved, including pain. However, although psychosocial well-being after surgery was slightly affected, these adverse effects were not different from those noted by controls [145].

Finally, several studies have assessed hysterectomy as compared with minimally invasive or medical treatments. Kupperman et al. compared hysterectomy with estrogen and/or progesterone, and/or prostaglandin synthesis inhibitor to treat abnormal uterine bleeding and noted that hysterectomy was better than medical treatment in this regard with half the women randomized to medical treatment choosing to undergo hysterectomy [146]. Hehenkamp et al. compared sexual function and body image following hysterectomy or uterine arterial embolization in a randomized study with a validated questionnaire. Sexual function and body image improved in both groups, but significant increases were noted more often in the embolization group [147]. In summary, most studies generally report improvement of sexual function, quality of life, and body image after hysterectomy. Although a few studies suggested better outcomes following subtotal hysterectomy, this was not a solid conclusion. The literature also suggests that uterine arterial embolization could be a better therapeutic option, because of less pain and preservation of ovarian function. Nonetheless, currently available evidence is very limited to support any solid conclusions.

FSD After Treatment of Pelvic Malignancies

Quality-of-life issues have become important endpoints in patients undergoing pelvic cancer surgery, not only gynecologic, but also vesical and rectal malignancies. The introduction of the Papanicolaou smear evaluation as a cervical screening program has contributed to early detection of cervical cancer at a younger age, thereby making sexual function a potential major postoperative variable in gynecologic cancer surgery. Older studies of sexual function did not use standardized, validated questionnaires, study designs, and definitions, leading to a wide variation in outcome reports (Table 2).

Surgical treatment of cervical cancer can induce significant problems of vaginal lubrication, vaginal length, dyspareunia, and loss of libido. These complications can be further exacerbated by bilateral oophorectomy, especially after radical surgery. Postoperative sexual pain is mostly associated with vaginal dryness and short vaginal vault. Several studies have shown reduced sexual satisfaction, dyspareunia as the main source of symptomatic distress following

Table 2 Validated questionnaires used in the evaluation of FSD

Name of PRO	Number of questions	Domain names	Developed in accordance with FDA guidance	Primary goal of PRO
Female Sexual Function Index (FSFI)	19	Sexual desire, arousal, lubrication, orgasm, satisfaction, pain	No	Self-administered questionnaire assessing key dimensions of sexual function in women
Profile of Female Sexual Function (PFSF)	37	Desire, arousal, orgasm pleasure, sexual concerns, responsiveness and sexual self-image	Yes	Self-administered questionnaire measuring loss of sexual desire and related aspects of sexual function in oophorectomized women
Brief Version of the Profile of Female Sexual Function (B-PFSF)	7	No domains	Not relevant	Self-assessment tool for use by women who are experiencing low sexual desire to assist them in seeking help
Sexual Interest and Desire Inventory-Female (SIDI-F)	13	No domains	No	Clinician administered tool to quantify the severity of symptoms in women diagnosed with HSDD
Sexual Quality of Life Questionnaire (SQoL)	18		No	Self-administered questionnaire to assess the impact of FSD on a woman's sexual quality of life and to evaluate the benefits of therapeutic intervention
McCoy Female Sexuality Questionnaire (MFSQ)	19	No domains	No	Self-administered questionnaire to assess aspects of female sexual function in postmenopausal women
Female Sexual Distress Scale-Revised (FSDS-R)	13	No domains	No	Self-administered questionnaire that assess distress associated with female sexual dysfunction

multimodality treatments for cervical cancer. However, surgery alone was less commonly associated sexual dysfunction as compared to radiotherapy or brachytherapy as primary treatment or in combination with surgery [148–150]. Therefore, regardless of treatment protocol, sexual dysfunction is an important and prevalent concern associated with cervical cancer treatment, and it should be included in the informed consent before treatment.

Sexual dysfunction is also a prevalent and significant complication in women treated for ovarian cancer. Multimodality treatments include radical hysterectomy, or oophorectomy, and adjuvant chemotherapy. The reported incidence rates of sexual dysfunction are similar to those observed with cervical cancer treatment [151, 152]. The literature reports 50–57% of negative impact on sexual function, ranging from no or little desire (47%), vaginal dryness (80%), and dyspareunia (62%). Some women reported that their sexual inactivity was also related to lack of partner (44.1%), lack of interest (38.7%), other physical problems causing sex difficulties (23.4%), and fatigue (10.8%). Therefore, sexual rehabilitation should be discussed with both patients and partners. The literature on sexual dysfunction after treatment of endometrial and vulvar malignancies are negligible.

Radical cystectomy or anterior exenteration has been used as standard treatment for muscle-invasive bladder cancer [153]. Sexual dysfunction is also a major concern of many younger women treated with this radical surgical modality [154]. The neurovascular bundles on the lateral vaginal walls are often transected during radical cystectomy [155, 156]. Also, the clitoris usually suffers important devascularization during distal urethrectomy, impacting subsequent sexual arousal and desire [155–157]. The literature on the influence of the urinary diversion technique (orthotopic vs. heterotopic) on sexual function is scant and has not been consensual, with some authors reporting sexual dysfunction (loss of libido, vaginal dryness, and dyspareunia) after ileal conduit, and others not showing any significant difference between types of urinary diversion and sexual dysfunction [154, 158]. All these studies lacked a validated questionnaire and included only short series of women in each cohort, probably explaining the failure to demonstrate statistically significant differences between the types of urinary diversion.

Zippe et al. evaluated sexual function in 34 post-radical cystectomy females and found that the patients' most common complaints was difficulty or inability in achieving orgasm (45%), decreased vaginal lubrication (41%), diminished libido (37%), and sexual pain (22%), with 52% noting reduced satisfaction in overall sexual function parameters, and only 48% being able to maintain successful vaginal intercourse [158]. Therefore, it can be concluded that sexual dysfunction is a prevalent and important quality-of-life problem after radical cystectomy, affecting all domains of sexual activity.

The enormous impact of cystectomy on sexual function has given rise to modifications of the surgical technique in female anterior exenteration. Distal urethrectomy has been associated with important devascularization of the clitoris and compromised sexual arousal [155]. Importantly, urethral preservation did not carry an increased risk of local recurrence [155]. Later reports revealed that complete removal of the proximal two-thirds of the vagina implies the dissection of most autonomic nerves to the urethra and vagina. Yet, preserving the lateral vaginal walls keeps intact most of the plexus fibers to the urethra, which seems to preserve sexual function [159]. These observations and modifications of the surgical technique prompted surgeons to avoid sacrificing unnecessarily the proximal vaginal and urethral, enabling maximum preservation of vagina and urethra, thereby helping preserve sexual function [160].

Rectal cancer is also a predominant pelvic neoplasm in women. Sexual dysfunction is a common complication of rectal cancer surgery [161]. The reported incidence of sexual dysfunction following low anterior resection and abdominoperineal resection varies from 10% to 60% [162]. Similarly, this high impact on sexual function led colorectal surgeons to modify their operative technique, adopting a total mesorectal excision (TME) with preservation of the neurovascular bundle and subsequent reduction of sexual dysfunction rates [163]. In a study by Enker et al., 57% of women undergoing abdominoperineal resection and 85% of those undergoing sphincter-preserving procedures maintained their sexual function when these operations followed the principles of TME [164].

Minimally invasive mesorectal resection is gaining increased popularity [165, 166]. However, most of these studies showed comparable pathological results of minimally invasive procedures to those of open ones. Quah et al. noted that the impact of laparoscopic and open surgical approaches on sexual dysfunction was similar [163]. Rectal cancers are usually managed with multimodal treatment protocols, including neoadjuvant and adjuvant radiotherapy, which showed a significant adverse effect on sexual function [167]. Risk factors for sexual dysfunction, such as age older than 45 years, local tumor extension, abdominoperineal resection but predominantly radiotherapy, have been reported [167, 168].

Evidence shows that sexual dysfunction is a major problem after rectal cancer management and has been underreported in the literature, particularly in female patients. TME has shown some encouraging value in improving sexual function outcomes.

FSD with Aging

Sexual dysfunction is considered an age-related and progressive problem, affecting 30% to 50% of the general female population [4, 5]. The prevalence in postmenopausal women is even higher, ranging from 68% to 86.5%, depending on the study characteristics [169]. This increased prevalence is conditioned by several physiological and psychological factors that are linked with menopausal transition and aging, which have a negative effect on sexual function [170–172]. Hypoactive sexual desire disorder is the most common problem, which is estimated to occur in 40–50% of postmenopausal women vs. 15–25% of premenopausal women. Other sexual function parameters, such as sexual arousal, vaginal lubrication, orgasm, and dyspareunia are reported to be significantly higher in postmenopausal women, up to 25% vs. up to 45%, respectively [21, 170, 172]. Many women experience a change in their sexual activity in the years immediately before and after menopause, which are related to a decrease in estrogen and testosterone levels. Aging is usually associated with decreased blood flow to the genital organs. These changes may induce complaints such as low libido, diminished sexual arousal, orgasm problems, vaginal atrophy and dryness, and dyspareunia. Moreover, other dimensions may factor in the equation, such as general physical and mental health, quality of relationship, personal, social, and cultural issues, as well as the presence of a sexual partner. Therefore, the evaluation of the exact origin of FSD is a hard task due to its multifactorial nature.

Evaluation of Female Sexual Dysfunction

Ensuring that your patient feels comfortable and safe to discuss her sexuality with the physician is one of the most important aspects in terms of evaluating a patient with FSD. If the healthcare professional is embarrassed to discuss sexual function with the patient, the patient then also becomes wary of openly discussing these issues. It is also important not to assume the gender of the patient's partner, or that the patient is in a monogamous relationship. These generalizations may hinder the patient's ability to freely discuss her sexual dysfunction [173].

Due to the multifactorial nature of FSD, a comprehensive history is imperative. It is important to obtain a full medical and surgical history, as well as a gynecological history. All medication that the patient is on should be assessed as various drugs are known to have sexual side effects. As HSDD may be primary or secondary, temporality should be sought with regard to the onset of other sexual disorders such as dyspareunia, anorgasmia, or lubrication disorders relative to the onset of HSDD.

Questions that should form Part of a Sexual History [173]

- What is the patient's description of the problem?
- What is the duration of the problem and is the onset sudden or gradual?
- Is the problem specific to a situation/partner or is it generalized?
- Are there any precipitating events (biologic or situational)?
- Is there guilt, depression, or anger that is not being directly addressed?
- Is the patient experiencing pain?
- Which problems appear to be most significant: desire, arousal, or orgasm?
- Is there a history of physical, emotional, or sexual abuse?
- Does the partner have any sexual dysfunction?

Questionnaires regarding sexual function may be useful to assess the baseline characteristics of the FSD. A comparison may be made after initiation of a management plan to objectively assess for improvement in the patient's symptoms [173].

A thorough examination is necessary, including a general examination, a breast examination, and a gynecological examination. In the event of the main complaint being dyspareunia, a swab test should be carried out. This involves gentle pressure applied with a small swab or Q-tip to various areas in the vagina to elicit specific trigger points, especially vulvo-vestibulitis. A mono-manual vaginal examination may also be useful in determining any specific points causing pain. A bimanual examination may hinder the patient's ability to pinpoint the exact location of the pain.

Blood tests may be needed if a patient has HSDD with concurrent amenorrhea, oligomenorrhea, or galactorrhea. Prolactin levels, thyroid function tests, estradiol, progesterone, luteinizing hormone, testosterone, and sex hormone-binding globulin levels should be assessed. These may allude to the presence of a prolactinoma or thyroid disorder that is reversible.

The findings of the history, clinical examination, and questionnaire should be assimilated in order to fully evaluate a patient with FSD. Incongruous findings should be examined further to avoid missing key features of the pathology.

Treatment Options

The treatment of FSD is heavily dependent on an adequate workup of the patient. Underlying somatic causes should be managed and optimized accordingly. Any drugs that may be contributing to the FSD should be substituted if it is safe to do so. A good rapport with the patient will facilitate application of the biopsychosocial model of treatment. Management of dysmenorrhea, prolapse, and incontinence (urinary and/or fecal) must be initiated early. Cognitive behavioral therapy (CBT) can be a useful adjunct to managing FSD. Should the sexual dysfunction persist, there are various treatment options available depending on the type and cause of the FSD (Table 3) [174].

The options available include vaginal lubricant agents, vaginal estrogen replacement, or intravaginal dehydroepiandrosterone. Physical therapy for pelvic floor muscle release causing pain may also be beneficial. Once vaginal health and pain are optimized, it may lead to improved sexual desire without the need for further treatment [175]. Genitourinary Syndrome of Menopause (GSM), which was previously known as vulvovaginal atrophy (VVA) responds well to topical hormonal therapy [176]. Oral hormonal replacement therapy (ORT) should only be given if the risk/benefit ratio is favorable, and if the patient has more than just GSM/VVA; a patient with vasomotor symptoms and/or bone density loss should be considered for oral hormonal therapy [176]. Taylor et al. compared oral estrogen to transdermal estradiol using the FSFI questionnaire and found that transdermal estradiol significantly improved lubrication and pain in early postmenopausal women, but there was no clear difference in desire [177]. Intravaginal testosterone cream has shown some success in improving the symptoms of GSM/VVA without changes in circulating sex hormone levels [176]. In patients who do not respond to local therapy, ospemifene is an option. Ospemifene is a selective estrogen receptor modulator, with agonist effects in the vaginal epithelium and neutral or antagonist effects in breast tissue. It has been approved for use in GSM/VVA as it has been shown to improve all domains of sexual function [176].

Hypoactive sexual desire disorder is best managed initially with education and sex therapy. Failing that, options include hormonal therapy and/or centrally acting agents. Flibanserin (100 mg at bedtime) is a centrally acting agent that is FDA approved for use in premenopausal women with HSDD. It is a nonhormonal multifunctional serotonin antagonist and agonist. Clinical trials showed significant improvement in desire and sexually satisfying events [175]. Postmenopausal women have similar outcomes, but the drug is not FDA approved for this group of women. The side effects of flibanserin include dizziness, somnolence, nausea, and fatigue. The rate of adverse events is similar to that of other centrally acting agents. They are usually mild and transient. The use of alcohol concurrently does not increase the rate of adverse events when using flibanserin. However, the FDA requires risk mitigation by discussing the risks of

Table 3 Phamacological treatments under development for FSD (Reprinted from Jordan E, et al. Clinical Pharmacol Ther. 2011;89(1):137–41.)

Drug product	Mechanism of action	Indication	Outcome measures	Status
Intrinsa	Androgen receptor agonist, transdermal testosterone patch	HSDD in oophorectomized women	SAL, PFSF, and PDS	Approved in European Union. Application withdrawn in the United States
Flibanserin	5-HT1A agonist, 5-HT2A antagonist	HSDD premenopausal women	SSE and eDiary desire score, FSFI, and FSDS-R	Phase III complete application for approval submitted in the United States and European Union
LibiGel	Androgen receptor agonist, testosterone transdermal gel	HSDD in oophorectomized women	SSE and ISED desire score	Phase III ongoing; approval and launch expected in 2012
Tibolone	Androgen receptor agonist	Osteoporosis; relief of symptoms from menopause		New drug application withdrawn in the United States. Approved in European Union
Bremelanotide	Melanocortin 4 receptor agonist	FSAD postmenopausal women	FSEP, FSFI, and GAQ	Phase II
Viagra	PDE5 inhibitor	FSAD, FOD, and lubrication problems	GAQ, LSC, SFQ, FIEI, and sexual event logs	Discontinued
Alprostadil	Topical PGE-1	FSAD	FSEP, FSFI, and GAQ	Discontinued
Bupropion	Norepinephrine reuptake inhibitor and nicotinic acetylcholine receptor antagonist	Antidepressant; smoking cessation; seasonal affective disorder	Changes in Sexual Functioning Questionnaire (CSFQ); Arizona Sexual Experiences Scale (ASEX); Brief Index of Sexual Functioning; and a 10-point visual analog scale	Approved; used off-label for SSRI-induced sexual dysfunction

hypotension and syncope, and they suggest against the concurrent use of alcohol [176].

Bremelanotide has also been FDA approved for use in patients with HSDD in premenopausal women. It is a melanocortin receptor agonist, thereby increasing dopamine release in the hypothalamus. It is used on-demand, usually 45 min prior to sexual activity at a dose of 1.75 mg subcutaneously [176], but not more than once a day and/or 8 doses per month. A clinically significant increase in desire and decrease in anxiety around the sexual experience was noted during 2 Phase III trials [178]. Side effects include nausea, headache, and flushing in 10% of patients.

Bupropion is a centrally acting agent used in the management of serotonin reuptake inhibitor (SSRI)-induced sexual dysfunction [175]. Its use is off-label, but safety has been proven for use in other disorders such as generalized anxiety disorder. This drug enhances the effect of dopamine and norepinephrine. In a RCT it was found to improve sexual desire when compared to placebo. The effect was not, however, statistically significant. Buspirone is another drug used off-label for SSRI-induced sexual dysfunction. It acts to inhibit serotonin reuptake. It also acts centrally and has similar side effects to flibanserin and bupropion.

Phosphodiesterase 5 inhibitors (PDE5-I) have been used in pre- and postmenopausal women with low desire. This class of drugs increases circulating NO, thereby leading to increased clitoral engorgement. However, it is difficult to prove that this improves the sexual experience. It may be more useful in patients with an arousal disorder secondary to diabetes mellitus, multiple sclerosis, or antidepressant use [176].

Unfortunately, a meta-analysis in 2018 by Weinberger et al. showed that 67.7% of treatment effect in patients with FSD can be attributed to the placebo effect [179]. Female sexual dysfunction is a complex problem, which is yet to be clearly understood and is largely multifactorial in its etiopathogenesis. Combination therapies are likely to be the most beneficial options for patients, but individualized care requires time and patience from the healthcare provider. It is imperative to continue researching this disorder to improve treatment options and overall patient outcomes.

Conclusion

The etiology of FSD is complex and multifactorial. The ideal approach to this disorder should be a collaborative effort involving therapists and physicians through an extensive medical and psychosocial evaluation with the inclusion of the spouse or partner in the diagnostic and therapeutic processes. Despite important anatomic and embryologic similarities between men and women, the multifaceted nature of FSD is unquestionably and definitely distinct from that of the male counterpart. This may be in part since the disease process involves multiple symptom complexes that respond to distinct therapeutic modalities. However, no single therapeutic modality addresses the totality of the underlying problem.

Significant advances in the female sexual anatomy and physiology that were obtained recently have led to an increased understanding of the female sexual function, which formed a crucial basis for an international consensus classification of FSD. This general consensus enabled the development of validated questionnaires illustrating the different domains of the female sexual function, culminating in a clearer understanding of the problem.

The development of new therapies should follow the strict rules of large, randomized, controlled clinical trials to assess efficacy and safety and to obtain regulatory approval. A better understanding of the complexity of the female sexual response cycle (and its dysfunction) is critical. Another area that still needs further improvement is an adequate measurement of therapeutic efficacy and an adequate risk-to-benefit ratio, as well as what constitutes a "normal" sexual response.

In short, treatment of FSD is also multifactorial, and it should be kept in mind that isolated medications will not be effective because of the important psychological component of the disorder involved. Therefore, a therapeutic algorithm that addresses all the four domains of the female sexual function is needed.

References

1. Aslan E, Fynes M. Female sexual dysfunction. Int Urogynecol J. 2008;19(2):293–305.
2. Kinsey A. Voices from the past – sexual behavior in the human male. Am J Public Health. 2003;93(6):894.
3. Masters WH, Johnson VE. Human sexual response. Bantam Books; 1966.
4. Spector IP, Carey MP. Incidence and prevalence of the sexual dysfunctions: a critical review of the empirical literature. Arch Sex Behav. 1990;19(4):389.
5. Rosen RC. Prevalence and risk factors of sexual dysfunction in men and women. Curr Psychiatry Rep. 2000;2(3):189–95.
6. Read S, King M, Watson J. Sexual dysfunction in primary medical care: prevalence, characteristics and detection by the general practitioner. J Public Health Med (United Kingdom). 1997;19(4):387–91.
7. Berman JR, Berman L, Goldstein I. Female sexual dysfunction: incidence, pathophysiology, evaluation, and treatment options. Urology. 1999;54(3):385–91.
8. Basson R, Berman J, Burnett A, Derogatis L, Ferguson D, Fourcroy J, et al. Report of the international consensus development conference on female sexual dysfunction: definitions and classifications. J Urol. 2000;163(3):888–93.
9. Kaplan HS. Hypoactive sexual desire. J Sex Marital Ther [Internet]. 1977;3(1):3–9. Available from: http://www.ncbi.nlm.nih.gov/pubmed/864734
10. Association AP. Diagnostic and statistical manual of mental disorders: DSM-IV-TR. LK – https://sun.on.worldcat.org/oclc/43483668 [Internet]. 4th ed., t. TA – TT -. Washington, DC SE – xxxvii, 943 pages; 26 cm: American Psychiatric Association; 2000. Available from: http://dsm.psychiatryonline.org/doi/pdf/10.1176/appi.books.9780890420249.dsm-iv-tr
11. Berman JR, Berman LA, Werbin TJ, Goldstein I. Female sexual dysfunction: anatomy, physiology,

evaluation and treatment options. Curr Opin Urol. 1999;9:563.
12. Basson R. Using a different model for female sexual response to address women's problematic low sexual desire. J Sex Marital Ther. 2001;27(5):395–403.
13. Basson R, Leiblum S, Brotto L, Derogatis L, Fourcroy J, Fugl-Meyer K, et al. Definitions of women's sexual dysfunction reconsidered: advocating expansion and revision. J Psychosom Obstet Gynaecol [Internet]. 2003;24(4):221–9. Available from: http://www.ncbi.nlm.nih.gov/pubmed/14702882
14. Segraves RT. Female sexual disorders: psychiatric aspects. Can J Psychiatr. 2002;47(5):419–25.
15. Bachmann GA, Leiblum SR. The impact of hormones on menopausal sexuality: a literature review. Menopause. 2004;11(1):120–30.
16. Rosen RC, Lane RM, Menza M. Effects of SSRIs on sexual function: a critical review. J Clin Psychopharmacol. 1999;19(1):67–85.
17. Fry RPW, Crisp AH, Beard RW. Sociopsychological factors in chronic pelvic pain: a review. J Psychosom Res. 1997;42(1):1–15.
18. Pauls RN, Berman JR. Impact of pelvic floor disorders and prolapse on female sexual function and response. Urol Clin North Am. 2002;29(3):677–83.
19. Salonia A, Zanni G, Nappi RE, Briganti A, Dehò F, Fabbri F, et al. Sexual dysfunction is common in women with lower urinary tract symptoms and urinary incontinence: results of a cross-sectional study. Eur Urol. 2004;45(5):642–8.
20. Rosen R, Brown C, Heiman J, Leiblum S, Meston C, Shabsigh R, et al. The female sexual function index (FSFI): a multidimensional self-report instrument for the assessment of female sexual function. J Sex Marital Ther [Internet]. 26(2):191–208. Available from: http://www.ncbi.nlm.nih.gov/pubmed/10782451
21. Laumann EO, Paik A, Rosen RC. Sexual dysfunction in the United States: prevalence and predictors. J Am Med Assoc. 1999;281(6):537–44.
22. Diokno AC, Brown MB, Brock BM, Herzog AR, Normolle DP. Prevalence and outcome of surgery for female incontinence. Urology. 1989;33(4):285.
23. Goldmeier D, Judd A, Schroeder K. Prevalence of sexual dysfunction in new heterosexual attenders at a Central London genitourinary medicine clinic in 1998. Sex Transm Infect. 2000;76(3):208–9.
24. Lewis RW, Fugl-Meyer KS, Bosch R, Fugl-Meyer AR, Laumann EO, Lizza E, et al. Epidemiology/risk factors of sexual dysfunction. J Sex Med. 2004;1(1):35–9.
25. Nazareth I, Boynton P, King M. Primary care London general practitioners: cross sectional study. 2003;327:1–6.
26. Mercer CH, Fenton KA, Johnson AM, Wellings K, Macdowall W, McManus S, et al. Sexual function problems and help seeking behaviour in Britain: national probability sample survey. Br Med J. 2003;327(7412):426.
27. Lindau ST, Schumm LP, Laumann EO, Levinson W, O'Muircheartaigh CA, Waite LJ. A study of sexuality and health among older adults in the United States. N Engl J Med. 2007;357(8):762–74.
28. Dennerstein L, Alexander JL, Kotz K. The menopause and sexual functioning: a review of the population-based studies. Annu Rev Sex Res. 2003;14:64–82. PMID: 15287158.
29. Shifren JL, Monz BU, Russo PA, Segreti A, Johannes CB. Sexual problems and distress in United States women. Obstet Gynecol. 2008;112(5):970–8.
30. Dennerstein L, Wood C, Burrows GD. Sexual response following hysterectomy and oophorectomy. Obstet Gynecol. 1977;49(1):92.
31. Nathorst-Böös J, Von Schoultz B. Psychological reactions and sexual life after hysterectomy with and without oophorectomy. Gynecol Obstet Investig. 1992;34(2):97.
32. Bellerose SB, Binik YM. Body image and sexuality in oophorectomized women. Arch Sex Behav. 1993;22(5):435–59.
33. Aziz A, Brännström M, Bergquist C, Silfverstolpe G. Perimenopausal androgen decline after oophorectomy does not influence sexuality or psychological well-being. Fertil Steril. 2005;83(4):1021–8.
34. Reed SD, Newton KM, LaCroix AZ, Grothaus LC, Ehrlich K. Night sweats, sleep disturbance, and depression associated with diminished libido in late menopausal transition and early postmenopause: baseline data from the herbal alternatives for menopause trial (HALT). Am J Obstet Gynecol. 2007;196(6):593.e1–7.
35. Kostis JB, Jackson G, Rosen R, Barrett-Connor E, Billups K, Burnett AL, et al. Sexual dysfunction and cardiac risk (the second Princeton consensus conference). J Urol. 2006;175:1452.
36. Schwarz ER, Kapur V, Bionat S, Rastogi S, Gupta R, Rosanio S. The prevalence and clinical relevance of sexual dysfunction in women and men with chronic heart failure. Int J Impot Res. 2008;20(1):85–91.
37. Fatemi SS, Taghavi SM. Evaluation of sexual function in women with type 2 diabetes mellitus. Diab Vasc Dis Res. 2009;6(1):38–9.
38. Newman AS, Bertelson AD. Sexual dysfunction in diabetic women. J Behav Med. 1986;9(3):261.
39. Panicker R, Pandurangan T. Cosmetic surgical procedures on the vulva and vagina – an overview. Indian J Med Ethics. 2022;07(01):54–7.
40. Brody S. Vaginal intercourse orgasm consistency accounts for concordance of vaginal and subjective sexual arousal. Arch Sex Behav. 2012;41:1073–5.
41. Angelou K, Grigoriadis T, Diakosavvas M, Zacharakis D, Athanasiou S. The genitourinary syndrome of menopause: an overview of the recent data. Cureus. 2020;12:e7586.
42. Patnam R, Edenfield A, Swift S. Defining normal apical vaginal support: a relook at the POSST study. Int Urogynecol J. 2019;30(1):47–51.
43. Kim-Fine S, Antosh DD, Balk EM, Meriwether KV, Kanter G, Dieter AA, et al. Relationship of postoperative vaginal anatomy and sexual function: a

systematic review with meta-analysis. Available from: https://doi.org/10.1007/s00192-021-04829-4
44. De Lancey JOL. What's new in the functional anatomy of pelvic organ prolapse? Curr Opin Obstet Gynecol. Lippincott Williams and Wilkins. 2016;28:420–9.
45. Rantell A, Srikrishna S, Robinson D. Assessment of the impact of urogenital prolapse on sexual dysfunction, vol. 92. Maturitas. Elsevier Ireland Ltd; 2016. p. 56–60.
46. Aydın S, Cavide Sönmez F, Filiz A, Karasu G, Gül B, Arıoğlu Ç. Search for the G spot: microvessel and nerve mapping of the paraurethral anterior vaginal wall. Int Urogynecol J. Available from: https://doi.org/10.1007/s00192-020-04379-1
47. Li T, Liao Q, Zhang H, Gao X, Li X, Zhang M. Anatomic distribution of nerves and microvascular density in the human anterior vaginal wall: prospective study. PLoS One. 2014;9(11):1–6.
48. Song YB, Hwang K, Kim DJ, Han SH. Innervation of vagina: microdissection and immunohistochemical study. J Sex Marital Ther. 2009;35(2):144–53.
49. Yeung J, Pauls RN. Anatomy of the vulva and the female sexual response. Obstet Gynecol Clin North Am. W.B. Saunders. 2016;43:27–44.
50. Ostrzenski A, Krajewski P, Ganjei-Azar P, Wasiutynski AJ, Scheinberg MN, Tarka S, et al. Verification of the anatomy and newly discovered histology of the G-spot complex. BJOG [Internet]. 2014;121(11):1333–9. Available from: http://www.ncbi.nlm.nih.gov/pubmed/24641569
51. Hoag N, Keast JR, O'Connell HE. The "G-spot" is not a structure evident on macroscopic anatomic dissection of the vaginal wall. J Sex Med [Internet]. 2017;14(12):1524–32. Available from: http://www.ncbi.nlm.nih.gov/pubmed/29198508
52. Gravina GL, Brandetti F, Martini P, Carosa E, Di Stasi SM, Morano S, et al. Measurement of the thickness of the urethrovaginal space in women with or without vaginal orgasm. J Sex Med [Internet]. 2008;5(3):610–8. Available from: http://www.ncbi.nlm.nih.gov/pubmed/18221286
53. Wylie KR. Emerging evidence for a discrete genital site for orgasm? BJOG. 2016;123(9):1550.
54. Sivashoğlu AA, Köseoğlu S, Dinç Elibol F, Dere Y, Keçe AC, Çalışkan E. Searching for radiologic and histologic evidence on live vaginal tissue: does the G-spot exist? Turkish J Obstet Gynecol [Internet]. 2021;18(1):1–6. Available from: http://www.ncbi.nlm.nih.gov/pubmed/33715320
55. Lloyd J, Crouch NS, Minto CL, Liao L-M, Creighton SM. Female genital appearance: "normality" unfolds * [Internet]. Available from: www.blackwellpublishing.com/bjog
56. Schober J, Cooney T, Pfaff D, Mayoglou L, Martin-Alguacil N. Innervation of the labia minora of prepubertal girls. J Pediatr Adolesc Gynecol. 2010;23(6):352–7.
57. Lev-Sagie A, Witkin SS. Recent advances in understanding provoked vestibulodynia. F1000Research. F1000 Research Ltd. 2016;5:2581.
58. Cervigni M, Natale F. Gynecological disorders in bladder pain syndrome/interstitial cystitis patients. Int J Urol. 2014;21(S1):85–8.
59. Hayes RD. Circular and linear modeling of female sexual desire and arousal. J Sex Res [Internet]. 2011;48(2–3):130–41. Available from: http://www.ncbi.nlm.nih.gov/pubmed/21409710
60. Cain VS, Johannes CB, Avis NE, Mohr B, Schocken M, Skurnick J, et al. Sexual functioning and practices in a multi-ethnic study of midlife women: baseline results from SWAN. J Sex Res [Internet]. 2003;40(3):266–76. Available from: http://www.ncbi.nlm.nih.gov/pubmed/14533021
61. Meston CM, Stanton AM. Understanding sexual arousal and subjective-genital arousal desynchrony in women. Nat Rev Urol [Internet]. 2019;16(2):107–20. Available from: http://www.ncbi.nlm.nih.gov/pubmed/30664743
62. Chivers ML. A brief update on the specificity of sexual arousal. Sex Relatsh Ther. 2010;25(4):407–14.
63. Brotto LA, Heiman JR, Tolman DL. Narratives of desire in mid-age women with and without arousal difficulties. J Sex Res [Internet]. 46(5):387–98. Available from: http://www.ncbi.nlm.nih.gov/pubmed/19291528
64. Meston CM, Levin RJ, Sipski ML, Hull EM, Heiman JR. Women's orgasm. Annu Rev Sex Res [Internet]. 2004;15:173–257. Available from: http://www.ncbi.nlm.nih.gov/pubmed/16913280
65. Levin RJ. The pharmacology of the human female orgasm – its biological and physiological backgrounds. Pharmacol Biochem Behav [Internet]. 2014;121:62–70. Available from: http://www.ncbi.nlm.nih.gov/pubmed/24560912
66. Levin RJ, Wagner G. Orgasm in women in the laboratory – quantitative studies on duration, intensity, latency, and vaginal blood flow. Arch Sex Behav [Internet]. 1985;14(5):439–49. Available from: http://www.ncbi.nlm.nih.gov/pubmed/4062540
67. Domoney C. Sexual function in women: what is normal? Int Urogynecol J. 2009;20(SUPPL. 1):9.
68. Traish AM, Kim NN, Munarriz R, Moreland R, Goldstein I. Biochemical and physiological mechanisms of female genital sexual arousal. Arch Sex Behav. 2002;31:393.
69. Min K, Munarriz R, Kim NN, Goldstein I, Traish A. Effects of ovariectomy and estrogen and androgen treatment on sildenafil-mediated changes in female genital blood flow and vaginal lubrication in the animal model. Am J Obstet Gynecol [Internet]. 2002;187(5):1370–6. Available from: http://www.ncbi.nlm.nih.gov/pubmed/12439533

70. Hoyle CH, Stones RW, Robson T, Whitley K, Burnstock G. Innervation of vasculature and microvasculature of the human vagina by NOS and neuropeptide-containing nerves. J Anat [Internet] 1996;188 (Pt 3):633–644. Available from: http://www.ncbi.nlm.nih.gov/pubmed/8763480
71. Myers LS, Morokoff PJ. Physiological and subjective sexual arousal in pre- and postmenopausal women and postmenopausal women taking replacement therapy. Psychophysiology. 1986;23(3):283.
72. Park K, Goldstein I, Andry C, Siroky MB, Krane RJ, Azadzoi KM. Vasculogenic female sexual dysfunction: the hemodynamic basis for vaginal engorgement insufficiency and clitoral erectile insufficiency. Int J Impot Res. 1997;9(1):27–37.
73. Sipski ML, Alexander CJ, Rosen RC. Physiological parameters associated with psychogenic sexual arousal in women with complete spinal cord injuries. Arch Phys Med Rehabil. 1995;76(9):811–8.
74. Sipski ML, Alexander CJ, Rosen RC. Orgasm in women with spinal cord injuries: a laboratory-based assessment. Arch Phys Med Rehabil. 1995;76(12):1097–102.
75. Berard EJJ. The sexuality of spinal cord injured women: physiology and pathophysiology. A review. Paraplegia. 1989;27(2):99–112.
76. Sarrel PM. Ovarian hormones and vaginal blood flow: using laser Doppler velocimetry to measure effects in a clinical trial of post-menopausal women. Int J Impot Res. 1998;10(Suppl. 2):S91–3.
77. Carlson KJ. Outcomes of hysterectomy. Clin Obstet Gynecol. 1997;40:939.
78. Berman JR. Female sexual dysfunction. Urol Clin North Am. 2001;28(2):405–16. Available from: http://www.urologic.theclinics.com/article/S0094-0143(05)70148-8/pdf
79. Davison SL, Davis SR. Androgens in women. J Steroid Biochem Mol Biol. 2003;85(2–5):363–6.
80. Rako S. Testosterone supplemental therapy after hysterectomy with or without concomitant oophorectomy: Estrogen alone is not enough. J Womens Health. 2000;9:917–23.
81. Rosenbaum TY. Pelvic floor involvement in male and female sexual dysfunction and the role of pelvic floor rehabilitation in treatment: a literature review. J Sex Med. 2007;4(1):4–13.
82. Wright JB, Wright AL, Simpson NAB, Bryce FC. A survey of trainee obstetricians preferences for childbirth. Eur J Obstet Gynecol Reprod Biol. 2001;97(1):23–5.
83. Mc Gurgan P, Coulter-Smith S, O'Donovan PJ. A national confidential survey of obstetrician's personal preferences regarding mode of delivery. Eur J Obstet Gynecol Reprod Biol. 2001;97(1):17–9.
84. MacDonald C, Pinion SB, MacLeod UM. Scottish female obstetricians' views on elective caesarean section and personal choice for delivery. J Obstet Gynaecol (Lahore). 2002;22(6):586–9.
85. Wu JM, Hundley AF, Visco AG. Elective primary cesarean delivery: attitudes of urogynecology and maternal-fetal medicine specialists. Obstet Gynecol. 2005;105(2):301–6.
86. Hicks TL, Forester Goodall S, Quattrone EM, Lydon-Rochelle MT. Postpartum sexual functioning and method of delivery: summary of the evidence. J Midwifery Womens Health. 2004;49(5):430–6.
87. Bogren LY. Changes in sexuality in women and men during pregnancy. Arch Sex Behav. 1991;20(1):35.
88. Sayle AE, Savitz DA, Thorp JM, Hertz-Picciotto I, Wilcox AJ. Sexual activity during late pregnancy and risk of preterm delivery. Obstet Gynecol. 2001;97(2):283–9.
89. Glazener C. Br J Obstet Gynecol. 1997;104(3):330–5.
90. Johanson R, Wilkinson P, Bastible A, Ryan S, Murphy H, O'Brien S. Health after childbirth: a comparison of normal and assisted vaginal delivery. Midwifery. 1993;9(3):161–8.
91. Buhling KJ, Schmidt S, Robinson JN, Klapp C, Siebert G, Dudenhausen JW. Rate of dyspareunia after delivery in primiparae according to mode of delivery. Eur J Obstet Gynecol Reprod Biol. 2006;124(1):42–6.
92. Signorello LB, Harlow BL, Chekos AK, Repke JT. Postpartum sexual functioning and its relationship to perineal trauma: a retrospective cohort study of primiparous women. Am J Obstet Gynecol. 2001;184(5):881–90.
93. Barrett G, Pendry E, Peacock J, Victor CR. Sexual function after childbirth: Women's experiences, persistent morbidity and lack of professional recognition. BJOG. 1998;105(2):242–3.
94. Robson KM, Brant HA, Kumar R. Maternal sexuality during first pregnancy and after childbirth. BJOG. 1981;88(9):882–9.
95. Moran PA, Dwyer PL, Ziccone SP. Burch colposuspension for the treatment of coital urinary leakage secondary to genuine stress incontinence. J Obstet Gynaecol (Lahore). 1999;19(3):289–91.
96. Yip SK, Chan A, Pang S, Leung P, Tang C, Shek D, et al. The impact of urodynamic stress incontinence and detrusor overactivity on marital relationship and sexual function. Am J Obstet Gynecol. 2003;188(5):1244–8.
97. Gordon D, Groutz A, Sinai T, Wiezman A, Lessing JB, David MP, et al. Sexual function in women attending a urogynecology clinic. Int Urogynecol J. 1999;10(5):325–8.
98. Handa VL, Cundiff G, Chang HH, Helzlsouer KJ. Female sexual function and pelvic floor disorders. Obstet Gynecol. 2008;111(5):1045–52.
99. Weber AM, Walters MD, Piedmonte MR. Sexual function and vaginal anatomy in women before and after surgery for pelvic organ prolapse and urinary incontinence. Am J Obstet Gynecol. Mosby Inc. 2000;182:1610–5.
100. Maaita M, Bhaumik J, Davies AE. Sexual function after using tension-free vaginal tape for the surgical treatment of genuine stress incontinence. BJU Int. 2002;90(6):540–3.

101. Ward KL, Hilton P. A prospective multicenter randomized trial of tension-free vaginal tape and colposuspension for primary urodynamic stress incontinence: two-year follow-up. Am J Obstet Gynecol. 2004;190(2):324–31.
102. Yeni E, Unal D, Verit A, Kafali H, Ciftci H, Gulum M. The effect of tension-free vaginal tape (TVT) procedure on sexual function in women with stress incontinence. Int Urogynecol J. 2003;14(6):390–4.
103. Mazouni C, Karsenty G, Bretelle F, Bladou F, Gamerre M, Serment G. Urinary complications and sexual function after the tension-free vaginal tape procedure. Acta Obstet Gynecol Scand. 2004;83(10):955–61.
104. Aslan E, Ugurlucan FG, Bilgic D, Yalcin O, Beji NK. Effects of transobturator midurethral sling surgery on sexual functions: one-year follow-up. Gynecol Obstet Investig. 2018;83(2):187–97.
105. Paul F, Rajagopalan S, Doddamani SC, Mottemmal R, Joseph S, Bhat S. Effect of midurethral sling (transobturator tape) surgery on female sexual function. Indian J Urol. 2015;31(2):120–4.
106. Alwaal A, Tian X, Huang Y, Zhao L, Ma L, Lin G, et al. Female sexual function following mid-urethral slings for the treatment of stress urinary incontinence. Int J Impot Res. 2016;28(4):121–6.
107. Hsiao SM, Lin HH. Impact of the mid-urethral sling for stress urinary incontinence on female sexual function and their partners' sexual activity. Taiwan J Obstet Gynecol [Internet]. 2018;57(6):853–7. Available from: https://doi.org/10.1016/j.tjog.2018.10.015
108. Spinosa JP, Dubuis PY, Riederer BM. Transobturator surgery for female stress incontinence: a comparative anatomical study of outside-in vs inside-out techniques. BJU Int. 2007;100(5):1097–102.
109. Weber AM, Walters MD, Piedmonte MR, Ballard LA. Anterior colporrhaphy: a randomized trial of three surgical techniques. Am J Obstet Gynecol. 2001;185(6):1299–306.
110. Shen T, Song LJ, Xu YM, Gu BJ, Lu LH, Li F. Sexual function and health-related quality of life following anterior vaginal wall surgery for stress urinary incontinence and pelvic organ prolapse. Int J Impot Res. 2011;23(4):151–7.
111. Jeffcoate TN. Posterior colpoperineorrhaphy. Am J Obstet Gynecol. 1959;77(3):490.
112. Komesu YM, Rogers RG, Kammerer-Doak DN, Barber MD, Olsen AL. Posterior repair and sexual function. Am J Obstet Gynecol. 2007;197(1):101.e1–6.
113. Kenton K, Shott S, Brubaker L. Outcome after rectovaginal fascia reattachment for rectocele repair. Am J Obstet Gynecol. 1999;181(6):1360–4.
114. Glavind K, Madsen H. A prospective study of the discrete fascial defect rectocele repair. Acta Obstet Gynecol Scand. 2000;79(2):145–7.
115. Maher CF, Qatawneh AM, Baessler K, Schluter PJ. Midline rectovaginal fascial plication for repair of rectocele and obstructed defecation. Obstet Gynecol. 2004;104(4):685–9.
116. Holley RL, Varner RE, Gleason BP, Apffel LA, Scott S. Sexual function after sacrospinous ligament fixation for vaginal vault prolapse. J Reprod Med Obstet Gynecol. 1996;41(5):355–8.
117. Paraiso MFR, Ballard LA, Walters MD, Lee JC, Mitchinson AR, Shull B. Pelvic support defects and visceral and sexual function in women treated with sacrospinous ligament suspension and pelvic reconstruction. Am J Obstet Gynecol. 1996;175(6):1423–31.
118. Goldberg RP, Tomezsko JE, Winkler HA, Koduri S, Culligan PJ, Sand PK. Anterior or posterior sacrospinous vaginal vault suspension: long-term anatomic and functional evaluation. Obstet Gynecol. 2001;98(2):199–204.
119. Baumann M, Salvisberg C, Mueller M, Kuhn A. Sexual function after sacrospinous fixation for vaginal vault prolapse: bad or mad? Surg Endosc. 2009;23(5):1013–7.
120. Maher CF, Qatawneh AM, Dwyer PL, Carey MP, Cornish A, Schluter PJ. Abdominal sacral colpopexy or vaginal sacrospinous colpopexy for vaginal vault prolapse: a prospective randomized study. Am J Obstet Gynecol. 2004;190(1):20–6.
121. Baessler K, Schuessler B. Abdominal sacrocolpopexy and anatomy and function of the posterior compartment. Obstet Gynecol. 2001;97(5):678–84.
122. Virtanen H, Hirvonen T, Makinen J, Kiiholm P. Outcome of thirty patients who underwent repair of posthysterectomy prolapse of the vaginal vault with abdominal sacral colpopexy. J Am Coll Surg. 1994;178(3):283–7.
123. Benson JT, Lucente V, McClellan E, Cornella J. Vaginal versus abdominal reconstructive surgery for the treatment of pelvic support defects: a prospective randomized study with long-term outcome evaluation. Am J Obstet Gynecol. 1996;175(6):1418–22.
124. Papa Petros PE. Vault prolapse II: restoration of dynamic vaginal supports by infracoccygeal sacropexy, an axial day-case vaginal procedure. Int Urogynecol J. 2001;12(5):296–303.
125. de Tayrac R, Devoldere G, Renaudie J, Villard P, Guilbaud O, Eglin G, et al. Prolapse repair by vaginal route using a new protected low-weight polypropylene mesh: 1-year functional and anatomical outcome in a prospective multicentre study. Int Urogynecol J. 2007;18(3):251–6.
126. Nieminen K, Hiltunen R, Takala T, Heiskanen E, Merikari M, Niemi K, et al. Outcomes after anterior vaginal wall repair with mesh: a randomized, controlled trial with a 3 year follow-up. Am J Obstet Gynecol [Internet]. 2010;203(3):235.e1–8. Available from: https://doi.org/10.1016/j.ajog.2010.03.030
127. Weber MA, Lakeman MME, Laan E, Roovers JPWR. The effects of vaginal prolapse surgery using synthetic mesh on vaginal wall sensibility, vaginal

128. Syed KK, Consolo MJ, Gousse AE. Anterior vaginal wall prolapse repair and the rise and fall of transvaginal mesh. Did we come full circle? A historical perspective. Urology [Internet] 2021;150:110–5. Available from: https://doi.org/10.1016/j.urology.2020.08.015

127. vasocongestion, and sexual function: a prospective single-center study. J Sex Med. 2014;11(7):1848–55.

129. Shi C, Zhao Y, Hu Q, Gong R, Yin Y, Xia Z. Clinical analysis of pain after transvaginal mesh surgery in patients with pelvic organ prolapse. BMC Womens Health [Internet]. 2021;21(1):1–9. Available from: https://doi.org/10.1186/s12905-021-01192-w

130. Mokate T, Wright C, Mander T. Hysterectomy and sexual function. J Br Menopause Soc. 2006;12(4):153–7.

131. Bradford A, Meston C. Sexual outcomes and satisfaction with hysterectomy influence of patient education. J Sex Med. 2010;4(1):106–14.

132. Helström L. Sexuality after hysterectomy: a model based on quantitative and qualitative analysis of 104 women before and after subtotal hysterectomy. J Psychosom Obstet Gynecol. 1994;15(4):219.

133. Lycke KD, Kahlert J, Damgaard R, Mogensen O, Hammer A. Trends in hysterectomy incidence rates during 2000-2015 in Denmark: shifting from abdominal to minimally invasive surgical procedures. Clin Epidemiol. 2021;13:407–16.

134. Dennerstein L, Wood G, Burrows GD. Sexual dysfunction following hysterectomy. Aust Fam Physician. 1977;6(5):535.

135. Dodds DT, Potgieter CR, Turner PJ, Scheepers GP. The physical and emotional results of hysterectomy; a review of 162 cases. S Afr Med J. 1961;35:53–4.

136. Rhodes JC, Kjerulff KH, Langenberg PW, Guzinski GM. Hysterectomy and sexual functioning. J Am Med Assoc. 1999;282(20):1934–41.

137. Roussis NP, Waltrous L, Kerr A, Robertazzi R, Cabbad MF. Sexual response in the patient after hysterectomy: total abdominal versus supracervical vesus vaginal procedure. Am J Obstet Gynecol. 2004;190(5):1427–8.

138. El-Toukhy TA, Hefni MA, Davies AE, Mahadevan S. The effect of different types of hysterectomy on urinary and sexual functions: a prospective study. J Obstet Gynaecol (Lahore). 2004;24(4):420–5.

139. Dragisic KG, Milad MP. Sexual functioning and patient expectations of sexual functioning after hysterectomy. Am J Obstet Gynecol. 2004;190(5):1416–8.

140. Goetsch MF. The effect of total hysterectomy on specific sexual sensations. Am J Obstet Gynecol. 2005;192(6):1922–7.

141. Kilkku P. Supra vaginal uterine amputation vs. hysterectomy: effects on coital frequency and dyspareunia. Acta Obstet Gynecol Scand. 1983;62(2):141–5.

142. Kilkku P, Gronroos M, Hirvonen T, Rauramo I. Supra vaginal uterine amputation vs hysterectomy: effects on libido and orgasm. Acta Obstet Gynecol Scand [Internet]. 1983;62:147–52. Available from: https://doi.org/10.3109/00016348309155779

143. Thakar R, Ayers S, Clarkson P, Stanton S, Manyonda I. Outcomes after total versus subtotal abdominal hysterectomy. N Engl J Med. 2002;347(17):1318–25.

144. Zobbe V, Gimbel H, Andersen BM, Filtenborg T, Jakobsen K, Sørensen HC, et al. Sexuality after total vs. subtotal hysterectomy. Acta Obstet Gynecol Scand. 2004;83(2):191–6.

145. Flory N, Bissonnette F, Amsel RTBY. The psychosocial outcomes of total and subtotal hysterectomy: a randomized controlled trial. J Sex Med. 2006;3(3):483–91.

146. Kuppermann M, Varner RE, Summitt RL Jr, Learman LA, Ireland C, Vittinghoff E, et al. Effect of hysterectomy vs medical treatment on health-related quality of life and sexual functioning. JAMA. 2004;291(12):1447.

147. Hehenkamp WJK, Volkers NA, Bartholomeus W, De Blok S, Birnie E, Reekers JA, et al. Sexuality and body image after uterine artery embolization and hysterectomy in the treatment of uterine fibroids: a randomized comparison. Cardiovasc Intervent Radiol. 2007;30(5):866–75.

148. Bergmark K, Åvall-Lundqvist E, Dickman PW, Henningsohn L, Steineck G. Patient-rating of distressful symptoms after treatment for early cervical cancer. Acta Obstet Gynecol Scand. 2002;81(5):443.

149. Jensen PT, Groenvold M, Klee MC, Thranov I, Petersen MA, Machin D. Early-stage cervical carcinoma, radical hysterectomy, and sexual function: a longitudinal study. Cancer. 2004;100(1):97–106.

150. Auchincloss SS. After treatment. Psychosocial issues in gynecologic cancer survivorship. Cancer. 1995;76(10 S):2117–24.

151. Carmack Taylor CL, Basen-Engquist K, Shinn EH, Bodurka DC. Predictors of sexual functioning in ovarian cancer patients. J Clin Oncol. 2004;22(5):881–9.

152. Stewart DE, Wong F, Duff S, Melancon CH, Cheung AM. "Hat doesn't kill you makes you stronger": an ovarian cancer survivor survey. Gynecol Oncol. 2001;83(3):537–42.

153. Stein JP, Skinner DG. Results with radical cystectomy for treating bladder cancer: a "reference standard" for high-grade, invasive bladder cancer. BJU Int. 2003;92(1):12–7.

154. Nordström GM, Nyman CR. Male and female sexual function and activity following ileal conduit urinary diversion. Br J Urol. 1993;72(2):1–267.

155. Stenzl A, Colleselli K, Poisel S, Feichtinger H, Pontasch H, Bartsch G. Rationale and technique of nerve sparing radical cystectomy before an orthotopic neobladder procedure in women. J Urol. 1995;154(December):2044–9.

156. Stenzl A, Colleselli K, Poisel S, Feichtinger H, Bartsch G. Anterior exenteration with subsequent ureteroileal urethrostomy in females. Anatomy, risk of urethral recurrence, surgical technique, and results. Eur Urol. 1998;33:18.

157. Berman L, Berman J, Felder S, Pollets D, Chhabra S, Miles M, et al. Seeking help for sexual function complaints: what gynecologists need to know about the female patient's experience. Fertil Steril. 2003;79(3):572–6.

158. Zippe CD, Raina R, Shah AD, Massanyi EZ, Agarwal A, Ulchaker J, et al. Female sexual dysfunction after radical cystectomy: a new outcome measure. Urology. 2004;63(6):1153–7.
159. Kessler TM, Burkhard FC, Perimenis P, Danuser H, Thalmann GN, Hochreiter WW, et al. Attempted nerve sparing surgery and age have a significant effect on urinary continence and erectile function after radical cystoprostatectomy and ileal orthotopic bladder substitution. J Urol. 2004;172(4 I):1323–7.
160. Schoenberg M, Hortopan S, Schlossberg L, Marshall FF. Anatomical anterior exenteration with urethral and vaginal preservation: illustrated surgical method. J Urol. 1999;161(2):569–72.
161. Desnoo L, Faithfull S. A qualitative study of anterior resection syndrome: the experiences of cancer survivors who have undergone resection surgery. Eur J Cancer Care (Engl). 2006;15(3):244–51.
162. Banerjee AK. Sexual dysfunction after surgery for rectal cancer. Lancet. 1999;353(9168):1900–2.
163. Enker WE. Total mesorectal excision – the new golden standard of surgery for rectal cancer. Ann Med. 1997;29(2):127–33.
164. Enker WE, Havenga K, Polyak T, Thaler H, Cranor M. Abdominoperineal resection via total mesorectal excision and autonomic nerve preservation for low rectal cancer. World J Surg. 1997;21(7):715–20.
165. Morino M, Parini U, Giraudo G, Salval M, Contul RB, Garrone C. Laparoscopic total mesorectal excision: a consecutive series of 100 patients. Ann Surg. 2003;237(3):335–42.
166. Conticchio M, Papagni V, Notarnicola M, Delvecchio A, Riccelli U, Ammendola M, et al. Laparoscopic vs. open mesorectal excision for rectal cancer: are these approaches still comparable? A systematic review and metaanalysis. PLoS One. 2020;15 (7 July):e0235887.
167. Bruheim K, Tveit KM, Skovlund E, Balteskard L, Carlsen E, Fosså SD, et al. Sexual function in females after radiotherapy for rectal cancer. Acta Oncol (Madr). 2010;49(6):826–32.
168. Li K, He X, Tong S, Zheng Y. Risk factors for sexual dysfunction after rectal cancer surgery in 948 consecutive patients: a prospective cohort study. Eur J Surg Oncol [Internet]. 2021;47(8):2087–92. Available from: https://doi.org/10.1016/j.ejso.2021.03.251
169. Addis IB, Van Den Eeden SK, Wassel-Fyr CL, Vittinghoff E, Brown JS, Thom DH. Sexual activity and function in middle-aged and older women. Obstet Gynecol. 2006;107(4):755–64.
170. Fugl-Meyer A, Fugl-Meyer K. Sexual disabilities, problems and satisfaction in 18–74 year old swedes. Scand J Sexol. 1999;2(2):79–105.
171. Dennerstein L, Hayes RD. Confronting the challenges: epidemiological study of female sexual dysfunction and the menopause. J Sex Med. 2005;2 (Suppl. 3):118–32.
172. Castelo-Branco C, Blumel JE, Araya H, Riquelme R, Castro G, Haya J, et al. Prevalence of sexual dysfunction in a cohort of middle-aged women: influences of menopause and hormone replacement therapy. J Obstet Gynaecol (Lahore). 2003;23(4)
173. Kingsberg S, Althof SE. Evaluation and treatment of female sexual disorders. Int Urogynecol J. 2009;20 (SUPPL. 1):33–43.
174. Jordan R, Hallam TJ, Molinoff P, Spana C. Developing treatments for female sexual dysfunction. Clinical. Pharmacol Ther. 2011;89(1):137–41. https://doi.org/10.1038/clpt.2010.262. PMID: 21085115.
175. Clayton AH, Goldstein I, Kim NN, Althof SE, Faubion SS, Faught BM, et al. The International Society for the Study of Women's sexual health process of care for management of hypoactive sexual desire disorder in women. Mayo Clin Proc. 2018;93(4):467–87.
176. Nappi RE, Tiranini L, Martini E, Bosoni D, Righi A, Cucinella L. Medical treatment of female sexual dysfunction. Urol Clin North Am [Internet]. 2022;49(2): 299–307. Available from: https://doi.org/10.1016/j.ucl.2022.02.001
177. Taylor HS, Tal A, Pal L, Li F, Black DM, Brinton EA, et al. Effects of oral vs transdermal estrogen therapy on sexual function in early postmenopause: ancillary study of the Kronos early estrogen prevention study (KEEPS). JAMA Intern Med [Internet]. 2017;177 (10):1471–9. Available from: http://www.ncbi.nlm.nih.gov/pubmed/28846767
178. Kingsberg SA, Clayton AH, Portman D, Williams LA, Krop J, Jordan R, et al. Bremelanotide for the treatment of hypoactive sexual desire disorder: two randomized phase 3 trials. Obstet Gynecol [Internet]. 2019;134(5):899–908. Available from: http://www.ncbi.nlm.nih.gov/pubmed/31599840
179. Weinberger JM, Houman J, Caron AT, Patel DN, Baskin AS, Ackerman AL, et al. Female sexual dysfunction and the placebo effect: a meta-analysis. Obstet Gynecol. 2018;132(2):453–8.

Part VIII

Fecal Incontinence and Defecatory Dysfunction

Pathophysiology, Diagnosis, and Treatment of Defecatory Dysfunction

55

Amythis Soltani, Domnique Malacarne Pape, and Cara L. Grimes

Contents

Introduction	998
Definitions	998
Epidemiology	999
Physiology	999
Approach to Care	1000
Anatomy	1000
Differential Diagnosis	1000
Evaluation	1002
History Taking	1002
Physical Exam	1003
Correlation Between Anatomy and Function	1003
Testing	1004
Management	1007
Behavioral Modification and Biofeedback	1007
Conclusion	1010
Cross-References	1011
References	1011

A. Soltani
Department of Obstetrics and Gynecology, Westchester Medical Center, Valhalla, NY, USA
e-mail: amythis.soltani@wmchealth.org

D. M. Pape · C. L. Grimes (✉)
Departments of Obstetrics and Gynecology and Urology, New York Medical College, Valhalla, NY, USA
e-mail: dominique.malacarnepape@wmchealth.org; caragrimesmd@gmail.com; cara.grimes@wmchealth.org

Abstract

Defecatory dysfunction describes any difficulty with defecation, excluding anal incontinence. An important distinction is to separate out defecatory dysfunction due to motility issues (stool consistency or colonic inertia) and obstructed defecation (difficult getting stool out once it reaches the rectum). Given the involvement of various anatomical components and the complex coordinated physiology

© Springer Nature Switzerland AG 2023
F. E. Martins et al. (eds.), *Female Genitourinary and Pelvic Floor Reconstruction*,
https://doi.org/10.1007/978-3-031-19598-3_56

required for normal defecation, various subspecialties in medicine are involved in the care of those with defecatory dysfunction with an array of approaches. Evaluation includes history, physical examination, and testing such as anal manometry, defecography, and more. Treatment modalities range from medication and biofeedback to surgical intervention by urogynecologists and/or colorectal surgeons.

Keywords

Defecatory dysfunction · Constipation · Obstructed defecation · Pelvic organ prolapse · Urogynecology

Introduction

Anorectal dysfunction encompasses both anal incontinence and defecatory dysfunction. Anal incontinence, also called accidental bowel leakage, consists of both fecal and flatal incontinence. Fecal incontinence is the involuntary passage of liquid or solid feces. Flatal incontinence is the involuntary passage of flatus. Defecatory dysfunction, however, is a term describing any difficulty with defecation, excluding anal incontinence. Defecatory dysfunction is usually related to anatomic dysfunction and presenting symptoms are splinting, straining, and manual evacuation. The remainder of this chapter will focus on the pathophysiology, evaluation, and treatment of defecatory dysfunction. Various subspecialties in medicine are involved in the care of these patients, each with their own approaches for the evaluation and treatment of this condition.

Definitions

Across specialties, defecatory dysfunction is described in many ways, including constipation or obstructed defecation. An important distinction is to separate out defecatory dysfunction due to motility issues, which is commonly labeled constipation (stool consistency, colonic inertia) and obstructed defecation (difficult getting stool out once it reaches the rectum and is often accompanied by splinting, straining, and/or manual evacuation). Patients often use both of these terms to refer variously to infrequent bowel movements, hard stool consistency, difficult defecation (straining), or behaviors needed to defecate (splinting, manual evacuation). Straining refers to the need for increased intraabdominal pressure through Valsalva maneuvers in order to achieve defecation. Splinting refers to the insertion of a finger in the vagina to apply pressure on the perineum, the wall between the vagina and the rectum, in order to defecate.

Similarly, constipation and difficult defecation are defined differently across specialties. The American College of Gastroenterology Chronic Constipation Task Force and the American Society of Colon and Rectal surgeons define constipation as unsatisfactory defecation characterized by infrequent stool (motility), difficult stool passage (obstructed defecation), or both [1, 2]. The International Continence Society and International Urogynecological Association define constipation as the complaint that bowel movements are infrequent and/or incomplete (motility) and/or there is a need for straining or manual assistance to defecate (obstructed defecation) [3]. The American Urogynecologic Society maintains a symptom-based understanding of defecatory dysfunction.

There are various definitions of forms of defecatory dysfunction by the Rome Foundation. Per the Rome IV criteria, functional constipation is a diagnosis based on the following symptoms for at least 3 months (with symptom onset at least 6 months prior to diagnosis). Patients must experience two or more of the following symptoms: straining during at least 25% of defecation, lumpy or hard stools (Bristol stool scale type 1–2, described further later in this chapter) in at least 25% of defecations, the sensation of incomplete evacuation for at least 25% of defecations, the sensation of anorectal obstruction/blockage for at least 25% of defecations, manual maneuvers to facilitate at least 25% of defecations (e.g., digital evacuation and support of the pelvic floor), or fewer than three defecations per week. Additionally, loose stools must rarely be present in the absence of laxatives and there must be insufficient criteria for a diagnosis of irritable bowel syndrome [4].

To be diagnosed with functional defecation disorders, the patient must meet diagnostic criteria for functional constipation and/or irritable bowel syndrome with constipation. Additionally, during repeated attempts to defecate, there must be features of impaired evacuation, as demonstrated by two of the following three tests: 1-abnormal balloon expulsion tests; 2-abnormal anorectal evacuation pattern with manometry or anal surface EMG; and 3-impaired rectal evacuation by imaging.

Dyssynergic defecation is characterized by the inappropriate contraction of the pelvic floor as observed on office physical exam, measured with anal surface EMG or with manometry with adequate propulsive forces during attempted defecation. Inadequate defecatory propulsion is defined as inadequate propulsive forces as measured with manometry with or without inappropriate contraction of the anal sphincter and/or pelvic floor muscles.

As urogynecologists, we focus on the subset of defecatory dysfunction that includes the symptoms of straining, incomplete emptying, splinting, manual evacuation, digitation that make up obstructed defecation. These can often be attributed to rectal or colon defects, pelvic organ support defects, or defecatory dyssynergia.

Epidemiology

Estimates of the prevalence of chronic constipation in North America have varied between 2–27% depending in part upon the criteria used to define it. A global prevalence of 12–19% (average 15%) has been reported [5, 6]. Among women with pelvic floor disorders, the prevalence of defecatory dysfunction was 60%, compared with 32% of unaffected women. Defecatory dysfunction was associated with neurologic disorders, pelvic floor disorders, depression, pulmonary disease, and pelvic surgery [7]. Given the prevalence and association with pelvic floor disorders and various comorbidities, providers caring for those with defecatory dysfunction should perform a thorough pelvic floor evaluation.

The prevalence of defecatory dysfunction increases with age. In fact, approximately 34% of females over 65 years of age report symptoms of constipation. Severe constipation is more common in elderly women, with rates of constipation two to three times higher than in men [8]. Given this context, it is unsurprising that there is a higher rate of laxative use in the elderly, particularly those living in nursing homes [9]. When adjusting for age, defecatory dysfunction appears to occur more commonly in those with little physical activity, low income, and poor education (defined as having less than 12 years of education) [10]. Additionally, constipation has been shown to frequently affect more nonwhites than whites [11].

Physiology

Before further discussions surrounding the evaluation and management of defecatory dysfunction, it is imperative to approach defecatory dysfunction in a multidisciplinary manner. After stool enters the rectosigmoid, the physical and social settings must be deemed appropriate. Next, the puborectal angle and pelvic floor must become relaxed and the intra-abdominal pressure becomes increased via normal straining efforts. Finally, as the rectum relaxes, defecation can occur voluntarily. In order for this process to occur, a competent anal sphincter complex, intact anorectal sensation, adequate rectal capacity, and conscious control of pelvic floor muscles are required. Given the involvement of all these components, the subspecialties in medicine involved in the care of those with defecatory dysfunction have various approaches for the evaluation and treatment of defecatory dysfunction. The pathophysiology of defecatory dysfunction is also complex. There may be autonomic and pelvic nerve dysfunction, with attenuation of voluntary motor control or impaired anorectal sensation and reflexes. In some cases, there are generalized systemic factors (such as changes in diet and behavior, impaired mobility, psychological issues, or medication side effects) [12]. These are further explored below.

Approach to Care

The focus of the American Urogynecologic Society (AUGS) is on providing guidelines for the diagnosis and treatment of conditions affecting people with the female reproductive system. Their approach to the diagnosis of defecatory dysfunction is based on symptomatology and physical exam. Typically, AUGS does not emphasize imaging modalities as a diagnostic method and takes on a more open-ended approach. The specialty, however, does not emphasize clear management guidelines. In the world of gastroenterology, both male and female patients are considered. Their diagnoses are similarly based on symptoms and physical examinations, mainly the digital rectal exam, but also consider anal manometry, a test that measures how well the rectum and anal sphincters work together to coordinate defecation. Urogynecologists and gastroenterologists manage defecatory dysfunction by utilizing pelvic floor retraining and biofeedback. Given the complicated aforementioned physiology of defecation, it is imperative to consider the evaluation of pelvic floor disorders when considering management routes for those suffering from defecatory dysfunction. Pelvic floor disorders are typically managed by multidisciplinary organizations of colorectal surgeons, urogynecologists, urologists, gynecologists, gastroenterologists, physiotherapists, etc., who collaborate on clinical care as well as research to develop and evaluate educational programs, management guidelines, and algorithms, and promote quality care.

Anatomy

To understand the diagnostic and management approach to defecatory dysfunction, it is important to understand the anatomical structures involved, starting with the posterior vaginal compartment. The posterior vaginal compartment is comprised of the posterior vaginal wall, fibromuscular layers comprising the rectovaginal septum, the levator ani complex, the uterosacral/cardinal ligament complex, perineal body, and associated vasculature and nervous system. Cardinal musculoskeletal components relevant to our discussion of defecatory dysfunction are the internal and external anal sphincters and the puborectalis muscle. The internal anal sphincter (IAS) is a 3–4 cm extension of the colon's smooth muscle; innervated by the autonomic nervous system, it providers 70–85% of the anal canal's resting tone [13]. The external anal sphincter (EAS) consists of striated muscles and is primarily innervated by the somatic nervous system arising from the inferior rectal branch of the pudendal nerve. The EAS contributes to approximately 25% of anal resting pressure. Part of the levator ani muscle group, the puborectalis muscle, is innervated by efferens from S3-S5 nerve roots and the inferior rectal branch of the pudendal nerve, contributing to the prevention of fecal incontinence [14]. Both the EAS and puborectalis muscle can be contracted either voluntarily or as a result of an increase in abdominal pressure. Therefore, contraction of the puborectalis muscle during defecation may lead to impaired evacuation and is a cause of one subset of defecatory dysfunction. When considering the anatomy, it is important to note that for purposes of this discussion the relationship between posterior compartment prolapse and defecation is incompletely understood and is further explored in a different section of this text.

Differential Diagnosis

Causes of defecatory dysfunction vary widely and are often multifactorial. They include systemic issues, obstructive intestinal diseases, as well as medication side effects, which are most commonly related to opioids and anticholinergics. Prior to further exploration of this topic, it is important to recognize that malignancy may also be a cause of chronic defecatory dysfunction Therefore, patients must have colorectal malignancy screening when appropriate. Any patient with alarm symptoms, further discussed under "History," should be referred to GI or colorectal surgery for further evaluation and to rule out malignancy. Chronic defecatory dysfunction not related to systemic issues is either caused by functional disorders (motility) (such as slow transit

Table 1 Causes of chronic defecatory dysfunction

Systemic/drugs	Motility (constipation)	Obstructed defecation

Peripheral nervous system
  Autonomic neuropathy
  Hirschsprung disease
  Chagas disease
Central nervous system
  Multiple sclerosis
  Parkinson's disease
Endocrine
  Hypothyroidism
  Panhypopituitarism
  Diabetes Mellitus
  Hypokalemia
  Hypercalcemia
Psychosocial
  Anorexia nervosa
  Anxiety disorders
  Post-traumatic stress
Drugs
  Opiates
  Anticholinergic
  Cation-containing agents
  Antihypertensives (calcium channel blocks, diuretics)
	Constipation-predominant irritable bowel syndrome
	Functional constipation
	Slow-transit constipation
	Stool consistency
		Posterior compartment prolapse
		Dyssynergic defecation
		Rectal lesions including trauma
		Central nervous system damage
		  Spinal cord injury or lesions
		    Low spinal anesthesia
		    Meningomyelocele

constipation) or anatomical disorders with normal transit (obstructed defecation). Etiologies of defecatory dysfunction can be found in Table 1.

Systemic causes include endocrine (such as hypothyroidism), neurological (such as multiple sclerosis), metabolic disorders (such as hypokalemia), and psychiatric disorders (such as post-traumatic disorder). Medications that can contribute to constipation and decreased bowel motility include antihistamines, antispasmotics, antidepressants, antipsychotics, iron supplements, aluminum-containing agents (i.e., antacids, sucralfate), barium, opiates, antihypertensives, calcium channel blockers, Ganglionic blockers, Vinca alkaloids, and 5HT3 antagonists.

To better understand the causes of decreased colonic motility as they relate to the spinal cord, it is imperative to discuss the nerve supply to the bowel. The distal colon receives its parasympathetic innervation from sacral nerve roots. Transection of these nerves or lesions in the cauda equina may produce decreased colonic motility. These injuries are typically associated with hypomotility, colonic dilatation, decreased rectal tone, and sensation. These findings may also be present in those with injury to the lumbosacral spine, meningomyelocele, or following spinal anesthesia. High spinal cord damage can also cause defecatory dysfunction; however, in these cases, colonic reflexes are intact and defecation can often be triggered by digital stimulation [15].

Functional gastrointestinal disorders refer to various motility issues that may contribute to defecatory dysfunction. These include constipation-predominant irritable bowel syndrome (IBS-C), functional constipation, and colonic inertia (slow transit constipation). Irritable bowel syndrome (IBS) is defined by the Rome IV criteria as recurrent abdominal pain on average occurring at least 1 day per week in the last 3 months and associated with two or more of the following criteria: pain is related to defecation, pain is associated with a change in frequency of stool or associated with a change in form or appearance of stool. When >25% of bowel movements are Bristol stool types 1 and 2 and < 25% of bowel movements are Bristol stool types 6 or 7, this is defined as constipation-predominant IBS [4]. Colonic inertia, another cause of functional constipation, is defined as the delayed passage of radiopaque markers through the proximal colon in the absence of a defecation abnormality. Diagnosis of this condition and explanation of the use of radiopaque markers is further discussed below. Colonic inertia is thought to be related to enteric nerve plexus dysfunction. Decreased volume of interstitial cells of Cajal in the myenteric plexus has been observed in resected colon specimens from patients with colonic inertia who have undergone colon resections and are therefore believed to play a role in colonic motility [16].

Obstructed defecation is defined as incomplete rectal evacuation, which can be related either to dyssynergic defecation or anatomic abnormalities. Obstructed defecation often occurs due to anatomical and structural defects with associated symptoms of straining, incomplete evaluation, splinting, manual evacuation, or digitation. These anatomic disorders are most commonly either caused by gastrointestinal anatomical issues or pelvic floor prolapse. A subset of these defects includes defecatory dyssynergia, which is inadequate propulsion of stool caused by failure of relaxation or increased muscle tone of the external anal sphincter and puborectalis muscles and often occurs in patients with normal transit, colonic inertia, or outlet delay [17].

Gastrointestinal culprits of obstructed defecation include rectal prolapse, neoplasia, anal strictures, anal fissures, prolapsing hemorrhoids, fecal impaction, and trauma. Pelvic organ support defects include posterior compartment prolapse, i.e., posterior vaginal wall prolapse, which is any defect in the posterior vaginal support and can include perineal descent. Posterior compartment prolapse includes rectoceles and enteroceles, which can further be divided into traction and pulsation enteroceles. The term rectocele refers to posterior vaginal wall defects, which allow prolapse of posterior vaginal wall tissue into the lumen of the vagina. The term enterocele refers to posterior apical defects, which are prolapse of the apical portion of the posterior vaginal wall adjacent to the small or large intestine. These include traction enteroceles, where the posterior cul-de-sac is pulled down with the prolapsed cervix or vaginal cuff but is not distended by the intestines and pulsation enterocele, where the intestinal contents of the enteroceles distend the rectovaginal septum and result in a protruding mass. Often the difference between a rectocele and enterocele cannot be positively determined on exam (but can on imaging), thus the term posterior vaginal wall prolapse is preferred over rectocele. Perineal descent refers to the perineum descending greater than or equal to 2 cm below the level of ischial tuberosities at rest or with straining [18]. Traumatic causes of obstructed defecation are beyond the scope of this chapter.

Evaluation

History Taking

An evaluation of any patient with defecatory dysfunction should start with a complete medical and surgical history, including a thorough review of prescribed and over-the-counter medication, family history, and obstetric history. Alarm symptoms concerning for malignancy should further be investigated by GI or colorectal surgery. They include blood in stool, rectal bleeding, unintentional weight loss, bloating, family history of colon cancer or inflammatory bowel disease, anemia, positive fecal occult blood tests, and acute onset of constipation in the elderly [1].

When obtaining patient history, the frequency of bowel movements, stool consistency, ease of defecation, and behaviors surrounding the act of defecation should be further elicited. A helpful tool can be the Bristol stool chart, shown in Table 2, to allow patients to characterize stool consistency. A patient's symptoms can be divided into motility disorder symptoms or obstructed defecation symptoms. Motility disorders are best evaluated and managed by gastroenterologists, as they are functional disorders in nature, while obstructed defecation is best managed by urogynecology or colorectal surgery given these are often anatomical problems with possible surgical solutions. Motility symptoms include bloating and pain, whereas obstructed symptoms include splinting, incomplete defecation, and straining. Straining is defined as making the effort to initiate, maintain, or improve defecation via abdominal straining or Valsalva maneuver to increase

Table 2 Bristol stool chart

Type	Description	Interpretation
Type 1	Severe hard lumps	Very constipated
Type 2	Lumpy and sausage-like	Slightly constipated
Type 3	A sausage shape with cracks in the surface	Normal
Type 4	Smooth, soft sausage or snake	Normal
Type 5	Soft blobs with clear cut edges	Lacking fiber
Type 6	Mushy consistency with ragged edges	Inflammation
Type 7	Liquid consistency with no solid components	Inflammation, diarrhea

intraabdominal pressure. Incomplete emptying or evacuation is when the patient senses the rectum is not empty after attempted defecating. Splinting describes behavior or the need to digitally replace prolapse or apply manual pressure to the vagina or perineum and achieve manual evacuation. Those with prolapse may report vaginal bulge, pelvic pressure, or a dragging sensation. Patients may even experience anorectal pain, incontinence with leakage of liquid feces around areas of hardened stool, or have post-defecatory soiling.

Physical Exam

The physical exam is the most important step in the evaluation of defecatory dysfunction related to posterior vaginal wall prolapse. The physical exam must include a full abdominal, pelvic, and rectal exam. The pelvic exam begins with careful inspection of the anus and perineum. This serves as the first step to assess for any anatomical abnormalities such as scarring, assessment of perineal body length, presence of hemorrhoids, anal warts, or rectal prolapse. An asymmetric anal opening may suggest a neurologic disorder. The rectal examination allows for the assessment of pelvic floor motion during simulated evacuation and is ideally performed before referral to further testing by means of anorectal manometry. The digital rectal exam (DRE) allows the provider to assess for anal sphincter resting tone, sample for blood in the rectum, palpate masses, or assess for fecal impaction. Additionally, subjective assessment is used to judge squeeze pressure while the patient voluntarily contracts the EAS around a gloved finger inserted into the anorectum. Responses of the puborectalis and external anal sphincter muscles may be evaluated by asking the patient to strain. The DRE is reasonably accurate relative to manometry for assessing anal resting tone, squeeze function, and for identifying dyssnergia [19]. Anal reflex can be assessed with a light stroke of a cotton swab to the perineal area, which results in circumferential contractions of the anal skin and external anal sphincter (EAS) in those without nervous system dysfunctions. This aspect of the physical exam allows for the assessment of pudendal nerve injury. Asking the patient to Valsalva by increasing intra-abdominal pressure can allow the provider to observe perineal body descent, vaginal wall prolapse, rectal prolapse, or muscular incoordination. Rectal or vaginal prolapse may also be identified with Valsalva in a squatting position if none is apparent when the patient strains while supine.

There are few standardized assessments of pelvic floor support and prolapse. POP-Q system is an objective system for describing and staging pelvic organ prolapse (POP) [20]. The POP-Q system involves quantitative measurements of various points to assess anterior, apical, and posterior vaginal wall prolapse. The importance of physical examination in assessing patients is further emphasized when discussing the various testing options for assessment of these patients. As discussed below, many of these tools do not correlate well to physical exam findings.

Correlation Between Anatomy and Function

The correlation between specific defecatory symptoms and physical exam findings is not clear. Although they may be present with any anatomic site of prolapse, defecatory symptoms are more commonly associated with posterior or apical prolapse [21]. In one study, those with stage I prolapse were the least likely to require splinting to defecate (8–15%), but the likelihood of splinting did not increase with advanced prolapse. For example, those with stage II prolapse were 21–38% likely to splint and those with stage III-IV prolapse were only 26–29% likely to splint [22].

In another study, women with posterior prolapse greater than or equal to stage 2 were older with higher BMI, higher numbers of births, and overall POP-Q stage than those with stage <2. There was no difference between the groups in terms of defecatory dysfunction, pelvic floor muscle strength, quality of life, or sexual impact. Given the POP-Q stage did not correlate with the degree of defecatory dysfunction the authors concluded that posterior vaginal prolapse is likely not an independent cause of defecatory dysfunction [23].

More recently, a study investigated the prevalence of true rectocele and obstructed defecation in those with pelvic organ prolapse, as well as the correlation between the two. A true rectocele was defined by this study as a discontinuity in the anterior contour of the internal anal sphincter and anterior anorectal muscularis noted on translabial ultrasound. Patients scheduled for surgical intervention for their pelvic organ prolapse without prior history of prior surgery for pelvic reconstruction or posterior vaginal wall repair were included in the study. The presence of posterior vaginal wall prolapse and increased levator-ani hiatus were independent risk factors of obstructed defecation. The presence of posterior vaginal wall prolapse was significantly correlated with straining, digitation, and incomplete emptying [24].

Testing

In order to further delineate the cause of defecatory dysfunction and therefore in order to find the right treatment path, testing beyond the physical exam may be helpful. These include colonoscopy, motility studies, radiography, colonic transit studies, and others.

Colonoscopy

The American Society for Gastrointestinal Endoscopy recommends GI endoscopy for the evaluation of constipation be reserved to the following settings: the presence of alarm symptoms when excluding organic disease if patients have rectal bleeding, heme-positive stool, iron deficiency anemia, weight loss, patients aged 50 years presenting with constipation who have not previously had colon cancer screening, or to allow dilation of benign colon strictures and creation of percutaneous cecostomy when clinically appropriate and feasible [25]. Per the American Society of Colon and Rectal Surgeons, "routine use of blood tests, radiographic examinations, or endoscopy is not typically needed in patients with constipation in the absence of alarming symptoms, screening recommendations, or other significant comorbidities" [26].

Motility Studies

Motility studies such as anal manometry and balloon expulsion should be performed in patients with suspected dyssynergia and/or those whose symptoms are refractory to laxatives.

Anorectal manometry provides a comprehensive understanding of the anal sphincter function at rest and during defecation. Anal sphincter function, maximal resting anal pressure, maximum squeeze pressure, functional anal canal length, rectoanal reflex activity, rectal sensation, and changes in anal and rectal pressures during attempted defecation can be evaluated by this study. Generally, anorectal manometry helps with the diagnosis of dyssynergic defecation (defined as paradoxical contraction or failure of anal relaxation with attempts to empty the rectum of contents), rectal sensory problems, and the assessment of response to biofeedback therapy [27]. It is important to distinguish between diagnoses, as dyssynergic defecation and sensory problems are rarely treated surgically.

Prior to testing, the patient empties their lower gastrointestinal tract with one to two enemas 2 h prior to the start of the study. In the left lateral position with their knees and hips bent, a lubricated pressure-sensitive probe is inserted into the rectum. To assess reflex pathways, a small balloon attached to a catheter is inflated in the rectum. The anal sphincter muscle pressures are measured during the patient's attempted "squeezing, relaxing, and pushing" efforts. Pressures recorded by the rectal balloon indicate intraabdominal pressures and pressures of the anal sphincter transducers indicate relaxation or contraction of the external anal sphincter [28]. Normally, an increase in intrarectal pressure and a decrease in external sphincter pressure occur during expulsion. In those with dyssynergic defecation, however, there is an increase in external sphincter pressure during expulsion.

Manometric diagnostic criteria for dyssynergic defecation include inappropriate contraction of the pelvic floor or more clearly defined as when there is less than 20% relaxation of the resting sphincter pressure with adequate propulsive forces during defecation [29]. With pelvic floor dyssynergia, patients are unable to straighten the anorectal angle during attempted defecation due to failed relaxation of the puborectalis muscle and the EAS. Four types of dyssynergic defecation are recognized: type 1 (increase in anal sphincter pressure with normal pushing), tyle 2 (inadequate pushing with paradoxical anal contraction), type 3 (adequate pushing with absent or incomplete (<20%) sphincter relaxation), and type 4 (inadequate pushing with inadequate anal sphincter relaxation (<20%)).

The balloon expulsion test, which can be performed in conjunction with anal manometry, is performed when a balloon is inserted into the rectum and inflated with water. Balloon expulsion simply assesses a subject's ability to expel stool. Although its methodology has yet to be standardized, it typically involves the expulsion of a 50 mL water-filled balloon to stimulate defecation while measuring the time it takes for balloon expulsion. Given the simplicity of this test, it can be utilized as an independent office screening tool even without anal manometry. If the balloon is expelled in less than 1 min, it is unlikely that dysfunction exists. The sensitivity of the test is 90% and its results are ideally interpreted along with the results of other evaluations [30].

There is no-to-weak correlation between the presence/extent of posterior vaginal wall prolapse and anorectal testing. Artifact due to psychologic factors may affect test results, reflected by the fact that in 20% of healthy controls, the anal sphincter does not relax during attempted defecation as in those with pelvic floor dyssynergia. In issues related to decreased sensation, patients can tolerate higher volumes of stool in the rectum prior to reporting or experiencing any pressure or pain and prior to the desire to defecate. This is associated with increased rectal compliance, seen in those with fecal impaction.

Colonic manometry evaluates intraluminal pressure activity of the colon and rectum. This study can be combined with a barostat apparatus to assess colonic tone, compliance, and sensation [28]. Although there is no evidence of the added value of this test to the management of defecatory dysfunction, it allows patients to be categorized as having normal, myopathic, or neuropathic colon.

Defecography
According to AUGS, although imaging is not a routine part of the evaluation, it may be considered when symptoms do not correlate to physical exam findings or when surgical intervention does not provide symptomatic relief. A few modalities exist in the realm of imaging for the evaluation of defecatory dysfunction and are discussed in detail here. Defecography is a radiological examination most helpful when investigating potential anatomic causes of symptoms (such as enteroceles and intussusceptions) in the event of obstructed defecation or when anal manometry is inconclusive.

One form of defecography is fluoroscopic defecography. It is performed by placing approximately 150 mL of barium into the rectum and asking the patient to squeeze, cough, and Valsalva while sitting on a commode. Evacuation is then monitored by fluoroscopy or videotape, which allows for assessment of the anorectum at rest and during expulsion. During this exam, the anorectal junction (ARJ) and the anorectal angle (ARA) are measured. ARJ is defined as the uppermost point of the anal canal and is measured in relationship to a bony part of the pelvis (i.e., ischial tuberosity or the pubococcygeal line). The migration of the ARJ is thought to indirectly represent the elevation and descent of the pelvic floor, which is considered normal when it is <3.5 cm relative to its resting position. ARA is an angle between the longitudinal axis of the anal canal and the longitudinal axis of the rectum, averaging 90°. The ARA is an indirect indicator of puborectal muscle activity, becoming more acute with muscle contraction (75°) and more obtuse with relaxation [31]. Pelvic floor dyssynergia is diagnosed by the presence of insufficient descent of the perineum (<1 cm) and less than a normal change in the anorectal angle (<15°).

A Consensus Definitions and Interpretation Templates for Fluoroscopic Imaging of Defecatory Pelvic Floor Disorders by the Pelvic Floor Disorders Consortium was recently published with varying points of consensus [32]. The relevant points are summarized in the following statements in this text. Given findings of defecography are highly dependent on patient effort, the quality of effort should be reported to provide context. A radiopaque marker on the perineal body can serve as an anatomic reference. While static images at rest should be obtained, the examination is ideally performed under fluoroscopic evaluation rather than static radiographs. While vaginal contrast is recommended, bladder contrast is not routinely needed. Small-bowel contrast (i.e., oral contrast) can be used to identify enterocele.

Another form of defecography is the dynamic MRI defecography. It is obtained in the supine position and assesses a patient's global pelvic floor anatomy. This imaging modality provides information about muscles and fibromuscular tissue of the pelvic floor at rest, during squeezing, straining, and/or defecation. However, it has been shown that MRI defecography has uncertain clinical value compared to fluoroscopic defecography described above. A meta-analysis comparing dynamic MRI imaging and POP-Q stage concluded that MRI has not yet been properly validated but may be able to more accurately assess the posterior compartment, particularly when considering enterocele and rectal intussusceptions [33].

A Consensus Definitions and Interpretation Templates for Magnetic Resonance Imaging of Defecatory Pelvic Floor Disorders by the Pelvic Floor Disorders Consortium was also recently published [34]. The relevant points are summarized in the following statements. Similar to fluoroscopic defecography, the quality of MRI defecography is highly dependent on patient cooperation and effort. As such, patients should be educated on the steps of this diagnostic tool. Patient effort should be reported to better assess in interpretation of the data and provide the appropriate clinical context. Rectal contrast and defecation are essential for MRI defecography. Therefore, patients should be coached to attempt defecation. Following defecation, the degree of evacuation should be assessed subjectively as a function of initial rectal volume. The presence and location of contrast retention during maximal defecatory effort should be described.

Unfortunately, definitions of rectocele based on defecography vary widely with 48% of nulliparous asymptomatic women demonstrating rectocele on defecography. This, in general, has a weak correlation between POP-Q and function/patient symptoms [35]. It is important to note that defecography should be used in tandem with a thorough examination in order to arrive at the appropriate treatment options for the patient.

Colonic Transit Studies

Colon transit studies are indicated if patients are refractory to conservative management or if anorectal testing does not show defecatory disorder. The radiopaque marker study, mentioned above during the explanation and definition of colonic inertia, is commonly performed by measuring the movement of radiopaque markers through the bowel. The patient is instructed to ingest a high fiber diet (20–30 g/day) while abstaining from any medications that may affect bowel function for 2–3 days prior to the study. Radiopaque markers are swallowed and their passage monitored by radiographs over the course of multiple days. In those with slow transit constipation, movement of markers in the right or left colon is delayed, while in those with outlet delay, markers stagnate once in the rectum. Retention of more than five markers on day 6 of the study is considered abnormal and suggestive of slow transit constipation, although this diagnosis should only be made after excluding dyssynergia via the use of anal manometry [36].

Wireless motility capsule is a well-tolerated study for the analysis of colonic transit. The test has good compliance from patients and avoids the risks of radiation exposure. Similar to the radiopaque marker study, the wireless motility capsule allows the provider to differentiate slow from normal colonic transit. The test is validated against the radiopaque marker test in patients with chronic constipation [37].

Others

Other studies include barium enemas, EMG, or transperineal ultrasonography. These studies are yet to be validated due to the lack of control groups and precise definitions of physical anatomy. Pelvic floor ultrasonography, an inexpensive imaging modality available in the outpatient office setting, allows for imaging of the bladder, cervix or vaginal vault, and rectum. Ultrasonography can be done at rest and maximal strain in order to differentiate between rectoceles and enteroceles. However, a poor correlation exists between perineal ultrasonography and POP-Q [38].

While these modalities may be useful in understanding the anatomy of the posterior compartment, the cost of these techniques needs to be considered against their clinical utility. Other tests include a breath test for intestinal methanogen overgrowth. Although it's unclear if treatment can improve constipation, there is an association between methane-producing organisms and constipation [39]. Another test that can be performed is the rectal barostat test, where a compliant balloon is inserted into the rectum and connected to a computerized pressure distending device, which can detect rectal hypersensitivity in patients with IBS-C. However, clinical significance remains uncertain.

Management

As previously discussed, the gastroenterology approach to the understanding of defecatory dysfunction is systemic and functional, colorectal surgery's approach is focused on the mechanical function of the rectum, and the gynecologist's approach is on the relationship of the pelvic organs, ligaments, and pelvic floor muscle function. Often patients benefit from a multidisciplinary approach. Despite these differences, conservative first-line management starts with dietary modification and medications for all specialties. Management options range from medications, behavioral, biofeedback, and surgical intervention. The approach to management should remain focused on symptoms rather than on findings found from imaging studies as some imaging findings, such as rectoceles or enteroceles, do not require treatment when found in asymptomatic patients.

Behavioral Modification and Biofeedback

Among management methods for defecatory dysfunction are behavior modification and biofeedback therapy, which can be a first-line treatment for symptomatic dyssynergia [26]. Due to the physiology of eating, defecation, and the gastrorectal reflex, patients should be advised to attempt defecation after eating, especially in the morning, and to take advantage of this physiological response to benefit from the timely increased colonic motility to aid in successful defecation [40]. An important aspect of behavioral modification to encourage defecation is positioning. Patients should be encouraged to use stools to correctly position themselves with their knees slightly more elevated than the hips, allowing the puborectalis muscle to relax and straighten the rectum. Finally, patients can splint or manually evacuate stool if needed. Although habit training has been used in children, a modified program may also be helpful in adults with neurogenic constipation, dementia, or those with physical impairments.

Treatment plans utilizing biofeedback techniques teach patients to better identify, contract, and relax their pelvic floor muscles by using anorectal manometry as a tool. Although this tool is not standardized, the general focus is on the patient watching recordings of sphincter activity or pressure and modifying inappropriate responses through trial and error. Biofeedback can alleviate inappropriate contraction of pelvic floor muscle groups including the external anal sphincter, with success rates as high as 70–80% in alleviating symptoms of chronic constipation. Compared to patient education, nutritional counseling, exercise combined with laxative use, laxative use alone, biofeedback has been shown to be the best treatment for those with at least a component of defecatory dyssynergia [28, 41]. While biofeedback benefits two-thirds of patients with dyssynergic defecation who have coexisting slow transit constipation, it does not appear to benefit patients with slow transit constipation without some component of dyssynergic defecation [41].

Medications

Per the American Society of Colon and Rectal Surgeons, the initial management of symptomatic constipation/hard stools is dietary modification, including fiber and fluid supplementation [26]. Dietary modifications, such as the incorporation of fiber supplementation, can improve symptoms of constipation/hard stools. For example, the fiber found in citrus fruits and legumes stimulates the growth of colonic flora, thereby increasing fecal mass. Wheat bran is one of the more effective fiber laxatives. The recommended amount of dietary fiber is 20–35 grams per day. However, for some patients (and especially almost all those with slow transit constipation or irritable bowel syndrome that is constipation-predominant), fiber increases bloating and distention, leading to poor compliance.

Bulk forming agents may be used for the treatment of constipation. They are natural or synthetic polysaccharides or cellulose and absorb water, therefore increasing fecal mass. Side effects of these drugs include impaction above structures, fluid overload, gas, and bloating. Examples include Psyllium (Metamucil), methylcellulose (Citrucel), Polycarbophil (FiberCon), and wheat dextrin (Benefir). Objective evidence for the use of these medications is insufficient [42, 43].

Surfactants are stool softeners and work by lowering the surface tension of stool such that more water enters the stool. These drugs are well tolerated. However, there is little evidence to support their use. Docusate sodium (Colace) and docusate calcium are examples [42, 43]. The use of stimulant laxatives, such as bisacodyl (Dulcolax) or senna (Senokot), for chronic constipation/hard stools is reasonable in the short term as a second-line treatment [26]. They work by altering the electrolyte transport within intestinal mucosa and increasing intestinal motility.

Osmotic laxatives, such as polyethylene glycol and lactulose, are also appropriate for the management of constipation/hard stools. They work by increasing intestinal water secretion and increasing stool frequency. These medications should be used with caution in those with renal or cardiac dysfunction as they may cause electrolyte derangements and fluid overload. Agents in this class include polyethylene glycol (GoLYTLEY, MiraLAX), lactulose (Enulose), Sorbitol, Glycerin, magnesium sulfate (milk of magnesia), and magnesium citrate. Some of these drugs may cause abdominal bloating, cramping, nausea, and watery stools [42, 43].

The use of newer agents, such as lubiprostone and linaclotide, may be considered in those refractory to osmotic and stimulant laxatives [26].

Surgery

Surgical management of defecatory dysfunction is targeted toward the cause of defecatory dysfunction. As previously discussed, defecatory dysfunction can be viewed as either a motility issue (constipation) or as a result of pelvic floor anatomy (obstructed defecation). Defecatory dysfunction related to obstructed defecation can be managed by urogynecologists or colorectal surgeons through repair of the posterior compartment or repair of rectal prolapse. Constipation thought to be related to motility that is chronic, severe, and refractory to medication may be managed by colorectal surgery via bowel resections in the most extreme cases. These are further discussed in this section.

For the patient with obstructed defecation, they may be evaluated by urogynecologists for the repair of the posterior compartment. Despite the weak correlation between defecatory dysfunction symptoms and posterior vaginal wall prolapse, patients with posterior vaginal prolapse who report splinting or straining do benefit from surgical repair of their prolapse. The goal of surgery is often to correct a posterior vaginal wall defect that may be contributing to pocketing and/or trapping of stool. A systematic review of posterior compartment surgery to treat bulge and obstructed defecation demonstrated that surgery of the posterior compartment, especially a native tissue posterior colporrhaphy, typically has a high rate of success for obstructed defecation and bulge symptoms. However, long-term data is limited [44].

Repair of the posterior compartment involves the repair of the fibromuscular layer of the posterior vaginal wall. Transvaginal approaches to the repair of posterior prolapse include traditional posterior colporrhaphy, site-specific repair, and graft augmentation.

Traditional native tissue posterior colporrhaphy is the midline plication of the fibromuscular layer of the posterior vaginal wall with sutures. Posterior colporrhaphy has success rates for anatomic restoration of 76–98% [45]. Lidocaine with epinephrine or vasopressin is typically injected under the vaginal mucosa for hydrodissection and hemostasis. This is often accompanied by a perinorrhaphy. For this, the bulbocavernosus muscles and transverse perineal muscles are plicated in the midline of the perineal body with interrupted 0 polyglactin sutures. Although a perineorrhaphy can slightly increase the functional length of the posterior vaginal wall, if performed aggressively, it can constrict the introitus, resulting in dyspareunia. To finish the posterior colporrhaphy, the vaginal epithelium is opened in the midline, extending the incision to an area superior to the defect. The posterior vaginal epithelium is dissected from the fibromuscularis layer until the levator muscles are visualized. The posterior vaginal wall now stripped of its epithelium is then plicated in the midline with interrupted vertical or transverse sutures that incorporate the fibromuscularis, beginning proximally and working toward the hymen. A rectal examination should be performed in order to ensure no rectal injury. The vaginal epithelium is trimmed if necessary and closed with a running 2–0 absorbable suture [46].

Site-specific posterior vaginal repair is the repair of the fibromuscular layer while also identifying and repairing individual-specific defects. Site-specific repairs have a success rate for anatomic restoration of 56–100% [45]. Defects in the posterior vaginal wall may occur as an isolated defect in the lateral, midline, or superior portions of the wall. Some occur as a combination of these defects. The vaginal epithelial is exposed in the same fashion as in a posterior colporrhaphy as described above. The posterior vaginal epithelium is dissected away from the underlying fibromuscularis, which is then carefully inspected to identify any defects. Irrigation and/or a rectal exam may be considered to aid in ease of identification of these defects, which are then individually isolated and repaired with a delayed-absorbable 0 or 2–0 suture [46].

Another method to repair the posterior compartment is a levator plication or levatorrhaphy. This is the plication of the levator ani muscle toward the midline, incorporating a portion of the lateral fibromuscular layer of the posterior vaginal wall [47]. Posterior vaginal wall prolapse repair can include a levator myorrhaphy or a plication of the levator ani muscles. Sutures are placed into the levator ani muscles, incorporating a portion of the lateral posterior fibromuscularis. This is typically a better option for older adult women with a wide levator hiatus who do not desire future sexual intercourse.

Posterior vaginal repair with graft is the reinforcement of the fibromuscular layer of the posterior vaginal wall with implanted graft material [47]. There is no evidence, however, to support the routine use of grafts (biologic or mesh) in the posterior compartment to improve anatomical or symptomatic outcomes [45]. Pre-cut mesh kit procedures have been developed by commercial companies for the repair of posterior vaginal wall prolapse and other prolapse sites. However, transvaginal mesh kits for the treatment of prolapse are now off the market in many countries.

Previously, a double-Stapled Trans-Anal Rectal Resection (STARR) procedure, where a device is inserted rectally and used to excise the rectal mucosa and area of the rectocele with anastomose of the edges, was used by colorectal surgeons for chronic refractory defecatory dysfunction related to rectoceles. However, most recently, as per The American Society of Colon and Rectal Surgeons' guidelines, transrectal stapled repair of rectoceles and rectal intussusception is typically not recommended because of the high rate of complications including rectovaginal fistula, painful defecation, and strictures [26].

For patients with concomitant rectal prolapse or herniation of the sigmoid colon, sigmoidectomy, and/or rectopexy can be considered by colorectal surgeons. Rectopexy is the fixation of the rectum to the sacrum to restore its anatomic position and improve mechanical functioning. This can be performed with suturing, staples, or biologic or synthetic mesh. If a redundant sigmoid is found to be prolapsing into the posterior compartment, a sigmoid resection can be performed at the time of rectopexy., which can be performed with suturing, staples, or biologic or synthetic mesh [45]. Typically, fixing the anatomic defect has been shown to improve, not completely resolve, defecatory symptoms [45].

Patients with refractory colonic slow-transit constipation (i.e., an issue of motility) may benefit from total abdominal colectomy with ileorectal anastomosis. Surgical repair of rectal intussusception may be considered in these patients. Although not a common management strategy, antegrade colonic enema with appendicostomy or cecostomy may also be effective in patients with refractory constipation. Completion proctectomy, on the other hand, is typically not recommended. Another option for patients who either failed or are not candidates for available treatment methods for intractable constipation due to decreased motility is fecal diversion with an ileostomy or colostomy [26].

Subtotal colectomy with ileorectal anastomosis has been used in certain cases and shown to alleviate incapacitating constipation [48]. In one study, 74 patients with severe slow-transit constipation underwent colectomy and ileorectostomy. Postoperative complications included, most commonly, small bowel obstruction (found in 9% of participants) and prolonged ileus (found in 12% of participants). Most of the patients, 97% specifically, in the study were satisfied with the results and 90% even reported improved quality of life during a mean follow-up of 56 months. In general, it is understood by most colorectal surgeons that some criteria should be met prior to consideration of these kinds of complex, high-risk surgical interventions as these patients must be carefully selected. The following five criteria must be met; patients must 1) have chronic, severe, and disabling symptoms that are refractory to medication, 2) have slow colonic inertia, 3) not have intestinal pseudo-obstruction based on radiologic or manometric studies, 4) not have pelvic floor dysfunction based on any of the diagnostic tools mentioned above, and 5) not have abdominal pain as the prominent symptom.

Others

Other forms of treatment for defecatory dysfunction include acupuncture and neuromodulation. At least one non-blinded randomized trial supports the use of acupuncture for chronic functional constipation using the Rome criteria, though long-term benefit has yet to be determined [49]. Sacral neuromodulation may also be effective for patients with chronic constipation when patients have a successful peripheral nerve evaluation test and conservative measures have failed. However, in one long-term study, the benefit was only observed in a minority of patients. The study also noted high dropout rates and high complication rates during the follow-up period. Adverse events reported included abdominal pain, constipation, implant site pain, device dislocation, as well as musculoskeletal and nerve pain [50].

Conclusion

Due to the various anatomical components and complex coordinated physiology required for normal defecation, multiple specialties are involved in the care of patients with defecatory dysfunction. Defecatory dysfunction can be split into two generalized categories, either related to motility or obstructed defecation. Motility issues are related to stool consistency or colonic inertia (constipation) whereas obstructed defecation is related to anatomical abnormalities. Evaluation includes the physical examination and if symptoms do not resolve with medications, anorectal manometry, defecography, or colonic transit studies may be conducted to better delineate the cause of dysfunction. Treatment modalities range from conservative measures with biofeedback and medication to surgical intervention by urogynecologists for the repair of the posterior compartment. Colorectal surgeons may also be involved in the care of these patients with treatment plans as extensive as bowel resection and colostomy creation. With an interdisciplinary approach to patient care, patients can be optimally evaluated and educated about the etiologies behind their symptoms, and in turn, can be offered a comprehensive approach to optimal treatment modalities.

Cross-References

► Clinical Evaluation of the Female Lower Urinary Tract and Pelvic Floor
► Management of Vaginal Posterior Compartment Prolapse: Is There Ever a Case for Graft/Mesh?
► Management of Fecal Incontinence, Constipation, and Rectal Prolapse
► Neuroanatomy and Neurophysiology

References

1. Brandt LJ, Prather CM, Quigley EMM, Schiller LR, Schoenfeld P, Talley NJ. Systematic review on the management of chronic constipation in North America. Am J Gastroenterol. 2005;100:s5–s21.
2. Ternent CA, Bastawrous AL, Morin NA, Ellis NC, Hyman NH, Buie DW. Practice parameters for the evaluation and management of constipation. Dis Colon Rectum. 2007;50:2013–22.
3. Haylen BT, de Ridder D, Freeman RM, et al. An International Urogynecological Association (iuga)/international continence society (ICS) joint report on the terminology for female pelvic floor dysfunction. Neurourol Urodyn. 2009;29:4–20.
4. Rome IV criteria. In: Rome foundation. Appendix A: Rome IV Diagnostic Criteria for FGIDs; 2020. https://theromefoundation.org/rome-iv/rome-ivcriteria/
5. Higgins PD, Johanson JF. Epidemiology of constipation in North America: a systematic review. Am J Gastroenterol. 2004;99(4):750–9.
6. Suares NC, Ford AC. Prevalence of, and risk factors for, chronic idiopathic constipation in the community: systematic review and meta-analysis. Am J Gastroenterol. 2011;106(9):1582–91.
7. Whitcomb EL, Lukacz ES, Lawrence JM, Nager CW, Luber KM. Prevalence of defecatory dysfunction in women with and without pelvic floor disorders. J Pelvic Med Surg. 2009;15:179–87.
8. Talley NJ, Weaver AL, Zinsmeister AR, Melton LJ. Functional constipation and outlet delay: a population-based study. Gastroenterology. 1993;105:781–90.
9. Harari D, Gurwitz JH, Avorn J, Choodnovskiy I, Minaker KL. Constipation: assessment and management in an institutionalized elderly population. J Am Geriatr Soc. 1994;42:947–52.
10. Sandler RS, Jordan MC, Shelton BJ. Demographic and dietary determinants of constipation in the US population. Am J Public Health; 1990.
11. Johanson JF, Sonnenberg A, Koch TR. Clinical epidemiology of chronic constipation. J Clin Gastroenterol. 1989;11:525–36.
12. Preziosi G, Emmanuel A. Neurogenic bowel dysfunction: pathophysiology, clinical manifestations and treatment. Expert Rev Gastroenterol Hepatol. 2009;3:417–23.
13. Frenckner B, Euler CV. Influence of pudendal block on the function of the anal sphincters. Gut. 1975;16:482–9.
14. Barber MD, Bremer RE, Thor KB, Dolber PC, Kuehl TJ, Coates KW. Innervation of the female levator ani muscles. Am J Obstet Gynecol. 2002;187:64–71.
15. Rao SSC, Camilleri M. Approach to the patient with constipation. In: Yamada's textbook of gastroenterology; 2015, pp. 757–780.
16. He CL, Burgart L, Wang L, Pemberton J, Young–Fadok T, Szurszewski J, Farrugia G. Decreased interstitial cell of Cajal volume in patients with slow-transit constipation. Gastroenterology. 2000;118:14–21.
17. Voderholzer WA, Neuhaus DA, Klauser AG, Tzavella K, Müller-Lissner SA, Schindlbeck NE. Paradoxical sphincter contraction is rarely indicative of anismus. Gut. 1997;2:258–62.
18. Grimes CL, Lukacz ES. Posterior vaginal compartment prolapse and defecatory dysfunction: Are they related? Int Urogynecol J. 2012;23:537–51.
19. Tantiphlachiva K, Rao P, Attaluri A, Rao SSC. Digital rectal examination is a useful tool for identifying patients with Dyssynergia. Clin Gastroenterol Hepatol. 2010;11:955–60.
20. Bump RC, Mattiasson A, Bø K, Brubaker LP, DeLancey JOL, Klarskov P, Shull BL, Smith ARB. The standardization of terminology of female pelvic organ prolapse and pelvic floor dysfunction. Am J Obstet Gynecol. 1996;1:10–7.
21. Ellerkmann RM, Cundiff GW, Melick CF, Nihira MA, Leffler K, Bent AE. Correlation of symptoms with location and severity of pelvic organ prolapse. Am J Obstet Gynecol. 2001;6:1332–8.
22. Tan JS, Lukacz ES, Menefee SA, Powell CR, Nager CW. Predictive value of prolapse symptoms: a large database study. Int Urogynecol J. 2004;6:203–9.
23. Augusto KL, Bezerra LR, Murad-Regadas SM, Vasconcelos Neto JA, Vasconcelos CT, Karbage SA,

Bilhar AP, Regadas FS. Defecatory dysfunction and fecal incontinence in women with or without posterior vaginal wall prolapse as measured by pelvic organ prolapse quantification (pop-Q). Eur J Obstetr Gynecol Reprod Biol. 2017;214:50–5.
24. Tan C, Geng J, Tang J, Yang X. The relationship between obstructed defecation and true rectocele in patients with pelvic organ prolapse. Sci Rep. 2020;10:1.
25. Cash BD, Acosta RD, Chandrasekhara V, Chathadi KV, Eloubeidi MA, Fanelli RD, Faulx AL, Fonkalsrud L, Khashab MA, Lightdale JR, Muthusamy VR, Pasha SF, Saltzman JR, Shaukat A, Wang A. The role of endoscopy in the management of constipation. Gastrointest Endosc. 2014;4:563–5.
26. Paquette IM, Varma M, Ternent C, Melton-Meaux G, Rafferty JF, Feingold D, Steele SR. The American Society of Colon and Rectal Surgeons' clinical practice guideline for the evaluation and management of constipation. Dis Colon Rectum. 2016;6:479–92.
27. Rao SSC. Dyssenergic defecation and biofeedback therapy. Gastroenterol Clin N Am. 2008;3:569–86.
28. Rao SSC, Singh S. Clinical utility of Colonic and anorectal manometry in chronic constipation. J Clin Gastroenterol. 2010;9:597–609.
29. Bharucha AE, Wald A, Enck P, Rao S. Functional anorectal disorders. Gastroenterology. 2006;5:1510–8.
30. Minguez M, Herreros B, Sanchiz V, Hernandez V, Almela P, Añon R, Mora F, Benages A. Predictive value of the balloon expulsion test for excluding the diagnosis of pelvic floor dyssynergia in constipation. Gastroenterology. 2004;1:57–62.
31. Ridgeway BM, Weinstein MM, Tunitsky-Bitton E. American urogynecologic society best-practice statement on evaluation of obstructed defecation. Female Pelvic Med Reconstr Surg. 2018;6:383–91.
32. Paquette I, Rosman D, Sayed RE, Hull T, Kocjancic E, Quiroz L, Palmer S, Shobeiri A, Weinstein M, Khatri G, Bordeianou L. Consensus definitions and interpretation templates for fluoroscopic imaging of defecatory pelvic floor disorders. Tech Coloproctol. 2021;1:3–17.
33. Broekhuis SR, Fütterer JJ, Barentsz JO, Vierhout ME, Kluivers KB. A systematic review of clinical studies on dynamic magnetic resonance imaging of pelvic organ prolapse: the use of reference lines and anatomical landmarks. Int Urogynecol J. 2009;6:721–9.
34. Gurland BH, Khatri G, Ram R, Hull TL, Kocjancic E, Quiroz LH, El Sayed RF, Jambhekar KR, Chernyak V, Mohan Paspulati R, Sheth VR, Steiner AM, Kamath A, Shobeiri SA, Weinstein MM, Bordeianou L. Consensus definitions and interpretation templates for magnetic resonance imaging of defecatory pelvic floor disorders. Dis Colon Rectum. 2021;10:1184–97.
35. Shorvon PJ, McHugh S, Diamant NE, Somers S, Stevenson GW. Defecography in normal volunteers: results and implications. Gut. 1989;12:1737–49.
36. Hinton JM, Lennard-Jones JE, Young AC. A new method for studying gut transit times using Radio-opaque markers. Gut. 1969;10:842–7.
37. Tran K, Brun R, Kuo B. Evaluation of regional and whole gut motility using the wireless motility capsule: Relevance in clinical practice. Ther Adv Gastroenterol. 2012;5:249–60.
38. Broekhuis SR, Kluivers KB, Hendriks JC, Fütterer JJ, Barentsz JO, Vierhout ME. Pop-Q, dynamic MR imaging, and perineal ultrasonography: do they agree in the quantification of female pelvic organ prolapse? Int Urogynecol J. 2009;5:541–9.
39. Pimentel M, Saad RJ, Long MD, Rao SS. ACG clinical guideline: small intestinal bacterial overgrowth. Am J Gastroenterol. 2020;2:165–78.
40. Gosselink MJ, Schouten WR. The gastrorectal reflex in women with obstructed defecation. Int J Color Dis. 2001;2:112–8.
41. Chiarioni G, Whitehead WE, Pezza V, Morelli A, Bassotti G. Biofeedback is superior to laxatives for normal transit constipation due to pelvic floor dyssynergia. Gastroenterology. 2006;3:657–64.
42. Ramkumar D, Rao SSC. Efficacy and safety of traditional medical therapies for chronic constipation: systematic review. Am J Gastroenterol. 2005;4:936–71.
43. Bharucha AE, Pemberton JH, Locke GR. American Gastroenterological Association technical review on constipation. Gastroenterology. 2013;1:218–38.
44. Grimes CL, Schimpf MO, Wieslander CK, Sleemi A, Doyle P, Wu Y. Surgical interventions for posterior compartment prolapse and obstructed defecation symptoms: a systematic review with clinical practice recommendations. Int Urogynecol J. 2019;9:1433–54.
45. Brown H, Grimes C. Current trends in management of defecatory dysfunction, posterior compartment prolapse, and fecal incontinence. Curr Obstetr Gynecol Rep. 2016;2:165–71.
46. Hoffman BL, Schorge JO, Bradshaw KD, Halvorson LM, Schaffer M, Corton MM. Williams gynecology. McGraw-Hill, New York; 2016.
47. Joint Writing Group of the American Urogynecologic Society and the International Urogynecological Association. Female Pelvic Med Reconstr Surg. 2020;3:173–201.
48. Nyam DC, Pemberton JH, Ilstrup DM, Rath DM. Long-term results of surgery for chronic constipation. Dis Colon Rectum. 1997;5:529.
49. Liu Z, Liu J, Zhao Y, Cai Y, He L, Xu H, Zhou X, Yan S, Lao L, Liu B. The efficacy and safety study of electro-acupuncture for severe chronic functional constipation: study protocol for a multicenter, randomized, controlled trial. Trials. 2013;1:176.
50. Maeda Y, Kamm MA, Vaizey CJ, Matzel KE, Johansson C, Rosen H, Baeten CG, Laurberg S. Long-term outcome of sacral neuromodulation for chronic refractory constipation. Tech Coloproctol. 2017;4:277–86.

Management of Fecal Incontinence, Constipation, and Rectal Prolapse

56

Johannes Kurt Schultz and Tom Øresland

Contents

Introduction	1014
Multidisciplinary Approach	1014
Pathophysiological Considerations During Workup	1015
Taking the Patient History	1016
Clinical Examination by Nonspecialists	1016
Clinical Examination by the Proctologist	1016
Imaging	1017
Special Investigations	1019
The Use of Special Investigations	1021
Primary Treatment	1021
Further Treatment Options in Incontinence	1022
Further Treatment Options in Constipation	1025
Rectal Prolapse	1025
Conclusion	1027
Cross-References	1027
References	1028

Cartoons are by courtesy of Jansen Pharma Sweden and by the authors

J. K. Schultz (✉)
Department of GI Surgery, Akershus University Hospital, Lørenskog, Norway
e-mail: josc@ahus.no

T. Øresland
Faculty of Medicine University of Oslo, Oslo, Norway
e-mail: tom.oresland@medisin.uio.no

Abstract

The management of fecal incontinence, constipation, and rectal prolapse needs to be based on a thorough patient history since there is an abundance of causes and hence treatments for these problems. Fecal incontinence and constipation are the most challenging of the three conditions to treat whereas rectal prolapse is a more confined entity where surgery is the treatment of choice for the majority of patients, although there are numerous surgical options. The vast majority of patients seeking advice for fecal incontinence or constipation will not be advised surgery. There are a multiple of factors and organ systems that may be involved in these conditions and the role of the therapist is first to seek out these factors in the individual patient. One should also note that urinary and sexual dysfunction is often present concomitantly and a multidisciplinary team approach is therefore often indicated. The management often needs to be directed toward multiple causes. The treatment options include behavioral or cognitive therapies, dietary interventions, pharmacological options, toilet habit instructions, physical activity, bio-feedback interventions, nerve modulation, and, in some cases, of fecal incontinence surgical interventions on the pelvic floor and sphincter muscles. In a very limited number of constipated patients, surgery may be an option. Possible surgical solutions are pelvic nerve modulation, appendicostomy, or resections (most frequently colectomy and ileorectal anastomosis). One of the essential components of management of incontinence and constipation is to give the patient a realistic goal of what can be achieved. Part of this is to undertake the necessary investigations, to give the patients a feeling of being fully understood, and enable them to better cope with their condition.

Keywords

Fecal incontinence · Constipation · Rectal prolapse · Conservative management · Surgery

Introduction

In this chapter on management of fecal incontinence, constipation, and rectal prolapse the layout is first to give information on the essential need of taking a good and comprehensive patient history. For constipation and incontinence this needs to be in depth and cover all aspects of the bowel function. Furthermore, the use of investigations will be discussed. Treatment options are manifold and have to be individualized depending on the symptoms and findings.

Patients with defecation disorders are often reluctant to seek health care; there is still a lot of shame associated with problems related to bowel emptying. Public knowledge in this area is scarce and patients often lack words to describe their concerns. When a patient seeks your help for problems with hemorrhoids, hemorrhoids frequently are not the cause of the complaints. History and physical examination might reveal anything from a rectal cancer to perianal dermatitis. Many patients have a very long history of meandering through the health care system without getting adequate help. This is on part of the doctors that do not understand the conditions and lack the ability to put themselves in the patient's situation. A typical scenario is that patients first towards the end of a consultation for something else dare to mention their "hemorrhoids" and the stressed doctor who accepts this as a fact prescribes an ointment. In the worst case, the patient shows up with an incurable rectal cancer some month later. Another scenario is that the doctor "downgrades" the severity of the problem due to lack of knowledge how to do or request the right investigations and consequently fails to act upon the patient's problem. The patient is disappointed and lives on until she meets the next doctor who just may "supplement" with some investigation without addressing the problem and so on... These patients tend not only to be devoid of adequate treatment but they also accumulate quite large costs to society due to health care consumption and working disabilities.

Multidisciplinary Approach

The fact that a good proportion of patients with defecation disorders also has urinary dysfunction with or without sexual dysfunction makes it necessary to handle many of them in multidisciplinary teams or pelvic floor centers [1, 2]. These centers can be organized in different ways. The optimum might be that all involved parties are working in the same physical unit with direct communication across the corridor. Another variant is to have regular conferences involving all parties, the aim being to organize investigations and treatment at the involved departments in a "one stop model" if possible. Depending on the resources available, the centers might include urologists, gynecologists, colorectal surgeons, gastroenterologists, psychiatrists, sexologists, physiotherapists, neurologists, enterostoma therapists, uro-therapists, and sociologists. Usually the patient is initially referred to one of the involved parties for a first visit, it can then be decided if a multidisciplinary approach is needed. Such centers are now established in tertiary care hospitals in many countries. Their mission is not only to treat individual patients but also to educate health care workers and the public. Modern media is most often utilized to spread their messages. Another big task is to promote and conduct research in the fields of pelvic floor problems. Multidisciplinary research spanning all or at least more than one part of the pelvic floor functions is indeed very rare. Studies on pelvic floor, functioning has not been a very hot subject for upcoming researchers and our knowledge compared to other parts of the body is scarce.

Pathophysiological Considerations During Workup

Figure 1 depicts the major causative factors in incontinence but also to a large degree in the case of obstipation; all these have to be addressed when taking the patient history. Some factors might have to be addressed by doing rectoanal physiology testing and endoscopies. However, the patient can give hints of physiology abnormalities, e.g., do you feel rectal filling and urge before emptying your bowels or does it just happen without any warning? This gives an indication of whether rectal sensation is normal or not. If you go very often to the toilet, is this because of urge and/or tenesmus or is it to avoid episodes of leakage? The answer might be indicative of a low rectal volume/non-compliant rectum, an overactive rectum as seen in proctitis. Passive leakage of fecal matter or extensive soiling in the elderly is a common indicator of a fecaloma in the ampulla recti. The fecaloma not only causes irritation and secretion from the rectal mucosa but it is a constant driver for the rectoanal inhibitory reflex causing a low resting anal sphincter tone.

Childbirths especially in multiparous women might also cause a neuropathy of the pudendal nerves [3]. Stool quality has to be assessed, loose, semisolid, hard, etc. The Bristol stool scale with pictures of different stool qualities might be helpful if the patient has difficulties in describing their stools [4]. This scale might also be an adjunct in follow-up and research. In constipation it is of importance to take a history well back in time down to childhood as bowel, functioning has often been impaired for a long time. The need for perineal support or to support the posterior vaginal wall is indicative of an obstructed defecation where possibly involving a rectocele. A diary registering bowel frequency, consistency, straining, and time

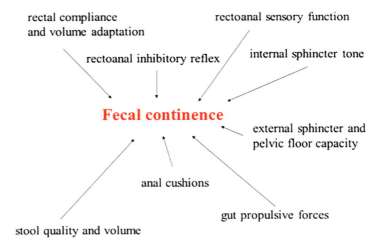

Fig. 1 Most important factors influencing fecal continence and defecation

spent at the toilet may be very helpful, especially to allow later assessment of treatment outcome.

Taking the Patient History

A complete history is essential in the workup of this patient group. It may take more than one visit to get the full picture of a patient's complete history. To induce confidence in your ability to help is essential. Try early on to explain to the patients that this is what you deal with in your clinic and that they are in no way unique. It is not until you have induced trust that a patient will reveal traumas like sexual abuse in childhood that may have a huge impact on pelvic floor functioning. The famous surgeon and later on psychologist Gislain Devrouede (Canada) had a favorite story on this. In short, the young woman with a very long history of severe constipation that had resisted all therapies until the death of her father. She then wrote down her story of him abusing her sexually throughout her childhood. The letter was buried with the father and her constipation resolved.

Taking the individual patient history includes a full history of previous illnesses and surgeries, a comprehensive gynecological and obstetric history focusing on childbirths, time in labor, perineal ruptures, etc. Special attention should be directed toward previous anorectal or perianal surgeries and treatments for hemorrhoids and fistulas as such interventions may harm the sphincters and or the anal cushions (see below). A list of medicines taken by the patient is essential as many drugs affect bowel functioning. Table 1 includes a list over items that a normal history of patients with defecation disorders should include.

Table 1 Important aspects in the history of patients with defecation disorders

Important points in the history	Specifications
Current problem	Short description
Comorbidity	Especially neurological disease, connective tissue disease...
Previous operations	Especially pelvic, spinal, and abdominal operations
Medication	Especially medications with influence on bowel function
Dietary habits	Type of nutrition, fiber intake, regularity
Stool frequency	Number of bowel movements per day/week
Stool consistency	Constant or varying/fluid, soft or hard
Incontinence or constipation score	Different scores can be used
Other symptoms	Descensus, itching, pain
Aggravation or alleviation by life situations	Actions with influence on the problem (activities, intake for certain foods/fluids, other)

Clinical Examination by Nonspecialists

The first outpatient visit should, apart from a general physical examination of course, include an anal inspection and palpation. Look for skin disorders, malformations, scars, asymmetries, and mucosal prolapse. A trained finger will be able to assess anal resting tone and squeeze pressure and the length of the anal canal. Notably some patients are unable to increase anal pressure indicating neurological defects or that the person is disconnected from her pelvis for other reasons. A pinprick test and sensation test for touch with a swab can give an indication for neurological disorders.

Depending on the patient's age and history, a complete examination of the colon by colonoscopy is most usually indicated especially if the patient has diarrhea or a recent change in bowel habits. This is to rule out other organic disease, mainly neoplasia and inflammation, which might be causing the complaint. Referring doctors should be aware that this is mandatory before referral to a pelvic floor specialist.

Clinical Examination by the Proctologist

In addition to the above mentioned, a proctologist will normally perform an anoscopy and a proctoscopy with possibility for biopsies. The proctoscopy, either with a rigid proctoscope or with a flexible sigmoidoscope, will give some information on rectal volume and sensation. Further, inflammation of the mucosa can be evaluated. A patient with IBS will usually indicate severe pain when trying to pass the valves of Huston or on insufflation of air at some pressure. A solitary ulcer on the anterior rectal wall is indicative of severe straining that might be caused by an intussusception or a pathologic puborectalis contraction [5]. Taking a biopsy from the ulcer will confirm this as a solitary ulcer and differentiate it from a neoplastic lesion. Rectal sensibility can be tested by inflating a balloon in the patient's rectum and registering the volume at first sensation, urge to defecate, and at discomfort.

Another informative test is to seat the patient on a toilet commode with a mirror underneath (Fig. 2), which will give valuable information on pelvic floor functioning at rest and on squeeze.

A weak pelvic floor will show as an extensive movement downward when the patient is asked to bear down. A rectal prolapse will easily be diagnosed; it does not always show on an examination in the left lateral (Sims) or in lithotomy position. Having a finger in the anal canal on this maneuver might also reveal an intussusception or an inability to relax the sphincter/pelvic floor during straining. However this paradoxical muscle response must be interpreted with caution, as it may be the result of the very unnatural and for many a bit shameful situation. Notably a patient with a rectal prolapse will not regularly tell you about this as to nonprofessionals something coming out on straining mostly is known as hemorrhoids.

Imaging

In a specialist, setting an anal ultrasound may well be included in the primary assessment. The ultrasound can give useful information about sphincter damage, fistulas, or abscesses. It is mostly done with a probe in the anal canal; the probe has a rotation crystal that also can move up or downward within the probe sheath. This will produce 3 D pictures of the sphincter muscles and surrounding pelvic floor muscles (Fig. 3). The depth of vision and the resolution can be varied by using different ultrasound frequencies. Defects in the muscles and their extension are readily displayed. The disadvantage of this method is the distortion of the anal canal imposed by the probe. An alternative is to use perineal ultrasound looking at the anal canal from the outside; this gives a more dynamic picture, it is even possible to see the rectoanal inhibitory reflex. However, outlining of sphincter defects may be difficult with a perineal probe.

Defecography is sometimes indicated in both incontinence and constipation mainly to visualize a weak pelvic floor with inability to maintain an

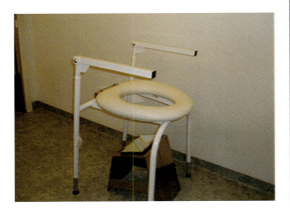

Fig. 2 A toilet commode with a mirror underneath is a very good tool for the study of pelvic floor function

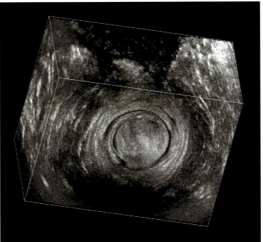

Fig. 3 A 3D picture of the anal sphincters showing a tear in the anterior aspect

anorectal angle and perineal descent when coughing or bearing down. It will also give information on whether the emptying process is obstructed or inefficient, e.g., by a paradoxical puborectalis contraction, blockage by an intussusception, or a large enterocele. A substantial rectocele can also be a part of an obstructed defecation but it can equally well explain fragmented emptying and incontinence (Fig. 4). Defecography can be done either by conventional X-ray cinegraphy or by dynamic MRI. Both methods have advantages and disadvantages; conventional cineradiography induces irradiation to the pelvis, which should be avoided in the younger patients. Conventional X-ray defecography includes contrast media in the rectum of a consistency similar to feces but also small bowel and vaginal contrast to assess these structures during bowel emptying. The MRI defecography gives a much better visualization of the surrounding structures including the pelvic floor. However, usually the dynamic MRI is performed with in a supine position, a definite abnormal position for emptying your stools whereas during barium proctography, the patient is seated on a radiolucent commode trying to imitate the normal position for defecation. Consequently, MRI may underreport pelvic floor disorders [6].

However, both methods are probably burdened by the unphysiological situation in which they are

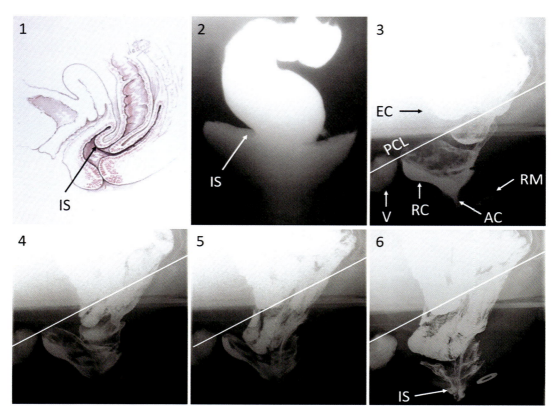

Fig. 4 Illustration of rectal intussusception (IS) and findings on defecography
1: Illustration; 2: Anterior posterior projection; 3–6: Sagittal projections with a radiomarker of known size and a contrast soaked swab in the vagina (V). During defecation the pelvic floor moves far below the pubococcygeal line (PCL) and an intussusception, which reaches the anal canal (AC) at the end of defecation can be seen. Note the movement of the enterocele (EC) and the large rectocele (RC), which empties nearly completely at the end

performed. Normality is also not defined; performing defecographies on people without bowel complaints will reveal both intussusceptions, rectoceles, enteroceles, and other presumed abnormalities. This makes the findings of these investigations difficult to interpret and as stand-alone investigations, they are of limited value.

The constipated patient should have a colonic transit time investigation. In our practice this is done according to Abrahamson [7]. Ten radiopaque markers are swallowed every day for 6 days and on the seventh day; a plain abdominal X-ray will reveal the remaining number of markers and their distribution. The number of markers divided by 10 will give an approximate measure on whole bowel transit time in days, which should be less than five for women and a bit shorter for men. This will hopefully give a confirmation on the patient's bowel habits but it is not very unusual with a patient denying having had any bowel movements and the X-ray displaying substantially less markers than the 60 ingested. In such cases, the history need better penetration. The investigation also gives information on whether the markers are evenly distributed in the colon or if they all remain in the recto sigmoid region; this indicates either a slow transit constipation or an outlet obstruction.

Special Investigations

Anorectal manometry is an investigation that can be performed in a variety of settings, some measuring overall anal canal pressures, and some graded pressures along the anal canal and yet others do this in 3D. These measurements are combined with rectal volume and compliance measurements with either gradual filling or incremental filling of a rectal balloon. This balloon can be of latex with an inherent compliance and uncertain lengthwise expansion, which is often used but not so good. A flaccid balloon with a defined length and maximal volume is better in the sense that you know better what is measured. Simultaneous measurement of rectal volumes and anal pressures are needed to assess the rectoanal inhibitory reflex. The optimal equipment for rectoanal physiology measurements is in our opinion the barostat (Fig. 5), which under predefined rectal pressure measures volume and motility in the rectum with simultaneous display of anal

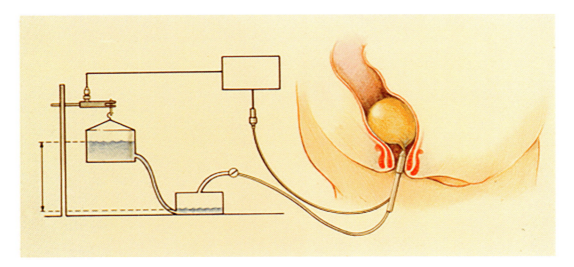

Fig. 5 The principle of a barostat
Air is pressed into the rectum at a preset constant pressure allowing the measurement of rectal volumes at preset pressure levels. Anal pressure can be measured simultaneously. Rectoanal inhibition reflex, anal pressures, rectal motility, and sensory function can be assessed

pressures. With this equipment resting anal pressures, squeeze pressures, rectal sensitivity, motility, volumes, and also thresholds for the rectoanal inhibitory reflex can be defined [8]. A simplified method is the balloon expulsion test that can be used for diagnoses of an obstructed defecation whereas an inability to retain the balloon indicates gross pelvic floor/sphincter insufficiency.

Rectoanal manovolumetry is mostly used in research and in complicated cases where as much information as possible has to be gathered. Variants of the equipment can be used in biofeedback training where measurements are displayed so the patient either sees or hears what is going on in their pelvis. For incontinence, it could be simple muscle training exercises or in combination with rectal sensory training when reduced rectal sensibility is involved in the problem. For obstructed defecation, biofeedback can be very effective provided the setup gives the patient simultaneous information on both pelvic/sphincter tone and rectal pressures [9]. This gives the patient the ability to bear down and increase rectal pressures while simultaneously learning to relax the muscles (Fig. 6).

Neurophysiology studies are rarely used in the clinical setting, apart from routine testing of perineal reflexes like the perineal and bulbocavernosus reflexes. Singel fiber EMG was more frequently used some decades ago. It implies using a fine bipolar needle picking up signals from single motor units and will give information on reinervation phenomena, i.e., diagnosis of proximal nerve damage. This could be used to map the whole sphincter circumference but is cumbersome and above all painful. Mapping of the sphincter anatomy is better done by endoanal sonography. A later more used investigation is the pudendal terminal nerve motor latency investigation, which is done by having an electrode attached to your index finger when palpating per rectum (Fig. 7) [9]. The top of the finger is covered by a stimulation electrode and at the finger base there are two receiving electrodes that will pick up contraction of the external sphincter muscle.

By pointing the finger at the spina ischiadica anterior the stimulating current will excite the pudendal nerve at this point. The time taken to elicit the muscle response can then be measured. It will normally be less than two msec. The motor latency is usually temporarily increased after childbirth but in multipara, this will be a lasting phenomenon [10]. An increased latency is thus an indication of nerve damage to the pelvic floor and sphincter and could have a manifold of causes. One example is the constipated patient with an outlet obstruction that has lasted over time with lots of straining on the pelvic floor and when this nerve damage is marked, the symptoms might change from outlet obstruction to incontinence.

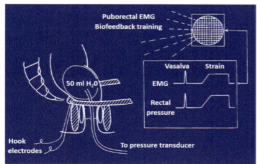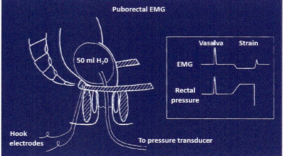

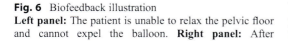

Fig. 6 Biofeedback illustration
Left panel: The patient is unable to relax the pelvic floor and cannot expel the balloon. **Right panel:** After biofeedback training, the patient has learnt to relax the pelvic floor and simultaneously increase rectal pressure, the balloon can be expelled

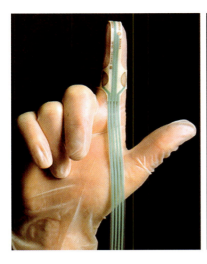
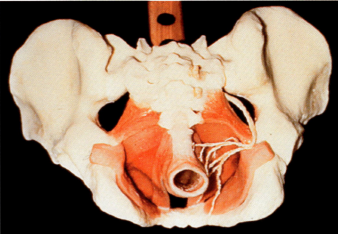

Fig. 7 Pudendal nerve terminal motor latency (PNTML)
The stimulating and recording electrode (left panel), the pudendal nerve anatomy (right panel)

The Use of Special Investigations

In routine practice, advanced manometric investigations and neurophysiological testing are rarely indicated. These methods have a place in research and very special cases with therapeutic challenges.

Primary Treatment

The typical patient with complaints of incontinence is the middle-aged multiparous woman. One should always consider underlying causes such as colorectal cancer especially for complaints that occur within a short time frame. Apart from that conservative therapy should be instituted before any further investigations are indicated. For incontinent and obstipated patients bulking agents (psyllium or equivalent) are used. The rationale is to regulate bowel function. The slight volume increase of the rectal content might facilitate rectal sensation, which combined with softened stool consistency may alleviate the complete emptying of stools. The addition of loperamide tablets may be of benefit in incontinence in patients with loose stools whereas its use in patients with normal stool consistency is questionable [11]. Loperamide regulates stool consistency in those with a tendency for loose stools and may in addition have a slight strengthening effect on internal sphincter tone [12]. The sensitivity to loperamide differs widely and it is wise to start the patients on a low dose (1–2, 2 mg tablets), which is increased gradually until the desired effect is reached to up to 16 mg per day. A specialist nurse could very well be in the frontline for primary treatment, which includes dietary advice, hints on pelvic floor muscle training, and proper seating at the toilet with as much hip flexing as possible. For a majority of patients with incontinence these measures will give substantial symptom relief. If the patient displays a very weak sphincter or pelvic floor, formalized muscle training under the governance of a physiotherapist or a specialist nurse is indicated. This training might use biofeedback or electrical stimulation as an adjunct. The evidence for efficacy is weak but as a part of the general care and treatment, we believe it is of benefit to the patients [13].

If simple laxatives like bulking agents or osmotic laxatives are ineffective, a constipated patient should in our view be handled by a gastroenterologist who can rule out all the different illnesses and medications that may cause constipation. The great flora of alternative laxatives and when indicated the new prokinetic drugs (5-Ht4 receptor agonists) are also best administered by gastroenterologists. When medication and the other measures above do not suffice and especially if an outlet obstruction is suspected the patient should be referred to a colorectal surgeon at a pelvic floor center.

Further Treatment Options in Incontinence

If first-line treatment does not give satisfactory symptom relief one has several choices.

In the young woman with a distinct postpartum sphincter defect, secondary sphincter repair still is the treatment of choice. The sphincter tear is often combined with a very short distance between the anus and the vagina because of the disruption of the perineal body and in these cases, the indication for surgery is strong. An inverted V-incision (with the patient in the stirrups) extending about 3–4 cm to each side of the midline is used. The scar of the torn muscle ends are identified and divided, and the muscle ends are mobilized laterally. Some argue that one should separate the internal sphincter from the external but there is no compelling evidence that this is necessary [14, 15].The muscle ends are mobilized so they can be overlapped in the midline. A sphincteroplasty is done using standing mattress sutures in two layers, 4–6 sutures in total, with slow resorbing suture material (PDS). Then if necessary, the perineal body should be restituted with a couple of stitches reaching out to the split levator edges. This should not be overdone to avoid dyspareunia. The subcutaneous tissue and the skin are then adapted toward the midline in two layers, this will elongate the perineum. The skin is adapted in an inverted Y fashion leaving the wound center open for drainage (Fig. 8).

Perioperative antibiotics and a stool softener for the first postoperative weeks are prescribed. The expected result after a successful sphincteroplasty is that the patient now should be able to defer defecation to a socially acceptable extent; there should be no leaks of formed stools. However only few remain fully continent at long-term follow-up, especially uncontrollable gas leaks are very common [16]. If symptom management is dissatisfactory, the next step could be a sacral nerve modulation procedure.

In the case with a minor sphincter defect or when a defect is detected in a middle aged to elderly woman who has not had any problems in the immediate years following childbirth, one should consider a sacral nerve modulation (SNM) procedure as the first option. The SNM was first developed for use in urinary incontinence but has been shown to work in fecal incontinence as well [17]. The mechanism of action is by large unknown but the general idea is that by placing an electrode with a weak pulsating current next to the sacral nerves (usually S2 – S4) the impulse traffic in these nerves is enhanced. Most of the nerve signals are afferent, which can be demonstrated by functional brain MRI or PET imaging [18, 19]. This implies that the whole nerve circuit to the pelvis is affected by this and that nerve traffic is modulated. The details of this operation are described in ▶ Chap. 15, "Bladder Dysfunction and Pelvic Pain: The Role of Sacral, Tibial, and Pudendal Neuromodulation." The debate in colorectal surgery has been whether one should first implant a test electrode for a few weeks to evaluate the efficacy of the nerve modulation and then in the next step withdraw this electrode and implant a permanent electrode and a nerve stimulator. The main reasoning behind this is that if not effective not much money has been spent and the removal of the test electrode is very simple. However there is no guarantee that when changing a test, electrode for permanent electrode this will be in exactly the same position. Due to a reduction in cost difference, the preferred method now is to implant the permanent electrode at first surgery and stimulate with an external stimulator during the trial period. Depending on the test result, the electrode is then either removed or connected to a permanent stimulator implanted in the subcutaneous fat. During the test period, the patients register the number of leak episodes and defecation

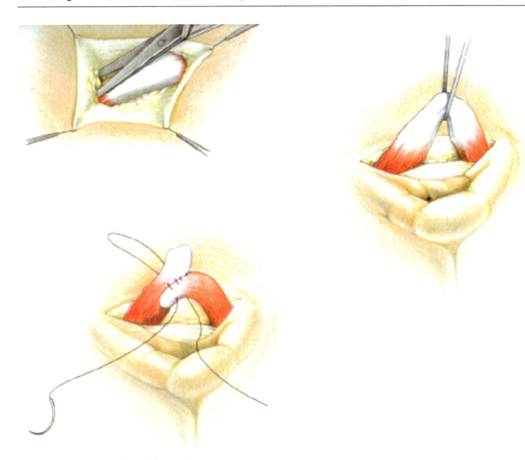

Fig. 8 The principle of a sphincteroplasty

frequency in a diary. If there is a 50% reduction in leaks, a permanent system is usually implanted. With optimal placement of the electrode low current is required for adequate stimulation and the battery than lasts up to 8 years to be replaced in a new operation. A rechargeable system has recently become available. Of all patients who have had an SNM test, approximately half of the patients still benefit from SNM after some years [20]. It is controversial whether SNM should be tried before sphincteroplasty also in the younger patients [21].

For patients with the main symptom being passive leakage, a number of devices to tighten the anal canal are available. Injectable bulking agents based on hyaluronic acid may be beneficial [22]. Deposits of the bulking agent are injected under the mucosa at the entrance of the anal canal a cm above the dentate line. They can also be injected in four or more sites around the circumference. With time, the bulking effect will diminish and if initially beneficial, the injections might be repeated. Other devices using the same principle are rod formed prosthesis implanted vertically around the anal canal [23]. The insertion is made possible with a special instrument. A third option is the magnetic ring; a string filled with magnets is inserted around the anal canal to keep it closed. On pushing and increasing rectal and upper canal pressure the magnetic forces holding the ring will disrupt and the anal canal opens up for emptying [24]. The documentation for these two options is rather scarce and time will tell if they will have a place in the therapeutic armamentarium.

The artificial sphincter that is commonly used in urology has also been modified for use in fecal incontinence. The system is in principle identical to the version used in urology but the inflatable cuff is modified to fit around the anal canal on the outside of the sphincters. The interest for this device has never been very high, migration of the cuff and infectious complications are common problems.

The dynamic graciloplasty is a yet more complicated procedure with the potential to help patients who lack sphincter continuity if a sphincteroplasty is not possible. One of the gracilis muscles is mobilized from the pes anserinus and upward to the insertion of the nerves and the main artery, taken great care not to damage these structures. A subcutaneous canal from the ipsilateral groin to the anus and around the anal canal is created in which the muscle is transposed. The tendon end of the muscle that thus lies in a circle around the anus it attached to the bony structures on the opposite side of the pelvis. In the developmental phase, this was all done with the hope that the transposed muscle would continue to be active and act as a sphincter. However, this was not the case, as the muscle atrophied into a tendinous rather ineffective sling. The solution to this was to continuously activate the muscle with inserted electrodes attached to a pacemaker. By gradually increasing the stimulus cycles the muscle transforms from a type 1 into a type 2 muscle that is characterized by the ability to have a continuous tone without accumulation of lactic acid. This makes the muscle physiologically like the rest of the pelvic floor muscles that are constantly active. The patient remotely controls the pacemaker to inactivate the muscle upon defecation. The operation takes some experience to learn, the main problem being the interface between biology and electronics gradually losing the effect of the stimulus, which will demand increased current to the electrodes, and sometimes re-siting of electrodes to improve efficacy of the stimulation. As for most new methods, the enthusiasm was big when this method was introduced some 25 years ago. As the initial enthusiasts are not active anymore, by now few surgeons are in command of this operation [25]. The long-term results are not that good but for few, this can be a very good solution [26] (Fig. 9).

For those with severe incontinence where other options have failed or are not considered as realistic a colostomy is the optimal solution. A colostomy is not protruding very much and if the patient can manage an irrigation system, the colon can be flushed clean in 30–45 min every

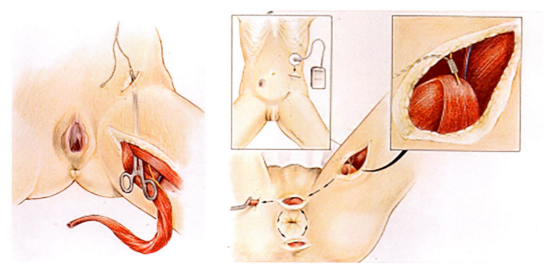

Fig. 9 The principles of a dynamic graciloplasty

or every other day. In the intervals between these irrigations, the bowel will be inactive and a simple stoma-cap appliance can be used. The acceptance of a stoma varies among patients, with less enthusiasm the further south Europe the patients live [27]. However, the general impression is that once a patient has the stoma they are generally very content with this solution. Although parastomal hernias occur frequently (around 50% of colostomies), severe complications are not very common [28].

Further Treatment Options in Constipation

Before undertaking more extensive, i.e., interventional treatment in constipated patients exhaustive conservative measures should have been tried often including dieticians and if necessary psychologists. A clear-cut distinction between slow transit constipation and outlet obstruction is not always possible. Few patients have a distinct slow transit as their only problem. Some decades ago, they were often offered a colectomy with an ileorectal anastomosis. The reported results are variable reaching from good to rather bad. The existing evidence is hampered by selection bias and heterogeneity in the reporting of the functional outcomes [29]. Today, with the advent of better pharmacological therapies, the option of an ileorectal anastomosis is indeed rare.

Outlet obstruction is definitely best treated by biofeedback and behavioral therapies. Surgeons have been tempted to operate patients with radiological proof of intussusception often with dismal results. Division of the puborectalis muscle has also been an option with doubtful results, injection of Botox in the puborectalis muscle is another option not very well documented. Some have found that the sigmoid might fall into the pelvis and cause obstructive symptoms [30]. There are some patients with an intussusception of the rectum that reaches all the way into the anal canal giving symptoms of either obstructed defecation or incontinence if the condition has lasted for a while. In these patients, a surgical correction of the disrupted anatomy is often indicated. Another effect of an intussusception or prolonged straining in outlet obstruction is the solitary rectal ulcer most often located approximately 7 cm from the anal verge on the anterior aspect of the rectum. The solitary ulcer may mimic a carcinoma but biopsies will reveal its nature. Symptoms are most often bleeding and obstruction and if conservative measures are inadequate, an operation is warranted. There are many surgical options available and these will be covered in the following chapter on rectal prolapse.

A rectocele, bulging of the lower rectum into the vagina, can cause a variety of symptoms. The gynecologist might refer to this as a posterior prolapse and the patient has a feeling of a lump in the posterior vagina. The rectocele may also affect bowel emptying with the forces of defecation directed anterior more than downward. Typically, the patient will report that she has to support the posterior vaginal wall to achieve complete emptying. The rectocele may also give symptoms of incomplete emptying and/or fractioned emptying. The patient may have to return to the toilet several times or she may have leaks of fecal matter a while after the defecation when she rises and the residue in the rectocele is forced into the anal canal. An enterocele alone is rarely causing obstructed defecation. Gynecologists do sometimes treat enteroceles when they bulge into the vagina. For rectoceles there is an abundance of surgical treatment options, transvaginal, perineal, and rectal approaches can be used and there is no consensus on which is the optimal operation [31, 32]. Probably gynecologists are most familiar with correcting rectoceles although they seldom do it on the indication of obstructed defecation. In our view, an operation of a rectocele causing obstructed defecation is best performed as a joint venture by gynecologist and colorectal surgeon.

Rectal Prolapse

This is a condition where the rectum falls out of the anal canal, the differential diagnoses is mucosal prolapse that does not extend as far and upon palpation can be felt to be thinner, i.e., not the full rectal wall. Rectal prolapse can affect both sexes and all ages, it is very rarely seen in men, it can be seen in infants but then it is usually self-correcting. Both younger adult females and older females may be affected, most frequently the elderly. The cause of prolapse is not fully established. It is as common in nulliparous as in multipara. In the younger it might be associated with extreme weight loss as in anorexia nervosa [33]. The relationship between a rectal intussusception and an overt rectal prolapse is not clarified. Some authors are of the opinion that they are separate disorders. A rectal prolapse most often appears as a more or less sudden event without any long history pointing toward a previous intussusception. This opinion is supported by radiological findings in a study that followed several hundred of patients with various degrees on intussusception on defecography. Some 10 years later almost none of them had presented with a rectal prolapse [34].

Diagnoses of a rectal prolapse is easy when the patient is seated on a commode as displayed in Fig. 1 above and asked to strain. In the left lateral position or even in the lithotomy position it is not always evident and it might not be so easy to provoke. One must bear in mind that the prolapse is the doctor's diagnosis, but most patients will not give the name of their condition rather refer to it as hemorrhoids or incontinence. A prolapse that does not retract spontaneously will give a lot of discomfort with mucus discharge and incontinence, pain is not so common but may be present. The treatment is surgical and there are several options, is his book from the 1970s "Diseases of the colon, rectum and anus" the former colorectal guru Goligher points out that there are 102 different methods described for the correction of a rectal prolapse [35]. This of course tells us that none of them is perfect; there is a balance between keeping the rectum in the pelvis and preserving continence and defecation functions.

In principal, there are two ways to approach the problem, an operation from the perineal side or an abdominal operation. The two most used perineal approaches are the Delorme and the Altemeier operations [36, 37]. The Delorme method is based on a plication of the prolapsing rectal musculature, which is then pushed up above the anal canal. The first step is then to remove the redundant mucosa, which is dissected off the muscle from a cm above the dental line down to the apex of the prolapse and then further on the inside of the prolapse up to the corresponding level on the inner aspect of the prolapse. The musculature of the prolapse is plicated with several standing sutures and then the mucosa is sutured as end-to-end anastomoses before the bulk is pushed up above the anal canal [38]. The problem is that the sphincter musculature is often weak in these patients and recurrence of the prolapse is most often seen. The Altemeier operation incurs a rectal resection from below. The full bowel wall is transected just below the dentate line, after this the redundant rectum can be pulled further down and the mesenteric vessel ligated stepwise. Usually the whole rectum and a bit of the sigmoid can be pulled out of the anus. Finally, the oral bowel is gradually transected while suturing it as a full wall anastomosis to the anal remaining bowel. This "pull though" rectal resection has been much favored in the USA even for younger patients. The recurrence rates are lower compared to the Delorme procedure but one can have doubts on the functional outcome. Removing the rectum and anastomosing the sigmoid to the upper anal canal is by default a prerequisite for a low anterior resection syndrome. The major problems will be urge and incontinence. In southern Europe, much attention has been devoted to variants of "internal Delorme" operation, which is to remove redundant mucosa in the lower rectum ether by using specially developed stapling devices [32] or doing it as a transanal operation [39]. The stapling mucosectomy technique mostly used for hemorrhoid disease has been burdened by cases of intractable anal pain and overall the benefit of the transanal mucosectomies is not all clear.

The operations through the abdominal route are considered to have greater risks and that is why the perineal procedures at least in Europe have been used mostly in the old and frail patients. The abdominal operations are based on different methods to secure the rectum from falling out through the anus. Usually, meshes have been used in different positions; some also advocate only suturing the mesorectum to the presacral periosteum. The methods also incur that the rectum has to be mobilized from its surrounding structures to allow it to be pulled up and secured. This entails damage to the rectal nerve supply especially if the lateral rectal ligaments are divided as was done in the Ripstein procedure that was popular some 40 years ago. The Ripstein operation also included a mesh, secured to the promontory, and wrapped around the upper rectum. Recurrence rates were low but functional outcome dismal. Later methods have used a posterior lateral mesh covering only parts of the rectal circumference and some also abandoned the mesh and only sutured the rectum to the presacral fascia. These latter methods had less negative functional sequel but this was only achieved on accepting higher recurrence rates. A variant of this is the Frykman-Goldberg operation introduced in the USA; this procedure combines a sutured presacral rectopexy with a sigmoid resection. The resection has a twofold rationale in that it is hoped that it will alleviate the outlet obstruction often seen after rectopexies and it might help to keep the rectum from meandering down into the lower pelvis. The latest development in rectal prolapse surgery is the anterior mesh rectopexy preferably done as a laparoscopic procedure. This method was introduced by Andre D'Hoore from Leuven and has gained widespread popularity during the last decade. The rectum is mobilized to avoid dividing the lateral ligaments but incising the peritoneum and dissecting anteriorly all the way down to the pelvic floor muscles between the posterior vagina and the anterior rectal wall. Then a narrow mesh (4–5 cm) is fixed to the pelvic floor and gradually to the anterior aspect of the rectum and the upper posterior aspect of the vagina. The mesh is drawn on the right side of the upper rectum and then secured to the bony structures at the promontory. Finally, the mesh is buried when the peritoneum is sewn together in front of it. This method addresses not only the rectal prolapse or intussusception but also prevents or deals with a rectocele. It also deals with the pelvic floor decent so often being a part of the

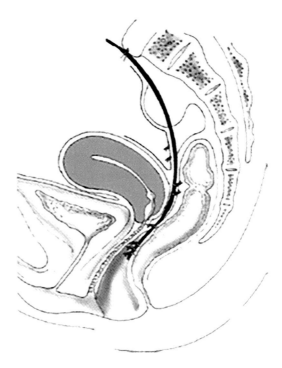

Fig. 10 Ventral mesh rectopexy. (courtesy of Jansen Pharma Sweden)

problem complex. The hitherto reported outcomes are very favorable in terms of both recurrence rates and functional outcomes although the overall quality of the evidence is low [40] (Fig. 10).

Conclusion

When dealing with anorectal functional disorders and to some extent rectal prolapses one should be extremely cautious to fully understand the pathophysiology of the patient's complaint and furthermore understand that surgery might do more harm than good.

Cross-References

▶ Female Sexual Dysfunction
▶ Indications and Use of Bowel in Female Lower Urinary Tract Reconstruction: Overview

References

1. Schluter PJ, Askew DA, Jamieson HA, Arnold EP. Urinary and fecal incontinence are independently associated with falls risk among older women and men with complex needs: a national population study. Neurourol Urodyn. 2020;39(3):945–53.
2. Cichowski SB, Komesu YM, Dunivan GC, Rogers RG. The association between fecal incontinence and sexual activity and function in women attending a tertiary referral center. Int Urogynecol J. 2013;24(9):1489–94.
3. Snooks SJ, Swash M, Henry MM, Setchell M. Risk factors in childbirth causing damage to the pelvic floor innervation. Int J Color Dis. 1986;1(1):20–4.
4. Koppen IJN, Velasco-Benitez CA, Benninga MA, Di Lorenzo C, Saps M. Using the Bristol stool scale and parental report of stool consistency as part of the Rome III criteria for functional constipation in infants and toddlers. J Pediatr. 2016;177:44–48.e1.
5. Gouriou C, Chambaz M, Ropert A, Bouguen G, Desfourneaux V, Siproudhis L, et al. A systematic literature review on solitary rectal ulcer syndrome: is there a therapeutic consensus in 2018? Int J Color Dis. 2018;33(12):1647–55.
6. Pilkington SA, Nugent KP, Brenner J, Harris S, Clarke A, Lamparelli M, et al. Barium proctography vs magnetic resonance proctography for pelvic floor disorders: a comparative study. Color Dis. 2012;14(10):1224–30.
7. Abrahamsson H, Antov S. Accuracy in assessment of colonic transit time with particles: how many markers should be used? Neurogastroenterol Motil. 2010;22(11):1164–9.
8. Akervall S, Fasth S, Nordgren S, Oresland T, Hulten L. Rectal reservoir and sensory function studied by graded isobaric distension in normal man. Gut. 1989;30(4):496–502.
9. Koh CE, Young CJ, Young JM, Solomon MJ. Systematic review of randomized controlled trials of the effectiveness of biofeedback for pelvic floor dysfunction. Br J Surg. 2008;95(9):1079–87.
10. Snooks SJ, Setchell M, Swash M, Henry MM. Injury to innervation of pelvic floor sphincter musculature in childbirth. Lancet. 1984;2(8402):546–50.
11. Jelovsek JE, Markland AD, Whitehead WE, Barber MD, Newman DK, Rogers RG, et al. Controlling faecal incontinence in women by performing anal exercises with biofeedback or loperamide: a randomised clinical trial. Lancet Gastroenterol Hepatol. 2019;4(9):698–710.
12. Hallgren T, Fasth S, Delbro DS, Nordgren S, Oresland T, Hulten L. Loperamide improves anal sphincter function and continence after restorative proctocolectomy. Dig Dis Sci. 1994;39(12):2612–8.
13. Norton C, Chelvanayagam S, Wilson-Barnett J, Redfern S, Kamm MA. Randomized controlled trial of biofeedback for fecal incontinence. Gastroenterology. 2003;125(5):1320–9.
14. Briel JW, de Boer LM, Hop WC, Schouten WR. Clinical outcome of anterior overlapping external anal sphincter repair with internal anal sphincter imbrication. Dis Colon Rectum. 1998;41(2):209–14.
15. Deen KI, Kumar D, Williams JG, Grant EA, Keighley MR. Randomized trial of internal anal sphincter plication with pelvic floor repair for neuropathic fecal incontinence. Dis Colon Rectum. 1995;38(1):14–8.
16. Barbosa M, Glavind-Kristensen M, Moller Soerensen M, Christensen P. Secondary sphincter repair for anal incontinence following obstetric sphincter injury: functional outcome and quality of life at 18 years of follow-up. Color Dis. 2020;22(1):71–9.
17. Leroi AM, Parc Y, Lehur PA, Mion F, Barth X, Rullier E, et al. Efficacy of sacral nerve stimulation for fecal incontinence: results of a multicenter double-blind crossover study. Ann Surg. 2005;242(5):662–9.
18. Bari AA, Pouratian N. Brain imaging correlates of peripheral nerve stimulation. Surg Neurol Int. 2012;3(Suppl 4):S260–8.
19. Lundby L, Møller A, Buntzen S, Krogh K, Vang K, Gjedde A, et al. Relief of fecal incontinence by sacral nerve stimulation linked to focal brain activation. Dis Colon Rectum. 2011;54(3):318–23.
20. Leo CA, Thomas GP, Bradshaw E, Karki S, Hodgkinson JD, Murphy J, et al. Long-term outcome of sacral nerve stimulation for faecal incontinence. Color Dis. 2020;22(12):2191–8.
21. Muñoz-Duyos A, Lagares-Tena L, Ribas Y, Baanante JC, Navarro-Luna A. Critical appraisal of international guidelines for the management of fecal incontinence in adults: is it possible to define what to do in different clinical scenarios? Tech Coloproctol. 2021;26(1):1–17.
22. Graf W, Mellgren A, Matzel KE, Hull T, Johansson C, Bernstein M. Efficacy of dextranomer in stabilised hyaluronic acid for treatment of faecal incontinence: a randomised, sham-controlled trial. Lancet. 2011;377(9770):997–1003.
23. Litta F, Parello A, De Simone V, Campenni P, Orefice R, Marra AA, et al. Efficacy of Sphinkeeper™ implant in treating faecal incontinence. Br J Surg. 2020;107(5):484–8.
24. Jayne DG, Williams AE, Corrigan N, Croft J, Pullan A, Napp V, et al. Sacral nerve stimulation versus the magnetic sphincter augmentation device for adult faecal incontinence: the SaFaRI RCT. Health Technol Assess. 2021;25(18):1–96.
25. Mege D, Omouri A, Maignan A, Sielezneff I. Long-term results of dynamic graciloplasty for severe fecal incontinence. Tech Coloproctol. 2021;25(5):531–7.
26. Rongen MJ, Uludag O, El Naggar K, Geerdes BP, Konsten J, Baeten CG. Long-term follow-up of

dynamic gracioplasty for fecal incontinence. Dis Colon Rectum. 2003;46(6):716–21.
27. Holzer B, Matzel K, Schiedeck T, Christiansen J, Christensen P, Rius J, et al. Do geographic and educational factors influence the quality of life in rectal cancer patients with a permanent colostomy? Dis Colon Rectum. 2005;48(12):2209–16.
28. Malik T, Lee MJ, Harikrishnan AB. The incidence of stoma related morbidity – a systematic review of randomised controlled trials. Ann R Coll Surg Engl. 2018;100(7):501–8.
29. Knowles CH, Grossi U, Chapman M, Mason J. Surgery for constipation: systematic review and practice recommendations: results I: colonic resection. Color Dis. 2017;19(Suppl 3):17–36.
30. Jorge JM, Yang YK, Wexner SD. Incidence and clinical significance of sigmoidoceles as determined by a new classification system. Dis Colon Rectum. 1994;37(11):1112–7.
31. Planells Roig M, Sanahuja Santafe A, Miranda G, de Larra JL, Garcia Espinosa R, Serralta SA. Prospective analysis of marlex mesh repair for symptomatic rectocele with obstructive defecation. Rev Esp Enferm Dig. 2002;94(2):67–77.
32. Tsar'kov PV, Sandrikov VA, Tulina IA, Darinov AA, Brindar NG, Kartashova OV, et al. Surgical treatment of rectocele with the use of mesh implants by the obstructive defecation syndrome. Khirurgiia (Mosk). 2012;8:25–33.
33. Mitchell N, Norris ML. Rectal prolapse associated with anorexia nervosa: a case report and review of the literature. J Eat Disord. 2013;1:39.
34. Broden B, Snellman B. Procidentia of the rectum studied with cineradiography. A contribution to the discussion of causative mechanism. Dis Colon Rectum. 1968;11(5):330–47.
35. H.H. GJCDHLN. Surgery of the anus, rectum, and colon. 2nd ed. London: Baillière Tindall & Cassell; 1967.
36. Watts AM, Thompson MR. Evaluation of Delorme's procedure as a treatment for full-thickness rectal prolapse. Br J Surg. 2000;87(2):218–22.
37. Altemeier WA, Culbertson WR, Schowengerdt C, Hunt J. Nineteen years' experience with the one-stage perineal repair of rectal prolapse. Ann Surg. 1971;173(6):993–1006.
38. Samalavicius NE, Klimasauskiene V, Simcikas D, Stravinskas M, Eismontas V, Dulskas A. The Delorme procedure for full-thickness rectal prolapse – a video vignette. Color Dis. 2021;23(3):762–3.
39. Trompetto M, Clerico G, Realis Luc A, Marino F, Giani I, Ganio E. Transanal Delorme procedure for treatment of rectocele associated with rectal intussusception. Tech Coloproctol. 2006;10(4):389.
40. Maeda Y, Espin-Basany E, Gorissen K, Kim M, Lehur PA, Lundby L, et al. European Society of Coloproctology guidance on the use of mesh in the pelvis in colorectal surgery. Color Dis. 2021;23(9):2228–85.

Part IX

Use of Bowel in Genitourinary and Pelvic Reconstruction and Other Complex Scenarios

Indications and Use of Bowel in Female Lower Urinary Tract Reconstruction: Overview

57

Warren Lo and Jun Jiet Ng

Contents

Introduction	1034
Historical Perspective	1036
Physics of Bowel	1036
Surgical Anatomy and Bowel Selection	1037
Stomach	1037
Jejunum	1037
Ileum	1037
Ileocolonic Segment	1038
Colon	1039
Evaluation of Patient	1040
Preoperative Preparation	1040
Surgical Techniques	1041
Bowel Anastomosis	1041
Ureterointestinal Anastomosis	1041
Urinary Stoma	1042
Urinary Diversion	1042
Malignancy	1042
Bladder Dysfunction	1044
Congenital Urogenital Anomaly	1045
Other Conditions	1046
Conduit	1046
Ileal Conduit	1046
Jejunal Conduit	1046
Colon Conduit	1047

W. Lo (✉)
Urology, Hospital Kuala Lumpur, Kuala Lumpur, Malaysia

J. J. Ng
Urogynecology, Hospital Kuala Lumpur, Kuala Lumpur, Malaysia

© Springer Nature Switzerland AG 2023
F. E. Martins et al. (eds.), *Female Genitourinary and Pelvic Floor Reconstruction*,
https://doi.org/10.1007/978-3-031-19598-3_58

Cutaneous Catheterizing Pouch	1047
Orthotopic Neobladder	1049
Continence	1052
Urinary Retention	1052
Quality of Life	1052
Ureterosigmoidostomy	1052
Augmentation Cystoplasty	1053
Non-neurogenic	1053
Neurogenic	1054
Ureter Substitution	1055
Neovaginal Reconstruction (Vaginoplasty)	1055
Complications of Bowel Use in Female Genitourinary Reconstruction	1056
Early Complications	1057
Late Complications	1057
Conclusion	1060
References	1060

Abstract

With an increased level of collaboration among urologists, gynecologists, and colorectal surgeons, the indications and use of bowel in female reconstructive surgery have expanded from urinary diversion to vaginoplasty. From congenital urogenital anomalies in newborns to bladder cancer in the older age group, from different inflammatory or infectious disorders to the trauma of the urogenital tract, the bowel is of use when replacement is needed for the urinary tract that is no longer functional. Even though the bowel is close to ideal as a substitute, it does not replace the role of the urothelium which has its own unique properties. Therefore, clinicians need to be aware of the long-term implications and complications that can potentially occur.

The right patient selection, the right method of urinary diversion, the right bowel segment selection, long-term follow-up, and understanding of the unique female urogenital anatomy are the key principles in the use of the bowel in female reconstructive surgery. To date, there is still no optimal material to replace the innate bladder, ureter, and urethra. Until newer biomaterials or scaffolds are available, the bowel is still the material of choice to be used as a substitute in female genitourinary reconstruction.

Keywords

Reconstructive urology · Bowel · Anastomosis · Urinary diversion · Neobladder · Metabolic changes · Augmentation Cystoplasty · Bowel vaginoplasty · Conduit · Reservoir

Introduction

The gastrointestinal system has had a significant role in the field of urology for many years. It serves as a substitute when replacement is needed for the ureter, bladder, or urethra which is no longer functional. The use of the bowel in female genitourinary reconstruction is on the rise in uro-oncology, reconstructive urology, pediatric and adolescent urology, female pelvic floor medicine, and reconstructive surgery. Improved anesthetic and intraoperative monitoring, intensive postoperative care, newer radiographic imaging, contemporary endoscopic technology, intermittent catheterization, and the emergence of regenerative medicine are some of the factors that have contributed to this development [1].

The stomach, small bowel (jejunum, ileum), and large bowel (cecum, appendix, ascending colon, transverse colon, descending colon, sigmoid colon, rectum) are among the parts of the gastrointestinal tract that are employed in female genitourinary reconstruction. They are used to reconstruct reservoirs, conduits, augmentations, continence mechanisms, and vaginoplasty (Fig. 1). In comparison to males, the female urogenital system is distinct in that the female urethra is shorter, and the presence of a vaginal opening contributes to weaker pelvic floor support. This must be taken into consideration during female reconstructive surgery.

The advantage of the bowel is that it is tubular in shape and it has the ability to form hollow reservoirs of various shapes that structurally can substitute diseased or resected parts of urinary

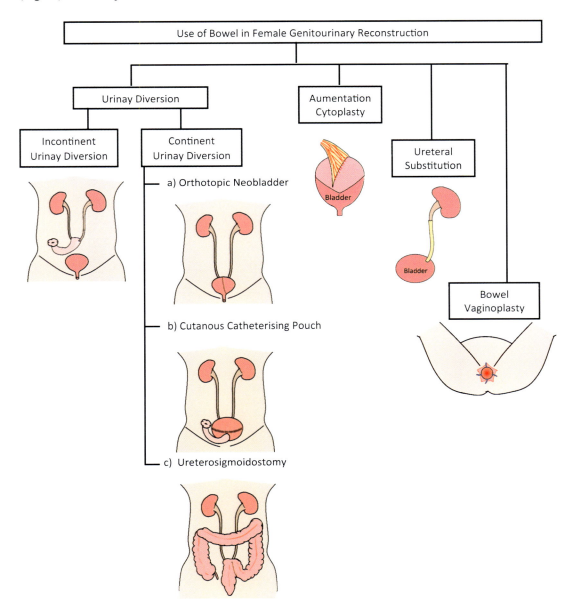

Fig. 1 Use of bowel in female genitourinary reconstruction: overview

tract. Additionally, the bowel is a well-vascularized autologous material with little potential for extensive fibrosis, rejection, or adverse immune reactions. However, bowel segment that is removed for reconstruction procedures retains its absorbing and secreting abilities, which results in various metabolic disorders that may be lethal.

In separate chapters of this book, each of these procedures will be covered in depth. This chapter will give a general overview of the subject, emphasizing the indication, use, surgical anatomy, and technical aspects of the use of the bowel in female genitourinary reconstruction. Early and long-term complications of the use of bowel segments will also be described.

Historical Perspective

For more than 150 years, urologists have used the bowel as the material of choice to divert the course of normal urine flow. The use of the bowel dated back to 1852 when Simon attempted the first urinary diversion by performing ureterosigmoidostomy in a patient with bladder exstrophy. Since then, there has been an increase in the use of urinary diversion in children with neurogenic bladder and congenital malformations, as well as bladder cancer survival requiring reconstructive surgery. In 1898, Thomas Smith did the first direct ureterointestinal implantation in London. Due to leakage and stricture, Nesbit, Cordonnier, Ledbetter, Le Duc, and Wallace subsequently made numerous modifications to the reimplantation technique. Augmentation ileocystoplasty was first described by Mikulicz in 1939. In 1950, Bricker described ileal conduit in patients after radical pelvic surgery. Camey and Le Duc created orthotopic neobladder in 1979. In addition to introducing the idea of continent cutaneous diversion in 1982, Kock also demonstrated the importance of detubularization of the bowel segment and using the double folding method to form a sphere [2].

Physics of Bowel

According to Laplace's law, the radius is inversely proportional to pressure. As the radius increases, the volume increases and the pressure decreases.

$$P = \frac{2TW}{R}$$

P – pressure, T – tension, W – wall thickness, and R – radius of reservoir

The sphere meets all three criteria for an optimal reservoir to safeguard the upper urinary tract: high compliance, high capacity, and low pressure. As a result, bowel segments that are naturally cylindrical in shape need to be detubularized and reconstructed to a spherical reservoir (Fig. 2).

Detubularization means splitting the bowel on its antimesenteric border. In addition, the sphere has the least surface area, which means that fewer bowel segments will be needed to reconstruct a reservoir and fewer metabolic complications due

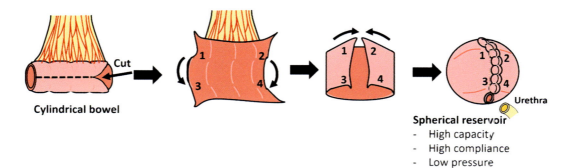

Fig. 2 Detubularization of bowel

to the exchange of electrolytes. Detubularized bowel segments also have less peristaltic activity, which improves continence. A mature reservoir should have a volume capacity of between 300 and 500 ml at low pressure. The reservoir needs to be filled frequently to gradually raise the volume capacity. Over time, a nonfunctional reservoir will shrink.

Surgical Anatomy and Bowel Selection

The anatomy and physiology of each bowel segment are unique, which explained the different complications caused. Each bowel segment has its advantages and disadvantages when employed in various reconstructive surgeries. Understanding this information will be crucial for surgeons when they are selecting the appropriate bowel segment. In addition, surgeons need to be familiar with the blood supply of the bowels to know which bowel segments to choose and which arteries can and cannot be ligated safely (Fig. 3).

Stomach

The stomach is a hollow, muscular organ where food is stored and mixed with gastric juices and digestive enzymes. Parietal cells of the stomach produce intrinsic factor, a glycoprotein that is necessary for vitamin B12 absorption in the small intestine. The stomach is rarely used in female genitourinary reconstructive surgery. It is only used in patients with severe adhesion, history of pelvis radiation, short bowel syndrome, and inflammatory bowel disease and patients with renal insufficiency who cannot tolerate metabolic acidosis. The stomach gets its blood supply from the celiac trunk which branches into the left gastric artery, splenic artery, and common hepatic artery. The left and right gastroepiploic arteries join to make the greater curvature anastomosis, whereas the left and right gastric arteries join to form the lesser curvature anastomosis. Due to its lengthy pedicle that might extend to the pelvis, the right gastroepiploic artery is frequently used, and occasionally, the left gastroepiploic artery might be atretic. The stomach can be used in both continent and incontinent urinary diversion in the form of stomach conduits, orthotopic neobladders, and continent cutaneous diversions.

The stomach is less permeable to solutes and has less risk of acidosis. Less mucus production also means less risk of bacteriuria. The stomach is not prone to adhesions, therefore more accessible. Its thick seromuscular layer makes it more suitable for submucosal ureteric reimplantation.

Hematuria-dysuria syndrome is a painful complication when a stomach segment is used due to its ongoing acid production. This acid production increases the risk of ulceration. In the remnant stomach, dumping syndrome occurs when rapid gastric emptying results in a hyperosmolar load in the small bowel. Vitamin B12 deficiency may occur due to the reduced production of intrinsic factors. Bilious vomiting may occur because of the reflux of duodenal content due to the loss of pylorus. Hypochloremic hypokalemic metabolic alkalosis, steatorrhea, and iron deficiency anemia are possible complications.

Jejunum

Due to severe complications such as hypochloremic hyponatremic hyperkalemic metabolic acidosis, azotemia, and malabsorption, the jejunum is only used when no other segment of the bowel is available. Excessive loss of sodium chloride can lead to severe dehydration.

Ileum

The small bowel is the main part of the gastrointestinal tract where digestion and absorption take place. The ileum is involved in water, electrolyte, bile salt, and vitamin B12 absorption and is the most commonly used bowel segment in female genitourinary reconstructive surgery. Compared to the jejunum, the ileum has a smaller diameter, multiple artery arcades with smaller vessels, and thicker mesentery. Like the jejunum, it receives its

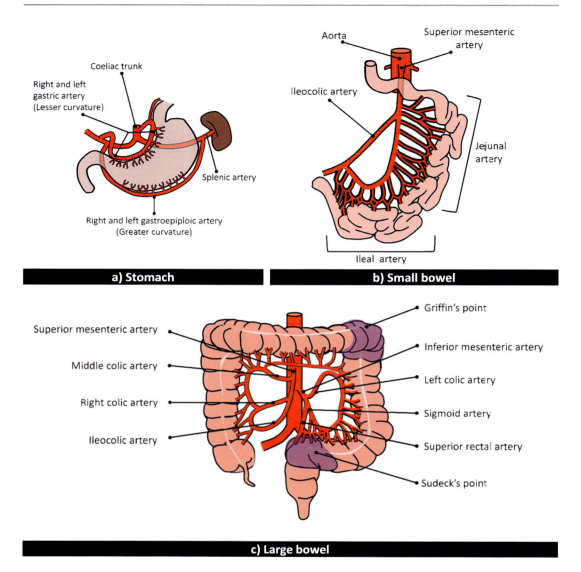

Fig. 3 Blood supply of the bowel segments. (**a**) Stomach, (**b**) small bowel, and (**c**) large bowel

main blood supply from the superior mesenteric artery. It has great mobility but, occasionally, excessive fat and a short mesentery might make the ileum less mobile. To ensure adequate intestinal perfusion and to lower the risk of bowel necrosis, no more than 8 cm of mesentery should be removed from the end of a small bowel segment [3]. Use of ileum for female reconstructive surgery may result in hypokalemic hyperchloremic metabolic acidosis, fat malabsorption, diarrhea, and vitamin B12 deficiency.

Ileocolonic Segment

The ileocolonic segment is referred to the terminal ileum, ileocecal valve, and proximal colon. The ileocolonic segment is frequently used to construct urinary reservoir as the ileocecal valve and the appendix can be used to create continence and antireflux mechanisms.

However, using the ileocolonic segment for diversion is at a higher risk of diarrhea and metabolic complications due to the removal of the terminal ileum and ileocecal valve, which are important for nutrient absorption and control of stool passage into the colon.

Colon

The colon serves as a reservoir to store feces and is responsible for absorbing water to make solid stools. The colon is typically used in patients with a history of pelvic radiation (transverse colon) or patients undergoing pelvic exenteration where bowel anastomosis is not required (sigmoid colon). The colon receives its blood supply from the superior mesenteric artery, inferior mesenteric artery, and internal iliac artery. The superior mesenteric artery branches into the ileocolic artery, right colic artery, and middle colic artery. The inferior mesenteric artery gives rise to the left colic artery, sigmoid artery, and superior rectal artery.

Watershed areas are parts of the colon that receive dual blood supply from the most distal branches of two larger arteries. The risk of ischemia during hypotension or a thromboembolic event is higher in these areas because of the small vessel caliber of these distal branches. They are also known as the weak point of blood supply. There are two watershed areas in the colon where anastomosis should be avoided at these areas: the junction between the middle colic artery and left colic artery near the splenic flexure (Griffith's point) and the junction between the sigmoid artery and superior rectal artery near the rectosigmoid junction (Sudeck's point). It is important to perform colonoscopic assessment of the entire colon prior to being used for reconstructive procedures.

The colon has great mobility and is less prone to bowel obstruction. Technically, it is easier to construct antireflux mechanisms due to its thickness. Because of its function, there are less metabolic and malabsorptive complications. However, it has a large caliber which may require tapering. There is also significant mucus production. Diarrhea and hyperchloremic hypokalemic metabolic acidosis may occur.

The selection and use of different bowel segments in female genitourinary reconstruction are summarized in Fig. 4.

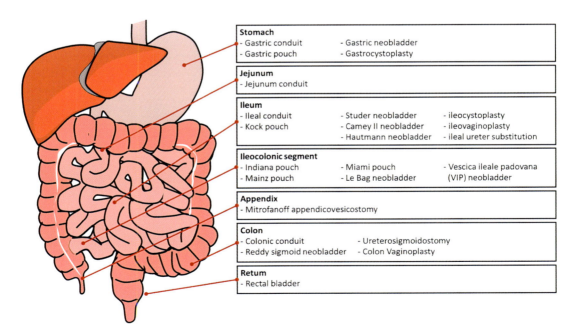

Fig. 4 Different bowel parts used in female genitourinary reconstruction

Evaluation of Patient

The use of the bowel in female genitourinary reconstruction involves three organ systems that have different roles and functions. The bowel is for digestion, nutrient absorption, and elimination of waste product in the form of feces, while the urinary tract is responsible for elimination of waste product in the form of urine and regulation of blood volume, electrolytes, and metabolites and serves as a buffer system to regulate blood pH. The female genitalia is part of the reproductive system that enables sexual intercourse, reproduction, pregnancy, and childbirth. Since the bowel is used to replace the function of the female genitourinary system, proper preoperative assessment is important to ensure that some of the requirements are fulfilled before using the bowel for female genitourinary reconstructive surgery. Preoperative evaluation can be divided according to the organ systems.

The upper urinary tract consists of the kidney and ureter. Ultrasound is a valuable tool to assess the kidney. Upper urinary tract deterioration may manifest as hydronephrosis, hydroureter, pyelonephritis, and renal atrophy, and these are well picked up by ultrasound. It is also important to evaluate renal function before urinary diversion because renal reserve is needed to buffer the metabolic and electrolyte disturbances caused by the bowel segments used. A GFR >40 ml/min/1.73 m^2 and serum creatinine <2.0 mg/dl are usually used as the cutoff for urinary diversion. Rarely, radioisotope imaging such as mercaptoacetyl-triglycyl (MAG3) renogram and dimercaptosuccinic acid (DMSA) scan will be needed.

The lower urinary tract consists of the bladder and urethra. Urodynamic study will be a useful tool to assess the bladder function: storage phase and voiding phase. Bladder capacity, bladder compliance, bladder sensation, presence of detrusor overactivity, and leak point pressure are important information prior to reconstructive surgery. Uroflowmetry and residual urine provide information on voiding phase which is important because patient might experience emptying problem after reconstructive surgery. Therefore, it is crucial to make sure that patients and family members are trained and committed to performing clean intermittent catheterization. Failure to do so will lead to a myriad of complications such as urinary tract infection, hydronephrosis, renal failure, and bladder rupture which can be life-threatening. For patients with physical and social limitations who are not able to perform clean intermittent catheterization, incontinent urinary diversion will be preferred over continence urinary diversion. The bladder neck and external urinary sphincter are important for continence mechanism. For example, if the continence mechanism is not functioning, continent cutaneous catheterizing pouch will be chosen over orthotopic neobladder.

Assessment to ascertain the suitability of bowel segments includes a thorough history of concomitant bowel conditions and any previous bowel surgery. Patients with inflammatory bowel disease or those who have shortened gut because of previous bowel surgery may not be suitable candidates. Colonic contrast study and colonoscopy are important to rule out bowel pathology such as polyps, diverticulum, inflammatory bowel disease, and malignancy when large bowel segments are used.

Other patient factors such as age, survival rate, and comorbidities must be taken into consideration when selecting suitable urinary diversion procedures. Incontinent urinary diversion may be more suitable in patients who cannot withstand prolonged surgery. Factors influencing the selection of urinary diversion are shown in Table 1.

Preoperative Preparation

Urine analysis and urine culture should be performed to rule out infection. Any positive urine culture should be treated with antibiotics according to local antibiotic sensitivity profile. Moreover, patients who are undergoing urinary diversion often have conditions such as neurogenic bladder, radiation cystitis, or fistula that put them at higher risk of urinary tract infection. After a complex reconstructive surgery, postoperative infection is the complication that we would least desire.

Table 1 Factors influencing urinary diversion selection

Disease factors	• Urethral margin
	• Continence mechanism
	• Bowel condition
Patient factors	• Age and survival rate
	• Comorbidities
	• Kidney function (GFR >40 ml/min/1.73 m^2 or serum creatinine <2.0 mg/dl)
	• Liver function
	• Manual dexterity and performance status
	• Patient preference and motivation
Surgeon factors	• Available expertise
	• Surgeon preference

Bowel preparation can be divided into mechanical bowel preparation and antibiotic bowel preparation. By utilizing polyethylene glycol or sodium phosphate, mechanical preparation lowers the amount of feces and bacteria concentration. However, it might lead to metabolic and electrolyte abnormalities. Antibiotic prophylaxis reduces bacterial concentration in feces; however, it has been known to cause pseudomembranous colitis by *Clostridium difficile*. The Best Practice Statement on Urologic Procedures and Antimicrobial Prophylaxis by the American Urological Association classified procedures using the bowel segments as contaminated procedures (Class III) and stated that:

> Preoperative mechanical bowel preparation and oral antibiotics for colorectal procedures are recommended by the WHO, consistent with most urologic practices using colorectal segments and associated with reduced complication rates. The use of small bowel segments for diversion does not necessitate a bowel prep." (Wolf et al. [4])

Coverage for both aerobic and anaerobic organisms is necessary since the bacterial flora in the colon is predominately composed of anaerobic organisms. It is recommended to use a first-generation cephalosporin and metronidazole for anaerobic coverage. According to one study, using the appropriate antibiotic prophylaxis reduced the likelihood of periprocedural infection complications from 39% to 13%, in line with the majority of the literature [5]. Clinicians need to be aware that many institutions have different protocols, regimes, and antimicrobial sensitivities, all of which influence how antibiotic prophylaxis is administered.

Surgical Techniques

Bowel Anastomosis

Bowel anastomosis is an important component of reconstructive urology. Sutures and staples can be used for end-to-end or side-to-side bowel anastomoses. Due to their simplicity, reliability, and wide availability, staples are frequently used nowadays. A successful bowel anastomosis requires adherence to several factors. As a general principle, avoid using irradiated bowel. Adequate bowel mobilization allows good exposure. Good vascularity is ensured by choosing the appropriate vascular arcade, avoiding excessive tension, and overuse of electrocautery. Measures must be taken to avoid spillage of bowel contents in the operative field and segments of the bowel to be used are irrigated with normal saline. Apposition of the bowel is usually done in single-layer anastomosis by using either absorbable sutures or staples. The apposition of serosa to serosa and mucosa to mucosa should be watertight and tension-free. The mesentery window is usually closed to avoid any potential herniation of the bowel through it. The use of indocyanine green fluorescence imaging is an effective method to assess bowel perfusion and to prevent anastomotic leak [6].

Ureterointestinal Anastomosis

The ureter can be implanted either to the small bowel or the large bowel. There are two types of ureterointestinal anastomosis: refluxing and antirefluxing. The benefits of antireflux mechanisms are controversial; numerous studies have found no conclusive advantages of one over the other. Antirefluxing anastomosis is at higher risk of stricture than refluxing anastomosis and does not prevent bacterial colonization of the renal pelvis. Additionally, refluxing anastomosis is easier to perform.

Regardless of the kind of anastomosis, long-term renal impairment is seen as a result of complications such as urolithiasis, infection, anastomotic stricture, and leakage [7].

Even though there are numerous techniques for constructing the various types of ureterointestinal anastomosis, certain fundamental surgical principles apply when performing them. Minimal mobilization of the ureter is important to preserve the periadventitial tissue in which ureter's blood supply courses. The bowel should be brought to the ureter and not otherwise to reduce mobilization of the ureter. Fine absorbable sutures are used to create a tension-free, watertight mucosa-to-mucosa anastomosis. Whenever possible, it is ideal to retroperitonealize the anastomosis. The use of temporary soft silastic stents across ureterointestinal anastomoses may prevent anastomotic leaks and strictures.

In Bricker technique, ureters are implanted individually to the bowel in an end-to-side fashion. In Wallace technique, ureters are spatulated, connected, and implanted to the bowel in an end-to-end fashion. Utilizing the Nipple method, the ureter is spatulated and flipped back on itself. The most common antireflux technique is submucosal tunneling where ureters are implanted submucosally with sufficient muscle support to act as a flap valve. As the reservoir fills, the implanted ureter's lumen is sealed off by the increase in intrareservoir pressure. Taenia colon is utilized as a muscle backboard because it has a firmer consistency than other intestinal segments. The submucosal tunneling concept is applied by Strickler, Pagano, and Goodwin transcolonic techniques with a few methodological modifications. In Leadbetter-Clarke technique, the ureter is spatulated and implanted to the bowel mucosa with the seromuscular layer of the bowel being sutured over the ureter. It is important not to occlude the ureter [3] (Fig. 5).

Urinary Stoma

A stoma is a urine-draining orifice above the abdominal wall. There are two types of stomas: flush stoma and protruding stoma. Flush stoma is flushed to the skin and is preferable for continent cutaneous urinary diversion where intermittent catheterization is performed. The protruding stoma is preferable in incontinent urinary diversion where a collecting device is worn. Marking of the stomal site is important and is often done with the patient in sitting and supine position. It is done over the rectus muscle at least 5 cm away from the planned incision site. Bony prominences, skin creases, scars, umbilicus, and belt line should be avoided. To prevent parastomal hernia, the stoma should be placed through the rectus muscle and positioned at the apex of the infraumbilical fat roll. Stomal complications include bowel necrosis, bleeding, stomal prolapse, stomal retraction, stomal stenosis, and parastomal hernia [8].

Urinary Diversion

Urinary diversion is the re-routing of urine from its natural pathway, which is the bladder and urethra. The aim of urinary diversion is to offer a practical, convenient, and reliable drainage system when the native bladder is no longer able to serve this function.

The following are the indications for urine diversion:

Malignancy

Bladder Cancer

Bladder cancer is one of the most common indications for urinary diversion as bladder cancer is the tenth most common malignancy worldwide and the sixth most common malignancy in men [9]. The American Cancer Society estimates that in 2022, there are 81,180 new cases of bladder cancer and 17,100 deaths from bladder cancer [10]. Bladder cancer is four times more common in men than women and 90% of the bladder cancer diagnosis are made in those 55 years of age and older. The etiology of bladder cancer is multifactorial, a combination of genetic factors, demographic factors, environmental factors, and chronic bladder irritation. Tobacco smoking, exposure to chemical carcinogens, and

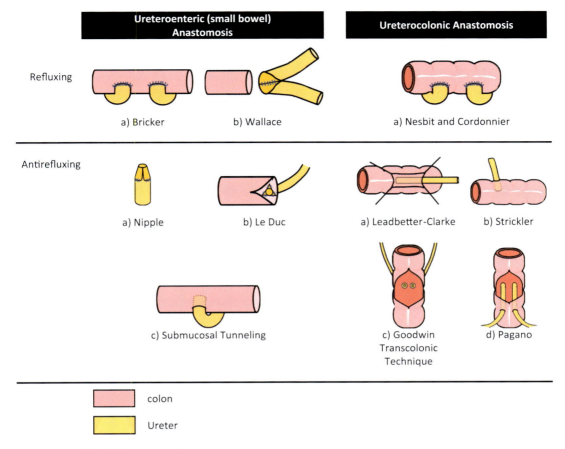

Fig. 5 Ureterointestinal anastomosis

schistosomiasis are among the main risk factors for bladder cancer. Based on the depth of invasion, bladder cancer can be divided into non-muscle-invasive and muscle-invasive diseases. While most bladder cancers are low-grade, are of early stage, and can be treated minimally invasively, radical cystectomy with urinary diversion is the standard treatment for patients with muscle-invasive bladder cancer or recurrent high-grade non-muscle-invasive bladder cancer. Radical cystectomy should also be considered in patients with concerning variant histology and high-grade T1 with concerning features such as CIS and in those with Bacillus-Calmette-Guerin (BCG) failure [11]. In these cohorts of patients who undergo radical cystectomy, bowel segments will be used for urinary diversion. The American Urology Association (AUA) guidelines on the treatment of nonmetastatic muscle-invasive bladder cancer recommend that different methods of urinary diversion should be discussed with patients, and in patients receiving orthotopic neobladder, a negative urethral margin needs to be verified. The 5-year relative survival is 77% in all stages combined, 96% in carcinoma in situ, 70% with localized disease, 38% with regional disease, and 6% with a distant-stage disease [10].

Nonurological Pelvic Tumor

Due to the proximity of the genitourinary system and gastrointestinal tract in the pelvic cavity, tumor from any one of the systems may interfere with the function of another system by infiltration, compression, and displacement. Colorectal cancer, gynecological malignancies, soft tissue sarcoma, and bone sarcoma are the common nonurological pelvic tumors that infiltrate the urinary system. Endometrial cancer, cervical cancer, ovarian cancer, and vaginal and vulvar cancer are examples of gynecological malignancies. Frequently, the urinary tract system is included in the staging of gynecological malignancies. For example, in stage IIIB of cervical cancer, it extends to the pelvic sidewalls causing hydronephrosis. The bladder and urethra are infiltrated in stage IV vulvar cancer. Multiple modalities of diagnosis are available and they are disease-specific. To achieve a clear tumor margin, treatment may involve ureteral reconstruction, cystectomy, and pelvic exenteration in which urinary diversion will be needed [12].

Bladder Dysfunction

Urinary diversion for benign conditions is not commonly performed and it is usually used as the last resort when medical treatments and other less invasive therapy have failed. Neurological bladder dysfunction is caused by various conditions in all ages such as multiple sclerosis, Parkinson's disease, spinal cord injury, and spina bifida. Non-neurological bladder dysfunction is caused by inflammatory contracted bladder. Although it is not included in the current standardization of terminology of lower urinary tract function reported by the subcommittee of the International Continence Society (ICS), inflammatory contracted bladder is defined as a volumetric capacity of less than 50 ml by Cantu et al. [13]. It usually manifests as end stage of a disease where irreversible damage had occurred. Among the benign causes of inflammatory contracted bladder are infection, inflammatory condition, neurogenic bladder, drugs, and radiation-induced and decompensated bladder outlet obstruction. All these conditions will lead to impaired urothelium permeability, detrusor hypertrophy, and reduction of collagen, elastin, and proteoglycan matrix in the bladder stroma.

Urogenital Tuberculosis

Mycobacterium tuberculosis, which causes tuberculosis, is a major public health issue in developing nations. There are two types of tuberculosis: pulmonary and extrapulmonary. Risk factors for extrapulmonary tuberculosis include immunosuppression, such as HIV infection, alcoholism, smoking, malnutrition, chronic kidney disease, and autoimmune disease. Genitourinary tuberculosis occurs in 15–20% of cases of pulmonary TB with a prevalence of 400/100,000 population [14]. It is the second most common form of extrapulmonary tuberculosis only after tuberculous lymphadenopathy, and it happens when the bacteria are spread through the bloodstream to the adjacent organs from the foci in the lung. The kidney is usually the first organ to be affected and then it spreads to the ureters and bladder. It is equally prevalent in both sexes and is most common in the fourth decade of life [15]. The clinical manifestation of tuberculosis is rather not specific, which results in late diagnosis, delayed treatment, irreversible organ damage, and severe complications. The pathophysiology of tuberculosis includes chronic inflammation, granulomatous inflammation, and caseation necrosis leading to fibrosis and stricture. In genitourinary TB, this will manifest as hydronephrosis, hydroureter, reduced bladder capacity, urinary outflow tract obstruction, distortion of renal pelvis and calyces, and renal failure. In advance stage of genitourinary tuberculosis where gross anatomy distortion leads to irreversible organ dysfunction, there is a role of reconstructive surgery such as bladder augmentation and ileal ureter substitution. The aim of reconstructive surgery is to restore the normal or near-normal function of the urinary system.

Urogenital Schistosomiasis

In Africa and the Middle East, schistosomiasis, also known as bilharzia, is endemic. It is a parasitic disease caused by blood fluke, *Schistosoma haematobium*. It is transmitted through contaminated water where the parasite enters the human body through the skin and subsequently travels to the liver to mature and produce eggs that are spread hematogenously. It has tropism for the lower urinary tract, such as the bladder and distal ureter because of the rich venous supply. With globalization and the advancement of transportation, clinicians from all around the world might encounter patients with schistosomiasis. It is an important differential diagnosis when a patient complains of hematuria. Patient demographics and travel history are important parts of the workup. Clinical presentation of the genitourinary tract includes hematuria, dysuria, urinary retention, intermenstrual bleeding, and pelvic pain. The body's immune response to the *Schistosoma* ova leads to inflammation, mucosal erosion, granuloma formation, fibrosis, scarring, and calcification. Damage to the urinary tract includes ureteric stricture, bladder neck stenosis, contracted bilharzial bladder, detrusor damage, periurethral abscess, and fistula formation. All these changes will subsequently lead to obstructive uropathy, vesicoureteric reflux, and renal failure. Besides that, it also increases the risk of urolithiasis and bladder cancer. In females, *Schistosoma haematobium* has been found in the cervix, vagina, and vulva, which can lead to subfertility. Because of the long latency of the disease with unspecific symptoms, patients usually present at an advanced stage with irreversible damage to their genitourinary system, which requires surgical treatments such as segmental resection, augmentation cystoplasty, or even radical cystectomy with urinary diversion [16].

Drugs and Radiation-Induced Cystitis

The incidence of ketamine cystitis is on the rise as it is abused as a recreational drug rather than for anesthetic purposes. It is characterized by lower urinary tract symptoms (LUTS), hematuria, and contracted bladder. Although the mainstay of treatment is cessation of ketamine use, unfortunately, due to addiction and chronic abuse of ketamine, some patients end up with severe ketamine cystitis involving upper tract deterioration that needs to revert to augmentation cystoplasty or urinary diversion. BCG, mitomycin C, and epirubicin are used as intravesical adjuvant agents for the treatment of non-muscle-invasive cancer. However, contracted bladder has been reported as a result of the extravasation of these agents [17]. Radiation therapy is one of the therapeutic modalities commonly used for pelvic malignancies that can lead to a spectrum of complications from mild LUTS to contracted bladder and life-threatening hemorrhagic cystitis. Conservative treatments for radiation cystitis include bladder irrigation, systemic and intravesical agents, endoscopic procedures, and hyperbaric oxygen therapy. Failure of these conservative measures may warrant surgical treatment such as cystectomy and urinary diversion. Newer pelvic radiotherapy techniques such as stereotactic body radiation therapy, image-guided radiotherapy, intensity-modulated radiation therapy, and brachytherapy have reduced the toxicity of radiation therapy [18].

Congenital Urogenital Anomaly

Congenital urogenital anomalies such as bladder exstrophy, posterior urethral valve, and prune belly syndromes constitute a huge burden and challenging field for pediatric and adolescent urology. Not only does the etiology is not well understood, but treatment for these conditions also requires complex reconstructive surgery and involves multidisciplinary teams. Not seldom, urinary diversion using bowel segments will be needed. Prune belly syndrome is a rare congenital anomaly with an incidence of 1 in 40,000 live births, characterized by the absence of abdominal musculature, urinary tract abnormalities, and cryptorchidism [19]. Dysplasia of the smooth muscles of the renal pelvis, ureters, and urethra will lead to renal dysplasia, hydronephrosis, mega-ureters, mega-vesicles, and renal failure. Treatment consists of orchidopexy and abdominal wall and urinary tract reconstruction. Bladder exstrophy or ectopia vesicae is a rare yet serious congenital anomaly with an incidence of 1 in 30,000 live births [20]. Incomplete fusion of the mesoderm, which forms the tubercle genitalia, bladder, and anterior abdominal wall, will lead to rectus muscle separation, symphysis pubis diastasis, eversion of the bladder into the anterior abdominal wall, and genitalia deformities. The surgical treatment of bladder exstrophy comprises not only bladder closure but also epispadias repair, bladder neck reconstruction, bladder augmentation, and ureteric reimplantation.

Other Conditions

Trauma of the ureters, bladder, and urethra and incurable urogenital fistula.

The ideal urinary diversion should mimic the physiologic urinary tract, which is a low-pressure reservoir with non-refluxing and continent mechanism. This principle is important to protect the upper urinary tract. Because of this, orthotopic neobladder has evolved into the most ideal form of urinary diversion available today compared to other forms of urinary diversion and should be considered the gold standard in fit and young patients. Technically, urinary diversion should be simple to construct, should avoid using excessive length of bowels, and should have low risk of surgical revision and have good cosmetic appearance and functional outcome [1]. Despite the large variation in the techniques used, urinary diversion can be divided into two general categories: continent and incontinent. Continent urinary diversion can be subdivided into three types depending on how the urine is drained. In cutaneous catheterizing pouch, the stoma is used to drain the urine, while in an orthotopic bladder, the urethra is used. In ureterosigmoidostomy, urine is drained through the anus. Each type of urinary diversion has its advantages and disadvantages.

Conduit

Conduit is when a segment of the bowel is anastomosed to the ureters at one end and opened through the abdominal wall via the stoma on the other end to excrete urine. An external appliance is applied to the stoma to collect urine. It is the simplest diversion to construct with the least complications and is usually used as palliative urinary diversion in patients with short life expectancy or patients who are frail and not fit for long extensive surgery. No bladder retraining is required and there is no issue of nocturnal incontinence as compared to continent pouches and neobladders. Compared with cutaneous ureterostomy, where the ureter is brought out directly to the abdominal wall, the conduit has a lower risk of ureteral stricture, stoma stenosis, infection, and renal deterioration. Typically, conduit only needs 15–25 cm segment of the bowel, as opposed to reservoirs, which need 40–80 cm of the bowel to construct. The conduit's length is important because if it is too short, the blood supply will be compromised. On the other hand, if the conduit is excessively long, it will cause greater metabolic difficulties by increasing the absorption of electrolytes. Other disadvantages of conduits are the need for stoma bags and stoma-related complications such as parastomal hernia and urinary leakage around the stoma, leading to skin excoriation. Conduits come in three different varieties: ileal, jejunal, and colonic.

Ileal Conduit

The ileum, which makes up 2/5 of the length of the small bowel, is easily accessible, and the majority of its segments can be easily mobilized to the pelvis. It is the most common and simple type of conduit with the least complication. However, it is not suitable for patients with short bowel syndrome, inflammatory bowel disease, and extensive pelvic radiation. A 10–15 cm length of the ileum 10–15 cm from the ileocaecal valve is harvested and the remaining bowel segment is brought cephalad to it for bowel anastomosis. The left ureter is brought to the right lower quadrant retroperitoneally under the mesentery and both ureters are spatulated and implanted into the ileum using the Bricker or Wallace technique. The proximal end of the ileal conduit is fixed to the posterior peritoneum to prevent volvulus of the conduit, and the distal end is brought through the abdomen rectus muscle, fixed to the fascia, and everted into a stoma. It is important to ensure the ileal conduit is in isoperistaltic fashion to prevent reflux. Due to the length of the ileal mesentery, stoma is usually located over the right lower quadrant of the abdomen rather than the left. To prevent bowel herniation lateral to the ileal conduit, the ureter is fixed to the peritoneum.

Jejunal Conduit

It is used only if no other bowel segment is available because of the severe metabolic complications caused.

Colon Conduit

It is used in patients who underwent extensive pelvic radiation limiting the use of the small bowel. The transverse colon is least likely to be exposed to radiation in patients who underwent pelvic irradiation. However, colon conduit is not suitable for patients with inflammatory large bowel disease and severe chronic diarrhea. Due to the proximity of the transverse colon and the upper ureter, transverse colon conduit is a good choice for patients with short ureter segments. The transverse colon conduit stoma is usually placed high on the patient's abdomen. The sigmoid colon conduit is a good option for patients who are undergoing total pelvic exenteration with colostomy placement because no bowel anastomosis will be needed.

Specific complications for conduit are parastomal hernia and conduit deformities. Parastomal hernia is an abnormal protrusion of intra-abdominal contents through an abdominal wall defect, near or within the site of stoma. Risk factors for parastomal hernia are advanced age, obesity, poor nutritional status, connective tissue disorder, and increased intra-abdominal pressure as in constipation, chronic cough, and heavy lifting. Most of the patients are asymptomatic; however, it can cause pain, poor stomal bag fitting, bowel obstruction, strangulation, and incarceration. Treatment of parastomal hernia includes hernia belt, primary suture repair, mesh-based repair, or relocation of the stoma. Conduit deformities can be in the form of conduit stricture or conduit elongation.

Cutaneous Catheterizing Pouch

Cutaneous catheterizing pouch is a type of continent urinary diversion where a small catheterizable stoma on the anterior abdominal wall is used to empty urine from an intra-abdominal reservoir (pouch). The reservoir can be made from the ileum, ileocolonic segment, or colon. Cutaneous catheterizing pouch is a blend of orthotopic neobladder and ileal conduit and shares some similar characteristics with the two methods. It has a low-pressure storage reservoir made of bowel segments, similar to the orthotopic neobladder; however, the reservoir is ectopically placed in the abdomen. Like the ileal conduit, it has a stoma on the anterior abdominal wall for the drainage of urine. It is used in patients who desire continence and are able to perform clean intermittent catheterization, but the urethra cannot be incorporated into reconstructive surgery due to stricture or malignancy.

With the increasing concern about body image and the need for a urinary diversion without external appliances, continent urinary diversion has become more popular for the benefit of psychological and functional well-being. Patients are able to achieve both daytime and nighttime continence. Continent catheterizing pouch is secured to the anterior abdominal wall and usually located at the umbilicus for ease of catheterization or at the lower abdominal quadrant below the bikini line so that the stoma can be concealed.

However, continent catheterizing pouch surgery is technically difficult and there is a significant risk of revision. Metabolic complications may occur due to the length of the bowel used. Patients need to have the dexterity to perform intermittent catheterization and the ability to follow a strict flushing and irrigation regime. Pouch rupture may occur if it is not catheterized and drained properly. Pouch urinary retention is also a urological emergency. Stomal stenosis and parastomal hernias are known complications. Intermittent catheterization may be difficult and cause false tracts.

Over the years, different types of cutaneous catheterizing pouches have been invented depending on the bowel segments used to construct the reservoir, the antireflux mechanism used in the afferent limb which connects to the ureter, and the continence mechanism used in the efferent limb which connects to the stoma (Fig. 6).

The Indiana pouch remains one of the most commonly performed cutaneous catheterizing pouches because it is easy to perform, reliable with a low complication rate, and able to withstand the trauma of catheterization through buttressed ileocaecal valve. Twenty centimeter length of cecum and ascending colon are detubularized

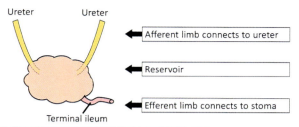

Cutaneous Catheterizing Pouch	Bowel Segment	Anti-reflux Mechanism	Continence Mechanism
Kock pouch	Ileum	Nipple valve	Nipple valve
Indiana pouch	Ileocolonic segment	Submucosal tunnelling (ureterotenial implant)	Imbricated ileocecal valve and tapering of ileum
Mainz pouch	Ileocolonic segment	Submucosal tunnelling (ureterotenial implant)	Nipple valve
UCLA pouch	Ileocolonic segment	Submucosal tunnelling (ureterotenial implant)	Nipple valve
Gastric pouch	Stomach	Any method	Flap valve

Fig. 6 Components and types of cutaneous catheterizing pouch

and constructed into a reservoir. The ureters are anastomosed to the reservoir at the taenia coli using the submucosal tunneling antireflux technique. Fifteen centimeter length of terminal ileum is used as the efferent limb and the ileocaecal valve is imbricated with sutures to improve continence. The Kock pouch was first developed by Nils Kock in 1975 to mimic the natural urinary system [21]. A 78 cm segment of the ileum is harvested 15 cm from the cecum. The ileum is divided into four smaller segments measuring 17, 22, 22, and 17 cm. The two 22 cm ileal segments are detubularized and sutured together to form a reservoir with larger volumes. The proximal 17 cm ileal segment is made into the afferent limb with nipple valve as the antireflux mechanism to which the ureters are attached. The distal 17 cm is made into the efferent limb with nipple valve as the continence mechanism and is brought to the abdominal wall. The Kock pouch is not commonly used in modern medicine because of the complications associated with the instability of the nipple valve needing revision surgery. The University of California, Los Angeles (UCLA) pouch uses the right colon as the reservoir with intussusception of the terminal ileum and ileocecal valve as the continence mechanism. The distal ileum is used as efferent limb. In the Miami pouch, the continence mechanism is provided by the circumferential suturing of the ileocecal segment. The Indiana, UCLA, and Miami pouches are simpler to construct than the Kock pouch but they hold a smaller volume of urine.

Figure 7 shows four continence mechanisms for the efferent limb where catheterization is performed:

a) In appendiceal tunneling or ileal tunneling (flap valve), part of the efferent limb is within the reservoir against a fixed wall. The increase in intra-reservoir pressure will compress the efferent limb during the filling phase. This mechanism is used in Mitrofanoff and Yang-Monti procedure.

b) In intussusception method (nipple valve), invagination of the efferent limb into the pouch results in nipple valve. Equivalent pressure inside the reservoir will be reflected on the outlet, preventing leakage. This mechanism is used in the Kock pouch.

c) Imbrication, plication, and tapering of the bowel (ileocaecal valve) will increase the resistance to urinary leakage by narrowing the

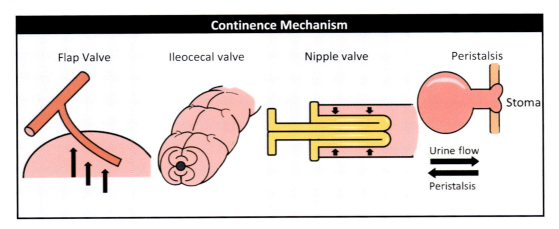

Fig. 7 Continence mechanism

efferent limb. This mechanism is used in the Indiana pouch.

d) Peristalsis is used as a continence mechanism. When the ileum is used as an efferent limb, the preceding peristalsis of the ileum which has higher contraction pressure compared to the colon will serve as a counteractive force to overcome leakage. This mechanism is used in the Studer pouch.

The Mitrofanoff procedure and Yang-Monti procedure are also using the same principle to divert urine. The difference is that these procedures usually use the bladder rather than the pouch as the reservoir. They are also called catheterizable urinary stomas. In the Mitrofanoff procedure (appendicovesicostomy), the appendix is used as a channel for catheterization to drain the urine. The stoma is usually located at the right lower quadrant of the abdomen or the umbilicus. The appendix is ideal for this use as it is a natural tubular structure with little known function and can be removed from the gastrointestinal tract without causing any complications. For patients who do not have an appendix or with a short appendix, the ileum may be used as a substitute (ileovesicostomy). A 2.5 cm length of the ileum with its vascular pedicle will be isolated, detubularized along the antimesenteric border, and transversally retubularized over a 12 F catheter. For other tubular structures such as the fallopian tube, the ureter has also been used as a channel. The goal of these procedures is to provide a continent urinary diversion that is easy to catheterize. The Mitrofanoff procedure and Yang-Monti procedure are usually performed in patients with neurogenic lower urinary tract dysfunction that have difficulty with standard urethral catheterization, such as the pediatric population, elderly population with limited dexterity, and wheelchair or bed-bound patients. These procedures are usually combined with augmentation cystoplasty. Children with prune belly syndrome, posterior urethral valves, or bladder exstrophy who have intact urethral sensation and are reluctant to catheterize through the urethra might benefit from these procedures as well. Besides that, these procedures are also performed in patients who have urethral stricture, urethral trauma, nonfunctional urethra, and severe autonomic dysreflexia, who require an alternative channel to drain the urine (Fig. 8).

Orthotopic Neobladder

Orthotopic neobladder is creating a new bladder in the pelvic cavity that is anastomosed to the urethra that allows volitional voiding. The neobladder should have the ideal properties of a natural intact bladder: good capacity of 300–500 ml, good compliance with low-pressure storage, anti-reflux mechanism, intact external urethral sphincter with continence mechanism, and minimal

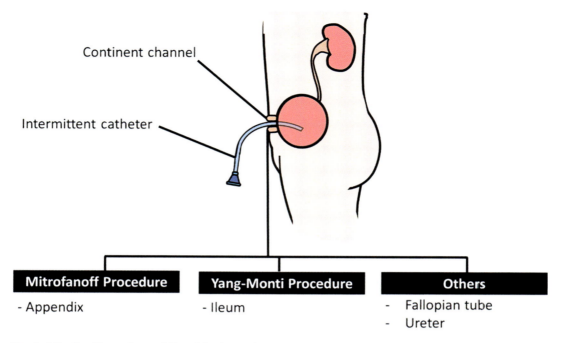

Fig. 8 Mitrofanoff procedure and Yang-Monti procedure

metabolic complications. There is no stoma involved and therefore patients have a better body image and better sexual function. An orthotopic bladder allows a physiological route of urination through the urethra with normal to near-normal continence. The urethra should be free from tumor and unobstructed and have adequate external urinary sphincter function. Patients must be highly motivated, have good dexterity, and be willing to do intermittent catheterization and irrigation. Seventy-five percent of females undergoing cystectomy are potential candidates for orthotopic neobladder. Contraindications of orthotopic neobladder are renal impairment (eGFR >40 ml/min), liver impairment, cognitive impairment, physical limitation with poor dexterity, lack of patient motivation and poor follow-up, and presence of metastatic disease and tumor at the bladder neck. Advanced age, obesity, and prior pelvic irradiation are not absolute contraindications, but should be taken into careful consideration.

There is a risk of urethral cancer recurrence when surgery is performed for the treatment of bladder cancer. The urethral margin for females will be the bladder neck. Female patients with palpable tumor at the anterior vaginal wall and cervix should be suspected of bladder neck involvement. Intraoperative frozen section will accurately identify the involvement of the bladder neck. Following radical cystectomy, it is crucial to monitor the retained urethra in individuals with orthotopic neobladders.

The orthotopic bladder is using the urethral sphincter for continence mechanism. To maintain continence mechanism, rhabdosphincter muscle fibers and innervation of the pudendal nerve in the area of the proximal urethra should be preserved. A Foley catheter balloon can be used to serve as a guide for defining the bladder neck. Endopelvic fascia and levator muscles should not be disturbed and the bladder is dissected completely off the anterior vaginal wall rather than excising it.

The orthotopic bladder consists of three components: reservoir, afferent limb connecting to the ureter, and efferent limb connect to the urethra. The ileum and ileocolonic segment appear to provide the best physiologic properties for orthotopic neobladder which are less contractility and better compliance. However, the disadvantages are diarrhea and decreased intestinal absorption of bile acid and vitamin B12. Mobilization of the bowel segments must be performed carefully to preserve the blood supply to the neobladder and bowel anastomosis. Bowel segments are detubularized and folded in different ways with the aim of constructing the cylindrical bowel segment into a spherical reservoir. The types of orthotopic bladder will depend on the types of bowel segments used, methods of folding (U-shaped, Z-shaped, W-shaped, spherical), and methods of ureterointestinal anastomosis (refluxing, antirefluxing). In the Studer, Hautmann and Camey II neobladder, 40–60 cm of ileal segment is used to construct the neobladder. All three techniques are commonly performed with good functional results. In the Mainz neobladder, a 15 cm length of the cecum and ascending colon and 30 cm segment of the distal ileum are used to construct the reservoir. The ureters are implanted to the reservoir and an opening is made at the inferior portion of the cecum and attached to the urethra. Different types of orthotopic neobladders are shown in Fig. 9.

Orthotopic neobladder is a technically difficult surgery. Although the use of ileal bowel segments is ideal, the disadvantages are diarrhea, decreased

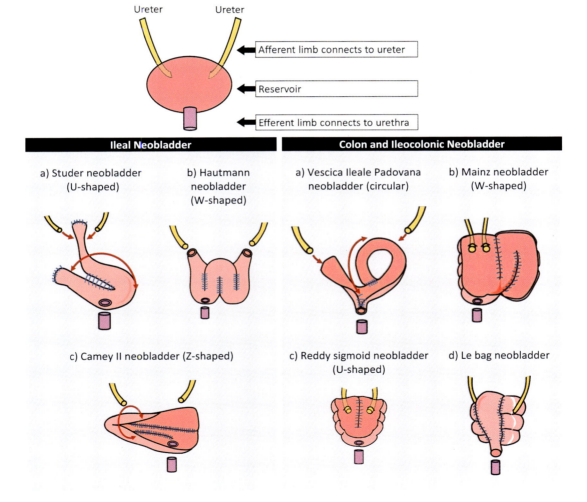

Fig. 9 Components and types of orthotopic neobladder

intestinal absorption of bile acid and vitamin B12, as well as metabolic complications. Postoperatively rigorous neobladder training is mandatory. There are risks of nocturnal urinary incontinence and urinary retention. Many studies are comparing orthotopic neobladders with other types of urinary diversion using different parameters and outcomes; however, the conclusion is heterogeneous. Some of the outcomes that are looked into are continence, urinary retention, quality of life, and complication rate.

Continence

Although orthotopic neobladder is classified under continent urinary diversion, patients should be warned regarding the risk of incontinence after surgery. Factors that influence continence are age, intestinal segment used, surgical techniques, and presence of incontinence before surgery. Published continence rates in large series range from 90% to 92% for daytime continence and 80% for nocturnal continence [22]. It is important to rule out other causes of incontinence such as fistula, urinary tract infection, or overflow incontinence due to urinary retention. Persistent nocturnal incontinence is observed in 20–50% of the patients. The mechanisms for nocturnal incontinence include decreased sensation leading to overdistension, failure of urethral closure, physiologic diuresis, and urinary sphincter relaxation during sleep. Urinary continence developed gradually over time and the evaluation and treatment of urinary incontinence after orthotopic diversion should be delayed until the neobladder has had time to expand and reach its functional capacity, which may take up to 12–18 months. As the treatment of urinary incontinence after orthotopic neobladder is challenging, it is best to avoid the development of urinary incontinence by careful patient selection, meticulous surgical technique, and good patient education to ensure good outcomes. Meticulous surgical technique in the form of urethral nerve-sparing and preserving the uterus has been shown to be crucial in maintaining continence and preventing urinary retention. Treatment will depend on the types of urinary incontinence and varies from conservative treatment such as lifestyle modification and behavioral therapy to medical treatment for urge urinary incontinence and surgical treatment for stress urinary incontinence such as urethral bulking agents, retropubic slings, and artificial urinary sphincter. Conversion to an incontinence or continent cutaneous diversion remains the last resort of treatment.

Urinary Retention

On the other spectrum, 20–60% of the patients do experience urinary retention after surgery. The mechanisms of urinary retention are acute angulation of the urethra, excess reservoir capacity, anastomotic stricture, pouchocele, and pelvic floor dyssynergia. It is important to rule out tumor recurrence by doing a vaginal and rectal examination. Self-catheterization is the most effective treatment for urinary retention. The incidence of chronic urinary retention could be decreased by transposing the omentum behind the neobladder to increase its support, preserving the uterus with its ligamentous support, preserving the vaginal wall's neurovascular bundle, and suspending the neobladder to the back of the rectus muscle [23].

Quality of Life

Patient's quality of life has been evaluated using different validated questionnaires and visual analog scales. Different aspects of life are being evaluated: general well-being, physical health, mental health, and psychosocial and sexual function. However, they are criticized for their methodologic flaws, limiting the ability to draw a uniform conclusion. Therefore, it is difficult to conclude which method of urinary diversion is the best.

Ureterosigmoidostomy

Ureterosigmoidostomy was the first urinary diversion performed in 1852 by Simon. A length of 20–25 cm of the sigmoid colon is harvested proximal to the rectosigmoid junction and folded into a

U-shaped pouch and ureters are implanted into it. It is also known as rectal bladder which results in a mixture of feces and urine, and it depends on the anal sphincter for urinary and fecal continence. Ureterosigmoidostomy is obsolete in modern medicine due to its high rate of serious complications such as secondary malignancy, urinary tract infection, urolithiasis, urinary and fecal incontinence, and renal failure. Different innovations had been invented, trying to reduce these complications by separating the fecal and urinary streams, and preventing the backflow of urine: folded rectosigmoid bladder, augmented valved rectum, sigma-rectum pouch, and hemi-Kock and T pouch procedures with valved rectum. However, these procedures are substituted by other better methods of urinary diversion that have fewer complications.

Augmentation Cystoplasty

Augmentation cystoplasty is a surgical procedure to increase bladder capacity by adding a bowel segment. The bladder is bivalved like a clam, through a coronal incision extending down close to the trigone, on either side of the ureteric orifices. A corresponding length of the bowel is harvested longitudinally along the anti-mesenteric border, preserving its blood supply. The bowel segment with its vascular pedicle is then patched and sutured onto the margins of the opened bladder. The goal of augmentation cystoplasty is to protect the upper urinary tract by converting a small, contracted, and high-pressure bladder to a low-pressure, compliant reservoir with effective continence and emptying mechanism. Besides increasing bladder compliance and capacity, it also lowers urinary tract symptoms and improves continence and patients' quality of life. The risk of pyelonephritis and renal impairment is also reduced with the resolution of vesicoureteral reflux.

Augmentation ileocystoplasty was first described by Mikulicz in 1989. Lemoine used colonic segment for colocystoplasty in 1912 and Couvelaire was the first to advocate the use of cecum in caecocystoplasty in 1950. The introduction of clean intermittent catheterization by Lapides in 1972 provided a solution to the problem of urine retention, and this has led to the increased utilization of bowel segments in urologic surgeries and the popularization of augmentation cystoplasty [24].

Different bowel segments are used to enlarge the bladder: the ileum (ileocystoplasty), colon (colocystoplasty), and stomach (gastrocystoplasty). Although each bowel segment has its advantages and disadvantages, the ileum is used the most due to its merits. The large bowel is at higher risk of metabolic complications and malignancy, and excessive mucus production. Like in any other graft, the ideal bladder augmentation material should have the following qualities: biologically inert, viable, easily shaped, capable of distention at low pressure, endoscopically accessible for routine examination, not absorbing urinary constituents, and not secreting mucus. With the advancement of technology, augmentation cystoplasty can now be performed not only using the open method but also laparoscopically and robotically. The indication for augmentation cystoplasty can be widely grouped into:

Non-neurogenic

Non-neurogenic bladder conditions that may require augmentation cystoplasty include infective conditions such as tuberculosis and schistosomiasis. Noninfective conditions include congenital urogenital anomalies, interstitial cystitis, radiation cystitis, and refractory overactive bladder (OAB). OAB is a clinical diagnosis defined by the International Continence Society (ICS) as the presence of "urinary urgency, usually accompanied by frequency and nocturia, with or without urgency urinary incontinence, in the absence of a urinary tract infection or other obvious pathology." Urgency is considered the hallmark symptom of OAB and it is defined by the ICS as the "complaint of a sudden, compelling desire to pass urine which is difficult to defer" [25]. To date, the pathophysiology of OAB is still not fully understood and there are various types of treatment available. First-line treatments are patient education and behavioral therapy, which include bladder training, bladder control strategies, pelvic floor muscle training, and fluid management. Second-line treatments consist of pharmacological treatment, which consists of anticholinergic drugs and beta-3 agonists. With the advancement of OAB treatment such as intradetrusor onabotulinum toxin A injection and sacral neuromodulation, the use of augmentation cystoplasty has declined. However, it remained as one of the surgical treatment modalities for refractory OAB where medical and other less invasive methods are exhausted. The American Urological Association (AUA) and European Urological Association (EAU) do not recommend surgery as the treatment for OAB patients. Augmentation cystoplasty should only be offered to patients after other modalities of treatment have failed. Patients should be counseled regarding the need for lifelong follow-up and the likely need for long-term clean intermittent self-catheterization and a small risk of malignancy [26, 27].

Neurogenic

Neurogenic lower urinary tract dysfunction (NLUTD) has replaced the prior commonly used terminology "neurogenic bladder" and is defined by AUA as "abnormal function of either the bladder, bladder neck, and/or its sphincters related to a neurologic disorder" [28]. The normal function of the lower urinary tract depends on the complex interplay between the central and peripheral nervous systems. Any neurological disorders can disturb the function of the urinary tract. The pattern of lower urinary tract dysfunction following neurological disorder will depend on the site, nature, and extent of the neurological lesion. Cerebral vascular accident, Parkinson's disease, Alzheimer's disease, multiple sclerosis, spinal cord injury, spina bifida, tethered spinal cord, and peripheral neuropathy are examples of neurological disorders that can cause NLUTD. According to AUA and EUA, clinicians may offer augmentation cystoplasty to NLUTD patients who are refractory to less invasive therapies for detrusor overactivity and/or poor bladder compliance [29].

Although many clinical conditions serve as the indication for augmentation cystoplasty, three parameters dictate the rationale for augmentation cystoplasty: bladder compliance, bladder capacity, and detrusor activity.

Bladder Compliance

Bladder compliance is the relationship between change in bladder volume and change in detrusor pressure ($\Delta V/\Delta P$). It is a measurement of bladder stiffness. Normal bladder is highly compliant and able to hold large amounts of urine at low pressure. For females, normal compliance will be >30 ml/ml H_2O for neurogenic bladder and >40 ml/cm H_2O for non-neurogenic bladder. Low bladder compliance is defined as bladder compliance <10 ml/cm H_2O for neurogenic bladder and <30 ml/cm H_2O for non-neurogenic bladder [30]. Low compliance bladder will lead to an increase in detrusor pressure causing vesicoureteral reflux and upper urinary tract deterioration. A decrease in bladder compliance may be seen in some pathological conditions such as infection or fibrosis such as radiation cystitis, tuberculous cystitis, interstitial cystitis, and neurogenic bladder. Augmentation cystoplasty has been proven to improve bladder compliance.

Bladder Capacity

Bladder capacity varies with age. There are many formulas for the calculation of bladder capacity. In a normal adult, the functional bladder capacity is 300–500 ml. Decreased bladder capacity can lead to lower urinary tract symptoms such as frequency, urgency, nocturia, and incontinence. This will affect the quality of life in many aspects: physically, psychologically, emotionally, socially, sexually, and financially. In addition, the bladder with a small capacity is at higher risk of urinary tract infection, vesicoureteral reflux, and upper tract deterioration. By expanding the bladder's capacity, augmentation cystoplasty is able to treat these problems.

Detrusor Overactivity

Detrusor overactivity is a urodynamic finding which is characterized by involuntary detrusor contractions during the filling phase that may be spontaneous or provoked. It can be divided into three subtypes: idiopathic where no identifiable cause for the involuntary detrusor contraction, neurogenic where there is evidence of neurologic disorder, and non-neurogenic where the causes are obstruction, infection, tumor, and stone [30].

Detrusor overactivity not only causes lower urinary tract symptoms but also is harmful to the upper urinary tract. Detrusor overactivity can be prevented in augmentation cystoplasty by increasing the bladder capacity and compliance and reducing the detrusor pressure.

Patients who require augmentation cystoplasty frequently will also have bladder outlet or emptying problems such as difficulty with catheterizing the urethra, urethral loss or incompetence due to scarring, and radiation or fistula formation. These patients will benefit from a continent catheterizable channel along with augmentation cystoplasty. Examples of continent catheterizable channels are the Mitrofanoff procedure and Yang-Monti procedure which have been discussed. Surgical closure of the bladder outlet, Burch colposuspension, or sling placement can also be carried out in the same setting if the patients have severe urinary leakage.

Patients undergoing augmentation cystoplasty must have the motivation and dexterity to perform intermittent urinary catheterization because perforation can occur due to overdistention and ischemia. A computed tomography cystogram should be performed if perforation is suspected and surgical exploration and repair need to be carried out if the patient's condition deteriorates. Long-term monitoring of patients is necessary due to the potential long-term complications associated with augmentation cystoplasty such as bladder perforation (1.9%), mucus production (12.5%), metabolic abnormalities (3.35%), bowel dysfunction (15%), and stone formation (10%) [31].

Ureter Substitution

Urologists have struggled with significant ureteral defect for a very long time. The integrity of the ureter is important to preserve the function of the kidney. Any lesions along the ureter can lead to urinary obstruction and reflux, causing hydronephrosis and the loss of renal function.

When there is significant ureteral loss or severe ureteral stricture, bowel segments can be used to substitute the ureter and to bridge the gap. This is usually seen in patients with extrapulmonary tuberculosis and malignancy and patients who sustained extensive ureteric injury. Ureter substitution using the ileum was first described by Shoemarker in 1909. The ileum is more commonly used than the colon because of its many advantages. Due to the availability of alternative procedures like renal autotransplantation and transureteroureterostomy, ureter substitution is not routinely performed. Additionally, the bowel mucosa differs from the urothelium in that it retains the capacity for secretion and absorption, which might result in mucus obstruction and various metabolic complications. Moreover, the urothelium is resistant to the inflammatory and potential carcinogenic effects of urine. To minimize the complication rate, we need to ensure that the kidney, bladder, and urethra are functioning normally prior to performing ileal ureter substitution. Combination with Boari flap or psoas hitch can also reduce the length of bowel used [32].

Neovaginal Reconstruction (Vaginoplasty)

Female pelvic medicine and reconstruction may involve any of the three female pelvic floor compartments: anterior (bladder, urethra), apical (uterus, vagina), and posterior (anal, rectum). A combination of these leads to a complex reconstruction. A multidisciplinary team involving the urologist, urogynecologist, colorectal surgeons, and plastic surgeons is important, and multiple reconstructive techniques are needed. Neovaginal reconstruction also known as vaginoplasty is a surgical procedure to create vagina. The function of the vagina is to allow penetration during sexual activity and, in women with a functioning uterus, to drain menstrual blood.

Among the common indications for vaginoplasty is vaginal agenesis in Mayer-Rokitansky-Kuster-Hauser (MRKH) syndrome, vaginal hypoplasia in congenital adrenal hyperplasia (CAH) and androgen insensitivity syndrome (AIS), and gender reassignment surgery in gender dysphoria. Other indications are urogenital sinus anomaly, cloacal anomaly, pelvic neoplasms, hermaphroditism, and post-traumatic/radiation vaginal stricture [33]. All these conditions may have great psychological impact on patients.

There are various methods for vaginoplasty, each with its advantages and disadvantages. It will depend on the patient's age, surgeon experience, vaginoplasty indication, and surgeon and patient preference. The ideal criteria for neovagina are adequate diameter and length, appropriate axis and position, self-lubricating, no need for regular dilatation, and good cosmetic outcomes. Vaginoplasty can be done using either a surgical or nonsurgical procedure. The Frank procedure and the Ingram procedure are examples of nonsurgical methods that apply the principle of regular dilatation to create a functional vagina. Different grafts are used for vaginoplasty surgery: the bowel, buccal mucosa, skin, peritoneum, and amniotic membrane.

In bowel vaginoplasty, laparotomy is performed to harvest a segment of the bowel with vascular pedicle for the creation of neovagina. The proximal end is closed to make a blind pouch and the distal end is pulled through the introitus. Bowel anastomosis is done to establish the continuity of the bowel. The advantages of bowel vaginoplasty are self-lubrication, adequate vaginal length, no regular dilatation needed, and reduced risk of neovaginal stenosis. The disadvantages of bowel vaginoplasty are excess mucus production with unpleasant smell, risk of colitis and malignancy, higher risk for sexually transmitted diseases and HIV, and necessitating abdominal surgery with bowel anastomosis. In gender reassignment surgery, bowel vaginoplasty is used when there is not adequate penile skin for penile skin flap vaginoplasty. With the increasing use of puberty suppression treatment, this condition is more commonly encountered. The sigmoid, right colon, and ileum are the frequently used bowel segments in bowel vaginoplasty.

A systemic review by Georgas et al. concluded that the bowel provides a great graft for vaginoplasty with positive results and few complications. Different outcomes such as sexual function, quality of life, psychological status, patient satisfaction, and complication rate are compared [34].

Complications of Bowel Use in Female Genitourinary Reconstruction

Female genitourinary reconstructive surgery is usually complex and requires interdisciplinary collaboration between urologists, gynecologists, and colorectal surgeons. Radical cystectomy with urinary diversion is considered one of the most difficult surgical procedures in urology. Therefore, it is not uncommon to encounter complications postoperatively. These complications can be life-threatening and have negative impacts on patient's health and quality of life. Prevention, close monitoring, early detection, and appropriate management are the key components in reducing the morbidity and mortality of these complications. Complications of bowel use in urinary diversion can be divided into early (<1 month after surgery) and late complications (≥ 1 month after surgery) [35]. However, there is a lack of standardization in the reporting of urinary diversion complications. According to the Clavien system, surgical complications are graded into five grades and early complication occurs within 90 days after surgery.

In grade 0, no complications are observed; in grade 1, oral medication and bedside intervention are required for the treatment of complication; in grade 2, intravenous pharmacological treatment, parenteral nutrition, or blood transfusion is required for the treatment of complication; in grade 3, surgical, radiological, or endoscopic intervention is required for the treatment of complication; in grade 4, life-threatening complication requiring ICU management and causing organ dysfunction and disability; and in grade 5, complications that lead to the death of patient [36].

Early complications are general perioperative complications that are the same as in any other surgery: anastomotic leakage, bleeding, thromboembolism, wound infection, fistula, fluid collection, bowel obstruction, and urinary obstruction. Late complications are complications that are long term and unique to urinary diversion: metabolic complications, urolithiasis, urinary tract infection, renal deterioration, and development of secondary malignancy. Late complications are more difficult to monitor, and the available data typically underestimate the true incidence and magnitude of problems because many patients are lost to follow-up or succumb to the primary disease, as the most common reason for urinary diversion is radical cystectomy for bladder cancer.

Besides that, some complications are specific only to each type of urinary diversion that has been discussed.

Early Complications

Anastomotic Leakage

Anastomotic leakage can happen in a few locations: bowel-bowel anastomosis, bowel-ureter anastomosis, and bowel-urethra anastomosis. Depending on the location, there can be fecal leakage, urinary leakage, or both. When there is increased output from the drainage system, the possibility of urinary leakage should be suspected. Continent urinary diversion has a higher rate of anastomotic leakage compared to incontinent urinary diversion due to the long suture lines [37]. Therefore, urinary catheters, stents, and drains have a role in the prevention and treatment of anastomotic leakage.

Fluid Collection

Differential diagnoses of postoperative fluid collection are urinoma, hematoma, lymphocele, or abscess [38]. Fluid collection is usually managed conservatively depending on the size, location, and nature of the collection, and the clinical course, rarely drainage will be needed. Conservative treatment includes observation, monitoring, and use of antibiotic. With the advancement of interventional radiology, percutaneous drainage can be done under ultrasound or CT guidance without the need to reenter the operation theatre for open surgical repair unless the collection is huge and multiloculated.

Alteration in Bowel Function

The bowel usually returns to its normal function within 5 days of surgery. Alteration in bowel function can be due to functional paralytic ileus or mechanical obstruction. Adhesion, intestinal edema, intestinal stricture, and external compression by fluid collection are causes of mechanical obstruction. Treatment of paralytic ileus includes bowel rest, intravenous fluid therapy, and nasogastric decompression if indicated. The underlying causes of paralytic ileus need to be investigated and treated such as infection and electrolyte imbalance. Enhanced recovery protocols, regional anesthesia, opioid-sparing analgesics, and early ambulation have all been shown to reduce the rate of paralytic ileus.

Urinary Obstruction

The urinary tract can be obstructed due to anastomotic stricture, external compression by fluid collection, or tumor recurrence. Compared to antirefluxing anastomosis, refluxing anastomosis has a lower rate of stricture. Anastomotic stricture can be avoided by adhering to the right surgical principles during ureterointestinal anastomosis construction, such as maintaining tension-free, watertight seals and using fine absorbable sutures. Anastomotic stricture can cause urinary obstruction, vesicoureteric reflux, upper urinary tract deterioration, and even renal failure if it is not detected early. Anastomotic stricture may develop many years after the surgery; therefore, lifelong follow-up is important.

Fistula

Fistula is one of the indications for urinary diversion. Contrary to this, urinary diversion itself can also lead to fistula formation. A fistula is an abnormal connection between organs. Fistula can occur in various forms depending on the size, location, and organs that are involved: intestino-urinary, intestino-genital, intestino-cutaneous, and genitourinary. Radiological investigations such as CT and MRI will assist in the diagnosis of fistulas. The use of contrast agent will increase the detection rate.

Late Complications

Urolithiasis

Patients with urinary diversion are at higher risk of urolithiasis. Ten percent of patients with urinary diversion have urolithiasis [39]. Major risk factors are hypercitraturia due to metabolic acidosis, hyperoxaluria due to short bowel syndrome, urinary stasis, and recurrent urinary tract infection. Preventive measures include high fluid intake with urine output target >2000 ml/day, correction of metabolic and electrolyte imbalance, ensuring adequate reservoir emptying, and treatment of urinary tract infection.

Urinary Tract Infection

Patients with urinary diversion are at higher risk of recurrent urinary tract infection, bacteremia, and sepsis. Bowel segments are colonized by bacteria and bowel mucosa in contrast to the urothelium is not capable of inhibiting bacterial proliferation. Bacterial colonization rate is highest in the colon and *Escherichia coli* is the most common isolated organism [40]. Since chronic asymptomatic bacteriuria is common among patients with urinary diversion, antibiotic treatment is not necessary. This helps to prevent antibiotic resistance. Antibiotic treatment is only needed for symptomatic urinary tract infection and those with positive urine culture for *Proteus* and *Pseudomonas* as these pathogens can often lead to struvite stones that can impair renal function.

Renal Deterioration

Renal deterioration has been observed in patients with urinary diversion. It has been demonstrated that GFR reduces by 15–25% following urinary diversion with an 11-year follow-up [41].

It is multifactorial and among the contributing factors are aging, comorbidities, anastomotic stricture, urinary tract obstruction, reflux uropathy, recurrent urinary tract infection, and urolithiasis. Patients should avoid nonsteroidal anti-inflammatory drugs and other nephrotoxic substances. Long-term follow-up with serum creatinine, renal ultrasound, and nuclear scans is advisable.

Development of Secondary Malignancy

It takes 10–20 years for secondary malignancy to develop. The incidence is highest when transitional epithelium of the bladder is in contact with the epithelium of the colon and both are bathed with urine and feces. Therefore, ureterosigmoidostomy and colonic neobladder are at higher risk than using other bowel segment parts. Different histopathology had been reported including adenocarcinoma, squamous cell carcinoma, sarcoma, and urothelial cell carcinoma. A multicenter analysis by Kälble et al. showed that a total of 32 secondary tumors occurred from 17,758 urinary diversions. The tumor risk in ureterosigmoidostomy is 2.58%, cystoplasty 1.58%, orthotopic colonic neobladder 1.29%, orthotopic ileal neobladder 0.05%, ileocecal pouches 0.14%, and ileal conduit 0.02% [42]. The pathophysiology is not well understood. One of the theories is that carcinogen is produced when nitrite in the urine combines with amine. Regular endoscopic evaluation after 5 years is recommended for this group of patients [43].

Metabolic Complications

Bowel segments retain their secretory and absorptive properties when they are used in reconstructive surgery, therefore leading to different metabolic complications when they are in contact with urine. Factors that influence metabolic complications are the segment of bowel used, the surface area of the bowel used, the duration of contact of urine with bowel segments, and the renal and hepatic function of the patient. For example, in urinary conduit, only 15–25 cm of bowel segments is harvested compared to the pouch or neobladder where 40–80 cm of bowel segments is used. Therefore, metabolic complications are higher in continent urinary diversion compared to urinary conduit due to more contact time between the urine and the bowel segment for metabolic exchange. Metabolic complications can be divided into electrolyte abnormalities, nutritional abnormalities, drug metabolism abnormalities, altered sensorium, osteomalacia, and growth retardation.

Electrolyte Abnormalities

Stomach

Complications are rare in patients who have normal renal function with good hydration. Stomach mucosa secretes hydrogen, chloride, and potassium into urine causing hypochloremic hypokalemic metabolic alkalosis and elevated aldosterone.

Clinical symptoms are lethargy, muscle weakness, seizures, and ventricular arrhythmia. Treatments include intravenous hydration, H2 blocker, and proton pump inhibitor. In life-threatening condition, arginine hydrochloride infusion can be used to restore acid-base balance and the gastric segment is removed.

Jejunum

Jejunum mucosa secretes sodium and chloride into urine with resorption of potassium and hydrogen causing hyponatremic hyperkalemic metabolic acidosis.

Hyponatremia will cause hypovolemia leading to activation of renin-angiotensin-aldosterone system. Clinical symptoms are lethargy, nausea, vomiting, and dehydration. Treatments consist of intravenous hydration and sodium bicarbonate to correct metabolic acidosis, and thiazide to correct hyperkalemia. In life-threatening condition, the bowel segment will need to be removed.

Ileum and Colon

The Ileum and colon mucosa secrete potassium and carbonic acid into the urine with reabsorption of ammonium chloride causing hyperchloremic hypokalemic metabolic acidosis, hypocalcemia, and total body potassium depletion. Clinical symptoms are fatigue, anorexia, and muscle weakness. Treatment includes alkalinizing agents, chloride transport blockers, and potassium replacement. Examples of alkalinizing agents are potassium citrate, sodium citrate, sodium bicarbonate, and citric acid, while examples of chloride transport blockers are nicotinic acid and chlorpromazine.

Nutritional Abnormalities

Resection of bowel segments used for urinary diversion will lead to short bowel syndrome where significant intestinal resorptive surface is lost. Resection of the ileum and colon can cause malabsorption of vitamin B12 and bile acid. Vitamin B12 deficiency will lead to megaloblastic anemia and neurological manifestations, while malabsorption of bile acid and fat will lead to diarrhea due to mucosal irritation. Cholestyramine which is a resin that binds bile salt and anti-diarrheal agents such as loperamide can be used in bothering diarrhea. Daily oral supplementation or monthly parenteral administration of vitamin B12 should be started in patients with vitamin B12 deficiency.

Drug Metabolism Abnormalities

This is due to the reabsorption of excreted drugs into the intestinal segment used for urinary diversion. Drugs that are absorbed unchanged by the gastrointestinal tract and excreted by the kidneys are likely to be problematic such as phenytoin, lithium, beta-lactamase, aminoglycosides, cisplatin, and methotrexate. This is important, especially in patients with urinary diversion receiving chemotherapy. Drug levels need to be monitored for dose adjustment and to prevent drug toxicity.

Altered Sensorium

Patients with urinary diversion can develop altered sensorium due to magnesium deficiency, drug intoxication, or hyperammonemia. Ammonia is a harmful byproduct of nitrogen metabolism which should be eliminated from the human body. In patients with normal liver function, the excess ammonia will be converted to urea in ornithine cycle and excreted through the kidneys. Patients with liver dysfunction have impaired capability of removing ammonia and are at higher risk of hyperammonemic encephalopathy and hepatic coma. Hyperammonemia can be caused by urinary tract obstruction and urinary tract infection. Urinary tract obstruction increases the absorption of urinary ammonia into the bloodstream. Urinary tract infection by urease-producing organisms such as *Proteus*, *Klebsiella*, *Pseudomonas*, and *Ureaplasma* further increases the ammonia load. Treatment includes limited protein intake, syrup lactulose, and neomycin to lower the level of ammonia. While drainage and diversion of the urine are essential in cases of urinary obstruction, antibiotics should be used to treat urinary tract infections.

Osteomalacia and Growth Retardation

Chronic metabolic acidosis can cause bone demineralization by increasing the level of osteoclast activity and reducing the activity of osteoblast. Besides that, metabolic acidosis impairs renal activation of vitamin D which is needed for bone mineralization. Absorption of vitamin D and calcium is also decreased due to short bowel syndrome. In children, this can lead to rickets and growth retardation. In adults, this can lead to osteopenia, pain at weight-bearing joints, and even fracture. Treatments include correction of acidosis and calcium and vitamin D supplementation.

Conclusion

The bowel is used in female urinary reconstructive surgery for urinary diversion, augmentation cystoplasty, ureter substitution, and bowel vaginoplasty. It is important to understand the indication, surgical anatomy, patient selection criteria, operative techniques, and associated complications. One of the most common uses is urinary diversion for the preservation of the upper urinary tract function: incontinent urinary diversion and continent urinary diversion.

Orthotopic neobladder is the most physiologic method of urinary diversion and should be performed whenever possible. However, every patient is different and many aspects such as patients' quality of life, procedure accessibility, and invasiveness need to be taken into consideration. Incontinent urinary diversion is reserved for frail elderly patients and patients with limited life expectancy who are not able to withstand long surgery. Evidence to support and compare types of urinary diversion is limited. A stepwise clinical algorithm should be in place to guide clinicians and surgeons in selecting the best urinary diversion for patients.

Comprehensive preoperative counseling is important to avoid regret and for better outcomes. A multidisciplinary team involving the urologist, gynecologist, colorectal surgeon, physiotherapist, occupational therapists, primary care physicians, and enterostomal therapists is required to improve communication and coordination of patient care.

To date, there is no ideal substitute for ureter and bladder replacement in terms of mechanical and biocompatibility properties. The bowel still retains its secretory and absorptive properties that may lead to different complications that need long-term surveillance. Surgeons and clinicians need to be familiar with diagnosing and managing these complications. With the advancement of tissue engineering technologies, newer materials such as stem cells, biomaterial scaffolds, synthetic grafts, or growth factor supplementation may emerge to provide a better material for urinary tract replacement with fewer complications.

References

1. Hendren WH. Historical perspective of the use of bowel in urology. Urol Clin N Am. 1997;24(4):703–13. https://doi.org/10.1016/S0094-0143(05)70412-2.
2. Pannek J, Senge T. History of urinary diversion. Urol Int. 1998;60(1):1–10. https://doi.org/10.1159/000030195.
3. Witner A, Dhal DM, McDougal WS. Use of intestinal segments in urinary diversion. In: Partin AW, Dmochowski RR, Kavoussi LR, Peters CA, editors. Campbell-Walsh urology. 12th ed. (pp.3160–3205). Philadelphia: Saunders; 2021.
4. Wolf JS Jr, Bennett CJ, Dmochowski RR, Hollenbeck BK, Pearle MS, Schaeffer AJ, Urologic Surgery Antimicrobial Prophylaxis Best Practice Policy Panel. Best practice policy statement on urologic surgery antimicrobial prophylaxis. The Journal of urology 2008; 179(4):1379–1390. https://doi.org/10.1016/j.juro.2008.01.068
5. Mangioni D, Rocchini L, Bandera A, Montanari E. Re. Best practice statement on urologic procedures and antimicrobial prophylaxis. J Urol. 2020;203(6):1214–5. https://doi.org/10.1097/JU.0000000000000789.
6. Su H, Wu H, Bao M, et al. Indocyanine green fluorescence imaging to assess bowel perfusion during totally laparoscopic surgery for colon cancer. BMC Surg. 2020;20:102. https://doi.org/10.1186/s12893-020-00745-4.
7. Pantuck AJ, Han KR, Perrotti M, Weiss RE, Cummings KB. Ureteroenteric anastomosis in continent urinary diversion: long-term results and complications of direct versus nonrefluxing techniques. J Urol. 2000;163(2):450–5. https://doi.org/10.1016/s0022-5347(05)67898-6.
8. Babakhanlou R, Larkin K, Hita AG, et al. Stoma-related complications and emergencies. Int J Emerg Med. 2022;15:17. https://doi.org/10.1186/s12245-022-00421-9.
9. World Cancer Research Fund International. Bladder cancer statistics. https://www.wcrf.org/cancer-trends/bladder-cancer-statistics/ (1999). Accessed 12 Oct 1999.
10. American Cancer Society. What is bladder cancer?. American Cancer Society, p. 17–18. https://www.

cancer.org/cancer/bladder-cancer/about/what-is-bladder-cancer.html/ (2019). Accessed 14 Oct 2022.
11. Igel DA, Chestnut CJ, Lee EK. Urinary diversion and reconstruction following radical cystectomy for bladder cancer: a narrative review. AME Med J. 2021;6:11. https://doi.org/10.21037/amj-20-76.
12. Falch C, Amend B, Müller S, et al. Management of nonurological pelvic tumors infiltrating the lower urinary tract. Curr Surg Rep. 2014;2:72. https://doi.org/10.1007/s40137-014-0072-z.
13. Cantu H, Maarof SNM, Hashim H. The inflammatory contracted bladder. Curr Bladder Dysfunct Rep. 2019;14:67–74. https://doi.org/10.1007/s11884-019-00507-w.
14. Bansal P, Bansal N. The surgical management of urogenital tuberculosis our experience and long-term follow-up. Urol Ann. 2015;7(1):49–52. https://doi.org/10.4103/0974-7796.148606.
15. Gupta NP, Kumar A, Sharma S. Reconstructive bladder surgery in genitourinary tuberculosis. Indian J Urol. 2008;24(3):382–7. https://doi.org/10.4103/0970-1591.42622.
16. Tsegaye S, Osman M, Bekele A, Tsegaye S, Hospital L. Surgically treated acute abdomen at Gondar University Hospital, Ethiopia. East Cent Afr J Surg. 2007;12(1):53–7.
17. Witjes J, Palou J, Soloway M, et al. Clinical practice recommendations for the prevention and management of intravesical therapy-associated adverse events. Eur Urol Suppl. 2008;7(10):667–74.
18. Majeed H, Gupta V. Adverse effects of radiation therapy. In: StatPearls [Internet]. Treasure Island: StatPearls Publishing; 2022. Available from: https://www.ncbi.nlm.nih.gov/books/NBK563259/
19. Zugor V, Schott GE, Labanaris AP. The Prune Belly syndrome: urological aspects and long-term outcomes of a rare disease. Pediatr Rep. 2012;4(2):e20. https://doi.org/10.4081/pr.2012.e20.
20. Ebert AK, Reutter H, Ludwig M, Rösch WH. The exstrophy-epispadias complex. Orphanet J Rare Dis. 2009;4:23. https://doi.org/10.1186/1750-1172-4-23.
21. Jonsson O, Olofsson G, Lindholm E, Törnqvist H. Long-time experience with the Kock ileal reservoir for continent urinary diversion. Eur Urol. 2002;40:632–40. https://doi.org/10.1159/000049849.
22. Zhang YG, Song QX, Song B, Zhang DL, Zhang W, Wang JY. Diagnosis and treatment of urinary incontinence after orthotopic ileal neobladder in China. Chin Med J. 2017;130(2):231–5. https://doi.org/10.4103/0366-6999.198012.
23. Puppo P, Introini C, Calvi P, Naselli A. Prevention of chronic urinary retention in orthotopic bladder replacement in the female. Eur Urol. 2005;47(5):674–8. https://doi.org/10.1016/j.eururo.2004.11.006.
24. Stewart JN, Boone TB. The contemporary indications for augmentation cystoplasty. Curr Bladder Dysfunct Rep. 2013;8(4):326–31. https://doi.org/10.1007/s11884-013-0204-9.
25. Haylen BT, de Ridder D, Freeman RM, Swift SE, Berghmans B, Lee J, Monga A, Petri E, Rizk DE, Sand PK, Schaer GN. An International Urogynecological Association (IUGA)/International Continence Society (ICS) joint report on the terminology for female pelvic floor dysfunction. Int Urogynecol J. 2010;21(1):5–26. https://doi.org/10.1007/s00192-009-0976-9.
26. Lightner DJ, Gomelsky A, Souter L, et al. Diagnosis and treatment of overactive bladder (non-neurogenic) in adults: AUA/SUFU guideline amendment 2019. J Urol. 2019;202:558.
27. Harding CK, Lapitan MC, Arlandis S, Bø K, Cobussen-Boekhorst H, Costantini E, Groen J, Nambiar AK, Omar MI, Phé V, van der Vaart CH, Farag F, Karavitakis M, Manso M, Monagas S, Nican Riogh A, O'Connor E, Peyronnet B, Sakalis V, Sihra N, Tzelves L. EAU guidelines on non-neurogenic female LUTS. Presented at the EAU annual congress, Amsterdam. Arnhem: EAU Guidelines Office; 2022. http://uroweb.org/guidelines/compilations-of-all-guidelines. ISBN 978-94-92671-16-5.
28. Ginsberg DA, Boone TB, Cameron AP, Gousse A, Kaufman MR, Keays E, Kennelly MJ, Lemack GE, Rovner ES, Souter LH, Yang CC, Kraus SR. The AUA/SUFU guideline on adult neurogenic lower urinary tract dysfunction: diagnosis and evaluation. J Urol. 2021;206(5):1097–105. https://doi.org/10.1097/JU.0000000000002235.
29. Blok B, Castro-Diaz D, Del Popolo G, Groen J, Hamid R, Karsenty G, Kessler TM, Pannek J, Ecclestone H, Musco S, Padilla-Fernández B, Sartori A. EAU guidelines on neuro-urology. Presented at the EAU annual congress, Amsterdam. Arnhem: EAU Guidelines Office; 2022. http://uroweb.org/guidelines/compilations-of-all-guidelines. ISBN 978-94-92671-16-5.
30. D'Ancona CD, Haylen BT, Oelke M, Herschorn S, Abranches-Monteiro L, Arnold EP, Goldman HB, Hamid R, Homma Y, Marcelissen T, Rademakers K, Schizas A, Singla A, Soto I, Tse V, de Wachter S. An International Continence Society (ICS) report on the terminology for adult male lower urinary tract and pelvic floor symptoms and dysfunction. Neurourol Urodyn. 2019; https://doi.org/10.1002/nau.23897.
31. Hoen L, et al. Long-term effectiveness and complication rates of bladder augmentation in patients with neurogenic bladder dysfunction: a systematic review. Neurourol Urodyn. 2017. https://pubmed.ncbi.nlm.nih.gov/28169459/
32. Xiong S, Zhu W, Li X, Zhang P, Wang H, Li X. Intestinal interposition for complex ureteral reconstruction: a comprehensive review. Int J Urol. 2020;27:377–86. https://doi.org/10.1111/iju.14222.
33. Chaudhary R, Dhama V, Singh S, Azad R. Vaginoplasty in Mayer Rokitansky-Kuster-Hauser syndrome using amnion: a case series. Int J Reprod Contracept Obstet Gynecol. 2016;5(11):3832–9. https://doi.org/10.18203/2320-1770.ijrcog20163849.

34. Georgas K, Belgrano V, Andreasson M, Elander A, Selvaggi G. Bowel vaginoplasty: a systematic review. J Plast Surg Hand Surg. 2018;52(5):265–73. https://doi.org/10.1080/2000656X.2018.1482220.
35. Hedgire SS, Tabatabaei S, McDermott S, Feldman A, Dahl DM, Harisinghani MG. Diversion ahead: imaging appearance of urinary diversions and reservoirs. Clin Imaging. 2014;38(4):418–27. https://doi.org/10.1016/j.clinimag.2014.01.017.
36. Hautmann RE, Hautmann SH, Hautmann O. Complications associated with urinary diversion. Nat Rev Urol. 2011;8(12):667–77. https://doi.org/10.1038/nrurol.2011.147.
37. Tan WS, Lamb BW, Kelly JD. Complications of radical cystectomy and orthotopic reconstruction. Adv Urol. 2015;2015:323157. https://doi.org/10.1155/2015/323157.
38. Onur MR, Sidhu R, Dogra VS. Imaging of urinary diversion and neobladder. In: Dogra V, MacLennan G, editors. Genitourinary radiology: male genital tract, adrenal and retroperitoneum. London: Springer; 2013. https://doi.org/10.1007/978-1-4471-4899-9_14.
39. Catalá V, Solà M, Samaniego J, Martí T, Huguet J, Palou J, De La Torre P. CT findings in urinary diversion after radical cystectomy: postsurgical anatomy and complications. Radiographics. 2009;29(2):461–76. https://doi.org/10.1148/rg.292085146
40. Symeonidis EN, Falagas ME, Dimitriadis F. Urinary tract infections in patients undergoing radical cystectomy and urinary diversion: challenges and considerations in antibiotic prophylaxis. Transl Androl Urol. 2019;8(4):286–9. https://doi.org/10.21037/tau.2019.07.12.
41. van der Aa F, de Ridder D, van Poppel H. When the bowel becomes the bladder: changes in metabolism after urinary diversion. Pract Gastroenterol. 2012;36(7):15–28.
42. Kälble T, Hofmann I, Riedmiller H, Vergho D. Tumor growth in urinary diversion: a multicenter analysis. Eur Urol. 2011;60(5):1081–6. https://doi.org/10.1016/j.eururo.2011.07.006.
43. Amini E, Djaladat H. Long-term complications of urinary diversion. Curr Opin Urol. 2015;25(6):570–7. https://doi.org/10.1097/MOU.0000000000000222.

Options for Surgical Reconstruction of the Heavily Irradiated Pelvis

58

Jas Singh, Margaret S. Roubaud, Thomas G. Smith III, and O. Lenaine Westney

Contents

Introduction	1064
Epidemiology and Clinical Presentation	1065
Pathophysiology of Radiation-Induced Cellular Injury	1065
Pelvic Radiation and Genitourinary Toxicity	1066
Genitourinary Complications of Pelvic Radiation	1067
Acute Complications	1067
Chronic Complications	1068
Initial Evaluation and Management of the Heavily Irradiated Pelvis	1070
Evaluation	1070
Management	1072
Urinary Tract Reconstruction	1073
Organ-Sparing Reconstruction	1073
Bladder Neck Reconstruction and Urethroplasty	1073
Anti-Iincontinence Surgery	1073
Bladder Neck Closure	1074
Bladder Augmentation	1074
Incontinent Urinary Channels	1075
Continent Urinary Channels	1075

J. Singh · T. G. Smith III · O. L. Westney (✉)
Department of Urology, Division of Surgery,
The University of Texas MD Anderson Cancer Center,
Houston, TX, USA
e-mail: Jsingh2@mdanderson.org;
TGSmith2@mdanderson.org; owestney@mdanderson.org

M. S. Roubaud
Department of Plastic Surgery, Division of Surgery,
The University of Texas MD Anderson Cancer Center,
Houston, TX, USA
e-mail: MSRoubaud@mdanderson.org

© Springer Nature Switzerland AG 2023
F. E. Martins et al. (eds.), *Female Genitourinary and Pelvic Floor Reconstruction*,
https://doi.org/10.1007/978-3-031-19598-3_59

Supravesical Diversion 1077

Non-organ-Sparing Reconstruction 1078
Pelvic Exenteration 1078
Urinary Diversion 1078

Abdominal Wall, Pelvic, and Genital Reconstruction 1080
Intraoperative Considerations 1080
Postoperative Considerations 1089

Conclusion 1092

Cross-References 1092

References 1092

Abstract

Pelvic cancers in which radiation therapy is frequently employed include gastrointestinal (i.e., colorectal, anal), genitourinary (i.e., bladder, urethral), gynecologic (i.e., cervical, endometrial, vaginal, and vulvar), and orthopedic cancers. Pelvic radiation can induce tissue toxicity and damage in the bowel, bladder, genitalia, and along the upper and lower urinary tracts. Factors associated with radiation-induced GU toxicity include the cumulative radiation dose, radiation modality, treatment volume, and prior pelvic surgery. Pelvic radiation is implicated in the development of several genitourinary complications which can have a devastating impact on patient QoL, bladder and sexual function, and even survival as recurrent infections, deterioration in renal function, and life-threatening hemorrhage contribute to increased morbidity and mortality. Prior to operation, preoperative consultation with a plastic and reconstructive surgeon is critical to establish a physiologic baseline and discuss postoperative expectations. Open discussion regarding postoperative functional and aesthetic changes, prior to surgery, dramatically reduces anxiety for the patient and sets realistic goals for both patient and surgeon. Numerous options for reconstruction are available depending on the severity and nature of the urinary tract and pelvic floor complications. Multidisciplinary co-management is often required, and a collaborative approach to surgical reconstruction allows for efficiency in care, improving outcomes, and minimizing patient morbidity and mortality.

Keywords

Radiation · Genitourinary toxicity · Reconstruction · Sexual function

Introduction

Radiation therapy (RT) has long represented a mainstay in the multimodality management of pelvic malignancy. It is estimated that greater than 50% of all cancer patients undergo radiation therapy at some point during their treatment course [1]. With improvements in therapeutic outcomes, patients have longer disease-free survival, and therefore the potential for radiation-induced complications is increasing. The treatment of pelvic cancers may include radiation treatment alone or in combination with surgery and/or systemic chemotherapy. RT has traditionally been administered to the pelvis using external beam radiation therapy (EBRT) or brachytherapy (BT). More recently, advances in radiotherapeutic modalities including 3D-conformal radiation therapy (3D-CRT), intensity-modulated radiation therapy (IMRT), 3D image-guided adaptive brachytherapy (IGABT), and proton beam therapy have allowed for improvements in tumor targeting in an attempt to deliver higher cumulative doses of radiation to the primary tumor, while sparing surrounding normal tissue. Despite these attempts at refinements in technique, considerable collateral damage to surrounding pelvic organs and structures is sustained during radiotherapy. Acute and chronic genitourinary (GU) toxicities represent problematic complications that negatively impact patient quality of life (QoL) and sexual function. With improvements in cancer-specific and overall survival, the number of cancer survivors is increasing and as a result the burden of radiation-induced toxicity along with it. Approximately 20–25% of cancer survivors report a decline in QoL as the result of the debilitating nature of cancer treatment [2].

The female genitourinary and pelvic floor provides a unique challenge to the reconstructive surgeon. Complex three-dimensional anatomy and functional requirements demand thoughtful and durable reconstruction. Aesthetic considerations, in particular regard to sexuality, are of great concern to many patients. Recent studies document the increasing trend of plastic surgery flap reconstruction of pelvic oncologic defects in the last 20 years, with decreasing risk of wound breakdown and secondary procedures for dehiscence [3–7]. Reconstructive plastic surgery is of paramount importance to patients undergoing challenging resections, for both physiologic and emotional healing.

The aim of this chapter is to provide an overview of the role of radiation therapy in the treatment of pelvic malignancy and the pathophysiologic effects of ionizing radiation on normal tissue and review potential early and late GU complications resulting from this treatment. Next, the chapter will delve into surgical options for reconstruction in the heavily irradiated pelvis from the perspective of the consultant urologic surgeon followed by options for pelvic floor reconstruction requiring tissue transfer and closure of extensive pelvic floor defects from the perspective of the consultant plastic surgeon.

Epidemiology and Clinical Presentation

Pelvic cancers in which radiation therapy is frequently employed include gastrointestinal (i.e., colorectal, anal), genitourinary (i.e., bladder, urethral), gynecologic (i.e., cervical, endometrial, vaginal, and vulvar), and orthopedic cancers. According to the American Cancer Society, in 2021, the incidence of lower gastrointestinal, genitourinary, and gynecologic cancers is estimated as 81,310, 29,130, and 108,580 cases, respectively [8]. By 2030, it is estimated that the total number of patients with irradiated pelvic tumors (excluding prostate cancer) will be about 450,000, and therefore the potential pool of patients with pelvic radiation disease is substantial given a 5–10% incidence of severe late complications [9].

About 50% of women presenting with acute GU toxicities may complain of low-grade urinary symptoms including urinary frequency, urgency, nocturia, hesitancy, and dysuria, following pelvic radiation. The incidence of low-grade acute GU toxicity during the treatment of cervical cancer is reported between 17 and 40%, while high-grade toxicity occurs less frequently in 2–5% of cases. Similarly, low-grade late GU toxicity has been reported in 28–45% of patients [10]. Patient-related factors that have been linked to an increased risk of pelvic radiation disease include age, BMI, hypertension, smoking history, diabetes, history of proinflammatory disease, and a history of collagen vascular disease [11].

In a report from the NRG Oncology RTOG 1203 study, 234 women with cervical or endometrial cancer requiring postoperative RT were randomly assigned to standard 4-field RT or IMRT. Patients then completed a 6-item questionnaire of patient-reported outcomes of the National Cancer Institute Common Terminology Criteria for Adverse Events (CTCAE) tool. While only gastrointestinal symptoms were evaluated, there was a reduction in symptoms associated with IMRT compared with standard RT, providing patient reported evidence of improvement in radiation toxicity following improvements in radiation technique [12].

Pathophysiology of Radiation-Induced Cellular Injury

The degree of cellular injury induced by ionizing radiation in normal tissue is influenced by the target organ and its respective cell types. Radiation-induced cellular damage is a chronic process beginning with an early inflammatory phase followed by late stromal changes resulting in chronic fibrosis. The entire spectrum of damage occurs hours to years following therapy [13]. Acute changes include increased endothelial cell swelling, changes in vascular permeability, the accumulation of mucosal edema, submucosal inflammation and congestion, progressive ulceration, and hemorrhage [14].

Cellular injury following radiation therapy begins with damage to vascular tissue within the target organ and surrounding normal tissue. The standard inflammatory pathway is induced with activation and infiltration of lymphocytes and other markers (neutrophils and macrophages) into the extravascular space followed by cellular apoptosis. These leukocyte-endothelial cell interactions are upregulated at the microvascular level rapidly within minutes to hours after exposure to 6 Gy [15]. These effects continue to persist thereafter for days to weeks following completion of radiotherapy. The second phase occurs over the proceeding months and includes capillary collapse, basement membrane thickening, scarring and fibrosis in the surrounding interstitial tissue, and telangiectasia. Capillaries are especially radiosensitive, and damage begins with separation of endothelial cells from the basement membrane, thrombosis, and tissue ischemia. As radiation-induced tissue injury progresses over the following months to several years, there is a depletion of tissue-specific stem cells followed by fibrosis, necrosis, and remodeling of normal tissues [11].

At the molecular level, radiation exposure induces tissue hypoxia and oxidative stress which in turn leads to the upregulation of transforming growth factor beta-1 (TGF-ß1) production by fibroblasts. Progenitor fibroblasts then undergo termination differentiation into post-mitotic fibrocytes, which are responsible for the deposition of high levels of collagen. TGF-ß1 also plays a role in maintaining extracellular matrix homeostasis through the synthesis of matrix proteins, decreasing the production of matrix degrading enzymes (i.e., matrix metalloproteinases), and increasing the production of inhibitors of these enzymes. As a result, this leads to both abnormal wound healing and concomitant tissue fibrosis [16, 17]. As well, hypoxia and oxidative stress contribute to the upregulation of transcription factors including hypoxia-inducible factor-1 (HIF-1) and nuclear factor kappa B (NF-kB) [18]. These transcription factors play a role in normal wound healing, and their dramatic upregulation by various factors including infection and radiation can lead to a chronic wound healing response resulting in fibrosis [11].

Pelvic Radiation and Genitourinary Toxicity

Pelvic radiation can induce tissue toxicity and damage in the bowel, bladder, genitalia, and along the upper and lower urinary tracts. Factors associated with radiation-induced GU toxicity include the cumulative radiation dose, radiation modality, treatment volume, and prior pelvic surgery [19]. The bladder and vagina are particularly radiosensitive organs owing to the rapid proliferation and turnover of epithelial cells. As a result, even small doses of radiation can precipitate bothersome genitourinary toxicity. On cross-sectional imaging, the bladder may demonstrate focal or diffuse bladder wall thickening with or without mucosal enhancement [20]. Bladder wall thickening from proliferative fibrosis and unimpeded deposition of collagen results in distortion of normal bladder mechanisms leading to impaired detrusor function and lower urinary tract symptoms. Concurrent systemic chemotherapy regimens can compound the potential for bladder fibrosis. Agents such as bleomycin, doxorubicin, cyclophosphamide, and other platinum-based agents have been implicated in chemotherapy-induced fibrosis [13, 21].

The classification of radiation toxicity is based upon criteria developed by both the Radiation Therapy Oncology Group (RTCG) and the European Organization for Research and Treatment of Cancer (EORTC) [22]. Patients with high-grade (grade 3–4) complications are those most likely to have genitourinary symptoms refractory to medical and conservative management, ultimately requiring extensive surgery with

Table 1 Radiation Therapy Oncology Group (RTOG)/European Organization for Research and Treatment of Cancer (EORTC) radiation therapy toxicity criteria for acute radiation morbidity

Organ/Complication	Grade 0	Grade 1	Grade 2	Grade 3	Grade 4	Grade 5
Genitourinary	No change	Frequency of urination or nocturia twice pretreatment habit/dysuria, urgency not requiring medication	Frequency of urination or nocturia that is less frequent than every hour. Dysuria, urgency, bladder spasm requiring local anesthetic	Frequency with urgency and nocturia hourly or more frequently/dysuria, pelvic pain or bladder spasm requiring regular, frequent narcotic/gross hematuria with/without clot passage	Hematuria requiring transfusion/acute bladder obstruction not secondary to clot passage, ulceration, or necrosis	Death

Table 2 Radiation Therapy Oncology Group (RTOG)/European Organization for Research and Treatment of Cancer (EORTC) radiation therapy toxicity criteria for late radiation morbidity

Organ/Complication	Grade 0	Grade 1	Grade 2	Grade 3	Grade 4	Grade 5
Bladder	No change	Slight epithelial atrophy; minor telangiectasia (microscopic hematuria)	Moderate frequency; generalized telangiectasis; intermittent macroscopic hematuria	Severe frequency and dysuria; severe telangiectasia (often with petechiae). Frequent hematuria; reduction in bladder capacity (<150 cc)	Necrosis/contracted bladder (capacity < 100 cc).	Death
					Severe hemorrhagic cystitis	

potential urinary diversion for symptom palliation (Tables 1 and 2).

Genitourinary Complications of Pelvic Radiation

Pelvic radiation is implicated in the development of several genitourinary complications which can have a devastating impact on patient QoL, bladder and sexual function, and even survival as recurrent infections, deterioration in renal function, and life-threatening hemorrhage contribute to increased morbidity and mortality. Overall, complications can be classified based upon their temporal development as either acute or chronic.

Acute Complications

Lower Urinary Tract Symptoms (LUTS)

Urinary symptoms related to voiding dysfunction can develop in the acute setting and persist chronically in some patients as bladder fibrosis develops. This leads to chronic changes within the bladder secondary to the proliferation of collagen resulting in impaired capacity and compliance. Acutely, patients may experience symptoms of cystitis including dysuria, urinary frequency, nocturia, and hesitancy [23]. Parkin et al. reported that 26% of women experienced severe symptoms of urgency, frequency, and incontinence 5–11 years after radiation therapy for cervical carcinoma. The most common symptoms were urgency and urge incontinence in 45% of women followed by significant frequency and nocturia in 35% [24].

In the Postoperative Radiation Therapy for Endometrial Cancer (PORTEC-2) trial, health-related quality of life (HRQOL) was examined in patients receiving vaginal BT versus EBRT. At 5 years of follow-up, there was no significant difference in urinary symptoms between these modalities in the first 12 months. After 1 year, there was a higher rate of storage symptoms and incontinence in the EBRT group, which was hypothesized to be the result of the long-term effects of EBRT on pelvic floor musculature with aging [25].

Hemorrhagic Cystitis

Hemorrhagic cystitis is estimated to occur in 5–9% of patients receiving full dose pelvic radiation therapy. Bleeding can develop anywhere from months to years and even decades following therapy [26]. Levenback et al. reported, in a series of 1784 patients undergoing treatment of cervical carcinoma with both intracavitary radiation and EBRT, a 6.5% rate of hemorrhagic cystitis. The mean time of onset was approximately 35 months with some cases of delayed onset bleeding at 20 years following treatment [27]. Initial treatment includes hydration, bladder irrigation, cystoscopic fulguration/ablation, and the intravesical instillation of agents including alum, formalin, or hyaluronic acid. Severe cases of hemorrhagic cystitis may warrant alternative therapies including hyperbaric oxygen therapy and more invasive treatments including selective embolization of the iliac arteries or rarely cystectomy and urinary diversion [28].

Chronic Complications

Urinary Fistulae

Urinary fistulae are abnormal communicative tracts of centrally epithelialized fibrosis that connect the lumens of separate organs or externally to the cutaneous surface. These fistulae can develop between any structures within the pelvis including the bony pelvis, bladder, urethra, ureters, vagina, bowel, rectum, and perineum. The most common postradiation urinary fistula in women is the vesicovaginal fistula (VVF) affecting up to 10% of women [29]. Fistulae may develop many years [20–30] following completion of treatment [30]. A history of genitourinary malignancy alone is a risk factor for urinary fistula as direct tumor invasion can precipitate fistula formation. Moore et al. reported on 23 patients with stage IVA cervical cancer with all demonstrating disease extension into the bladder. Chemoradiation was utilized in 60.8%, while radiation alone was used in 30.4%. Eleven patients (47.8%) developed a fistula at a median time of 2.9 months from cancer diagnosis. Smoking was significantly associated with risk of fistula formation [31]. The diagnosis of a fistula in the post-cancer treatment setting requires biopsy to rule out the local recurrence of malignancy which can present with both tissue necrosis and fistula development [32].

Recently a retrospective study evaluated post-radiation treatment biopsy in patients with a history of cervical cancer. A total of 89 patients underwent an invasive biopsy with only 28 (31.5%) patients demonstrating recurrent or residual cancer. Of the remaining 61 patients with no recurrent disease, 9 (14.8%) subsequently developed a fistula. Postradiation biopsy was associated with a low diagnostic yield and significant risk of fistula development [33]. Given the impact of radiation on local tissue vascularity, invasive procedures, such as biopsy on radiated tissue, needs to be considered carefully as the risk of fistula formation is not insignificant.

Urinary Strictures and Fibrosis

Radiation-induced fibrosis can lead to stricture formation within the distal ureters leading to upper urinary tract obstruction and renal failure if unrecognized or left unmanaged. The distal ureters lie directly anterior to the cervix and as a result are directly within the radiation treatment field [34]. Given the gradual and progressive nature of the obstruction, many patients may be asymptomatic. The mean latency period from treatment to diagnosis of obstruction is 16.8 years [35]. The risk of stricture is higher with preoperative RT given the higher cumulative dose and often multimodal radiation delivered. As well, intraoperative surgical dissection may contribute to additional interruption in the local tissue blood supply. In contrast, adjuvant RT and RT alone are associated with a reduced rate of ureteral stricture from more moderate dosage due to the dose-dependent local tissue toxicity of RT [10]. Another risk factor for ureteral stricture formation is intraoperative electron beam radiotherapy (IOERT). IOERT has been shown to increase the risk of ureteral stricture formation in patients undergoing treatment for recurrent rectal cancer [36]. As well, patients receiving treatment for rectal cancer in whom the ureter was contained within the IOERT field had an increased incidence of ureteral toxicity [37]. Most recently, the EMBRACE-I trial evaluated MRI-guided adaptive brachytherapy in locally advanced cervical cancer and revealed a 5-year actuarial cumulative incidence of ureteral strictures in 2.9% of patients [38].

Ureteral strictures are diagnosed using a combination of imaging modalities including ultrasonography, cross-sectional imaging (CT and MRI), retrograde ureteropyelography, and functional nuclear renography. Treatment may include renal decompression with retrograde ureteral stent placement or percutaneous nephrostomy. Minimally invasive endoscopic treatment options include balloon dilation and endoscopic incision (endoureterotomy). Surgical reconstruction may be considered for patients with a favorable surgical risk profile with no evidence of disease recurrence who are seeking definitive treatment. Surgical reconstruction involves ureteral reimplantation, graft ureteroplasty (e.g., buccal mucosal graft), complete ureteral replacement with intestinal segments, or nephrectomy in renal units with unsalvageable function following decompression [39]. See section on surgical reconstruction for additional details.

Urethral stricture disease following pelvic radiation in female patients is exceedingly rare and will not be reviewed further.

Sexual Dysfunction

Sexual dysfunction is estimated to occur in up to 50% of women following pelvic radiation for gynecologic malignancy. In addition to this, radiation-induced premature ovarian failure leads to premature menopause in these patients, typically within the first 6 months following treatment. Given their location within the pelvis, the ovaries are susceptible to radiation-induced dysfunction. Factors that influence the degree of dysfunction include dose, irradiation field, and age at the time of treatment [40]. The effective sterilizing dose (ESD) has been shown to decrease with increasing age (16.5 Gy at 20 years vs 14.3 Gy at 30 years) [41].

Vaginal stenosis is another potential complication of pelvic radiation, particularly in older patients (> 50 years of age) receiving high-dose vaginal brachytherapy with doses in excess of 80 Gy. This results in mucosal pallor, telangiectasia, and shortening and narrowing of the vaginal vault leading to vaginal dryness and dyspareunia. These changes are most likely to occur within the first year following treatment [42]. Treatment is aimed at limiting progressive stenosis and improving patency with vaginal dilators, topical estrogens, and frequent sexual activity. Occasionally, surgical reconstruction may be required [43]. A potentially devastating complication of high-dose vaginal brachytherapy is vaginal necrosis, particularly in patients who have undergone re-irradiation [44].

An evaluation of sexual functioning in women following radiotherapy for high-intermediate risk endometrial cancer was performed in the PORTEC-2 trial, which demonstrated no difference in sexual functioning between those receiving vaginal BT compared with EBRT. However, sexual functioning was lower in women in both treatment groups compared with nontreatment controls [25].

Secondary Malignancy

Overall, the risk of secondary malignancy following pelvic radiation is low, and most reported cases occur following a long latency period, beyond 5 years. The estimated risk rate is 17% to 19% which is in part related to improved survival and genetic susceptibility. Ionizing radiation leads to single-strand and double-strand DNA breaks which in turn results in the accumulation of genetic mutations followed by malignant transformation of irradiated cells. Additional factors that influence the development of secondary malignancies include age at radiation (higher in children), gender (greater in females), radiation technique (lower with proton beam), and the site of radiation [45].

In the Postoperative Radiation Therapy for Endometrial Cancer (PORTEC-1) trial, patients with stage I endometrial carcinoma were randomized to EBRT vs no additional treatment (NAT). The rate of secondary malignancies after 15 years of follow-up was 19% in the entire cohort (22% for EBRT and 16% for NAT). The most common secondary cancer types included breast cancer in 6%, cancers of the gastrointestinal tract in 5%, and other types in 8%. Breast cancer was more frequently reported in those receiving NAT, while GI cancers were more frequent in those receiving EBRT [46].

Initial Evaluation and Management of the Heavily Irradiated Pelvis

Evaluation

Urology

Clinical evaluation should begin with a careful medical history, physical examination, and laboratory studies including a complete blood count, electrolyte panel, renal and liver function studies, measurement of glycemic control (HbA1c), and coagulation parameters. In addition, urine studies with urinalysis and urine culture are critical to rule out infection prior to performing surgery on the urinary tract and will help direct additional investigations and therapies. Positive urine cultures should be treated preoperatively with an appropriate duration of culture-directed antibiotics. Coagulopathies should be corrected if possible, and anticoagulation may need to be held or reversed in the case of severe intractable hemorrhagic cystitis or preoperative planning.

Imaging studies including cross-sectional imaging with contrast-enhanced computed tomography (CE-CT) or magnetic resonance imaging (MRI) are helpful to evaluate the pelvic anatomy and identify potential surgical planes for dissection. Given the possibility of bladder dysfunction following radiation-induced injury, urodynamic studies (with or without fluoroscopy) can be considered to evaluate lower urinary tract function including bladder capacity, compliance, and bladder neck function. In selected cases, cystourethroscopy may be helpful to rule out urothelial malignancy, stones, and strictures and to facilitate pelvic examination under anesthesia for assessment of radiation-induced induration, tissue atrophy, and organ mobility. Parkin et al. reported on 40 patients who underwent urodynamic studies 5–11 years following radiation therapy and compared them with 27 patients receiving urodynamics prior to treatment. They found that following treatment, the mean volume of first bladder sensation and mean cystometric capacity were lower following RT. As well, mean filling detrusor pressure was higher, and detrusor instability was more frequently reported following RT [47]. In a prospective study of 36 consecutive patients undergoing urodynamics following EBRT and subsequent BT for cervical carcinoma who received a total dose administration of 46 Gy, 2 Gy per fraction, with 5 fractions per week, there were no significant changes in volume of residual urine, maximum bladder capacity, maximum flow rate, or volume of first bladder sensation. Detrusor instability and frequent small volume voiding were observed in 15–20% of patients [48].

Plastic Surgery

Prior to operation, preoperative consultation with a plastic and reconstructive surgeon is critical to establish a physiologic baseline and discuss postoperative expectations. Open discussion regarding postoperative functional and aesthetic changes, prior to surgery, dramatically reduces anxiety for the patient and sets realistic goals for both patient and surgeon. This conversation gives the patient a sense of ownership in their postoperative outcome and restores a sense of control.

In preparation for surgery, plastic surgeons predict a resection defect as much as possible and formulate the reconstructive plan accordingly. However, they also expect that this defect may be enlarged or changed based on intraoperative findings and formulate multiple flexible secondary plans. Neoadjuvant treatment, previous surgical history, comorbidities, and baseline sexual function all affect surgical outcome and are critical considerations for surgical plan formulations.

Both neoadjuvant chemotherapy and radiation dramatically alter wound healing ability. Certain types of chemotherapy will depress the immune system and predispose patients to infection. Nausea or fatigue-induced malnutrition will alter the protein and vitamins available for postoperative collagen formation and soft tissue healing. In the presence of open wounds or fistulas, protein deficiency is exaggerated. Due to the tantamount importance to wound healing, patients with preoperative malnutrition should be started on supplemental nutritional formulas and continued postoperatively if oral intake does not improve.

Neoadjuvant radiation is extremely common in cancers affecting the pelvis and genital tracts. While absolutely beneficial and required, it unequivocally makes tissue healing slower and delayed. Radiation therapy induces a cascade of cellular events that begins with the influx of inflammatory cells causing erythema, desquamation, and ulceration and results in chronic changes from fibroblast proliferation including inelastic and thickened skin [49–54]. At the time of preoperative consult, many patients present with ongoing stigmata of radiation treatment, including poor skin laxity, alopecia, decreased vascularity of soft tissue, and labial or introital strictures (Fig. 1). Jakowatz et al. found that patients receiving pelvic radiation before exenteration had a significantly higher complication rate (67%) compared to those who did not receive radiation (26%) [55]. When discussing reconstructive surgery, the patient should be advised early that their surgical sites will require careful attention to hygiene and positioning to prevent undue burden on physiologically stressed tissue.

Previous surgical history must be discussed in depth. Prior caesarian sections or pelvic surgeries may have damaged important vascular pedicles. The reconstructive workhorse flap, the omental flap, is often scarred and frozen due to previous exploratory laparotomies or prior debulking procedures. Diverting ostomies affect one half of the abdominal wall and may alter the use of important flaps such as the vertical rectus abdominis

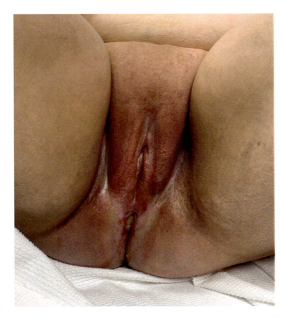

Fig. 1 Radiation stigmata

myocutaneous flap (VRAM). Liposuction, which is frequently considered "nonoperative" by patients, can disrupt superficial vascular perforators. In the thigh or abdomen, this may render a local flap unusable and must be a point of discussion.

Frequently, patients have comorbidities that have little time for correction before surgery. Even with a short amount of time, there are certain conditions that need immediate remediation. Smoking must be stopped, if possible, or decreased as much as possible, as nicotine will induce vasoconstriction that alters healing and reconstructive flap perfusion [56]. Patients should be referred to smoking cessation programs without delay. Elevated blood glucose levels in diabetics predispose to poor postoperative outcomes and infection [57]. Hyperglycemia should be strictly managed in the perioperative setting by an endocrine team and insulin therapy, if required. Poorly controlled hypertension may affect local flap survival and cause venous congestion of flaps, not to mention stress on the cardiovascular system [58]. Beta-blockers and other forms of antihypertensives should be discussed with anesthesiology [59].

Regarding comorbidities that are not readily correctable, such as obesity, the plastic surgeon must consider the degree of risk and discuss ahead of time with the patient. Obesity complicates any surgical treatment by increasing the risk of surgical adverse events, including nosocomial infections, readmissions, blood transfusion, would healing problems, surgical site infections, and abscess formation [60, 61]. Furthermore, obesity increases intrabdominal pressure and will make any abdominal reconstruction more likely to result in surgical site complications, bulging, or hernia [62–64]. Obesity may also affect the cutaneous thickness of local flaps. The VRAM flap may be prohibitively thick and difficult to inset. Some surgeons will consider a thigh-based flap over an abdominal flap based on fat distribution across the body. A pannus or redundant folds alter hygiene and personal care. In severe cases, a panniculectomy may be added to the consent in order to visualize certain structures within the pelvic region. Finally, obesity will absolutely place more stress on pelvic or perineal sutures, and careful sitting and activity protocols must be enforced.

Regardless of age or orientation, sexual function and activity must be discussed. Frequently, patients have ceased intimate relations due to pain, tumor-related discharge, or radiation changes and strictures. However, many patients, when carefully asked, will say that they wish to resume activity in the future if possible. In the author's experience, most have strongly charged and emotional reactions to the changes that have occurred to their genital and pelvic structures due to cancer. Most worry that their partner, or future partner, may find them undesirable based on surgical changes. Many are frightened when considering penetrating intercourse due to postradiation burning and pain. It is extremely important to tease out the patient's desire for sexual intercourse as they are now versus how they may feel when fully healed. Maintenance of sexual function and prevention of the psychologic sequelae of surgery are fundamental issues [65].

It is the author's opinion that for those who have any interest in penetrating intercourse in the future, surgery affecting the vagina or perineum should be reconstructed with adequate soft tissue to prevent scarring or stricture. Furthermore, the patients should be advised that postoperative maintenance, such as daily dilation or penetration, will be required to keep a reconstructed vault open. Patients must be told genital sensation changes are the rule, rather than the exception. Lastly, if the partner is present, it is important to consider their feelings regarding sexuality.

Management

Following a thorough evaluation, the initial management of the heavily irradiated pelvis is reliant upon treatment directed at managing patient symptoms, minimizing morbidity, and preventing additional complications. This may include conservative or nonsurgical options in most patients. Typically, these are managed by the consulting urologist. If conservative management has failed, then surgical reconstruction may be offered in a multidisciplinary manner.

Conservative/Non-reconstructive

Initial management may include pharmacologic therapy and catheter-based urinary diversion. Topical local anesthetic effects within the urinary tract can be provided using phenazopyridine (Pyridium), while antimuscarinic or β-3 adrenergic agonist therapy may be utilized for symptomatic relief of significant LUTS. Patients with incomplete emptying or dysfunctional voiding may require placement of an indwelling urinary catheter, suprapubic tube placement, or intermittent self-catheterization. Upper urinary tract obstruction is typically managed with retrograde ureteral stent placement or percutaneous nephrostomy (PCN). Pelvic floor muscle therapy (PFMT) may provide transient relief of LUTS and improve bladder function for patients who are not candidates or unable to tolerate more invasive therapy. Failure of pharmacologic therapy may require the introduction of more invasive therapies including intradetrusor onabotulinumtoxinA (Botox) injection or sacral neuromodulation. Chuang et al. evaluated botulinum toxin A (BoNT-A) injection in six patients with radiation cystitis and demonstrated a mean increase in bladder capacity from 104 mL to 250 mL and urinary frequency decrease from 14 episodes per day to 11 episodes per day [66].

Urinary Tract Reconstruction

Following careful clinical evaluation and patient counseling, options for urinary tract reconstruction can be offered to patients who fail to respond to initial conservative management and are appropriate surgical candidates based on performance status, life expectancy, and range of comorbidities. Options for reconstruction will depend upon the underlying clinical sequelae of the radiation therapy such as urinary fistulae or the presence of a severely contracted bladder. Broadly, reconstructive options can be categorized as organ-sparing reconstruction or pelvic exenteration with urinary diversion.

The management of genitourinary fistulae is reviewed elsewhere within this book. Discussion here will consist of reconstructive options for severe bladder/pelvic floor dysfunction and/or locally invasive pelvic malignancy (rectal, cervical, etc.).

Organ-Sparing Reconstruction

With organ-sparing approaches, the goal of reconstruction is to restore structure and function to dysfunctional pelvic organs impacted by severe radiation toxicity. With this approach, the aim is to maintain the bladder and urethra in their current capacity. Shared clinical decision-making will assist the surgeon in selecting the best option for the patient depending on whether the patient has the physical and cognitive capacity to perform self-catheterization or if the desire to avoid an external appliance is expressed. Otherwise, an incontinent diversion can be performed for patients who lack the ability to provide self-care or for those who lack the necessary social supports.

Bladder Neck Reconstruction and Urethroplasty

Patients with severe pelvic floor dysfunction, detrusor instability, and/or reduced bladder capacity and compliance may experience mild to severe levels of urinary incontinence. This is the result of radiation-induced ischemia and fibrosis of the pelvic floor which in turn leads to bladder neck and external urethral sphincter dysfunction. For these patients, management of the bladder neck may include either reconstruction with an anti-incontinence procedure or closure and urinary diversion. In general, female urethral stricture disease (FUSD) is most commonly related to instrumentation, recurrent infection, or traumatic injury with pelvic fracture [67]. Pelvic radiation as an etiologic factor is infrequently reported for female urethral stricture disease. Shin et al. reported on a single case of spontaneous urinary bladder rupture secondary to radiation-induced urethral stricture disease following treatment for cervical carcinoma 13 years prior [68]. In a small series of three cases of radiation-induced FUSD, Gupta et al. evaluated clinical outcomes following dorsal onlay buccal mucosal graft (BMG) urethroplasty. Mean IPSS improved from 27.33 +/− 1.15 to 3.33 +/− 1.5. Qmax improved from 6.46 +/− 0.6 mL/s to 23.33 +/− 6.1 mL/s. Post-void residual (PVR) improved from 56.67 +/− 16.07 mL to 15.67 +/− 8.14 mL. No patients reported bothersome LUTS or stricture recurrence at 12 months of follow-up [69].

In the authors' experience, when approaching radiation-induced FUSD, strictures located within the distal two-third of the urethra are typically most amenable to reconstruction, while strictures located within the proximal one-third may be complicated by dense fibrosis causing bladder neck fixation. Augmentation urethroplasty with graft placement is further complicated by the poor-quality graft bed from radiation-induced ischemia. For these reasons, FUSD in the post-radiation setting should be approached with caution and following a thorough evaluation.

Anti-lincontinence Surgery

Patients with a stabilized bladder neck and no further contracture with severe incontinence can be best managed with anti-incontinence therapy using conservative options such as continence pessary, vaginal inserts, or pelvic floor muscle exercises before moving on to surgical options in refractory cases. Currently approved surgical options include bulking agents, mid-urethral synthetic slings, autologous pubovaginal fascial slings, or the Burch colposuspension. However, the placement of synthetic mesh should be used with caution in the patient with prior pelvic irradiation due to an increased risk for mesh exposure following poor wound healing [70]. The artificial urinary sphincter (AUS) has been endorsed for use in the management of refractory SUI and neurogenic SUI in female patients by the European Association of Urology (EAU), International Continence Society (ICS), and the French Association of Urology (AFU). While studies have shown continence rates from 61% to 100%, a high rate of intraoperative bladder and vaginal injury has been reported along with moderately high rates of explantation, erosion, and mechanical failure [71]. However, AUS placement in female patients following pelvic radiation is contraindicated. As the series reported by Thomas et al., all patients who had AUS placed following pelvic RT for cervical carcinoma required explantation for erosion and subsequent urinary diversion [72]. At present, the AUS is not approved for use in female patients for any indication in the United States by the Food and Drug Administration (FDA) [73].

Bladder Neck Closure

When bladder neck reconstruction proves unsuccessful from either failed attempts or if the bladder neck tissue is deemed of poor quality, bladder neck closure and diversion can be attempted. Options for bladder neck closure include methods to increase bladder outlet resistance and achieve hypercontinence including the autologous pubovaginal fascial sling which leads to intentional obstruction of the bladder neck. Alternatively, closure can be achieved by surgical dissection, mobilization, and division of the bladder neck at the level of the proximal urethra followed by closure of the bladder neck with 2-0 absorbable suture such as PDS or Vicryl in an interrupted manner with 2-layer closure. This provides the optimal strength for closure in patients with a history of pelvic radiation and minimizes the risk of dehiscence and urine leak. Selection of technique is dependent upon patient-related factors and surgeon preference and familiarity. Coordination with the plastic reconstructive surgeon for placement of a vascularized pedicle flap to augment the bladder closure and fill dead space is paramount to the success of the closure and is discussed further later in this chapter.

Bladder Augmentation

Bladder augmentation may be considered in patients with a preoperative evaluation suggestive of reduced bladder capacity and/or compliance. This procedure can be performed as a solitary procedure if the only complaint is increased lower urinary tract symptoms related to poor storage. Often patients may have evidence of a high-pressure, poorly compliant, and contracted bladder with intrinsic sphincteric deficiency, in which a combination of techniques including augmentation and anti-incontinence surgery can be performed. The advantage of bladder augmentation over incontinent supravesical diversion is the preservation of urine flow and functionality of the native bladder which avoids the risks of pyocystis and the risks associated with ureteroenteric anastomoses. Preoperative counseling regarding the requirement for clean intermittent catheterization is mandatory to frame patient expectations and to avoid complications including anastomotic leak in the early recovery period along with recurrent UTIs, bladder stones, and metabolic disorders in the long term [74].

Bladder augmentation can be performed using distal ileum or colon (cecum, sigmoid), with the former being a more common source for bowel segment use given the location, mobility, and blood supply of the distal ileum being optimal for use in urologic reconstruction. Anytime the large bowel is considered for use within the urinary tract, thorough evaluation with contrast enema, sigmoidoscopy, or colonoscopy is recommended to rule out bowel disease including diverticulosis, inflammatory bowel disease, and occult colon cancer [75]. The use of the stomach (gastrocystoplasty) has been reported in the past but is rarely performed and not recommended in contemporary urologic reconstruction given potential complications including hypokalemic, hypochloremic metabolic alkalosis, hematuria-dysuria syndrome, and cases of gastric adenocarcinoma developing in the augmented bladder [76, 77]. Bowel tissue requires careful inspection for evidence of radiation enteritis, as this bowel is potentially associated with an increased risk of devastating complications, including bowel leak. Despite this historical assertion, data supports the safe and effective use of ileum in diversion following pelvic irradiation, and therefore the necessity of these other techniques has become less common [76].

Incontinent Urinary Channels

Urinary channels can be established between the native or augmented urinary bladder and the abdominal wall when the decision to proceed with bladder neck closure for a devastated outlet or severe refractory urinary incontinence is established. The decision to construct an incontinent versus continent channel once again is dictated based on patient preference and suitability to the clinical scenario.

Incontinent Ileovesicostomy

Incontinent ileovesicostomy first gained popularity in the 1990s as an option for urinary diversion in patients with neurogenic bladder dysfunction unable to perform intermittent self-catheterization. Most of the reported outcomes with this technique have been in the pediatric and adult neurogenic bladder/spinal cord injury (SCI) population. In this technique, urinary diversion is similar to the construction of an ileal conduit diversion except that the proximal ileal segment is anastomosed directly with the bladder while the distal end undergoes maturation at the abdominal wall. Stomal maturation is performed in a similar manner as in the ileal conduit following passage of the ileal limb through the rectus hiatus [78]. An external appliance is attached, and postoperative management is performed in the routine manner. Advantages include the lack of requirement for cystectomy and ureteroenteric anastomoses. If the patient is able to return to urethral catheterization, the procedure lends itself favorably to reversal [79]. Hellenthal et al. reported on 12 patients undergoing ileovesicostomy, with 58% showing reduced antibiotic usage and issues with chronic upper tract obstruction. However, 17% of the patients eventually required conversion to an ileal conduit. Of note, in the neurogenic/SCI population, the bladder neck is not routinely closed [80]. Tan et al. reported on 50 adult patients in which the average complication rate for stomal complications and mechanical obstruction was 1.47 and 2.09 events per patient, respectively [81].

Continent Urinary Channels

Continent urinary diversion is offered to patients who desire urinary continence, wish to avoid an external appliance, and have the physical and cognitive capacity to perform self-catheterization. There are several different techniques for catheterizable channel construction including appendix (appendicovesicostomy – APV), reconfigured ileum (Yang-Monti), or intussuscepted ileal nipple valve (Kock). In all examples, the continence mechanism is further enhanced through tapering and reinforcement with interrupted suture placement. Patients with underlying neurocognitive disorders that may impact their long-term cognitive capacity and ability to perform self-catheterization require special consideration prior to continent channel construction.

Mitrofanoff Appendicovesicostomy

First described by Mitrofanoff in 1980, the appendicovesicostomy has been an established technique for catheterizable channel construction in children with neurogenic bladders and adults requiring diversion from a defunctionalized bladder outlet or compromised urethra. When a suitable appendix with respect to length is available, it can serve as an ideal channel given its consistent blood supply, mobility, and diameter. In addition, given its vestigial nature, isolation from the remainder of the gastrointestinal tract has negligible metabolic consequences [82].

Yang-Monti Channel

The Yang-Monti channel was developed between 1993 and 1997 [83, 84]. This technique can be utilized when the appendix is either too short or has been previously surgically removed. The advantage with this technique is that if a coinciding bladder augmentation is required, then the ileum adjacent to that required for the channel can be isolated for the augmentation, in effect requiring a single bowel anastomosis. For both the appendix and reconfigured ileum channels, the continence mechanism is provided by formation of a detrusor tunnel flap valve. Overall continence rates exceed 95% for both the APV and Yang-Monti channels. The advantage of tubularized channel construction is in the use of shorter bowel segments to bridge long gaps between the bladder and abdominal wall. More recently, the Yang-Monti tube has been utilized in ureteral reconstruction for the management of stricture disease. Modifications of this technique include the double-tube Monti and the spiral Monti procedures which allow for longer channel construction, while minimizing the length of bowel required for construction [85].

Continent catheterizable channels are not without complications including incontinence and difficult catheterization. Difficult catheterization can develop secondary to stomal stenosis, false passage, diverticulum, channel redundancy, parastomal hernia, or fibrosis following ischemia. The rate of stomal stenosis varies between 5% and 10% in contemporary series and appears similar between APV and Yang-Monti [82]. However, several series have reported higher rates of surgical revision with Yang-Monti (2X) and spiral Monti (4X) when compared with APV [86]. Pagliara et al. reviewed 51 adult patients following revision or replacement of their catheterizable channel. At a median follow-up of 19 months, channel patency was achieved in 66%. Channel patency was significantly improved in patients undergoing "channel replacement" (89%) and "above fascia" (62%) repairs compared with "below fascia" (52%) repairs. However, the rate of new incontinence following revision was 40% overall (Mitrofanoff, 37%; Monti, 64%; tapered ileum, 17%) [87]. These results highlight the importance of patient selection and counseling during the perioperative period and that the possibility of requiring additional procedures for revision remains high.

Kock Nipple Valve

In the Kock procedure, a longer segment of ileum is utilized with intussusception of ileum to form a nipple valve. The technique was initially applied by Kock as part of construction of the efferent limb in his "Kock pouch" [88]. The concept was then utilized in isolation to serve as a standalone channel. However, this technique has failed to gain widespread adoption due to the increased amount of ileum required, technical complexity, difficulty in construction, and failure of the continence mechanism through detussusception [82].

Continent Catheterizable Ileal Cecocystoplasty (CCIC)

A CCIC is a form of urinary diversion that combines bladder augmentation with continent catheterizable channel construction as a single component based on the cecum, ascending colon, and utilization of the ileocecal valve and tapered terminal ileum as the continence mechanism and catheterizable channel, respectively. An additional bladder neck closure procedure using either urethral ligation or pubovaginal sling placement can be utilized for the patient with intrinsic sphincter deficiency and detrusor overactivity on preoperative urodynamics [89].

There are advantages and disadvantages to this technique. Advantages include excellent continence given the ileocecal valve and increase in functional bladder capacity. As well, the technique is faster to perform as a smaller segment of colon is required to achieve a satisfactory increase in capacity compared with ileocystoplasty which also requires more suturing to configure the appropriate bowel plate for anastomosis to the bladder. Also, only a single bowel anastomosis is required for the entire procedure as compared with creation of ileocystoplasty and a separate Monti or double-Monti channel. Finally, the terminal ileum is continuous with the augmented segment and therefore negates the risk of stenosis of the channel at the bladder [82]. Disadvantages include the requirement for preoperative colonoscopy in patients of screening age to rule out colonic malignancy and the potential for electrolyte dysfunction, malabsorptive disorders, chronic diarrhea, and the complications that arise from foreign body catheterization including urinary stones and infection [90]. Patient education and counseling are of the utmost importance to guide patient decision-making and to provide realistic expectations regarding these types of urinary diversion.

In a retrospective review by Redshaw et al., outcomes and complications were reviewed for CCIC compared with other tunneled cutaneous channels (i.e., APV and Monti channel). In total, 61 patients were evaluated including 31 with CCIC. The rate of secondary procedures was higher for tunneled channels compared with CCIC (50% vs 13%, OR 6.4, 95% C.I 1.8–28). As well, stomal leakage rates were higher for tunneled channels at 43% compared with 29% in CCIC. However, a high rate of postoperative complications was observed in both groups at 40% for tunneled channels and 51.7% in CCIC [91].

In a large multicenter retrospective review over a 10-year period, Cheng et al. evaluated 114 patients with a history of neurogenic bladder. The 90-day major complication rate was 15.8% with 21.1% of patients requiring readmission, most often for intra-abdominal abscess (3.5%) or bowel leak (3.5%). The channel revision rate was 20.2%, which was performed for obstruction (13.2%) and incontinence (3.5%). Revision procedures included superficial stomal revision, stomal dilation, injection of bulking agent, or major revision with replacement or revision below the fascia [92].

Supravesical Diversion

In some cases of severe pelvic irradiation and radiation-induced endarteritis of pelvic blood vessels, ischemia and fibrosis can lead to significant ureteral stricture development resulting in partial or complete ureteral obstruction. Most of the blood supply to the distal ureters arises from the internal iliac vessels and their branches, and therefore small vessels are particularly susceptible to radiation-induced injury in this region [93]. Initial management in these cases will necessitate renal decompression with either retrograde ureteral stent or PCN placement. At this point, management may consist of chronic stent or PCN exchange depending on patient preferences, comorbidities, and life expectancy. Otherwise, surgical reconstruction can be offered to the carefully selected and counseled patient with a desire to be "tube free."

Options for reconstruction will depend on the length and laterality of the ureteral stricture disease and the condition of the contralateral renal unit. Depending on the length of the stricture, options include ureteroneocystostomy, psoas hitch, Boari flap, ileal interposition, renal autotransplantation, and nephrectomy [94]. The presence of significant preoperative LUTS, reduced capacity and compliance, and poor bladder mobility will negatively impact the use of some of these techniques. Transureteroureterostomy is contraindicated in patients with a history of urolithiasis, urothelial carcinoma, contralateral reflux, retroperitoneal fibrosis, and bilateral ureteral stricture disease. Given the distribution of radiation over the entire pelvis in some treatments, bilateral disease is more likely, and therefore a history of pelvic irradiation precludes this technique [95].

Autotransplantation is infrequently performed and will depend on surgeon experience. As well, there are concerns of this technique in patients with a solitary kidney. Hedges et al. reported on a series of 54 autotransplants in 51 patients over a 27-year period. Ureteral stricture was the indication in 20.4% of patients. The early and late high-grade complication rates were 14.8% and 12.9%, respectively. Two graft losses occurred, and cold ischemia time was the only predictor of postoperative complications [96]. Nephrectomy can be offered for patient with evidence of reduced renal function or significant renal atrophy who are bothered by pain and or persistent infection. Otherwise, the best options for reconstruction in the case of unilateral or bilateral radiation-induced ureteral stricture disease with mild to moderate bladder dysfunction include ileal ureteral substitution with or without concomitant ileocystoplasty. Ileal interposition can be performed in a "seven" or "reverse-7" configuration to incorporate both proximal normal ureters into a single conduit that is then anastomosed directly to the bladder [97]. To perform an ileocystoplasty, the distal ileal segment is opened along the anti-mesenteric border, reconfigured into the appropriate bowel flap, and anastomosed to the bladder following longitudinal cystotomy [98].

For situations in which the bladder is unsalvageable and cystectomy or pelvic exenteration is not required, severe ureteral stricture disease can be managed with supravesical diversion using ileal conduit or transverse colon conduit diversion (see later).

Non-organ-Sparing Reconstruction

Pelvic Exenteration

Pelvic exenteration was first described by Brunschwig in 1951 for treatment in female patients with extensive irradiation necrosis of the pelvic viscera. Since that time, this technique has undergone little modification, and the emphasis has been on advancing techniques for reconstruction following extirpation. In his original description, urinary diversion with reimplantation was performed into the left colon just proximal to the colostomy, creating a "wet colostomy"; however complications including electrolyte disturbances and severe urinary tract infections reduced popularity of the technique until Bricker's concept of the ileal conduit in 1950 became more widely accepted [99, 100].

Patients in whom reconstruction and organ preservation are not possible secondary to severe radiation-induced necrosis/fibrosis, an end-stage bladder (contracted, <100 ml capacity), or complex genitourinary fistulae may benefit the most in achieving symptom palliation and improvement in QoL. Pelvic exenteration includes an extended en bloc resection of all pelvic visceral organs. Specifically, an anterior pelvic exenteration includes resection of all pelvic organs of the urinary and gynecologic systems including the bladder, urethra, uterus, cervix, fallopian tubes, and all or part of the vagina. In the case of pelvic exenteration for a non-malignancy-related indication, the ovaries can be left in situ in premenopausal women. In contrast, posterior pelvic exenteration involves removal of all pelvic organs of the gynecologic and gastrointestinal systems including the uterus, cervix, fallopian tubes, sigmoid colon, rectum, and anus. In this instance, if gastrointestinal resection is required, the patient will require a permanent end colostomy. Total pelvic exenteration includes resection of the anterior and posterior compartments of pelvic organs [101]. If symptoms are confined to the urinary tract, a simple cystectomy and urinary diversion may be all that is required, while more extensive resection including removal of the uterus, cervix, vagina, and bowel may be required if there are extensive fibrotic changes precluding safe separation and preservation of these organs. Sexual function preservation with vaginal-sparing techniques requires special consideration in female patients wishing to preserve sexual function and can be accomplished utilizing vaginal reconstruction techniques (see later) [102].

With advancements in perioperative care, anesthesia, critical care techniques, and access to tertiary-level care with nursing and ancillary service support, mortality following pelvic exenteration has fallen to less than 5%. However, treatment-related morbidity remains in excess of 50% as the consequence of poor healing following advanced and complex reconstruction in the heavily irradiated pelvis [103, 104].

Urinary Diversion

Options for urinary diversion following pelvic exenteration for the severely irradiated pelvis include incontinent and continent techniques. The most common technique is the ileal conduit which is the simplest and easiest form of urinary diversion and associated with relative ease of care and a reduced complication rate [105]. Conversely, patients may elect to maintain continence at all costs, in which case an ileocecal reservoir (i.e., Indiana pouch) or orthotopic ileal neobladder can be constructed. In a small retrospective case series by Chiva et al., orthotopic ileal neobladder construction was performed in six patients undergoing pelvic exenteration for recurrent cervical cancer following pelvic irradiation. All patients reported satisfaction with their decision to undergo continent diversion. Good daytime urinary continence was reported in 66% patients and good nighttime continence in 50% of the patients. Half of the patients developed an anastomotic urine leak, with two patients having spontaneous resolution with conservative treatment and one patient requiring surgery [106]. Hautmann et al. retrospectively reviewed a single institutional experience of 25 patients (7 male, 18 female) with a history of neobladder construction and prior pelvic irradiation. The 90-day complication rate was 76% (neobladder) and 52% (non-neobladder) but with less frequent grade 3–5 complications in the neobladder group. Total day and night continence was reported in 76% of the patients, while 16% of patients continued to have refractory severe stress incontinence [107]. Continent urinary diversion is relatively safe and effective and can be offered in select well-informed patients with end-stage bladders wishing to preserve urinary continence. Success of orthotopic neobladder reconstruction, as in patients with bladder cancer, depends on intact urethral rhabdosphincter and pelvic floor muscles which are more likely to be functionally impaired following pelvic irradiation [108]. Mannel et al. reported on ten women who underwent pelvic exenteration following a history of pelvic irradiation for cervical cancer. Eight of the women underwent pelvic exenteration for recurrent pelvic tumor, while two had urinary diversion for radiation-induced vesicovaginal fistula. All women achieved daytime continence with time between catheterization of 4.5 h and a median pouch capacity of 500 ml. There was no evidence of significant ureteral reflux or urinary obstruction. Minimal complications were reported [109].

The potential for urinary complications exists following pelvic exenteration, owing to the urinary diversion. Significant complications include urinary fistulae, ureteral obstruction, urinary leak, stomal stenosis, and complications related to the bowel anastomosis including anastomotic leak and obstruction. These complications have been reported to be higher in this patient group owing to the history of pelvic irradiation compared with patients undergoing urinary diversion following surgery for bladder cancer [110]. This highlights the selection of suitable segments of bowel, preferably without evidence of radiation enteritis, for incorporation in the reconstruction. However, given the recurrent and severe nature of complications previously incurred in this patient group, they may be more likely to opt for lower-risk and less complicated forms of diversion to minimize the rate of reoperation [111]. In a retrospective review, Smith et al. reported on postoperative outcomes in 34 women who underwent urinary diversion for the management of adverse effects related to gynecologic radiation. Incontinent diversion was performed in 76.5% of the women, and 79.4% of women experienced complications within 90 days. High-grade complications were reported in 26.5% with 32% requiring readmission within 30 days. The rate of high-grade complications was not significantly impacted by diversion type, concurrent cystectomy, or sarcopenia (based on preoperative CT scans) [112].

The jejunal conduit is not commonly utilized given the availability and suitability of the ileum, but it is worth mentioning as a potential option in the heavily irradiated pelvis as it is located out of the standard radiation field and may prove useful when the large bowel is unsuitable or unavailable. Golimbu et al. reported on 30 patients undergoing jejunal urinary diversion, and the primary indication was diversion for malignant disease in the heavily irradiated pelvis. Overall complications did not differ compared with the ileal conduit, but a high incidence of electrolyte abnormalities with hyperkalemic, hypochloremic, hyponatremic metabolic acidosis was reported requiring correction with salt tablets, sodium bicarbonate, and thiazide diuretics [113].

While less commonly performed in contemporary urologic practice, the transverse colon conduit provides an option for incontinent diversion when suitable ileum that is without severe radiation damage cannot be isolated. Given its high position within the abdomen, the transverse colon is relatively shielded from the radiation field of pelvic organs [114]. A particular advantage of the colonic conduit is a lower rate of bowel obstruction compared with small bowel conduits, at a rate of 4% and 10%, respectively [115, 116]. As well, shorter ureteral length is required for ureteroenteric anastomosis and may be advantageous when severe ureteral damage is also present. Another example of the colon conduit is the sigmoid conduit, which is useful in pelvic exenteration cases in which a colostomy will be fashioned as this avoids a bowel anastomosis. However, this technique is not recommended when there has been prior pelvic radiation or if there is disease in the segment [105]. Schmidt et al. reported on 22 patients with extensive pelvic irradiation who underwent primary supravesical diversion using the transverse colon conduit for management of radiation cystitis, vesicovaginal fistula, and ureteral obstruction. Minimal complications were reported with no evidence of upper tract obstruction or deterioration in renal function. An operative mortality rate of 4% was observed, and no cases of adenocarcinoma were reported after more than 10 years of follow-up, owing to the lack of a fecal stream [117]. Ravi et al. reported on their series of 30 patients with transverse colon conduits following very high-dose pelvic irradiation ($\geq$ 65 Gy) with an overall complication rate of 37% and reoperation rate of 20%. No bowel or urinary anastomotic leaks were reported, and renal function was normal or improved in 83% [118].

Abdominal Wall, Pelvic, and Genital Reconstruction

Depending on the nature and extent of urinary tract reconstruction, additional reconstruction of the abdominal wall, pelvic floor, and/or genitalia may be required to restore cosmesis and anatomic functionality and to fill and close dead space. Techniques in plastic reconstructive surgery are reviewed in this section.

Intraoperative Considerations

Defect size and defect location are the two biggest determinants of reconstructive selection.

Abdominal Wall

Abdominal wall reconstruction is typically reserved for cases requiring extensive pelvic reconstruction from either major extirpation surgery or abdominal wall flap-based closure of the pelvis. Given the degree of radiation-induced fibrosis typically present within the pelvis, a well-vascularized pedicle flap may be needed in which case the operative team should anticipate and be prepared for abdominal wall reconstruction to close the primary defect and prevent postoperative wound-related complications. In addition, abdominal wall stomal construction may need to be performed following a careful discussion with the plastic surgery team in order to delineate stomal positioning based on the anticipated abdominal wall closure technique and graft harvesting, particularly for myocutaneous flaps. Occasionally stomal complications may result postoperatively, such as peristomal herniation, in which plastic surgery consultation may be required for assistance with mesh-based repair.

If the abdominal wall resection has minimal fascial involvement, it may be possible to close the abdominal wall by primary closure alone. However, for patients with an existing stoma or a new conduit or stoma, the rate of parastomal herniation and infection significantly increases as patient morbidities increase. In 2010, the Ventral Hernia Working Group (VHWG) recommended a novel hernia grading system based on risk factor characteristics of the patient and the wound and the risk of surgical site occurrence [119]. Grade 1 (low risk) included younger patients without comorbidities. Grade 2 (comorbid) included patients with smoking, obesity, diabetes, immunosuppression, or COPD. Grade 3 (potentially contaminated) captured patients with previous infection, present stoma, or violation of the gastrointestinal tract. Lastly, grade 4 (infected) included all patients with existing infected mesh or septic dehiscence. The VHWG recommended prosthetic mesh placement for all hernias to reduce recurrence rates. As patients became more morbid, the group recommended transition from a synthetic to bioprosthetic mesh and consideration of adjunct procedures such as component separation.

The choice of mesh type and mesh location is highly dependent upon surgeon preference. Synthetic mesh is currently the most common repair material used for reinforcement of ventral hernias [120]. Synthetic meshes are known for their high tensile strength and lower cost but are extremely problematic if they become infected. In particular, draining infectious sinuses or fistulas may result in explantation and need for further abdominal wall [121–124]. Biologic meshes are more resistant to infection and extrusion, although they are more costly and may stretch over time [125, 126]. If the surgeon is working in a highly contaminated field or immunosuppressed patient, a biologic mesh is recommended. In a clean or minimally contaminated field, a prosthetic mesh may perform better.

In regard to mesh location, an incisional hernia may be repaired with an overlay (on top of the rectus fascia), retrorectus (between the rectus fascia and posterior rectus sheath), or underlay (posterior to the rectus sheath and peritoneum). In all cases, a segment of the mesh can be designed with a "keyhole" opening to reinforce a stoma. Alternatively, a parastomal repair or reinforcement can be done by the Sugarbaker technique, in which the mesh is sewn with a short tunnel protecting the intestinal segment against the posterior abdominal wall before it exits the stoma [127, 128]. This technique has proven effective against hernias that tend to "piston" through the fascial opening. Recent studies have demonstrated that concomitant abdominal wall reconstruction with ostomy-associated herniorrhaphy is safe to perform and does not lead to increased ventral hernia recurrence rates [129, 130]. Regardless of mesh placement, repair material should overlap with intact fascia by at least 3–5 cm [131–133].

In extreme cases, a bridged repair may be necessary to close the abdominal wall. In this instance, primary fascial approximation is not possible. Unfortunately, bridged repairs lead to higher recurrence rates due to the avascular and deneurotized reconstruction in the central abdomen [129, 134]. In these instances, it is recommended that the patient undergo unilateral or bilateral component separation. Pioneered by Ramirez, this technique involves a surgical release of the layers of the abdominal wall to allow centralization of vascularized muscle and fascia [135]. The original technique, open anterior release, releases the first layer of the linea semilunaris, thereby allowing the rectus muscle complex, internal oblique, and transversus muscles to slide medially away from the more fixated external oblique aponeurosis. This "component" muscle flap is based on the intercostal nerves and vasculature that run in the plane between the internal oblique and transversus muscles. The external oblique remains as a reinforcement of the lateral abdominal wall, while the remaining muscles serve as a vascularized, neurotized muscle complex centrally. Each unilateral release can provide up to 8–10 cm of advancement at the most central portion of the abdomen (Fig. 2).

Multiple variations of the component release now exist, including posterior and endoscopic releases. All releases demonstrate decreased ventral and incisional hernia rates when neurotized tissue is restored on the central abdominal wall [136–138]. Component releases may be easily performed in combination with mesh placement and are safe to perform near ostomies. Of note, case series have suggested that while component separation has utility in challenging cases and

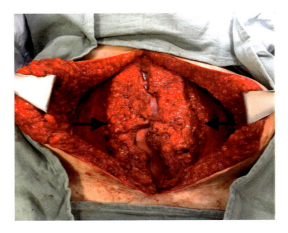

Fig. 2 Bilateral component release

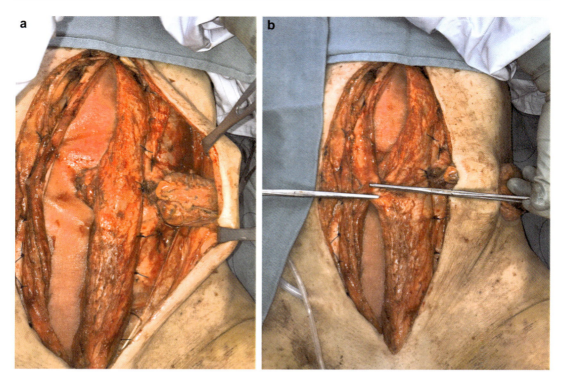

Fig. 3 (**a**) Component with stoma and mesh (**b**) Component with stoma and mesh primary approximation

reduce recurrence, patients still benefit from prosthetic repair material especially in complex defects [121, 137, 139]. Several studies have documented a reduced hernia rate when component separation is reinforced by biologic mesh, in either overlay or underlay fashion [139, 140]. In particular, biologic mesh is favored for this use in patients with a radiated abdominal wall [119, 129, 141]. See Fig. 3 for an example of component release near an ostomy and reinforcement with biologic mesh underlay.

Pelvic Dead Space

In many instances of pelvic reconstruction, the rectum, uterus, or bladder may be taken. If pelvic floor is left bereft of sufficient soft tissue, fluid collections and potential abscess may occur. Small bowel may migrate to the pelvic floor. In radiated patients, bowel adhesions near the pelvic floor may result in eventual fistula. If substantial pelvic floor musculature is removed, herniation of intra-abdominal contents is possible. For these reasons, sufficient vascularized soft tissue should be brought to the pelvis when more than one structure is removed.

The omental flap is a workhorse flap for obliteration of pelvic dead space. The omental flap is large and fan-shaped with a reliable arterial arcade supplied by three vascular branches: the right, middle, and left omental vessels. These vessels originate from the right and left gastroepiploic vessels. The flap may be isolated on one of its vascular pedicles, usually the right gastroepiploic as it is larger, and will retain sufficient vascular inflow to supply the entire flap [142]. Ligation of the additional pedicles allows the flap to be advanced deeper into the pelvis. As a free flap, it can be up to 40×60 cm in size, although as a pedicled flap it more commonly provides 20×30 cm at the target location [143]. Several studies have documented the favorable use of the omentum for pelvic dead space obliteration [144, 145]. However, its size may limit its use in larger defects and provides no cutaneous paddle. When a large or external defect is present, an abdominal-based flap may be preferred [146].

In cases where the omental flap is prohibitively scarred or small, alternative sources of tissue may come from the abdominal wall. The rectus muscle may be harvested alone or in combination with its fascia and overlying cutaneous tissue, also known as a vertical rectus abdominis myocutaneous (VRAM) flap. Both the rectus flap alone and the VRAM require isolation of the flap on the deep inferior epigastric artery and vein system. These vessels are readily isolated as they branch from the external femoral artery and vein prior to the inguinal canal. The rectus flap is helpful for small defects but may prove to be insufficient in a broad gynecoid pelvis. Furthermore, the muscle will undergo atrophy over time from ligation of the motor nerves. Alternatively, the VRAM flap can be designed with variable sizes of skin and subcutaneous tissue. Modifications such as the extended VRAM, which incorporates tissue near the costal cartilages, allow the flap to reach nearly 30–40 cm from its vascular pedicle and may be up to 10 cm wide. For the reconstructive surgeon, the VRAM provides extreme flexibility to reconstruct a variety of defects. Figure 4 demonstrates a large VRAM flap that is used to reconstruct an extremely large defect from a pelvic exenteration combined with sacrectomy.

Importantly, it must be discussed that the traditional VRAM does create an incisional hernia of the abdominal wall that requires repair. Fascial and muscle-sparing techniques have been popularized to avoid this comorbidity, but patients must be counseled regarding the potential for bulge, hernia, or weakness in the future. When a traditional VRAM is taken, or even a fascial-sparing VRAM, it is the author's preference in comorbid patients to reinforce the abdominal wall repair with biologic mesh, especially if an ostomy is present. Van Vliet et al. demonstrated that when a VRAM flap was used in pelvic defect reconstruction, defect size did not affect the risk of partial flap necrosis, complete flap loss, infection, abdominal fascial dehiscence, ventral hernia, or seroma but did increase the rate of wound complications regardless of age or BMI [147]. Techniques to minimize wound healing issues, such as perforator and fascial-sparing harvest, can improve outcomes. Figure 5 demonstrates a fascial-sparing harvest of the VRAM flap.

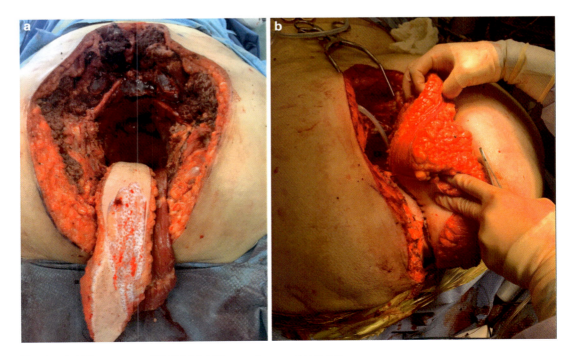

Fig. 4 (a) APR sacrectomy VRAM (b) APR sacrectomy vaginectomy

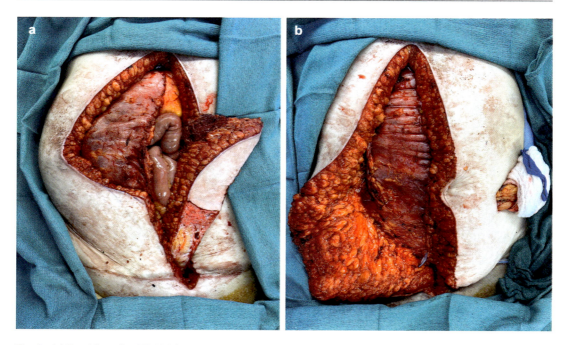

Fig. 5 (a) Fascial sparing VRAM for vagina (b) Primary fascial reapproximation after VRAM with stoma

Of note, it is important to know that as robotic and laparoscopic extirpative surgery advances, so does flap harvest. Several studies now demonstrate excellent results with the use of robotically harvested rectus abdominis muscle flap for pelvic dead space obliteration [148–150]. After a multidisciplinary robotic case, it is unfortunate to have to open and perform a laparotomy for flap harvest alone.

As an alternative to abdominal-based flaps, local tissue flaps from the thigh may be considered for pelvic dead space filling. However, these flaps remain second choice unless there is an external defect present. Even with certain external defects, the reach of such flaps at the gracilis or profunda artery perforator may be limited.

Vaginal Reconstruction

Vaginal defects after oncologic resection vary from mucosal excision to full circumferential loss. Cordeiro and Pusic describe an algorithmic approach to vaginal reconstruction based on defect classification [151, 152]. In these classifications, defects are described as partial (type 1) or total (type 2) and further subclassified based on location. The authors describe the use of three workhorse flaps for reconstruction of these defects, including the rectus abdominis, gracilis, and Singapore flaps. This algorithm demonstrates the choice of flap based on location as well as body habitus and is highly valuable as a reference.

With small defects of the vagina (less than one-third the circumference), primary repair of the vaginal wall may be possible. However, if a patient has previously undergone radiation or surgery, constriction and atrophy of the tissue may prevent sufficient laxity for repair. It is especially important to have asked a patient about their sexual activity preoperatively for this reason. If a patient desires a vagina sufficient for penetration, the vault must be reconstructed with enough depth and laxity for this purpose. Additionally, if the vaginal mucosa is intact but heavily thinned by the resection, reinforcement with a rotational flap such as the omentum or rectus may prevent ulceration or breakdown in high-risk patients.

In regard to vaginal repair over one-third of the circumference, such as a type IA or IB, several options exist. As previously discussed, the VRAM is an extremely reliable source of tissue with multiple design permutations available. For resections that are near or involve the cervix, such

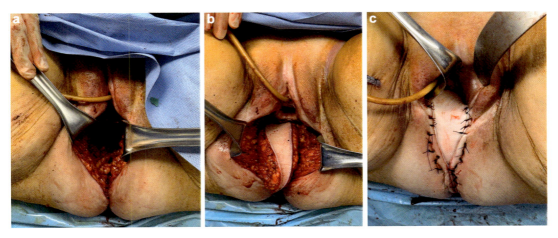

Fig. 6 (**a**) APR with vaginectomy (**b**) APR with vaginectomy and VRAM (**c**) APR with vaginectomy VRAM inset

as posterior vaginectomy, the cutaneous paddle of the VRAM provides exceptional lining of the vault, while the subcutaneous tissue provides posterior dead space obliteration for perineal reconstruction. Multiple authors cite the VRAM as the best choice for posterior vaginal defects (Fig. 6) [151, 153, 154]. In more involved vaginectomies or total vaginectomies, the VRAM may be tubularized and inset as a neovagina. For total vaginectomy, it is recommended to provide a cutaneous paddle at least 9 × 9 cm, as to allow a 3 cm circumference and 8–9 cm depth. In women who are obese or have significant central adiposity, the cutaneous paddle may be prohibitively thick for inset. In these instances, the rectus flap may be harvested with the anterior fascia or posterior peritoneum alone. This surface is then skin grafted or allowed to mucosalize secondarily. Skin grafting may decrease contraction but is prone to poor take given the difficulty of graft stabilization.

Alternatives to abdominal-based vaginal reconstruction include local rotational flaps from the thigh. The gracilis muscle, and/or its overlying cutaneous tissue, may be dissected as a rotational flap on the medial femoral circumflex artery and venae comitantes. The skin paddle may be designed vertically (for increased intrapelvic length) or transversely. The gracilis is located just posterior to the adductor longus muscle and anterior to the adductor magnus. In thin patients, the gracilis flap is exceptionally pliable and valued for ease of inset. It is very useful for treating vaginal fistulas when there is no laparotomy performed (Fig. 7). However, it may also be insufficient in size for larger defects. In these cases, bilateral gracilis flaps may be harvested and used in conjunction (Fig. 8). This is especially useful for low or total vaginectomy defects, such as Pusic type IIB. In high-volume centers, surgeons may need to reconstruct defects after recurrent cancer resection, which removes a previous flap. The gracilis can also serve as an important second-line flap for this purpose (Fig. 9).

An alternative to the gracilis flap is the profunda artery perforator (PAP) flap. This flap is based on perforators traveling through the adductor magnus muscle or between the adductor muscle septa. In the right patient, it has exceptional use for low vaginal or introital defects. It may also be designed vertically or horizontally. As with all flaps, body habitus will largely determine the bulk and reach of any of these local flaps.

An additional flap that is highly useful for anterior (Pusic type IA) or low vaginal defects is the Singapore flap. This flap incorporates thin, pliable fasciocutaneous groin tissue (lateral to labia) based on the posterior labial artery perforators, which is a continuation of the perineal artery. These flaps may be designed up to 6 × 15 cm [155]. The Singapore flap is raised unilaterally or bilaterally and rotated medially for repair of

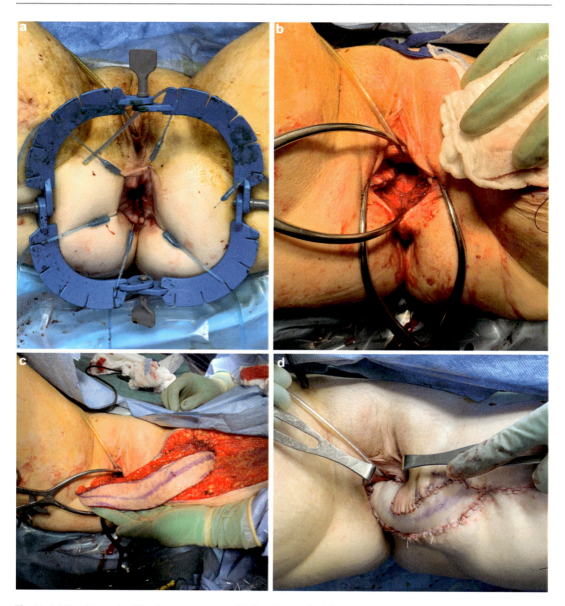

Fig. 7 (**a**) Gracilis vaginal fistula retractor set-up (**b**) Gracilis vagninal fistula exposure (**c**) Gracilis vaginal fistula pedicle flap transfer (**d**) Gracilis vaginal fistula flap inset

defects near the introitus. It is exceptionally useful in patients with vaginal fistulas that require healthy vascularized tissue for closure. Due to its proximity to the vagina, it may be less reliable in patients who have been radiated or undergone multiple previous local excisions. Ultrasound-guided (Doppler) investigation of available perforators is highly valuable in such instances.

Perineal Repair

All of the previously mentioned flaps may be used for perineal repair. In particular, the abdominal-based flaps are exceptional for repair of complex defects, such as those after pelvic exenteration or abdominoperineal resection. This is due to its ability to repair both internal and external components. In patients with defects limited to the external surface, such as the perineum or genitalia, the thigh-based and groin-based flaps are exceptionally versatile and avoid the donor morbidity of the abdomen.

In regard to perineal repair, especially if the vaginal introitus is involved, it cannot be overstated that sufficient soft tissue surface area must be restored. Without sufficient tissue, the perineal and introital tissues are prone to stricture, webbing, and excoriation. Painful tears and scar banding may occur and prohibit not only sexual activity but routine sitting and stair climbing. Scar release procedures, such as the "jumping man" z-plasty, are described later in the chapter.

Vulvar Repair

The vulva is a collective term for the female external genitalia that includes the mons pubis, labia majora, labia minora, clitoris, and vestibule. The vestibule is the triangular space between the labia minora where the urethra and vagina open. All structures are important considerations in peripelvic female reconstruction.

The labia majora and labia minora serve both functional and aesthetic purposes to the female genitourinary tract. As protection for sensitive structures, their loss may cause exquisite sensitivity or dyspareunia. In particular, the labia majora make up prominent folds of cutaneous tissue that protect the orifices of the urogenital triangle. The labia minora unite superiorly to protect the clitoris. Aesthetically, many patients feel disfigured or unattractive if these structures are removed.

Isolated vulvar cancer, including cancers of the labia, is rare, accounting for less than 5% of female genital cancers. However, resection of labial and vulvar structures is common in combination with other peripelvic cancers. Vulvar reconstruction attempts to restore genitalia, body image, sexual function, micturition, and defecation [156]. Several algorithms have been

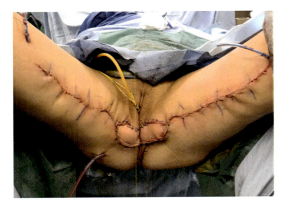

Fig. 8 Bilateral gracilis total vaginectomy

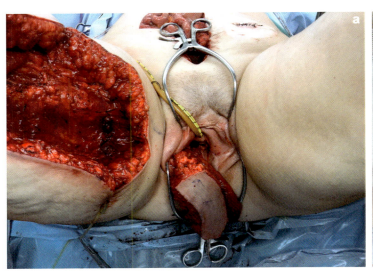
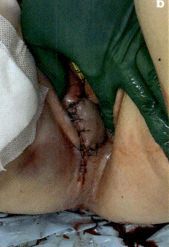

Fig. 9 (a) Gracilis after VRAM resected (b) Gracilis after VRAM resected and inset

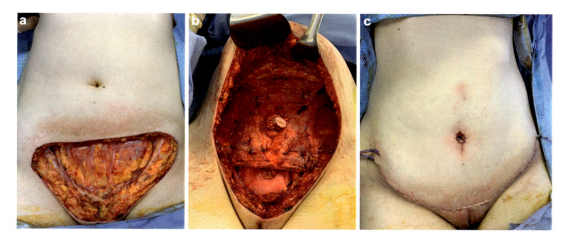

Fig. 10 (a) Abdominoplasty for mons exposure (b) Abdominoplasty with mesh for mons - component separation (c) Abdominoplasty result

proposed based on location and size of the defect [157–160]. The vulva is generally divided into the upper third (mons pubis to labia), the middle third (labia proper), and the lower third (vaginal orifice and perineum).

In general, upper third defects less than 20 cm² can be closed primarily or with adjacent tissue transfer [156]. In multiparous women, the upper abdomen may be recruited in "abdominoplasty fashion" to cover defects of the mons (Fig. 10). In larger defects, local rotational flaps, such as the anterolateral thigh flap, may be needed to restore adequate soft tissue [161, 162]. The anterolateral thigh flap is based on the descending branch of the lateral femoral circumflex artery and its associated venae comitantes. The pedicle travels in the septum between the vastus lateralis and rectus femoris muscles and gives several musculocutaneous or septocutaneous perforators to the overlying thigh skin. The flap can be designed with skin paddles up to 8 × 20 cm and still undergo primary closure of the donor site. It may be rotated above or below the rectus femoris muscle based on necessary pedicle length.

Middle third defect reconstruction, including those of the labia major and labia minora, is highly dependent on defect size. Small resections of the labia major (up to 2 cm) and labia minora (up to 1 cm) may be amenable to primary closure alone. Larger resections require local tissue flap coverage, including the previously mentioned Singapore, gracilis, and profunda artery perforator flaps. Several unique designs have been described in case series, including Sawada's lotus flap for vulvo-perineal reconstruction [163]. In elderly patients or those with significant gluteal laxity, random pattern gluteal fold flaps may be designed that advance buttock tissue from the lateral buttock and thigh toward the perineum. This flap was initially described by Yii and Niranjan and later modified by Hashimoto [164–166]. The flap is located in the triangle formed by the ischial tuberosity, anus, and vaginal orifice. The fascia is lifted over the gluteus maximus to preserve fasciocutaneous blood supply from the internal pudendal perforators (Fig. 11).

The lower third includes the vaginal orifice and perineum. This area is surrounded by a rich supply of vascular perforators. This region may be reconstructed using random pattern local flaps such as the previously described gluteal fold flap or by axial pattern flaps such as the Singapore flap. Again, it cannot be overstated that sufficient soft tissue is required in this area to prevent painful contraction or excoriation. Bilateral local flaps may be required in large defects. In defects that result from pelvic exenteration, the VRAM flap is still the gold standard due to the ability to obliterate pelvic dead space while relining the external surface area. A combination of flaps may be used in unique defects when different subunits of the pelvis and perineum are resected (Fig. 12).

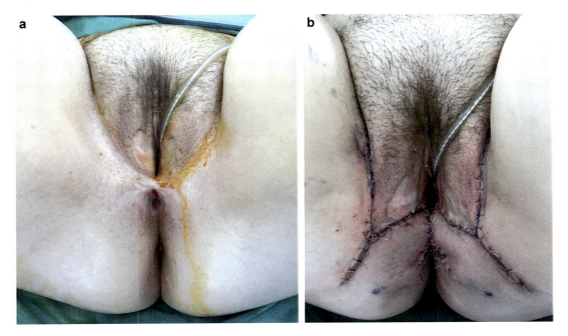

Fig. 11 (**a**) Contracture prior to gluteal fold flap (**b**) Gluteal fold flap

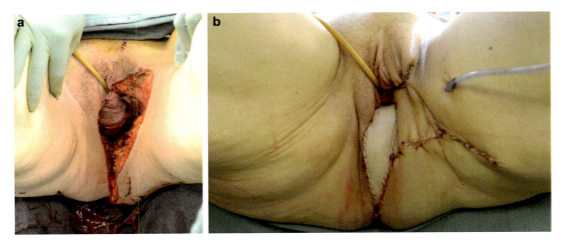

Fig. 12 (**a**) Combination vulvar and perineal defect (**b**) Combination vulvar and perineal defect with two flaps

Postoperative Considerations

While the reconstruction of the female genitourinary and pelvic area is largely a surgical maneuver, postoperative care determines final outcome. Without careful protection of surgical sites and graduated physical activity, reconstructive sites are prone to dehiscence and infection. Even with flap reconstruction, the risk of infection and pelvic abscess approaches 10%, and delayed wound healing may occur in 10–66% of patients [121, 167–170].

Sitting Protocols

After any rotational flap to the pelvis or perineum, it is recommended that sitting is limited for at least 5 days. Dependent pressure from body weight or positioning can cause ischemia and reconstructive flap loss. Furthermore, ischemia and bacterial contamination create a perfect environment for wound infection and dehiscence [171, 172]. Physical therapy is consulted and present postoperative day 1, so that the patient is taught to "log roll" out of bed and avoid shearing on the surgical site. Patients are allowed to ambulate short distances, such as 100 feet, up to 4 times a day, but are not allowed to sit at any time. This includes no sitting for transfers or toileting. As such, a foley catheter is recommended for 5 days to limit urination on the surgical sites and to avoid sitting to urinate. A bedpan may be used for bowel movements if an ostomy is not present. After 5 days, the patient begins a sitting protocol, which includes sitting 5 min four times daily (QID) the first day, 10 min QID the second day, 15 min QID the third day, and advancing as such every day until 1 h is reached. If a patient demonstrates signs of early dehiscence or surgical site strain, this is delayed.

Drains

Surgical drains are left in all surgical sites until less than 20 cc for 2 days in a row. In particular, no drains are removed while the patient is in the early postoperative period, when physical activity and sitting have yet to be fully resumed. The perineal region, secondary to the urogenital and anorectal systems, has been shown to have the highest counts of bacterial contamination in the body [173]. In the pelvic and perineal regions, simple fluid collections will break down suture lines and form abscesses. In areas of dependency, especially those that are previously radiated, seromas will persist up to 3 weeks after surgery. Avoiding wound contamination and/or subsequent infection by urine or stool creates an environment highly susceptible to complication. The use of abundant and reliable drainage is critical.

Lifting and Strenuous Activity

If any abdominal surgery has taken place, patients are advised to avoid lifting anything over 10 pounds for 6 weeks. This prevents undue pressure on the abdominal repair or early ostomy. Some surgeons prefer patients to wear an abdominal binder during this time period, although not required. Light walking or gentle stretching is recommended, but vigorous athletic activity is held until 6 weeks. This helps prevent shear and breakdown in difficult areas such as the perineum.

Vaginal Dilation and Sexual Activity

After reconstruction of the vaginal cavity or perineum, the area is highly prone to stricture. This is exacerbated in patients who have undergone radiation therapy. There is a careful balance between allowing sutures lines to strengthen and heal and starting scar massage and dilation to prevent contracture.

In general, if a patient has healed without complication, a speculum exam is performed at 4 weeks postoperatively. If the speculum exam reveals all sutures lines intact and all tissues viable, then the patient is advised to begin dilation. Medical-grade dilators are available from a variety of companies. In general, they are sized from smallest to largest with increasing length and width. If the speculum passes easily on an adult female, it is usually recommended to start with a mid-range size and advise dilation twice daily with water-based lubricant. The patient is advised to pass the dilator into the cavity three times, gently holding and removing at each pass. At the end of 2 weeks, if there is no tightness and no pain, they then advance to the next size. Once they are able to pass the maximal size dilator, they may resume intercourse. If the patient is not resuming penetrating intercourse at least once a week, then they need to maintain dilation at least three times a week.

Of note, many patients are frightened and scared by dilation. Some will have undergone dilation during radiation therapy and report that it was uncomfortable or painful due to inflamed and ulcerated tissue. It is important to encourage the patient that dilation should not be painful. Gently stretching is normal, but pain is uncommon. If the patient encounters pain, they are advised to downsize the dilator or increase lubrication and massage of the area. Occasional spotting is normal, but frank bleeding is not. Additionally, it is important to communicate to patients that the dilators are a medical-grade device that is part of normal postoperative care. This removes some of the stigma that may be associated with such devices. For improved compliance, it is recommended that they be given to the patient at the time of postoperative visit, rather than via a prescription.

Lastly, it is important to encourage the patient's partner that once the patient has completed dilation therapy, they cannot hurt their partner. Intercourse should be resumed slowly and will not feel completely normal to either the patient or the partner. If there is anxiety or stress regarding this, it is highly recommended that patients and their partners be given sexual counseling referrals [168]. Although a vagina may be anatomically reconstructed, the emotional and physiologic reconstruction is a more complicated process. Ratliff et al. investigated sexual adjustment after vaginal reconstruction with gracilis flaps and found that while 70% of patients were judged to have a physically adequate vagina, less than 50% resumed sexual activity [169]. For patients, the absence of pleasure (37%), vaginal dryness (32%), excess secretions (27%), self-consciousness about ostomies (40%), and body image concerns regarding nudity (30%) were all major issues.

Postoperative Revisions

Despite the goal of performing a "perfect" reconstruction at the time of resection, many patients will require revisions. These revision procedures are discussed preoperatively so they are expected by the patient.

The most common indication for revision is a sense of "bulkiness" in the perineum or vaginal area. If a patient has a thicker flap, the subcutaneous tissue may be thinned either directly or by liposuction. In the absence of redundant skin, liposuction is recommended as it reduces the subcutaneous fat, while preserving healthy skin. In general, the skin will contract once the bulk is removed, and therefore it is advised to be conservative at all times. Liposuction is not recommended until a minimum 6 months postsurgery, as this gives adequate time for neovascularization of the skin from the defect edges.

A second indication for revision is tightness or banding at the introitus. Due to the circular nature

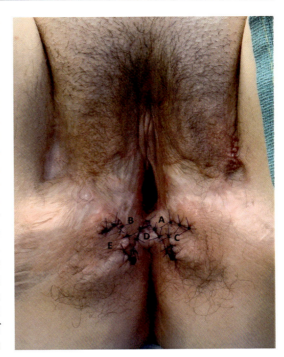

Fig. 13 Jumping man flap

of the area, scars will tend to contract in ring-like fashion, causing a web or tight opening. Using techniques borrowed from burn surgery, local tissue rearrangements are performed to lengthen scar bands and disrupt linear patterns. These local tissue rearrangements, frequently known as "z-plasties," take advantage of geometric principles to lengthen areas using laxity in perpendicular fields. The gain in length of a scar is related to the angles between the central and lateral limbs [174]. One extremely powerful local tissue rearrangement for introital stricture is known as a "jumping man" z-plasty [175, 176]. Variations of this flap combine double opposing z-plasties with a V-Y advancement. It is classically used in concave areas, such as finger web release or release at the medial canthus. See Fig. 13 for demonstration. Other z-plasties may be adopted for contractures across the groin crease or labia. If a patient is highly prone to hypertrophic scarring or keloid formation, judicial use of an intralesional steroid injection may be employed.

Conclusion

Pelvic radiation therapy has the potential for producing severe urinary tract and pelvic floor dysfunction in female patients. Understanding the nature of radiation therapy, the diversity of radiotherapeutic modalities, and radiation-induced genitourinary toxicity and developing an approach to the evaluation and management in these patients are essential. Numerous options for reconstruction are available depending on the severity and nature of the urinary tract and pelvic floor complications. Multidisciplinary co-management is often required, and a collaborative approach to surgical reconstruction allows for efficiency in care, improving outcomes, and minimizing patient morbidity and mortality.

Cross-References

▶ Management of Fecal Incontinence, Constipation, and Rectal Prolapse

References

1. Baskar R, Lee KA, Yeo R, Yeoh KW. Cancer and radiation therapy: current advances and future directions. Int J Med Sci. 2012;9(3):193–9.
2. Armes J, Crowe M, Colbourne L, Morgan H, Murrells T, Oakley C, et al. Patients' supportive care needs beyond the end of cancer treatment: a prospective, longitudinal survey. J Clin Oncol. 2009;27(36):6172–9.
3. Zeiderman MR, Nuno M, Sahar DE, Farkas LM. Trends in flap reconstruction of pelvic oncologic defects: analysis of the national inpatient sample. J Plast Reconstr Aesthet Surg. 2021;74:2085–94.
4. Chessin DB, Hartley J, Cohen AM, et al. Rectus flap reconstruction decreases perineal wound complications after pelvic chemoradiation and surgery: a cohort study. Ann Surg Oncol. 2005;12:104–10.
5. Shibata D, Hyland W, Busse P, et al. Immediate reconstruction of the perineal wound with gracilis muscle flaps following abdominoperineal resection and intraoperative radiation therapy for recurrent carcinoma of the rectum. Ann Surg Oncol. 1999;6:33–7.
6. Khoo AK, Skibber JM, Nabawi AS, et al. Indications for immediate tissue transfer for soft tissue reconstruction in visceral pelvic surgery. Surgery. 2001;130:463–9.
7. Buchel EW, Finical S, Johnson C. Pelvic reconstruction using vertical rectus abdominis musculocutaneous flaps. Ann Plast Surg. 2004;52:22–6.
8. Siegel RL, Miller KD, Fuchs HE, Jemal A. Cancer statistics, 2021. CA Cancer J Clin. 2021;71(1):7–33.
9. Bryant AK, Banegas MP, Martinez ME, Mell LK, Murphy JD. Trends in radiation therapy among cancer survivors in the United States, 2000–2030. Cancer Epidemiol Biomark Prev. 2017;26:963–70.
10. Viswanathan A. Uterine cervix. In: Halperin E, Wazer D, Perez C, Brady L, editors. Perez and Brady's principles and practice of radiation oncology. 6th ed. Lippincott, Williams and Wilkins: Philadelphia; 2013. p. 1355–446.
11. Huh JW, Tanksley J, Chino J, Willett CG, Dewhirst MW. Long-term consequences of pelvic irradiation: toxicities, challenges, and therapeutic opportunities with pharmacologic mitigators. Clin Cancer Res. 2020;26(13):3079–90.
12. Yeung AR, Pugh SL, Klopp AH, et al. Improvement in patient-reported outcomes with intensity-modulated radiotherapy (RT) compared with standard RT: a report from the NRG oncology RTOG 1203 study. J Clin Oncol. 2020;38(15):1685–92.
13. Morris KA, Haboubi NY. Pelvic radiation therapy: between delight and disaster. World J Gastrointest Surg. 2015;7(11):279–88.
14. Jensen PT, Froeding LP. Pelvic radiotherapy and sexual function in women. Transl Androl Urol. 2015;4(2):186–205.
15. Kimura H, Wu NZ, Dodge R, Klitzman BM, McIntyre TM, Dewhirst MW. Inhibition of radiation-induced up-regulation of leukocyte adhesion to endothelial cells with the platelet-activating factor inhibitor, BN52021. Int J Radiat Oncol Biol Phys. 1995;33:627–33.
16. Straub JM, New J, Hamilton CD, Lominska C, Shnayder Y, Thomas SM. Radiation-induced fibrosis: mechanisms and implications for therapy. J Cancer Res Clin Oncol. 2015;141(11):1985–94.
17. Mancini ML, Sonis ST. Mechanisms of cellular fibrosis associated with cancer regimen-related toxicities. Front Pharmacol. 2014;5:51.
18. Dewhirst MW, Cao Y, Moeller B. Cycling hypoxia and free radicals regulate angiogenesis and radiotherapy response. Nat Rev Cancer. 2008;8:425–37.
19. Viswanathan AN, Yorke ED, Marks LB, Eifel PJ, Shipley WU. Radiation dose-volume effects of the urinary bladder. Int J Radiat Oncol Biol Phys. 2010;76:S116–22.
20. Peterson CM, Menias CO, Katz DS. Radiation-induced effects to nontarget abdominal and pelvic viscera. Radiol Clin N Am. 2014;52(5):1041–53.
21. Pattanshetty R, Rao MS. Cancer related fibrosis: prevention or treatment? A descriptive review. Clin Oncol. 2021;6:1835.
22. Cox JD, Stetz J, Pajak TF. Toxicity criteria of the Radiation Therapy Oncology Group (RTOG) and

22. the European Organization for Research and Treatment of Cancer (EORTC). Int J Radiat Oncol Biol Phys. 1995;31(5):1341–6.
23. Nicholas S, Chen L, Choflet A, Fader A, Guss Z, Hazell S, et al. Pelvic radiation and normal tissue toxicity. Semin Radiat Oncol. 2017;27(4):358–69.
24. Parkin DE, Davis JA, Symonds RP. Long-term bladder symptomatology following radiotherapy for cervical carcinoma. Radiother Oncol. 1987;9(3):195–9.
25. Nout RA, Putter H, Jurgenliemk-Schulz IM, et al. Five-year quality of life of endometrial cancer patients treated in the randomized Post-Operative Radiation Therapy in Endometrial Cancer (PORTEC-2) trial and comparison with norm data. Eur J Cancer. 2012;48:1638–48.
26. Smit SG, Heyns CF. Management of radiation cystitis. Nat Rev Urol. 2010;7(4):206–14.
27. Levenback C, Eifel PJ, Burke TW, et al. Hemorrhagic cystitis following radiotherapy for stage Ib cancer of the cervix. Gynecol Oncol. 1994;55(2):206–10.
28. Chorbinska J, Krajewski W, Zdrojowy R. Urological complications after radiation therapy – nothing ventured, nothing gained: a narrative review. Transl Cancer Res. 2021;10(2):1096.
29. Angioli R, Penalver M, Muzii L, et al. Guidelines of how to manage vesicovaginal fistula. Crit Rev Oncol Hematol. 2003;48(3):295–304.
30. Zoubek J, McGuire EJ, Noll F, et al. The late occurrence of urinary tract damage in patients successfully treated by radiotherapy for cervical carcinoma. J Urol. 1989;141:1347–9.
31. Moore KN, Gold MA, McMeekin DS, Zorn KK. Vesicovaginal fistula formation in patients with stage IVA cervical carcinoma. Gynecol Oncol. 2007;106(3):498–501.
32. Narayanan P, Nobbenhuis M, Reynolds KM, et al. Fistulas in malignant gynecologic disease: etiology, imaging, and management. Radiographics. 2009;29(4):1073–83.
33. Feddock J, Randall M, Kudrimoti M, et al. Impact of post-radiation biopsies on development of fistulae in patients with cervical cancer. Gynecol Oncol. 2014;133(2):263–7.
34. Liberman D, Mehus B, Elliott SP. Urinary adverse effects of pelvic radiotherapy. Transl Androl Urol. 2014;3(2):186–95.
35. Gellrich J, Hakenberg OW, Oehlschläger S, et al. Manifestation, latency and management of late urological complications after curative radiotherapy for cervical carcinoma. Onkologie. 2003;26:334–40.
36. Suzuki K, Devine RM, Dozois RR, et al. Intraoperative irradiation after palliative surgery for locally recurrent rectal cancer. Cancer. 1995;75:939–52.
37. Gunderson LL, Nelson H, Martenson JA, et al. Intraoperative electron and external beam irradiation with or without 5-fluorouracil and maximum surgical resection for previously unirradiated, locally recurrent colorectal cancer. Dis Colon Rectum. 1996;39:1379–95.
38. Pötter R, Tanderup K, Schmid MP, et al. EMBRACE Collaborative Group. MRI-guided adaptive brachytherapy in locally advanced cervical cancer (EMBRACE-I): a multicentre prospective cohort study. Lancet Oncol. 2021;22(4):538–47.
39. Srikanth P, Kay HE, Tijerina AN, et al. Narrative review of the current management of radiation-induced ureteral strictures of the pelvis. AME Med J. 2021;1–17. https://doi.org/10.21037/amj-21-5
40. Meirow D, Nugent D. The effects of radiotherapy and chemotherapy on female reproduction. Hum Reprod Update. 2001;7(6):535–43.
41. Wallace WH, Thomson AB, Saran F, et al. Predicting age of ovarian failure after radiation to a field that includes the ovaries. Int J Radiat Oncol Biol Phys. 2005;62(3):738–44.
42. Viswanathan AN, Lee LJ, Eswara JR, et al. Complications of pelvic radiation in patients treated for gynecologic malignancies. Cancer. 2014;120(24):3870–83.
43. Denton AS, Maher EJ. Interventions for the physical aspects of sexual dysfunction in women following pelvic radiotherapy. Cochrane Database Syst Rev. 2003;(1):CD003750.
44. Nunns D, Williamson K, Swaney L, et al. The morbidity of surgery and adjuvant radiotherapy in the management of endometrial carcinoma. Int J Gynecol Cancer. 2000;10(3):233–8.
45. Dracham CB, Shankar A, Madan R. Radiation induced secondary malignancies: a review article. Radiat Oncol J. 2018;36(2):85–94.
46. Creutzberg CL, Nout RA, Lybeert ML, Wárlám-Rodenhuis CC, Jobsen JJ, Mens JW, PORTEC Study Group, et al. Fifteen-year radiotherapy outcomes of the randomized PORTEC-1 trial for endometrial carcinoma. Int J Radiat Oncol Biol Phys. 2011;81(4):e631–8.
47. Parkin DE, Davis JA, Symonds RP. Urodynamic findings following radiotherapy for cervical carcinoma. Br J Urol. 1988;61(3):213–7.
48. Lajer H, Thranov IR, Bagi P, Aage Engelholm S. Evaluation of urologic morbidity after radiotherapy for cervical carcinoma by urodynamic examinations and patient voiding schemes: a prospective study. Int J Radiat Oncol Biol Phys. 2002;54(5):1362–8.
49. Desmouliere A. Factors influencing myofibroblast differentiation during wound healing and fibrosis. Cell Biol Int. 1995;19:471–6.
50. Gabbiani G. Modulation of fibroblastic cytoskeletal features during wound healing and fibrosis. Pathol Res Pract. 1994;190:851–3.
51. Desmouliere A, Gabbiani G. Modulation of fibroblastic cytoskeletal features during pathologic situations: the role of extracellular matrix and cytokines. Cell Motil Cytoskeleton. 1994;29:195–203.
52. Martin M, Lefaix J, Delanian S. TGF-beta1 and radiation fibrosis: a master switch and a specific therapeutic target? Int J Radiat Oncol Biol Phys. 2000;47:277–90.

53. Malkinson FD, Keane JT. Radiobiology of the skin: review of some effects on epidermis and hair. J Invest Dermatol. 1981;77:133–8.
54. Thanik VD, Chang CC, Zoumalan RA, et al. A novel mouse model of cutaneous radiation injury. Plast Reconstr Surg. 2011;127:560–8.
55. Jakowatz JG, Porudominksy D, Riihimaki DU, et al. Complications of pelvic exenteration. Arch Surg. 1985;120:1261–5.
56. Chang DW, Reece GP, Wang B, et al. Effect of smoking on complications in patients undergoing free TRAM flap breast reconstruction. Plast Reconstr Surg. 2000;105(7):2374–80.
57. Van den Berghe G, Wouters P, Weekers F, et al. Intensive insulin therapy in critically ill patients. N Engl J Med. 2001;345(19):1359–66.
58. Mangano DT, Browner WS, Hollenberg M, Tarco IM. Long-term cardiac prognosis following non-cardiac surgery. JAMA. 1992;268:233–9.
59. Mangano DT, Layug EL, Wallace A, Tateo I. Effect of atenolol on mortality and cardiovascular morbidity after noncardiac surgery. N Engl J Med. 1996;335(23):1713–20.
60. Manilich E, Vogel JD, Kiran RP, et al. Key factors associated with postoperative complications in patients undergoing colorectal surgery. Dis Colon Rectum. 2013;56:64–71.
61. Wick EC, Hirose K, Shore AD, et al. Surgical site infections and cost in obese patients undergoing colorectal surgery. Arch Surg. 2011;146:1068–72.
62. Giordano SA, Garvey PB, Baumann DP, et al. The impact of body mass index on abdominal wall reconstruction outcomes: a comparative study. Plast Reconstr Surg. 2017;139:1234.
63. Tsereteli Z, Pryor BA, Heniford BT, et al. Laparoscopic ventral hernia repair (LVHR) in morbidly obese patients. Hernia. 2008;12:233–8.
64. Desai KA, Razavi SA, Hart AM, Thompson PW, Losken A. The effect of BMI on outcomes following complex abdominal wall reconstructions. Ann Plast Surg. 2016;76:S295–7.
65. Panici PB, Cutillo G, Angioli R. Modulation of surgery in early invasive cervical cancer. Crit Rev Oncol Hematol. 2003;48:263–70.
66. Chuang YC, Kim DK, Chiang PH, Chancellor MB. Bladder botulinum toxin a injection can benefit patients with radiation and chemical cystitis. BJU Int. 2008;102(6):704–6.
67. Keegan KA, Nanigian DK, Stone AR. Female urethral stricture disease. Curr Urol Rep. 2008;9(5):419–23.
68. Shin JY, Yoon SM, Choi HJ, Lee SN, Kim HB, Joo WC, et al. A case of post-radiotherapy urethral stricture with spontaneous bladder rupture, mimicking obstructive uropathy due to cancer metastasis. Electrolyte Blood Press. 2014;12(1):26–9.
69. Gupta P, Kalra S, Dorairajan LN, Manikandan R, Ks S, Jagannath A. Dorsal onlay buccal mucosal graft urethroplasty in post radiation female urethral stricture – a technical appraisal with outcomes. Urology. 2021;S0090-4295(21):00537–9.
70. Kobashi KC, Albo ME, Dmochowski RR, et al. Surgical treatment of female stress urinary incontinence: AUA/SUFU guideline. J Urol. 2017;198(4):875–83.
71. Peyronnet B, O'Connor E, Khavari R, et al. AMS-800 artificial urinary sphincter in female patients with stress urinary incontinence: a systematic review. Neurourol Urodyn. 2019;38(Suppl 4):S28–41.
72. Thomas K, Venn SN, Mundy AR. Outcome of the artificial urinary sphincter in female patients. J Urol. 2002;167(4):1720–2.
73. Peyronnet B, Greenwell T, Gray G, et al. Current use of the artificial urinary sphincter in adult females. Curr Urol Rep. 2020;21(12):53.
74. Hansen MH, Hayn M, Murray P. The use of bowel in urologic reconstructive surgery. Surg Clin North Am. 2016;96(3):567–82.
75. Ahlstrand C, Herder A. Primary adenocarcinoma of distal ileum used as outlet from a right colonic urinary reservoir. Scand J Urol Nephrol. 1998;32(1):70–2.
76. Parekh DJ, Donat SM. Urinary diversion: options, patient selection, and outcomes. Semin Oncol. 2007;34(2):98–109.
77. Tran THT, Melamed J, Deng FM. Gastric adenocarcinoma arising in gastrocystoplasty. Urology. 2021;148:270–3.
78. Chang SS, Alberts GL, Smith JA Jr, Cookson MS. Ileal conduit urinary diversion in patients with previous history of abdominal/pelvic irradiation. World J Urol. 2004;22(4):272–6.
79. Westney OL. The neurogenic bladder and incontinent urinary diversion. Urol Clin North Am. 2010;37(4):581–92.
80. Hellenthal NJ, Short SS, O'Connor RC, Eandi JA, Yap SA, Stone AR. Incontinent ileovesicostomy: long-term outcomes and complications. Neurourol Urodyn. 2009;28(6):483–6.
81. Tan HJ, Stoffel J, Daignault S, McGuire EJ, Latini JM. Ileovesicostomy for adults with neurogenic bladders: complications and potential risk factors for adverse outcomes. Neurourol Urodyn. 2008;27(3):238–43.
82. Levy ME, Elliott SP. Reconstructive techniques for creation of catheterizable channels: tunneled and nipple valve channels. Transl Androl Urol. 2016;5(1):136–44.
83. Yang WH. Yang needle tunneling technique in creating antireflux and continent mechanisms. J Urol. 1993;150(3):830–4.
84. Monti PR, Lara RC, Dutra MA, de Carvalho JR. New techniques for construction of efferent conduits based on the Mitrofanoff principle. Urology. 1997;49(1):112–5.
85. Leslie JA, Dussinger AM, Meldrum KK. Creation of continence mechanisms (Mitrofanoff) without appendix: the Monti and spiral Monti procedures. Urol Oncol. 2007;25(2):148–53.

86. Leslie JA, Cain MP, Kaefer M, Meldrum KK, Dussinger AM, Rink RC, et al. A comparison of the Monti and Casale (spiral Monti) procedures. J Urol. 2007;178(4 Pt 2):1623–7.
87. Pagliara TJ, Gor RA, Liberman D, Myers JB, Luzny P, Stoffel JT, (Neurogenic Bladder Research Group [NBRG]), et al. Outcomes of revision surgery for difficult to catheterize continent channels in a multi-institutional cohort of adults. Can Urol Assoc J. 2018;12(3):E126–31.
88. Kock NG, Nilson AE, Nilsson LO, Norlén LJ, Philipson BM. Urinary diversion via a continent ileal reservoir: clinical results in 12 patients. J Urol. 1982;128(3):469–75.
89. Sutton MA, Hinson JL, Nickell KG, Boone TB. Continent ileocecal augmentation cystoplasty. Spinal Cord. 1998;36(4):246–51.
90. Myers JB, Lenherr SM. Perioperative and long-term surgical complications for the Indiana pouch and similar continent catheterizable urinary diversions. Curr Opin Urol. 2016;26(4):376–82.
91. Redshaw JD, Elliott SP, Rosenstein DI, Erickson BA, Presson AP, Conti SL, et al. Procedures needed to maintain functionality of adult continent catheterizable channels: a comparison of continent cutaneous ileal cecocystoplasty with tunneled catheterizable channels. J Urol. 2014;192(3):821–6.
92. Cheng PJ, Keihani S, Roth JD, Pariser JJ, Elliott SP, Bose S, et al. Contemporary multicenter outcomes of continent cutaneous ileocecocystoplasty in the adult population over a 10-year period: a neurogenic bladder research group study. Neurourol Urodyn. 2020;39(6):1771–80.
93. Lescay HA, Jiang J, Tuma F. Anatomy, abdomen and pelvis, ureter. In: StatPearls [internet]. Treasure Island: StatPearls Publishing; 2021. [Updated 2021 May 8].
94. Burks FN, Santucci RA. Management of iatrogenic ureteral injury. Ther Adv Urol. 2014;6(3):115–24.
95. Iwaszko MR, Krambeck AE, Chow GK, et al. Transureteroureterostomy revisited: Long-term surgical outcomes. J Urol. 2010;183:1055–9.
96. Cowan NG, Banerji JS, Johnston RB, Duty BD, Bakken B, Hedges JC, et al. Renal autotransplantation: 27-year experience at 2 institutions. J Urol. 2015;194(5):1357–61.
97. Jeong IG, Han KS, Park SH, Song SH, Song G, Park HK, et al. Ileal augmentation cystoplasty combined with Ileal ureter replacement after radical treatment for cervical cancer. Ann Surg Oncol. 2016;23(5):1646–52.
98. Singh J, Smith TG III, Westney OL. Images – urinary tract reconstruction following ureteral coil embolization for ureterovaginal fistula in a young female patient. Can Urol Assoc J. 2022 16(1):E54–E56. https://doi.org/10.5489/cuaj.7223
99. Brunschwig A. Partial or complete pelvic exenteration for extensive irradiation necrosis of pelvic viscera in the female. Surg Gynecol Obstet. 1951;93(4):431–8.
100. Bricker EM. Bladder substitution after pelvic evisceration. Surg Clin North Am. 1950;30(5):1511–21.
101. Di Saia PJ, Morrow CP. Pelvic exenteration. Calif Med. 1973;118(2):13–7.
102. Grimes WR, Stratton M. Pelvic exenteration. In: StatPearls [internet]. Treasure Island: StatPearls Publishing; 2021. 2021 May 4.
103. Barber HR. Pelvic exenteration. Cancer Investig. 1987;5(4):331–8.
104. Höckel M, Dornhöfer N. Pelvic exenteration for gynaecological tumours: achievements and unanswered questions. Lancet Oncol. 2006;7(10):837–47.
105. Lee DJ, Tyson MD, Chang SS. Conduit urinary diversion. Urol Clin North Am. 2018;45(1):25–36.
106. Chiva LM, Lapuente F, Núñez C, Ramírez PT. Ileal orthotopic neobladder after pelvic exenteration for cervical cancer. Gynecol Oncol. 2009;113(1):47–51.
107. Hautmann RE, de Petriconi R, Volkmer BG. Neobladder formation after pelvic irradiation. World J Urol. 2009;27(1):57–62.
108. Bernard S, Ouellet MP, Moffet H, Roy JS, Dumoulin C. Effects of radiation therapy on the structure and function of the pelvic floor muscles of patients with cancer in the pelvic area: a systematic review. J Cancer Surviv. 2016;10(2):351–62.
109. Mannel RS, Braly PS, Buller RE. Indiana pouch continent urinary reservoir in patients with previous pelvic irradiation. Obstet Gynecol. 1990;75(5):891–3.
110. Bladou F, Houvenaeghel G, Delpéro JR, Guérinel G. Incidence and management of major urinary complications after pelvic exenteration for gynecological malignancies. J Surg Oncol. 1995;58(2):91–6.
111. Reed P, Osborne LA. Factors related to patient choice of bladder reconstruction following radical cystectomy. J Clin Urol. 2019;12(6):449–54.
112. Smith D, Albersheim J, Moses R, O'Dell D, Stoffel J, Myers J, et al. Outcomes of urinary diversion for late adverse effects of Gynecologic radiotherapy. Urology. 2020;144:214–9.
113. Golimbu M, Morales P. Jejunal conduits: technique and complications. J Urol. 1975 Jun;113(6):787–95.
114. Beckley S, Wajsman Z, Pontes JE, Murphy G. Transverse colon conduit: a method of urinary diversion after pelvic irradiation. J Urol. 1982;128(3):464–8.
115. Dahl DM. Use of intestinal segments in urinary diversion. In: Wein AJ, Kavoussi LR, Novick AC, Partin AW, Peters CA, editors. Campbell-Walsh urology. Philadelphia: Saunders Elsevier; 2015. p. 2281.
116. Varkarakis IM, Chrisofos M, Antoniou N, Papatsoris A, Deliveliotis C. Evaluation of findings during re-exploration for obstructive ileus after radical cystectomy and ileal-loop urinary diversion: insight into potential technical improvements. BJU Int. 2007;99(4):893–7.

117. Schmidt JD, Buchsbaum HJ. Transverse colon conduit diversion. Urol Clin North Am. 1986;13(2):233–9.
118. Ravi R, Dewan AK, Pandey KK. Transverse colon conduit urinary diversion in patients treated with very high dose pelvic irradiation. Br J Urol. 1994;73(1):51–4.
119. Breuing K, Butler CE, Ferzoco S, Ventral Hernia Working Group (VHWG), et al. Incisional ventral hernias: review of the literature and recommendations regarding the grading and technique of repair. Surgery. 2010;148:544–8.
120. Millennium Research Group. US markets for soft tissue repair 2009. Toronto: Millennium Research Group, Inc; 2008.
121. de Vries Reilingh TS, van Goor H, Charbon JA, et al. Repair of giant midline abdominal wall hernias: "components separation technique" versus prosthetic repair: interim analysis of a randomized controlled trial. World J Surg. 2007;31:756–63.
122. Paton BL, Novitsky YW, Zerey M, et al. Management of infections of polytetrafluoroethylene-based mesh. Surg Infect. 2007;8:337–41.
123. Kim H, Bruen K, Vargo D. Acellular dermal matrix in the management of high-risk abdominal wall defects. Am J Surg. 2006;192:705–9.
124. Patton JH Jr, Berry S, Kralovich KA. Use of human acellular dermal matrix in complex and contaminated abdominal wall reconstructions. Am J Surg. 2007;193:360–3.
125. Helton WS, Fisichella PM, Berger R, et al. Short-term outcomes with small intestinal submucosa for ventral abdominal hernia. Arch Surg. 2005;140:549–60.
126. Maurice SM, Skeete DA. Use of human acellular dermal matrix for abdominal wall reconstruction. Am J Surg. 2009;197:35–42.
127. Diaz JJ Jr, Conquest AM, Ferzoco SJ, et al. Multi-institutional experience using human acellular dermal matrix for ventral hernia repair in compromised surgical field. Arch Surg. 2009;144:209–15.
128. Losanoff JE, Richman BW, Jones JW. Enterocolocutaneous fistula: a late consequence of polypropylene mesh abdominal wall repair. Hernia. 2002;6:144–7.
129. Mericli AF, Baumann DP, Butler CE. Reconstruction of the abdominal wall after oncologic resection: defect classification and management strategies. Plast Reconstr Surg. 2018;142:187S.
130. Harth KC, Broome AM, Jacobs MR, et al. Bacterial clearance of biologic grafts used in hernia repair: an experimental study. Surg Endosc. 2011;25:2224–9.
131. Butler CE, Prieto VG. Reduction of adhesions with composite Alloderm/polypropylene mesh implants for abdominal wall reconstruction. Plast Reconstr Surg. 2004;114:464–73.
132. Klinge U, Conze J, Krones CJ, Schumpelick V. Incisional hernia: open techniques. World J Surg. 2005;29:1066–72.
133. Schumpelick V, Klinge U, Junge K, Stumpf M. Incisional abdominal hernia: the open mesh repair. Langenbeck's Arch Surg. 2004;389:1–5.
134. Stone HH, Fabian TC, Turkleson ML, et al. Management of acute full-thickness losses of the abdominal wall. Ann Surg. 1981;193:612–8.
135. Ramirez OM, Ruas E, Dellon AL. "Components separation" method for closure of abdominal wall defects: an anatomic and clinical study. Plast Reconstr Surg. 1990;86:519–26.
136. de Vries Reilingh TS, van Goor H, Rosman C, et al. "Components separation technique" for repair of large abdominal wall hernias. J Am Coll Surg. 2003;196:32–7.
137. DiBello JN Jr, Moore JH Jr. Sliding myofascial flap of the rectus abdominis muscles for the closure of recurrent ventral hernias. Plast Reconstr Surg. 1996;98:464–9.
138. Levine JP, Karp NS. Restoration of abdominal wall integrity as a salvage procedure in difficult recurrent abdominal wall hernias using a method of wide myofascial release. Plast Reconstr Surg. 2001;107:707–16.
139. Espinosa de los Monteros A, de la Torre JI, Marrero I, et al. Utilization of human cadaveric acellular dermis for abdominal hernia reconstruction. Ann Plast Surg. 2007;58:264–7.
140. Jin J, Rosen MJ, Blatnik J, et al. Use of acellular dermal matrix for complicated ventral hernia repair: does technique affect outcome? J Am Coll Surg. 2007;205:654–60.
141. Butler CE, Langstein HN, Kronowitz SJ. Pelvic, abdominal, and chest wall reconstruction with AlloDerm in patients at increased risk for mesh-related complications. Plast Reconstr Surg. 2005;116:1263–75.
142. Matros E, Disa JJ. Uncommon flaps for chest wall reconstruction. Semin Plast Surg. 2011;25:55–9.
143. Mathes SJ, Nahai F. Reconstructive surgery: principles, anatomy, and technique. 1st ed. New York: Churchill Livingstone; 1997.
144. Momoh AO, Kamat AM, Butler CE. Reconstruction of the pelvic floor with human acellular dermal matrix and omental flap following anterior pelvic exenteration. J Plast Reconstr Aesthet Surg. 2010;63:2185–7.
145. Mazzaferro D, Song P, Massand S, et al. The omental free flap – a review of usage and physiology. J Reconstr Microsurg. 2018;34:151–69.
146. Chaudhry A, Oliver JD, Vyas KS, et al. Comparison of outcomes in oncoplastic pelvic reconstruction with VRAM versus omental flaps: a large cohort analysis. J Reconstr Microsurg. 2019;35:425–9
147. Van Vliet A, Girardot A, Bouchez J, et al. How big is too big? The effect of defect size on postoperative complications of vertical rectus abdominis flap reconstruction. Ann Plast Surg. 2021;86:S571–4.
148. Asaad M, Pisters L, Klein GT, et al. Robotic rectus abdominis muscle flap following robotic extirpative surgery. Plast Reconstr Surg. 2021;148:1377.

149. Ibrahim AE, Sarhane KA, Pederson JC, Selber JC. Robotic harvest of the rectus abdominis muscle: principles and clinical applications. Semin Plast Surg. 2014;28:26–31.
150. Pedersen J, Song DH, Selber JC. Robotic, intraperitoneal harvest of the rectus abdominis muscle. Plast Reconstr Surg. 2014;134:1057–63.
151. Pusic AL, Mehrara BJ. Vaginal reconstruction: an algorithm approach to defect classification and flap reconstruction. J Surg Onc. 2006;94:515–21.
152. Cordeiro PG, Pusic AL, Disa JJ. A classification system and reconstructive algorithm for acquired vaginal defects. Plast Reconstr Surg. 2002;110:1058–65.
153. Bell SW, Dehni N, Chaouat M, et al. Primary rectus abdominis myocutaneous flap for repair of perineal and vaginal defects after extended abdominoperineal resection. Br J Surg. 2005;92:482–6.
154. D'Souza DN, Pera M, Nelson H, et al. Vaginal reconstruction following resection of primary locally advanced and recurrent colorectal malignancies. Arch Surg. 2003;138:1340–3.
155. Woods JE, Alter G, Meland B, et al. Experience with vaginal reconstruction utilizing the modified Singapore flap. Plast Reconstr Surg. 1992;90:270–4.
156. Weichman KE, Matros E, Disa JJ. Reconstruction of peripelvic oncologic defects. Plast Reconstr Surg. 2017;140:601e.
157. Mericli AF, Martin JP, Campbell CA. An algorithmic anatomical subunit approach to pelvic wound reconstruction. Plast Reconstr Surg. 2016;137:1004–17.
158. Tan BK, Kang GC, Tay EH, Por YC. Subunit principle of vulvar reconstruction: algorithm and outcomes. Arch Plast Surg. 2014.41:379–86.
159. John HE, Jessop ZM, Di Candia M, et al. An algorithmic approach to perineal reconstruction after cancer resection: experience from two international centers. Ann Plast Surg. 2013;71:96–102.
160. Salgarello M, Farallo E, Barone-Adesi L, et al. Flap algorithm in vulvar reconstruction after radical, extensive vulvectomy. Ann Plast Surg. 2005;54:184–90.
161. Gravannis AI, Tsoutsos DA, Karakitsos D, et al. Application of the pedicled anterolateral thigh flap to defects from the pelvis to knee. Microsurgery. 2006;26:432–8.
162. Zeng A, Qiao Q, Zhao R, Song K, Long X. Anterolateral thigh flap-based reconstruction for oncologic vulvar defects. Plast Reconstr Surg. 2011;127:1939–45.
163. Sawada M, Kimata Y, Kasamatsu T, et al. Versatile lotus petal flap for vulvoperineal reconstruction after gynecologic ablative surgery. Gynecol Oncol. 2004;95:330–5.
164. Yii NW, Niranjan NS. Lotus petal flaps in vulvo-vaginal reconstruction. Br J Plast Surg. 1996;49:547–54.
165. Hashimoto I, Murakami G, Nakanishi H, et al. First cutaneous branch of the internal pudendal artery: an anatomical basis for the so-called gluteal fold flap. Okajimas Folia Anat Jpn. 2001;78:23–30.
166. Hashimoto I, Nakanishi H, Nagae H, Harada H, Sedo H. The gluteal-fold flap for vulvar and buttock reconstruction: anatomic study and adjustment of flap volume. Plast Reconstr Surg. 2001;108:1998–2005.
167. de Haas WG, Miller MJ, Temple WJ, et al. Perineal wound closure with rectus abdominis musculocutaneous flap after tumor ablation. Ann Surg Oncol. 1995;2:400–6.
168. Small T, Friedman DJ, Sultan M. Reconstructive surgery of the pelvis after surgery for rectal cancer. Semin Surg Oncol. 2000;18:259–64.
169. Ratliff CR, Gershenson DM, Morris M, et al. Sexual adjustment of patients undergoing gracilis myocutaneous flap vaginal reconstruction in conjunction with pelvic exenteration. Cancer. 1996;78:2229–35.
170. Gleeson NC, Baile W, Roberts WS, et al. Pudendal thigh fasciocutaneous flaps for vaginal reconstruction in gynecologic oncology. Gynecol Oncol. 1994;54:269–74.
171. Larson EL, McGinley KJ, Foglia AR, Talbot GH, Leyden JJ. Composition and antimicrobic resistance of skin flora in hospitalized and healthy adults. J Clin Microbiol. 1986;23:604–8.
172. Robson MC, Heggers JP. Surgical infection: II. The beta-hemolytic streptococcus. J Surg Res. 1969;9:289–92.
173. Guarner F, Malagelada JR. Gut flora in health and disease. Lancet. 2003;361:512–9.
174. Rohrich RJ, Zbar PI. A simplified algorithm for the use of Z-plasty. Plast Reconstr Surg. 1999;103:1513.
175. Hirshowitz B, Karev A, Rousso M. Combined double z-plasty and Y-V advancement for thumb web contracture. Hand. 1975;7:291–3.
176. Mustarde JC. Epicanthus and telecanthus. Br J Plast Surg. 1963;16:346–56.

Use and Complications of Neobladder and Continent Urinary Diversion in Female Pelvic Cancer

59

Bastian Amend, Kathrin Meisterhofer, Jens Bedke, and Arnulf Stenzl

Contents

Introduction	1100
Indications and Forms of Female Cystectomy	1101
Specific Surgical Aspects of the Ablative Part Related to an Orthotopic or Heterotopic Urinary Diversion	1102
Patient Selection for Continent Urinary Diversion	1105
Preoperative Patient Preparation	1106
Important Intraoperative Surgical Steps	1106
General Aspects of Reservoirs	1106
Orthotopic Neobladder	1107
Continent Cutaneous Reservoir	1108
Types of Orthotopic Neobladders	1108
Studer Neobladder	1109
I-Pouch	1109
Hautmann Neobladder	1110
Kock Ileal Neobladder	1110
T-Pouch	1110
Pouch of Abol-Enein and Ghoneim	1111
Padua Ileal Neobladder	1111
Types of Heterotopic Continent Urinary Diversions	1111
Mainz I Pouch: Mixed Augmentation Ileum and Cecum	1112
Ileal Heterotopic Continent Cutaneous Pouches	1113
Specific Aspects of Robot-Assisted Surgery	1115
Immediate Postoperative Patient Care	1116

B. Amend · K. Meisterhofer · J. Bedke · A. Stenzl (✉)
Department of Urology, University Hospital of Tuebingen;
Eberhard Karls University, Tuebingen, Germany
e-mail: bastian.amend@med.uni-tuebingen.de;
kathrin.meisterhofer@med.uni-tuebingen.de;
jens.bedke@med.uni-tuebingen.de;
arnulf.stenzl@med.uni-tuebingen.de

© Springer Nature Switzerland AG 2023
F. E. Martins et al. (eds.), *Female Genitourinary and Pelvic Floor Reconstruction*,
https://doi.org/10.1007/978-3-031-19598-3_60

Early Risks of Continent Urinary Diversions 1118

Long-Term Risks of Continent Urinary Diversions 1118
General Long-Term Risks after Continent Urinary Diversion 1118
Orthotopic Neobladder 1119
Continent Cutaneous Reservoirs 1119

Outcome 1120
Outcome of Orthotopic Neobladders 1120
Outcome of Continent Cutaneous Reservoirs 1121

Recommendations for Follow-Up 1122

Conclusion 1123

References 1123

Abstract

Cancer of the female pelvis originates from organs of the three different pelvic compartments. The lower urinary tract is often also affected by the malignancy. Cystectomy is therefore part of treatment, especially in patients with extensive disease. Preservation of the urethra and the urethral sphincter complex is crucial for orthotopic neobladder placement. Various patient factors and disease-specific factors might lead to the decision of a heterotopic urinary diversion, either continent or incontinent. The current literature supports the use of orthotopic neobladders in female patients based on the oncological and functional outcomes. Over time, many different forms of neobladders have been described and modified by surgeons. To date, the use of the ileum is the most commonly accepted approach. If a patient is not eligible to receive an orthotopic urinary diversion, a continent cutaneous heterotopic reservoir is a useful option, to avoid an incontinent diversion and its negative effects on body image. Heterotopic pouches need regular catheterization by the patient and have a higher complication rate compared to other diversions. Furthermore, there are fewer and fewer centers that have surgical knowledge of the construction and the postoperative care of heterotopic pouches, including management of complications. This chapter reviews the indications for and different forms of urinary diversions, the surgical aspects of the ablative and reconstructive part of the surgery, and the complications and their management in female pelvic cancer patients.

Keywords

Lower urinary tract · Cystectomy · Orthotopic neobladder · Continent cutaneous urinary diversion · Nerve sparing · Rhabdosphincter · Urinary incontinence · Intermittent catheterization · Acid-base balance · Nutritional deficit

Introduction

Female pelvic cancer originates from various organs that are situated in the three pelvic compartments. The anterior compartment includes the urinary bladder, the urethra, and the urethral sphincter complex. Urothelial cancer of the urinary bladder is the most common cause of cancer in the anterior pelvis. The middle compartment consists of the vagina, the uterus, and the inner genitalia. Cervical cancer and ovarian cancer are the most common diseases affecting this anatomical region. The natural orifices of the anterior and middle compartments are part of the vulva and can be involved in infrequent cancers arising from the urethra, the vagina, or the vulva itself. Finally, the posterior compartment comprises the rectum and sphincter muscles. Therefore, rectal cancer, in contrast to anal cancer, is the most common malignant disease of the posterior female pelvis.

The selection of oncological treatment among surgery, radiotherapy, chemotherapy, or combinations of these options is mainly dependent on the origin and cell type of cancer. A multidisciplinary approach is essential for the patient to reach the goal of long-term survival and quality of life, especially in cases of extensive tumor growth that crosses the borders of different compartments. After the accurate diagnosis and staging of the disease, it is imperative to have a tumor board discussion to develop an interdisciplinary therapy plan.

From the urological point of view, the first question is whether we can spare major parts of the urinary bladder, with or without augmentation strategies and possible reimplantation of the ureters, or whether a complete removal of the urinary bladder is necessary. This decision is directly influenced by the extent of the tumor, the rules of oncological treatment, and patient-specific factors. For example, in muscle-invasive urothelial cancer of the urinary bladder, partial cystectomy is not the recommended treatment and should be limited to very selected subset of patients [1]. On the other hand, bladder sparing or orthotopic urinary diversion would not make sense in female patients suffering from treatment-resistant stress urinary incontinence, given considerations of postoperative quality of life.

If the urinary bladder will be removed, the question of urinary diversion arises. The various diversions are classified into orthotopic or heterotopic procedures. The latter are subdivided into continent and incontinent urinary diversion. For several decades, the use of orthotopic neobladder placement was neglected in female patients, and the use of an incontinent urinary diversion, such as an ileal conduit or a ureterocutaneostomy, was the most common. In younger patients, the use of a rectal urinary diversion or a catheterizable continent cutaneous reservoir was a useful option arising from new surgical techniques. In the early 1990s, the use of an orthotopic ileal neobladder became more and more accepted as a reasonable option for female patients with bladder cancer [2]. The initial concerns of tumor recurrence and urinary incontinence due to a compromised urethral sphincter have been overcome by increasing evidence of oncological and functional outcomes comparable to those of other diversions [3, 4]. Increased knowledge of female pelvic floor anatomy has also made an essential contribution to the breakthrough of orthotopic neobladders. In particular, findings on the profile and the localization of the U-shaped female urinary rhabdosphincter as well as the pelvic routes of relevant autonomic nerves have positively influenced the frequency and the results of the orthotopic neobladder procedure [5]. Consequently, increasing attention has been paid to the sexual function and satisfaction of female patients needing ablative pelvic surgery [6]. Increasing rates of orthotopic reservoirs have resulted in declining rates of heterotopic pouches. Accordingly, the number of centers with sufficient experience to offer heterotopic continent urinary diversions has continued to decrease.

This chapter presents the indications for and different forms of urinary diversions, the surgical aspects of the ablative and reconstructive part of the surgery, and the complications and their management in female pelvic cancer patients.

Indications and Forms of Female Cystectomy

The main indication for female cystectomy is still cancer of the urinary bladder, whereby urothelial cancer is the most common form, followed by squamous cell carcinoma. Radical cystectomy is indicated in patients with muscle-invasive bladder cancer (T2-T4a, N0-Nx, M0). Patients with high-risk situations and non-muscle-invasive bladder cancer might also be candidates for radical surgery. This includes patients who are Bacillus Calmette-Guerin (BCG)-refractory, BCG-relapsing, or BCG-unresponsive, as well as patients with a very extensive papillary disease that cannot be managed by endoscopic treatment. The use of a neoadjuvant cisplatin-containing combination chemotherapy has led to an overall survival benefit of 5–8% at 5 years without compromising the feasibility of cystectomy [1]. In these cases, recovery of bone marrow function is necessary, and it is typically present at two or more weeks after the end of the last chemotherapy cycle. The surgical team should expect a challenging cystectomy in patients with recurrence of bladder cancer after primary radio-chemotherapy and also in all other female patients with pelvic cancer and prior irradiation exposure to the urinary bladder.

In patients with bladder cancer, the extent of cystectomy depends on the localization and depth of tumor growth. Figure 1 illustrates different extents of surgical dissection during radical cystectomy. A urethra-sparing radical cystectomy (green line) includes the urinary bladder with bladder neck, the uterus with cervix, and the anterior third of the vaginal wall. In young patients, a genital- and urethra-sparing cystectomy (blue line) can be offered. Both approaches necessitate an absence of tumor at the dissection line below the bladder neck, which can be verified by intraoperative frozen section [1, 6].

In cases of bladder neck involvement or pre-existing stress urinary incontinence, a urethra-sparing technique is contraindicated. Figure 1 marks the surgical borders (red line) of an extended cystectomy including the entire urethra and (in cases of deep vaginal infiltration) major parts of the vaginal tissue.

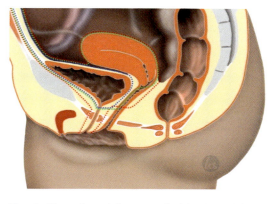

Fig. 1 Illustration of the anatomical borders of female cystectomy: genital- and urethra-sparing cystectomy (blue line), urethra-sparing radical cystectomy (green line), and extended radical cystectomy including the entire urethra, uterus, and major parts of the vagina (red line). (With permission by John Wiley and Sons [6])

Besides bladder cancer, all the female pelvic cancers summarized above can be an indication for an additive cystectomy with subsequent urinary diversion. The extent of this non-urologically indicated cystectomy depends mainly on the level of infiltration of the urinary tract as well as the previous function of the pelvic floor. Patients therefore should be thoroughly informed about the risk of bladder removal and about the various options of urinary diversion including risks and possible complications.

Several patients with gynecological tumors or rectal cancer have been treated with radiotherapy in advance. Patients who had radiotherapy a long time ago (non-neoadjuvant use) need special advising. In these patients, a partial cystectomy has a high risk of tissue necrosis, wound healing problems, or fistula development. Therefore, these patients might also be candidates for cystectomy, even though the extent of the tumor does not already make it necessary.

Besides these oncological indications, there are also benign diseases that can be an indication for bladder removal. These include post-radiogenic cystitis with bleeding, small-capacity bladder, or more rarely, interstitial cystitis.

Specific Surgical Aspects of the Ablative Part Related to an Orthotopic or Heterotopic Urinary Diversion

It is essential that the surgeon who performs the urinary diversion is also responsible for the ablative urological part. Both heterotopic and (even more so) orthotopic urinary diversions require paying attention to specific anatomical structures, to ensure an optimal postoperative outcome. The focus during ablative surgery should also be on autonomic innervation, pelvic floor muscles, bowel handling, and attention to the anterior abdominal wall in cases of heterotopic continent cutaneous pouches. In addition, close preoperative and intraoperative consultation with the anesthesia team is crucial for successful surgery. In particular, restrictive fluid management is needed to avoid increased swelling of the intestinal wall and the mesentery, because this might negatively influence the anastomosis to the urethra or the tightness of intestinal sutures [6].

Preservation of the autonomic nerve fibers is essential for urinary continence and sexual function. Although the external urinary sphincter (rhabdosphincter) is mainly innervated by the pudendal nerve (below the pelvic floor in the Alcock's channel), sympathetic nerves also innervate the proximal urethra. Preservation positively influences the phenomenon of first drop incontinence. Furthermore, parasympathetic and sympathetic nerves also contribute to the innervation of the inner and outer genitalia and contribute to sexual function [6, 7].

Sympathetic fibers originate from the sympathetic trunk (L1, L2) and reach the pelvis bilaterally, from the singular superior hypogastric plexus to the inferior hypogastric plexus. Additional sympathetic fibers (sacral splanchnic nerves) arise directly from the sacral nerves. Figure 2 shows the nerve pathway in front of the common iliac artery, medial to the ureter. These fibers should be respected, especially if a pelvic lymphadenectomy is performed. In this case, all tissue medial to the ureter should be preserved, unless there is an oncological indication for resection.

By contrast, the parasympathetic nerves derive mostly from the sacral nerves and merge to the inferior hypogastric plexus bilaterally through the pelvic splanchnic nerves.

Figure 3 shows the autonomic nerve routes deep in the female pelvis, as a three-dimensional reconstruction from a cadaver study. There are a substantial number of autonomic nerves in the paravaginal tissue, and they reach the bladder neck and the proximal urethra very distally. Therefore, if nerve preservation is intended, keeping the level of paravaginal dissection high and a close preparation to the bladder neck are essential [6–8].

In patients planned for an orthotopic ileal neobladder, preservation of the sphincter complex is imperative. The female urethral sphincter consists of a U-shaped striated muscle component (rhabdosphincter), located in the lower third of the urethra, and a smooth muscle component (lissosphincter), which comprises circular and longitudinal muscle layers [7]. Although one might think that maximum preservation of the bladder neck is crucial, it requires accurate identification of the ideal line of dissection. If the urethra is cut too far, there is a deficit of sphincter tissue with resulting incontinence. In cases of a left bladder neck, the risk of urinary retention increases with the need for catheterization. Figure 4 shows the identification of the optimal dissection below the bladder neck. Palpation of the Foley catheter under careful tension (left figure with projection of the catheter) helps to clearly identify the bladder neck. The urethra is then divided about 0.5 cm below the level of the bladder neck, which ensures preservation of the sphincter muscles (right figure) and avoids urinary retention [6].

As illustrated in Fig. 1, cystectomy might require the (partial) resection of the vagina, depending on the oncological situation. In cases of necessary vaginal resection with a vaginal closure with absorbable sutures, a direct neighborhood between the vaginal closure line and the

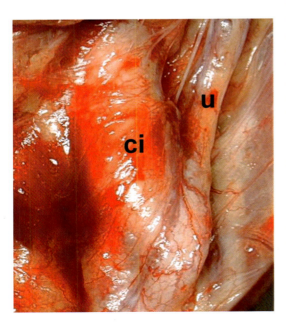

Fig. 2 Photograph of the course of sympathetic autonomic nerves crossing the common iliac artery (ci) medial to the left ureter (u). (With permission by John Wiley and Sons [6])

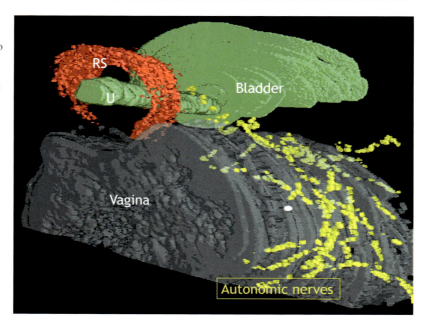

Fig. 3 3D reconstruction of the paravaginal autonomic nerves routing to the bladder neck and the proximal urethra based on histological sections. (With permission of Wolters Kluwer Health, Inc. [5])

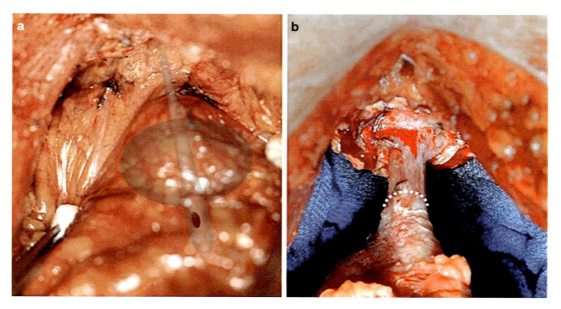

Fig. 4 Photographs of urethra-sparing cystectomy: Foley catheter (virtually superimposed) facilitates bladder neck identification (left). Dissection 0.5 cm below the bladder neck (right). (With permission by John Wiley and Sons [6])

anastomosis between the urethra and a neobladder should be avoided, due to the risk of fistulas between the anastomosis and the neobladder directly. In addition, (partial) preservation of the anterior vaginal wall increases the depth of the vagina and thus the possibility of sexual intercourse [6].

It goes without saying that careful intraoperative bowel handling should be routine, because it reduces swelling and postoperative adhesions and optimizes the construction of intestinal reservoirs for urinary diversion. Particularly in cases of continent cutaneous urinary diversion, attention should be paid to the anterior abdominal wall with the umbilicus when opening the abdomen. If anatomically possible, the efferent segment for catheterization is connected to the umbilicus. If this is not sufficiently cut around, complications can occur here.

Patient Selection for Continent Urinary Diversion

Correct patient selection is essential for excellent postoperative results with high patient satisfaction and outstanding quality of life [9]. As described above, preservation of a full-functional urethra and sphincter complex is the main factor to decide between an orthotopic (ileal) neobladder and a heterotopic continent urinary diversion [6, 8].

The following criteria are necessary for all patients:

- Oncological resection without negative margins. In most malignant diseases, positive margins are associated with a high risk of recurrence. In such cases, less complicated urinary diversion should be discussed instead.
- Sufficient physical and psychological health to handle a continent urinary diversion. In contrast to an ileal conduit or ureterocutaneostomy, patients with continent diversions must accept that their daily routine will be influenced by the diversion with catheterization, urinary incontinence, metabolic influences, and particularities regarding micturition.
- Renal function should be tested in all patients. Continent reservoirs bear a higher risk of renal function impairment compared to incontinence urinary diversion (e.g., ileal conduit). If the calculated glomerular filtration rate is inconclusive, creatinine clearance with urine collection over 24 h should be measured directly. A glomerular filtration rate of 50–60 is recommended for a continent urinary diversion. Reduced renal function increases the risk of metabolic imbalances.

- Acceptance of nutritional substitution in case of metabolic deviations or vitamin deficits (vitamin B12).
- Patients with chronic inflammatory bowel disease (e.g., Crohn's disease, ulcerative colitis, etc.) are not candidates for urinary diversions reconstructed by the intestine.
- Previous major bowel resection, especially of the ileocecal area, limits the use of additional intestinal segments for urological reconstruction and increases the risk of vitamin B12 deficiency, bile acid loss resulting in diarrhea, and short bowel syndrome.

Candidates for an orthotopic neobladder should be assessed according to the following aspects:

- Patients should be informed about and accept the risk of urinary incontinence, especially nighttime incontinence, which is more common in patients with orthotopic neobladder in contrast to male patients after prostatectomy.
- Patients with stress urinary incontinence greater than grade I should be excluded.
- Patients with clinically relevant genital descensus should be excluded.
- Patients should accept the risk of transurethral catheterization in case of residual urine or mucus obstruction.
- Intraoperative negative frozen section of the urethral margin or preoperative histological endoscopic histological evaluation (if a frozen section is not available) is recommended.

There is no defined age limit for an orthotopic neobladder, but the patient should have a good life expectancy and needs to accept a longer time period of postoperative rehabilitation. Obesity is also not a contraindication. In some of these patients, an orthotopic neobladder has advantages over an ileal conduit or a continent cutaneous reservoir, due the thickness of their anterior abdominal wall, which carries a higher risk of stomal problems [8].

Patients considering a continent cutaneous catheterizable reservoir should be evaluated for the following points:

- The patients need to be informed about and must accept the higher complication rates of this procedure compared to other urinary diversions: stone formation, stoma complications (incontinence, stricture, catheterization problems), and metabolic changes.
- The patients must catheterize themselves four to six times a day depending on the volume of the reservoir (max. 500 ml).
- The patients must be able to irrigate the pouch in case of an increased mucus production.
- In cases of planned use of colonic segments, a colonoscopy is mandatory.

Today, the use of a urinary diversion by implantation of the ureters into a rectosigmoidal reconfigured pouch (so-called Mainz II) is more and more uncommon, due to the risk of adenocarcinoma at the implantation side after several years. If patients are planned for this kind of urinary diversion, a colonoscopy and a test of the anal sphincter with irrigation of 500 ml of slightly thickened liquid are recommended.

Preoperative Patient Preparation

Besides intensive informing and decision-making (extent of cystectomy, planned urinary diversion, and alternative options) and informed consent, all patients should see a specialized nurse to mark the optimal point of the urological stoma if the preferred diversion is not possible. The decision of the stoma side should consider negative aspects of skin folds in upright and supine positions, skin abnormalities, and the patient's ability to take care of her stoma herself. Also, in patients with a planned continent cutaneous reservoir, it is helpful to mark a line for a possible side of the catheterizable stoma in the subumbilical part of the abdominal wall, in case the umbilicus is surgically not achievable. If stomal incontinence is present, this facilitates the placement of stoma plates.

Preoperative preparation includes the following important factors [10]:

- Blood typing and ordering of blood preparations
- Bowel preparation:
  - Only the small intestine used: fast track with only rectal suppositories or enema
  - Large intestine used: complete bowel preparation
- Prophylaxis of thrombosis with fractionated heparin
- Offering carbohydrate-containing clear fluids up to 2 h prior to surgery (depending on the anesthesiologist)
- Administering perioperative antibiotic prophylaxis 30 min prior to skin incision

Immediately before the procedure in the operating room, it makes sense to place a rectal tube, which facilitates accurate preparation in the rectovaginal space. It is also useful to insert a surgical instrument (e.g., a handle clamp) into the vagina under sterile conditions to establish the plane of the paravaginal dissection for nerve sparing. This is also helpful to define the vaginal resection line with the help of palpation of the distally positioned Foley catheter with identification of the bladder neck [6, 10].

Important Intraoperative Surgical Steps

This section discusses general surgical steps and aspects that are necessary for reservoir construction regardless of the specific type of orthotopic or heterotopic urinary diversion.

General Aspects of Reservoirs

The main goal of a continent reservoir, regardless of its location, is to provide an adequate storage volume (350 to 500 ml), preferably with low pressure in the pouch during the urine collection phase, in order to avoid deterioration of renal function and incontinence either transurethrally or through the efferent segment (stoma). Additionally, the metabolic influence of the reservoir on the whole organism should be as low as possible.

Generally, the large bowel is characterized by higher pressures due to reduced compliance (compared to the small intestine). The construction of a urinary reservoir from bowel segments includes two important techniques: detubularization (following Laplace's law) of the bowel segments and reconstitution of a spherical reservoir by folding. Goodwin described this technique with cross-folding of a U-shaped plate sutured from a detubularized bowel segment. Metabolic imbalances are less frequent and severe in reservoirs made from terminal ileal segments compared to those made from the proximal ileum, jejunum, or large bowel [11, 12].

If only the small intestine is used, a space of about 20–25 cm to the ileocecal valve is recommended. The use of parasympatholytics (e.g., butylscopolamine) is helpful to silence bowel movement and to avoid the recruitment of too much length of the intestine, especially if long intestinal small intestine segments are needed. This should be carefully communicated with the anesthesiology team, due to the resulting tachycardia [6].

The choice of the type of intestinal anastomosis should be based mainly on the experience of the surgeon. Typical anastomotic techniques include manual hand-sewn end-to-end or side-to-side anastomosis (single or multiple suture layers) and mechanical anastomosis with linear stapler devices. Currently, there are no data supporting the use of one anastomotic technique over the other. Special attention should be given to the closure of the mesenteric gap, in order to avoid inner hernias with intestinal obstruction.

A look into the specifics of various urinary diversion constructs demonstrates the different use of refluxing and non-refluxing implantation of the ureters into the reservoir. Anti-refluxing mechanisms should prevent the ascent of bacteria from the reservoir into the upper urinary tract. But on the other hand, they carry a higher risk of ureteral strictures (especially in techniques with long ureters) compared to a refluxing implantation, and ureteral strictures then negatively influence renal function [13]. Ureteral strictures for the Kock neobladder (afferent antireflux valve mechanism) and the T-Pouch have been reported at rates of 4.3 to 5% [14, 15], whereas other publications focusing on the Abol-Enein and Ghoneim pouch and on the I-Pouch have described slightly lower rates of ureteral implantation strictures of 2.1 to 3.8% [16–18]. Skinner et al. reported no significant differences of renal function impairment or incidence of urinary tract infection between the Studer neobladder (refluxing implantation but afferent ileal tunnel) and the T-Pouch (non-refluxing technique) [19]. This again supports the idea that the surgeon's experience is more important than the insistence of a non-refluxing implantation technique. Currently, both techniques, refluxing and non-refluxing implantation, are still in widespread use.

Typically, after spatulation of the ureters, they will be implanted separately (side-to-side, side-to-end) – the so-called Nesbit technique – or combined as described by Wallace as a sutured plate mostly side-to-end [20]. It is generally accepted that the ureterointestinal anastomosis is temporarily stented with mostly mono-J or double-J stents.

Orthotopic Neobladder

Although most surgeons use their preferred technique of neobladder formation, it is important that every surgeon should be able to perform at least one other alternative technique. Neobladder techniques differ between the level and the type of ureteral implantation. For example, the I-Pouch (as described in the next section) is characterized by ureteral dissection near the bladder, which results in easy access to the upper urinary tract [11, 18]. In patients with distal ureteral disease (ureteral cancer, positive surgical margins, ureteral stricture), the available ureteral length is not enough to fulfill the requirements of the I-Pouch. So in this situation, a surgeon who knew how to use the alternative technique of a Studer neobladder with a long ileal afferent segment would still be able to offer an orthotopic neobladder [8, 21, 22].

The optimal position of the neobladder outlet for anastomosis must be defined individually during surgery, especially in female patients. The pouch should have a plain contact area to the pelvic floor. If instead a pointed suture line end is used as the neobladder neck, the consequence will be a high risk of kinking with subsequent urinary retention or at least residual urine [8]. If available, an additional omental flap surrounding the neobladder neck might help to stabilize this region, thus minimizing emptying problems. If it is possible to prepare an omental flap, then the use of an omental flap is recommended, in order to cover the anterior aspect of the neobladder. This prevents direct adhesions of the intestinal neobladder wall to the symphysis pubis and the anterior abdominal wall. Such adhesions bring a high risk of direct injury upon midline revision surgery, so use of an omental flap facilitates future potential revision surgery.

Continent Cutaneous Reservoir

Heterotopic continent cutaneous reservoirs are characterized by a detubularized and folded intestinal reservoir with an afferent segment for ureteral implantation and an efferent segment for catheterization. In heterotopic pouches formed only out of the small intestine, the construction of the efferent segment is challenging. Usually, different combinations of invagination, intussusception, and tapering techniques of the small bowel are used to achieve continence of the stoma and a straight and narrow catheterization channel. Several pouches are based on the use of combined terminal ileum and cecum [23, 24]. The most popular ileocecal cutaneous continent reservoir consists of "mixed augmentation ileum and c (z)ecum" – the so-called MAINZ I pouch [23].

In heterotopic ileocecal pouches, the afferent segment is created through a direct submucosal tunneled implantation of the ureters into the colonic segment [25]. The terminal ileum can also be used as the afferent segment with the ileocecal valve as a reflux mechanism. If the appendix vermiformis is still present with sufficient diameter ($\geq$16F) and length (depends on the thickness of the abdominal wall of the patient), it represents the ideal efferent segment for catheterization, when embedded into the longitudinal muscular layer of the taenia libera to reinforce the continence mechanism [23]. The use of the appendix as a (neo)vesicocutaneostomy is also called a Mitrofanoff stoma/procedure [26]. In cases of an absent appendix, a possible alternative is the use of an intussuscepted terminal ileum pulled through the ileocecal valve and affixed with linear staples [25].

Besides the kind of ureteral implantation and the construction of the catheterizable efferent segment, the localization of the heterotopic pouch, especially the efferent segment, is of great importance. Easy and smooth catheterization of the efferent branch is essential for all patients postoperatively. Therefore, it is recommended to place absorbable sutures to connect the pouch and especially the efferent segment straight along the anterior abdominal wall to the side of the stoma (umbilicus or lower abdominal wall). An adequate incision of the fascia prevents stenosis of the efferent segment [23, 27].

Besides an indwelling catheter through the efferent segment, an additional indwelling pouch catheter analogous to a suprapubic tube (a "salvage" catheter with the possibility of circular irrigation) and bilateral percutaneous ureteral stents (mono-J stents) are generally used to reduce anastomotic insufficiencies with urinary leakage.

Types of Orthotopic Neobladders

Various orthotopic neobladders have been described in the literature. An orthotopic continent pouch should fulfill the criteria mentioned above of a physiological capacity of 350 to 500 ml, with low pressure during urine collection and sufficient emptying [11, 17, 18, 22]. The variants of neobladder reconstruction differ mainly in regard to the bowel segments used, the configuration of the reservoir itself, the afferent segment, and the kind of ureteral implantation (refluxing vs. non-refluxing). This section focuses on various commonly used orthotopic reservoirs. Data about the different forms of orthotopic pouches comes primarily from studies using an open surgical approach. Comments specifically about robot-assisted intracorporeal urinary diversions are summarized and discussed in section

"Specific Aspects of Robot-Assisted Surgery" of this chapter. The following subsections focus on the most important forms of orthotopic urinary diversion, with no claim to completeness, given the large number of available options.

Studer Neobladder

Studer and colleagues introduced the Studer neobladder, consisting of approximately 55 cm of the terminal ileum. The spherical reservoir is formed from the aboral 40 to 45 cm of the small intestine, while the proximal 10 to 15 cm model the afferent segment with ureteral implantation [8, 21, 22]. Figure 5 illustrates stepwise the formation of the Studer neobladder. The separated small intestine is positioned below the mesentery of the intestinal anastomosis, as is performed in typically all orthotopic diversions, with the proximal end in an upright fashion to include the ureters. The length of this chimney is tailored to the remaining length of the ureters, to use as much as possible of the bowel for reservoir composition. These parts need to be antimesenterically incised (Fig. 5, left), and a U-shaped plate is established by seromuscular suturing of the medial portions (Fig. 5, middle). Goodwin's principle is fulfilled by cross-folding of the U-shaped plate from left to right to obtain a spherical pouch (Fig. 5, middle and right). Ureteral implantation is performed in a refluxing manner, mostly side-to-side following the Nesbit technique. As discussed before, a separate opening for urethral anastomosis is imperative, to permit undisturbed micturition [21].

The main advantages of the Studer neobladder are the elementary implementation of the surgical technique, complete fulfillment of all principles of an orthotopic neobladder, and the guided peristalsis of the chimney, which partly reduces reflux. On the other hand, in patients who need upper tract instrumentation due to postoperative problems or patients who need oncological follow-up of the upper urinary tract, the entry to the ureters is very challenging and is often restricted. In such cases, a percutaneous approach is necessary.

I-Pouch

The I-Pouch is an interesting alternative to overcome the limitation of an entry to the upper urinary tract. Only 40 cm of the terminal ileum is used for this technique. After creating a U-shaped plate, the ureters are implanted with the Wallace technique of spatulated and combined ends into a vertical subserosal tunnel (about 8 cm length), which functions as a refluxing mechanism. Cross-folding finalizes formation of the pouch, which results in a spherical shape that fulfills all the necessary principles. In female patients, in accordance with Studer's technique, a separate hole is created for urethral

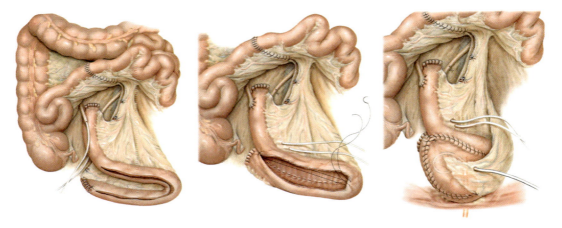

Fig. 5 Illustration of the formation of the Studer neobladder: detubularization (left), neobladder folding (middle), and final result (right). (With permission by John Wiley and Sons [22])

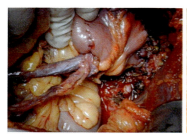 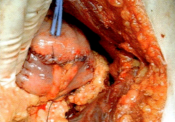 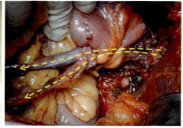

Fig. 6 Photographs of the I-Pouch: neobladder with antirefluxive implanted ureters in situ (left), omentum majus flap to support the bladder neck (middle), and visualization of the easy access to the upper urinary tract

anastomosis. Finally, an omental flap is helpful to stabilize the neobladder neck [18, 28, 29]. Figure 6 shows the intraoperative result with the neobladder attached to the urethra (left figure), the "omental wrap-up" of the bladder neck (middle figure), and the easy access to the upper urinary tract, if needed (right figure).

The main benefits of this technique are the relatively short ileal segment (approximately 40 cm) needed for the pouch and the access to the upper tract. Patients with insufficient length of preexisting bowel will be able to receive an orthotopic substitution. In cases of shortened ureters, it is not possible to create this pouch. Although long ureters might increase the risk of distal ureteral necrosis with resulting stenosis, studies have reported low incidences of this possible complication [18, 28].

Hautmann Neobladder

In contrast to the previous orthotopic solutions, the Hautmann neobladder uses a W-shaped ileal plate, which is formed and antimesenterically formed from 70 cm of the terminal ileum. On both sides, an approximately 4 cm tubular segment is spared for bilateral refluxing ureteric neo-implantation. The urethral opening is placed in the midline at the most distal part of the two U-shaped flaps, as illustrated in Fig. 7. Both flaps are then cross-folded to form the definite reservoir [30, 31].

Although 70 cm of the small intestine is needed, this type of neobladder avoids the crossing of the left ureter below the sigmoid mesentery to the right pelvic entry, as is required for the Studer neobladder and the I-Pouch.

Kock Ileal Neobladder

The Kock ileal neobladder was first intended as a heterotopic cutaneous continent reservoir with two distinct nipple valve mechanisms. With adaption to an orthotopic diversion, the afferent valve still functions as a non-refluxing mechanism, whereas the efferent segment is omitted [11]. This reservoir needs 60 cm of the terminal ileum, which is positioned in a U-shape with two 22 cm segments opposite each other forming the plate. The rest of the small intestine forms an intussuscepted nipple valve for ureteral implantation, which is secured with several rows of linear staplers, also to the pouch itself [15, 32].

The main problem of the Kock ileal reservoir is the negative impact of the staples on the blood supply of the afferent segment, which leads to ureteral stricture renal impairment and an increased risk of stone formation. Increasingly, this technique has been replaced by the T-Pouch ileal neobladder [15].

T-Pouch

Basically, the T-Pouch is founded on the same U-shaped configuration as the Kock ileal neobladder [33]. The primary difference addresses the weak point of the Kock pouch: the afferent segments. The stapler-configured nipple valve is replaced by a tapered ileal segment, which is embedded – preserving the segment's mesentery by creating small windows inside – into flaps at the upper end of the reservoir to create

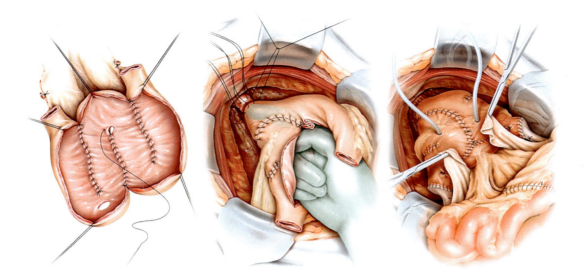

Fig. 7 Illustration of the formation of a Hautmann neobladder: Detubularization with two short chimneys (left), configured neobladder with urethral anastomosis (middle), and final result with the ureters anastomosed to the chimneys on both sides (right). (With permission by John Wiley and Sons [30])

an antireflux mechanism [14, 33]. Though the non-refluxing technique should prevent negative effects on renal function, a direct comparison to the Studer neobladder did not demonstrate relevant differences regarding renal protection [19]. Moreover, an increased frequency of revision surgery has been documented [19].

Pouch of Abol-Enein and Ghoneim

A serous-lined extramural tunnel technique for non-refluxing ureteral implantation was introduced by Abol-Enein and Ghoneim in 2001 [16]. The main principle of the reservoir is again a W-shaped form, comparable to the Hautmann neobladder, with about 60 cm of the terminal ileum. The medial parts of the plate are closed by a running suture; the lateral portions receive a seromuscular suture line for embedding of the ureters on both sides. This technique benefits from the direct implantation of the ureters without any additional need for afferent ileal segments. Yet in comparison to other forms of diversion, the question of the need for an antireflux mechanism is still raised [11, 19].

Padua Ileal Neobladder

Along with the Studer neobladder, the Padua ileal neobladder, also called the "Vescica Ileale Padovana," belongs to the group of the most frequently used orthotopic neobladder techniques worldwide [34]. The Padua ileal neobladder shares with the I-Pouch the main advantage of the reduced need of only 40 cm of the terminal ileum. In contrast to the I-Pouch, the Padua ileal neobladder forms a short funnel for urethral anastomosis, and the backwall plate consists of an S-shaped antimesenterically detubularized ileum, as shown in Fig. 12 (right two panels). Ureteral implantation is performed, analogously to the technique of Abol-Enein and Ghoneim, into bilaterally created serous-lined tunnels. The anterior wall of the ileal pouch is formed by downfolding of the primary created plate [34, 35].

Types of Heterotopic Continent Urinary Diversions

A variety of continent heterotopic urinary diversions also exist, and they have undergone many modifications over their history. The age of continent urinary diversions started early in the beginning of the nineteenth century, but relevant surgical progress with a positive influence on patient outcomes emerged only later around 1950 [25]. This section focuses on continent cutaneous urinary diversions, mainly the rectoileal Mainz I and heterotopic ileal reservoirs. The use of a rectal continent urinary diversion, in particular the Mainz II detubularized ureterosigmoidostomy [24, 25], is declining, due to other alternatives and the long-term risk of carcinoma if the ureter is implanted directly into the large bowel.

Continent cutaneous urinary diversions are composed of the reservoir itself, an afferent segment for ureter implantation, and an efferent segment, which facilitates emptying of the reservoir by intermittent (aseptic) catheterization. The diversion should offer enough capacity with low pressure, safety for the upper urinary tract, and a catheterization channel that is continent and easy to pass.

Mainz I Pouch: Mixed Augmentation Ileum and Cecum

The Mainz I pouch consists of a "mixed augmentation ileum and c(z)ecum," which, in addition to the location of the first description, is eponymous for the procedure. The use of the reservoir started in the 1980s with both an orthotopic and heterotopic placement, and it was subsequently improved regarding the efferent segment for a heterotopic application [23, 36]. Prior to surgery, it is essential to have information about the presence of the appendix, because it influences the continence rates of the cutaneous stoma. If large bowel segments are used for urinary tract reconstruction, a complete bowel preparation is essential to reduce postoperative complication rates, as discussed above.

The original technique used 10–12 cm of the cecum and 25 cm of the terminal ileum, including the ileocecal valve, as illustrated in Fig. 8 (left panel). Before transection of the intestine, it is essential to check if the appendix is present and useable as the efferent segment, because this directly influences the additional amount of the small intestine needed if the appendix is not suitable. After resection of the tip of the appendix, a 16F catheter should pass through, requiring only gentle dilation at most. The length of the appendix should allow enough space for embedding into the colonic wall (continence mechanism, Fig. 8 (middle panel)), and it should be long enough to reach the skin, mainly through the opened umbilicus. After bowel transection and assembly of an ileoascendostomy (by various possible techniques, depending on the surgeon's prior experience), the ileum is antimesenterially opened, and the incision follows the taenia libera after passage of the ileocecal valve. The ureters are implanted with submucosal tunnels straight through the upper dissection line of the colon. The detubularized ileum configures an ileal plate after both limbs have been sutured. This plate completes the spherical reservoir as a cap to the opened colonic part (Fig. 8 (middle panel)) [27, 36]. The use of the appendix for a continent catheterizable stoma was first described in 1980 by Mitrofanoff in pediatric patients needing continent cutaneous vesicostomies (appendicovesicostomies) [26, 37]. The continent catheterizable stoma based on the appendix has been adapted for use in heterotopic urinary diversions. It is also a good option for female cancer patients with an indication for urethrectomy and bladder neck closure.

In patients whose appendix is missing or not usable, an additional 12 cm segment of the ileum is necessary to create a continent efferent segment pulled through the conserved ileocecal valve, as shown in Fig. 8 (right panel) [23].

To facilitate a tension-free connection of the efferent segment (preferably to the umbilicus, which hides the urostomy best), it is essential to have good mobilization of the right hemi-colon. This is also essential in order to achieve sufficient anastomosis between the ileum and the ascending colon. Typically, the patient receives two ureteral stents with percutaneous routing: one catheter through the efferent segment (at least 16 F) and an additional safety catheter into the reservoir like a suprapubic tube. The ureteric stents stay in place for 9–10 days. Catheter removal with the beginning of intermittent catheterization is possible

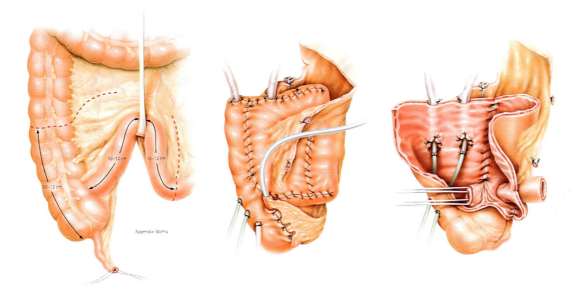

Fig. 8 Illustration of the Mainz I pouch: necessary intestinal segments if the appendix is present (left), configured pouch with ureteral implantation to the cecal wall and appendix embedded into the colonic wall for catheterization (middle). Alternative valve mechanism for catheterization in patients after appendectomy (right). (With permission by John Wiley and Sons [23])

after at least 3 weeks and inconspicuous radiography [23].

Figure 9 shows the use of a Mainz I pouch stepwise, with modification of the afferent segment. After complete exposition and mobilization of the right hemi-colon and terminal ileum, the segments needed are measured and marked with loops (upper left photo). The appendix is tested for usability, and a 16 F catheter is introduced (upper middle photo). Then the mesoappendix is fenestrated to facilitate incorporation of the appendix into the incised and laterally mobilized taenia libera (upper right photo). In this particular patient, 8–10 cm of the terminal ileum including the ileocecal valve was left in place to serve as a reflux mechanism for ureteral implantation (lower left photo). The mobility of the completed pouch with the 16 F catheter in place is shown in the last picture (lower right photo).

Ileal Heterotopic Continent Cutaneous Pouches

As described above, solitary ileal containing reservoirs (e.g., Kock ileal pouch or pouch of Abol-Enein and Ghoneim) have been used for heterotopic and orthotopic urinary diversion. Nowadays, the handling of the ileum is easier for many surgeons, because the surgical skills needed to use colonic segment have become more and more rare. Whereas ileocecal pouches might have the chance to use a present appendix as an excellent efferent segment, pure ileal continent cutaneous pouches always need distinct and modeled solutions for the afferent and the efferent segments. As discussed above, the Kock ileal pouch with two intussuscepted nipple valves had disadvantages, due to in increased use of staples, which led to stone formation.

Figure 10 shows the continent cutaneous pouch of Abol-Enein and Ghoneim with 40 cm of the terminal ileum used for the pouch configuration in a W-shaped form. In contrast to their orthotopic solution that uses direct ureteral implantation, their cutaneous pouch needs two additional 10 cm segments of the ileum to form an afferent non-refluxing segment with ureteral implantation and a continent efferent segment with a junction of this 10 cm segment to the skin. The use of staples with the risk of subsequent stone formation is here completely avoided [17].

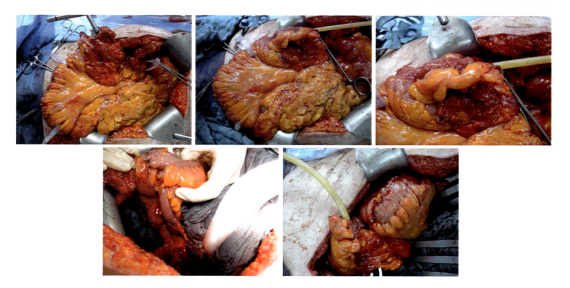

Fig. 9 Photographs of the Mainz I pouch: determination of the bowel segments (upper left), the appendix checked for catheterization mechanism (upper middle), the appendix incorporated into the colonic wall (upper right), ureteral implantation (Wallace technique) to the terminal ileum using the ileocecal valve as reflux mechanism (lower left), fully constructed pouch (lower right)

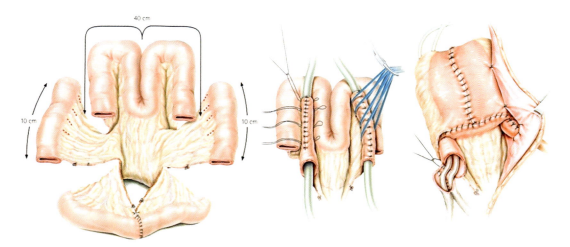

Fig. 10 Illustration of continent cutaneous ileal neobladder using serous-lined extramural valves, as described by Abol-Enein and Ghoneim: necessary intestinal segments (neobladder 40 cm, valve mechanism 2x 10 cm, left panel), incorporation of the valve mechanisms into the neobladder (middle panel), and final result with ureteral implantation through the left and catheterization through the right valve (right panel). (With permission by John Wiley and Sons [17])

Figure 11 shows a modified Kock ileal pouch. The left photo shows the mobile ileal pouch after assembly, with the oral ending of the ileum on the right side, and a modified intussuscepted nipple valve pointing in the upper right direction. Similar to the Studer neobladder, a tubularized afferent segment has been used for ureter implantation, and the invaginated nipple shows staples on the outside. The inner part of the nipple has been sutured with absorbable suture, even though the risk of "nipple sliding" is thereby increased. The end of the efferent segment has been tapered

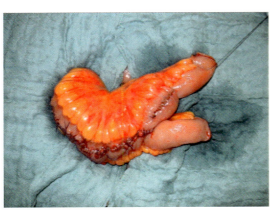
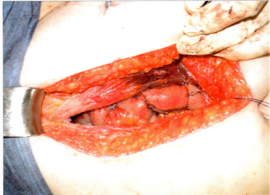

Fig. 11 Photographs of an ileal heterotopic cutaneous pouch with ureteral implantation to the oral ileal segment and catheterization through an invaginated and tapered aboral segment (left, before anastomosis; right, in situ)

to the size of a 16 F catheter (not shown). The right photo shows the straight arrangement of the efferent segment to the midline. It is recommended to fix the pouch itself and also the efferent segment to the anterior abdominal wall (using absorbable sutures), to avoid kinking and its risk of later catheterization problems.

Specific Aspects of Robot-Assisted Surgery

For a long time, radical prostatectomy was the focus of robot-assisted surgery in the urological field. The first robot-assisted radical cystectomy was reported in 2003, including nerve-sparing techniques to improve the functional outcomes [38]. Over the past two decades, the uses, techniques, and outcomes of robotic surgery have advanced tremendously for both the ablative portion of cystectomy and the reconstructive portion of urinary tract obstruction. In the beginning, robot-assisted surgery was used for radical cystectomy followed by an extracorporeal preparation of the urinary diversion with neobladder or ileal conduit. With increasing experience, novel robotic instruments (e.g., stapler devices) and the adaption of specific techniques for urinary diversion cleared the way for a total intracorporeal urinary diversion, with special attention to orthotopic neobladders [12, 39]. A recent retrospective multicenter analysis demonstrated a learning curve of 137 consecutive cases to reach a stable rate of serious complications [40].

Currently, it is still debated whether open surgery or robot-assisted surgery is better for cystectomy and urinary tract reconstruction. The guidelines of the European Association of Urology 2022 summarize the evidence as follows [41]:

- Robot-assisted radical cystectomy is characterized by longer operating times and higher costs but shorter length of stay and less blood loss in comparison to open surgery (level of evidence (LE) 1).
- Robot-assisted and open radical cystectomy may result in similar (major) complications (LE 2).
- Robot-assisted and open radical cystectomy do not differ in most endpoints including intermediate-term oncological outcome and quality of life (LE 2).
- The key factors for radical cystectomy are the surgeon's experience and the institutional volume, not the technique used (LE 2).

The European Association of Urology recommends informing the patient of the advantages and disadvantages of the two techniques to find the ideal decision for the patient. Additionally, the EAU guidelines emphasize that radical cystectomy and urinary diversion should be performed at centers with sufficient experience, regardless of which technique is used [41]. These recommendations are essential to avoid situations where less experienced surgical teams tend to prefer incontinent urinary diversion (ileum conduit) in the context of a total intracorporeal technique or situations where the previously explained principles of an orthotopic bladder replacement (Laplace's law, intestinal detubularization, cross-folding (Goodwin's principle)) are relaxed, in order to compensate for technical inadequacies. Although robotic surgery brings many technical advantages to this complex intervention, any surgeons using robotic assistance must always give careful attention to make all the necessary adjustments to the surgical technique with appropriate caution and compliance with medical rules and knowledge, in order to maintain patient safety [34]. Figure 12 illustrates some modified versions of the main orthotopic neobladders – the Studer neobladder and the Padua ileal neobladder – to adapt the techniques for use in robot-assisted surgery [34].

Immediate Postoperative Patient Care

It is generally accepted that patients benefit from standard operating procedures (SOPs), especially after extensive surgical procedures. The use of a fast-track concept belongs to the standard of care after radical cystectomy [6]. The following points address the most important areas of postoperative patient care [8]:

- Sufficient pain management is essential, including the possibility of epidural anesthesia, as well as patient and nurse-controlled analgesia. Close communication with specialized pain doctors, if available, is helpful.
- A preoperatively inserted stomach tube should be retrieved as soon as possible. Irritation from the tube might negatively influence bowel recovery.
- Patients should be offered clear fluids containing carbohydrates starting 4 h after surgery, with the aim of a continuous increase of nutrition. Cooperation with a nutrition support team, if available, is recommended.
- Bowel recovery should be supported by enteral and parenteral bowel stimulation (indirect parasympathomimetic drugs). The use of chewing gum positively influences directed bowel movement.
- Early mobilization is one of the essential factors for bowel recovery and for prophylaxis of thrombosis and pulmonary embolism. In addition, fractionated heparin should be administered for 4 weeks, as recommended for pelvic surgery.
- Surgical drains should be removed as early as possible, depending on the flow rate and the absence of urine, checked by the evaluation of creatinine levels in the drains in comparison to serum levels.
- Continent urinary diversions have a higher risk of metabolic imbalance, and this risk increases after catheter removal. Therefore, regular blood tests, including blood gas analysis, are recommended. Electrolyte deficits should be compensated accordingly.
- Irrigation of the reservoir is recommended three times per day, to prevent mucus obstruction of the catheter. Active aspiration is recommended preferentially above passive irrigation.
- Ureteric stents are typically removed on days 8 and 9 after surgery. In complex pouches, radiographic exclusion of reservoir leakage is helpful.
- In orthotopic neobladders, catheter removal can be performed after radiography on day 10. In patients with continent cutaneous reservoirs, 3 weeks of catheter drainage is recommended prior to radiography.

After catheter removal, patients need thorough advising by physical therapists (for both orthotopic and heterotopic pouches). Patients with continent cutaneous reservoirs need to be taught intermittent (aseptic) catheterization.

In neobladder patients, voiding is mediated by an active relaxation of the pelvic floor and an increase of the intra-abdominal pressure by Valsalva maneuver. It is strongly recommended to measure the residual urine, because it increases

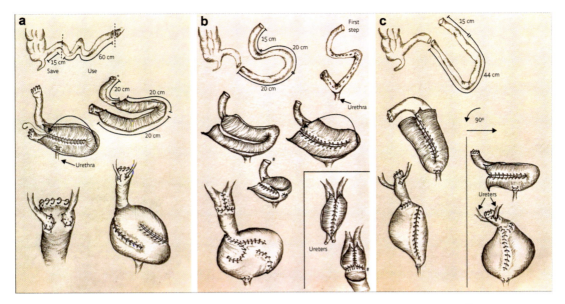
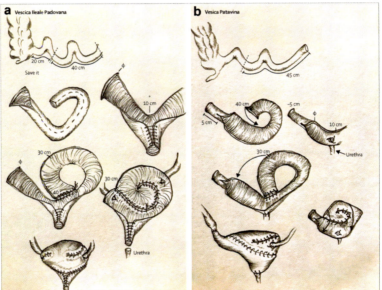

Fig. 12 Illustration of open surgery neobladders and their robot-assisted adaption: the three panels on the top (a, b, c) show classical Studer neobladder with modifications of Karolinska and University of Southern California, while the two panels below (a, b) show the classical Vescica Ileale Padovana and the adapted Vescica Patavina. (With permission by Elsevier [34])

the risk of metabolic changes. Blood gas analysis is therefore also essential at that time.

The recommended time interval for reservoir emptying is every 2 h while awake and every 3 h while sleeping. Within several weeks, the initially low volume increases to physiological amounts of up to 500 ml, compared to a healthy urinary bladder, due to continuous but slow dilatation of the reservoir. Patients should be advised that volumes higher than 500 ml should be avoided, because that would increase the risk of renal impairment and because rupture of the reservoir is possible.

Early Risks of Continent Urinary Diversions

The choice of urinary diversion directly influences surgical effort and operating time. The following specific risks and complications must be considered, with early detection being essential for patient outcome [6, 8].

- The use of bowel segments with the need of intestinal anastomosis increases the risk of protracted intestinal atony and ultimately paralytic or mechanical ileus. Early enteral nutrition and the use of enteral and parenteral stimulation positively influence bowel recovery. A mechanical ileus (which is more often reported by radiologists than clinically observable) that is refractory to conservative treatment will need surgical revision.
- Insufficiency of the intestinal anastomosis generally leads to acute abdominal pain and stool or air apart from the usual drain fluids is visible in the drains. Immediate revision is imperative to reduce the patient's risk of a devastating clinical course.
- Insufficiency of the various urological anastomoses (ureter to bowel, bowel to urethra, and bowel to skin) or the sutures of the reservoir itself must be considered in cases of increased fluid flow in the drainage. Creatinine measurement as described above can identify leakage. In many cases, subsequent drainage or reinsertion of already removed stents (e.g., ureteric stents or additionally nephrostomy tubes) facilitates conservative treatment. Refractory leakage sometimes needs surgical revision.
- Necrosis of parts of the continent urinary diversion might be occult for a long time and prolonged extravasation is the main symptom present. Necrosis of the efferent segment can be visualized on the abdominal skin anastomosis only in patients with a continent cutaneous reservoir. In cases of prolonged urine leakage, surgeons should be aware of (partial) reservoir necrosis, which can only be treated with surgical revision.
- Urinary tract infection is one of the most common problems after reconstructive urologic surgery. It is recommended to check for significant bacteria prior to the removal of catheters and stents, in order to reduce the risk of febrile urinary tract infections, which can be life-threatening.
- Obstruction of uretic stents or catheters is seen as frequently as urinary tract infections are, so prophylactic irrigation and active aspiration is strongly advised (irrigation volume: 20 ml for neobladder and continent heterotopic pouches, 2 ml for ureters).

Long-Term Risks of Continent Urinary Diversions

The complexity of urinary diversions directly influences the risk of long-term complications. This section focuses on specific long-term risks of orthotopic and heterotopic continent urinary diversions [6, 8, 41]. Examples of the incidences of long-term risks of specific continent urinary diversions are outlined in section "Outcome."

General Long-Term Risks after Continent Urinary Diversion

In patients with continent urinary diversion, the following general risks should be evaluated in follow-up.

Metabolic imbalance often occurs in the time period after catheter removal, but patients with acute health issues independent of the urinary tract are also at risk of acute metabolic changes. Therefore, regular blood gas analysis is recommended for all patients, not only for those who present in poor health. Patients with an ileal reservoir typically have hypochloremic acidosis, whereas patients with colonic segments typically have hyperchloremic acidosis. Sodium bicarbonate is used to treat acidosis. Patients with hyperchloremic situations often also need potassium substitution. Chronic metabolic acidosis carries the risk of bone demineralization and therefore osteoporosis.

The use of bowel segments is accompanied by the risk of negative effects on nutrition and fluid management. In patients with short bowel syndrome, nutrition and drug treatment (loperamide, opium tincture) focus on an increased stool consistency.

Patients are at risk of vitamin B12 deficiency, based on a reduced absorption of vitamin B12 in combination with intrinsic factor, especially patients with long segments of the terminal ileum for urologic reconstructions. Healthy persons have great storages of vitamin B12 in the liver. Therefore, screening of vitamin B12 deficiency is recommended lifelong.

Bile acids are normally reabsorbed in the terminal ileum. Extensive use of this small intestinal part might result in chologenic diarrhea. Colestyramine can bond bile acids and improve the amount and frequency of diarrhea.

Urinary tract infections (UTIs) are more frequent in patients with urinary diversions compared to healthy patients and are defined as complicated UTIs. Besides adequate microbiological examination, obstruction of the upper and lower urinary tract should be excluded by ultrasound or additional investigations if needed (e.g., renal scintigraphy).

Pelvic organ prolapse is a challenging situation after radical cystectomy. In cases of heterotopic urinary diversion, the current available surgical strategies can be applied, if conservative therapy including vaginal pessaries fails. In patients with an orthotopic neobladder, an individual approach is necessary, because there is no standardized recommendation. In sexually inactive patients, colpocleisis remains a possible salvage option.

Orthotopic Neobladder

In the case of patients with an orthotopic neobladder, the following special aspects must be observed during follow-up care.

Stress urinary incontinence is one of the relevant long-term risks for patients with an orthotopic neobladder. Preexisting urinary incontinence increases this risk. Whereas nighttime urinary incontinence is common in many patients, the chance of daytime continence after pelvic floor exercise is high and depends on the patient's compliance. Surgical treatment of female stress urinary incontinence after orthotopic neobladder is limited. Bulking agents might help temporarily. Only a few case reports exist of using tension-free vaginal tapes (TVT), and they seem to suggest a high risk of perforation. Oral treatment with duloxetine might be an option in selected patients. Refractory stress urinary incontinence can be treated by diversion into an ileal conduit or a catheterizable continent reservoir.

Reduced reservoir capacity can mimic stress urinary incontinence. Radiography with the determination of the maximum neobladder capacity is helpful to identify these patients. Surgical revision is able to increase pouch volume and thereby reduce urinary incontinence.

Anastomotic strictures, neobladder neck kinking, and intestinal folds can all lead to residual urine or acute urinary intention. Cystoscopic evaluation helps to identify the cause. Strictures and intestinal folds can be resected transurethrally, whereas longer kinking of the bladder neck often results in long-term intermittent catheterization.

Ureteric stricture, especially in cases of long distal ureters, results in hydronephrosis and a risk of renal insufficiency. Double-J stenting is the primary solution to prevent further damage. Long-term stents are under investigation, but a cure of the stricture is only possible with revision surgery, which is demanding.

Continent Cutaneous Reservoirs

Specific problems of continent cutaneous reservoirs can affect either the reservoir or the afferent and efferent segments.

Stone formation and mucus balls occur more often in patients with heterotopic reservoirs compared to patients with orthotopic neobladders. The main risk factors are the incomplete emptying of the pouch and the use of staples. Subsequent catheterization of the pouch and irrigation might reduce the frequency of this problem. In addition, off-label use of acetylcysteine (oral intake or irrigation) might reduce mucus production.

A stricture of the afferent loop inevitably leads to obstruction of the upper urinary tract. In most cases, this problem is not accompanied by symptoms. Chronic hydronephrosis will result in renal impairment of the affected renal unit. In some patients, renal scintigraphy helps to distinguish chronic ectasia without urodynamic problems from a significant hydronephrosis. Due to the nature of cutaneous continent reservoirs, a nephrostomy is the treatment of choice in acute situations. Definitive treatment requires surgical revision.

Problems of the efferent segment can be divided into stoma incontinence, stricture of the catheterizable channel, and kinking with difficult or impossible catheterization. The latter problem can only be treated by surgical intervention. Stoma incontinence can occur in different degrees. Mild incontinence can be treated with regular catheterization and specialized stomal caps. Data supports an off-label trial of bulking agents in patients with significant incontinence. If refractory incontinence is not acceptable, surgical revision might be offered, which is the same in patients with persistent obstruction after dilatation or incision of the efferent segment. Salvage options include the serosa-lined and tapered ileum (so-called Fulda nipple) [42, 43] or the intussuscepted ileal nipple valve [44].

In cases of stoma incontinence, it is of course necessary to exclude fixed reduced capacity of the heterotopic reservoir, prior to any open surgical revision. Surgical revision then follows the same principles described above for orthotopic neobladders.

In summary, given all these early and long-term risks and complications, these patients need and benefit from a close and lifelong urological consultation. Furthermore, although it is not a pouch-specific problem, patients should be informed about the high risk that ablative surgery will have negative effects on their sexual life. Sexual anamnesis should be routine during follow-up.

Outcome

With a brief look at the many various continent orthotopic and heterotopic urinary diversions, it becomes clear that a comprehensive presentation of the results is not possible here. Therefore, clinically relevant examples that underline the importance of the various continent urinary diversions are presented. Regrettably, most of the studies report their oncological and functional results for their entire study sample of men and women together. Although the portion of female versus male patients is reported by nearly all publications, sex-specific subgroup analysis is only rarely provided.

Radical cystectomy in patients with muscle-invasive bladder cancer has a 5-year recurrence-free survival of 58%, with a cancer-specific 5-year survival of 66% overall. Nodal-positive patients showed reduced recurrence-free survival between 34% and 43%, which directly influences life expectancy. Accordingly, a clinically or histopathologically positive nodal status should not exclude patients from receiving a continent form of urinary diversion [41]. It is precisely from this point of view that the need for excellent long-term functional results for the individual patients becomes evident.

Outcome of Orthotopic Neobladders

The orthotopic pouch described by Abol-Enein and Ghoneim was associated with early complications in 9% of the patients (97 female, 353 male patients), with surgical transvaginal correction of neovesicovaginal fistulas in three patients. Stone formation was reported in 10 patients, outflow obstruction in 11, mucus retention in 2, and hypercontinence in 9 female patients. Daytime continence was reported in 93.3% of patients, and nighttime continence was reported in 80% of patients. The integrity of the upper urinary tract was reported in 96.2% of the implanted renal units, with ureteral reflux documented in 3% of the cohort [16].

Functional results of the I-Pouch were published in 2015 for a patient cohort of 72 men and 25 women with a median oncological follow-up of 41 months and a median functional follow-up of 18 months. The 5-year cancer-specific survival rate was 67.9%. The complication rate was reported as 14.4% for the 30-day postoperative period and 17.5% for the 90-day postoperative period. Open surgical reimplantation of the ureter due to obstruction was necessary in 2.1% of the patients. Clean intermittent catheterization was necessary in 2.1%, which is comparably low to other studies. Ureteral reflux was documented in one patient, and the risk of UTI was not associated with residual urine [18]. Other studies showed no inferiority of the I-Pouch compared to the Studer neobladder regarding 30-day and 90-day major complication rates [28, 29]. Also, no significant influence on bowel function could be identified between the two procedures [29]. The need for intermittent catheterization was reported for 12% in female patients with an I-Pouch [45].

The first description of the Padua ileal neobladder reports a high capacity of 400 to 650 ml, with a low pressure of mean 17 cm H_2O and no pressure waves in 50% of the patients. Daytime continence in 16 patients was reported as 87%, and nighttime continence reduces to 81%, within a mean follow-up of 10 months [35].

In 2006, a paper reporting 20 years of experience using the Studer neobladder was published [21]. The authors reported on 482 patients (including 40 women) with this type of orthotopic urinary diversion. One-year continence was reported in 92% of the patients during the daytime and 79% at night. Ninety-three percent of the patients were able to void spontaneously. Ureteroileal stenosis was reported in only 2.7% of the patients. Metabolic evaluation showed vitamin B12 deficiency in 5% of the patients [21].

Intracorporeal neobladder in a Studer fashion has been described in a study on 12 female and 50 male patients, with a mean age of 63.6 years [39]. Continence was reported in 88% of the patients. The 90-day mortality was 0, but the 180-day mortality rate was 3.3%.

The investigation of the T-Pouch by Stein et al. consisted of 209 patients (40% women), with a mean follow-up of 33 months. Perioperative mortality was 1.4%, and early complications occurred in 30% of the patients (with 5% related to diversion). Urine leakage was the most common early complication. The 38 late complications included pouch calculi in 17 patients and ureteral ileal obstruction in 9 patients. T-limb-associated complications were documented in four patients (three of whom had prior radiotherapy). Reflux was present in 15 patients. Good daytime continence was reported by 87% of the patients, and good nighttime continence by 72% of the patients. Any kind of intermittent catheterization was necessary in 43% of the female patients [14].

Analysis of the importance of non-refluxing implantation was carried out by Shaaban et al. in 2006 [13]. The authors were not able to detect an advantage of non-refluxing implantation. Furthermore, antirefluxive implantation was associated with a higher stricture rate and increased risk of impairment of the upper urinary tract [13]. This is consistent with the data of Skinner et al. mentioned above, without any significant advantage of the T-Pouch over the Studer neobladder concerning renal function [19].

Outcome of Continent Cutaneous Reservoirs

Specific analysis of the Mitrofanoff stoma, independent of urinary diversions (appendicovesicostoma), in young patients demonstrated 96% continued catheterization of the stoma (instead of an indwelling catheter). Stoma stenosis developed in 10% of the patients, and four patients suffered from stenosis or perforation (two each) of the appendix. Surgical revision was needed for 16% of the patients, at a median of 7.3 months after the primary surgery. The median time to stomal stenosis was 13 months, and continence was reported in 98% of the patients, which underlines the main advantage of this kind of efferent segment [26].

In 1986, the inventors of the Mainz I pouch reported on 11 patients after orthotopic positioning with complete continence during the day and night in 10 patients [36]. In 2006, data was published on 800 patients with heterotopic positioning of Mainz I pouches, performed at two centers, with a considerable mean follow-up of 7.6 years [27]. The continence rate (overall) was 92.8%. Stomal stenosis was present in 23.5% of the patients with appendix stoma and 15.3% in patients with an intussuscepted ileal nipple. In contrast, calculi formation was higher in patients with an ileal nipple (10.8%) compared to patients with an appendix stoma (5.6%), which can be explained by the stapler lines used. Ureteral stricture was detected in 6.5% of the renal units with submucosal tunnel implantation and in 5% of the renal units with serosa-lined extramural tunnel. Reintervention due to necrosis of the continence mechanism was necessary in 11 patients [27].

High rates of stoma continence are also reported for other cutaneous continent diversions. Cheng et al. recently reported data of patients with the "Indiana" pouch (consisting of the ileum, cecum, and ascending colon), right colon pouch with appendico-umbilicostomy, and right colon pouch with neo-appendico-umbilicostomy. Most stoma complications (>60%) occurred at the level of the fascia and the skin [46]. The review of Moon et al. published in 2013 also reported continence rates of between 72.0% (Indiana pouch) and 96.0% (Mainz I with appendix stoma) [24].

Kälbe et al. investigated the use of their serosa-lined and tapered ileum as a primary and secondary option of an efferent segment in various reservoirs. They report on five patients with complete urinary continence and smooth catheterization through the umbilical connected "Fulda nipple" [43], which supports this technique as a salvage procedure for efferent segment difficulties. Comparable results of 92% success could be reached with the intussuscepted ileal valve described by Kalogirou et al. to salvage disturbed efferent segments [44].

In summary, both continent urinary diversions – orthotopic neobladder and heterotopic continent cutaneous reservoir – represent promising treatment options for patients who need a cystectomy in the context of treating carcinoma of the pelvis in women. Very good continence rates, acceptable postoperative morbidity, and manageable postoperative revisions due to long-term complications make continent urinary diversion an attractive alternative to incontinent urinary diversion for those affected. Patient-specific advising on the types, risks, and opportunities of the various urinary diversion options remains essential.

Recommendations for Follow-Up

Both orthotopic and heterotopic continent urinary patients need lifelong interdisciplinary follow-up [8, 10, 41]. The frequency and content of the follow-up are dependent on the type of pelvic cancer and the kind of urinary diversion. In fact, no general follow-up recommendations can be made.

In patients who had cystectomy due to bladder cancer, screening for distant metastasis, local recurrence, and secondary tumors of the upper urinary tract is recommended and is performed by either computed tomography or magnetic resonance imaging. Urine cytology or irrigation cytology of the persistent (inactive) urethra complements the oncological follow-up. Follow-up in these patients starts 3 months postoperatively, with increasing intervals thereafter. After 5 years, annual follow-up is recommended.

Functional follow-up of the urinary diversions should focus on the reservoir with attached segments and the upper urinary tract. Drinking and voiding/catheterization diaries help to identify capacity problems with the pouch. Regular ultrasound helps to identify hydronephrosis, residual urine of an orthotopic neobladder, or incomplete emptying of a heterotopic pouch. In cases of asymptomatic hydronephrosis, renal scintigraphy can distinguish between fixed ectasia of the renal collective system and obstructed hydronephrosis. Endoscopic or percutaneous intervention is indicated in patients with proven obstructed hydronephrosis. Blood tests should focus on hemoglobin (anemia), creatinine (renal function), electrolytes and venous blood gas analysis (metabolic imbalances), and vitamin B12 and folic acid (hyperchromic anemia). Urine culture should of course be performed if there is a complicated urinary tract infection. Sexual anamnesis should also be performed routinely, as explained above.

Conclusion

Pelvic cancer in female patients is associated with a high risk of involvement of the lower urinary tract. Depending on the extent and location of the infiltration of the bladder and urethra, the extent of the ablative surgery must be estimated preoperatively and discussed with the patient. The extent of the surgical intervention and also patient-specific factors, especially the patient's wishes, guides the decision-making process for the ideal urinary diversion. The prerequisites for a continent orthotopic urinary diversion are primarily the exclusion of preexisting, relevant stress urinary incontinence and the preservation of a functioning urethra, including the sphincter complex. Appropriate patient compliance is essential for both orthotopic and heterotopic continent diversion.

The structure of the reservoir should follow the established principles of a spherical reservoir made of detubularized intestine, with folds made according to Goodwin's principle, regardless of the surgical approach (open vs. laparoscopic vs. robot-assisted). Currently, the terminal ileum is used mainly to build up an orthotopic neobladder. In the case of heterotopic continent urinary diversion, the existence of an appendix plays a decisive role in the selection of the technique, as it enables an ideal access route for intermittent catheterization into the ileocecal pouch (Mainz I). Pure ileal heterotopic reservoirs avoid the use of the colon, but they have the difficulty of obtaining effective afferent and efferent segments. There is still no proof that non-refluxive implantation of the ureters into the neobladder is important.

In addition to all the technical features of the specific urinary diversion, the experience of the surgical team and surgical center plays a significant role. Consequently, it is increasingly recommended that such interventions be concentrated in specialized surgical centers. The experience needed becomes apparent not only in the primary intervention. Rather, postoperative care, including recognizing and eliminating complications, require a wealth of experience.

Patients should be aware that all forms of urinary diversion have risks, with the heterotopic cutaneous reservoir in particular having a higher probability of later reintervention than orthotopic bladder replacement. Yet even among patients for whom an orthotopic neobladder is not an option, the risks of later reintervention should not ultimately deter patients from choosing a continent catheterizable urinary diversion over an incontinent stoma.

References

1. Witjes JA, Bruins HM, Cathomas R, Comperat EM, Cowan NC, Gakis G, et al. European Association of Urology Guidelines on muscle-invasive and metastatic bladder cancer: summary of the 2020 guidelines. Eur Urol. 2021;79(1):82–104.
2. Stein JP, Stenzl A, Grossfeld GD, Freeman JA, Esrig D, Boyd SD, et al. The use of orthotopic neobladders in women undergoing cystectomy for pelvic malignancy. World J Urol. 1996;14(1):9–14.
3. Gerber WL. Is urethral sparing at cystectomy a safe procedure? Urology. 1990;36(4):303–4.
4. Le Duc A, Camey M. A procedure for avoiding reflux in uretero-ileal implantations during enterocystoplasty (author's transl). J Urol Nephrol (Paris). 1979;85(7–8):449–54.
5. Colleselli K, Stenzl A, Eder R, Strasser H, Poisel S, Bartsch G. The female urethral sphincter: a morphological and topographical study. J Urol. 1998;160(1):49–54.
6. Schilling D, Horstmann M, Nagele U, Sievert KD, Stenzl A. Cystectomy in women. BJU Int. 2008;102 (9 Pt B):1289–95.
7. Amend B, Stenzl A. In: Chapple CR, Steers WD, Evans CP, editors. Urologic principles and practice. Springer specialist surgery series. Gross and laparoscopic anatomy of the lower tract and pelvis. 2nd ed. Heidelberg: Springer; 2021.
8. Studer UE. Keys to successful orthotopic bladder substitution. Heidelberg: Springer; 2015.
9. Lee RK, Abol-Enein H, Artibani W, Bochner B, Dalbagni G, Daneshmand S, et al. Urinary diversion after radical cystectomy for bladder cancer: options, patient selection, and outcomes. BJU Int. 2014;113 (1):11–23.

10. Amend B, Schilling D, Bedke J, Stenzl A. Aktuelle Urol. 2020;51(2):202–16.
11. Gakis G, Stenzl A. Ileal neobladder and its variants. Eur Urol Suppl. 2010;9(10):745–53.
12. Tan WS, Lamb BW, Kelly JD. Evolution of the neobladder: a critical review of open and intracorporeal neobladder reconstruction techniques. Scand J Urol. 2016;50(2):95–103.
13. Shaaban AA, Abdel-Latif M, Mosbah A, Gad H, Eraky I, Ali-El-Dein B, et al. A randomized study comparing an antireflux system with a direct ureteric anastomosis in patients with orthotopic ileal neobladders. BJU Int. 2006;97(5):1057–62.
14. Stein JP, Dunn MD, Quek ML, Miranda G, Skinner DG. The orthotopic T pouch ileal neobladder: experience with 209 patients. J Urol. 2004;172(2):584–7.
15. Stein JP, Freeman JA, Esrig D, Elmajian DA, Tarter TH, Skinner EC, et al. Complications of the afferent antireflux valve mechanism in the Kock ileal reservoir. J Urol. 1996;155(5):1579–84.
16. Abol-Enein H, Ghoneim MA. Functional results of orthotopic ileal neobladder with serous-lined extramural ureteral reimplantation: experience with 450 patients. J Urol. 2001;165(5):1427–32.
17. Abol-Enein H, Ghoneim MA, Surgical atlas. A continent cutaneous ileal neobladder using the serous-lined extramural valves. BJU Int. 2006;98(5):1125–37.
18. Gakis G, Abdelhafez MF, Stenzl A. The "I-Pouch": Results of a new ileal neobladder technique. Scand J Urol. 2015;49(5):400–6.
19. Skinner EC, Fairey AS, Groshen S, Daneshmand S, Cai J, Miranda G, et al. Randomized trial of Studer pouch versus T-pouch orthotopic ileal neobladder in patients with bladder cancer. J Urol. 2015;194(2):433–9.
20. Wallace DM. Ureteric diversion using a conduit: a simplified technique. Br J Urol. 1966;38(5):522–7.
21. Studer UE, Burkhard FC, Schumacher M, Kessler TM, Thoeny H, Fleischmann A, et al. Twenty years experience with an ileal orthotopic low pressure bladder substitute – lessons to be learned. J Urol. 2006;176(1):161–6.
22. Studer UE, Varol C, Danuser H. Orthotopic ileal neobladder. BJU Int. 2004;93(1):183–93.
23. Thuroff JW, Riedmiller H, Fisch M, Stein R, Hampel C, Hohenfellner R. Mainz pouch continent cutaneous diversion. BJU Int. 2010;106(11):1830–54.
24. Moon A, Vasdev N, Thorpe AC. Continent urinary diversion. Indian J Urol. 2013;29(4):303–9.
25. Fisch M, Thuroff JW. Continent cutaneous diversion. BJU Int. 2008;102(9 Pt B):1314–9.
26. Harris CF, Cooper CS, Hutcheson JC, Snyder HM 3rd. Appendicovesicostomy: the mitrofanoff procedure-a 15-year perspective. J Urol. 2000;163(6):1922–6.
27. Wiesner C, Bonfig R, Stein R, Gerharz EW, Pahernik S, Riedmiller H, et al. Continent cutaneous urinary diversion: long-term follow-up of more than 800 patients with ileocecal reservoirs. World J Urol. 2006;24(3):315–8.
28. Izquierdo-Luna JS, Norz V, Bedke J, Aufderklamm S, Amend B, Mischinger J, et al. A modified neobladder technique: the "I-pouch" - illustration of surgical approach and tricks. Urology. 2021;147:318.
29. Mischinger J, Abdelhafez MF, Rausch S, Todenhofer T, Neumann E, Aufderklamm S, et al. Perioperative morbidity, bowel function and oncologic outcome after radical cystectomy and ileal orthotopic neobladder reconstruction: Studer-pouch versus I-pouch. Eur J Surg Oncol. 2018;44(1):178–84.
30. Hautmann RE. Surgery illustrated - surgical atlas ileal neobladder. BJU Int. 2010;105(7):1024–35.
31. Hautmann RE, Egghart G, Frohneberg D, Miller K. The ileal neobladder. J Urol. 1988;139(1):39–42.
32. Steven K, Poulsen AL. The orthotopic Kock ileal neobladder: functional results, urodynamic features, complications and survival in 166 men. J Urol. 2000;164(2):288–95.
33. Stein JP, Skinner DG. Surgical atlas: the orthotopic T-pouch ileal neobladder. BJU Int. 2005;98(2):469–82.
34. Dal Moro F. Tomorrow (and surgery) never dies. Lancet. 2019;393(10172):642–4.
35. Pagano F, Artibani W, Ligato P, Piazza R, Garbeglio A, Passerini G. Vescica Ileale Padovana: a technique for total bladder replacement. Eur Urol. 1990;17(2):149–54.
36. Thuroff JW, Alken P, Riedmiller H, Engelmann U, Jacobi GH, Hohenfellner R. The Mainz pouch (mixed augmentation ileum and cecum) for bladder augmentation and continent diversion. J Urol. 1986;136(1):17–26.
37. Mitrofanoff P. Trans-appendicular continent cystostomy in the management of the neurogenic bladder. Chir Pediatr. 1980;21(4):297–305.
38. Menon M, Hemal AK, Tewari A, Shrivastava A, Shoma AM, El-Tabey NA, et al. Nerve-sparing robot-assisted radical cystoprostatectomy and urinary diversion. BJU Int. 2003;92(3):232–6.
39. Schwentner C, Sim A, Balbay MD, Todenhofer T, Aufderklamm S, Halalsheh O, et al. Robot-assisted radical cystectomy and intracorporeal neobladder formation: on the way to a standardized procedure. World J Surg Oncol. 2015;13:3.
40. Wijburg CJ, Hannink G, Michels CTJ, Weijerman PC, Issa R, Tay A, et al. Learning curve analysis for intracorporeal robot-assisted radical cystectomy: results from the EAU Robotic Urology Section Scientific Working Group. Eur Urol Open Sci. 2022;39:55–61.
41. Witjes JA, Bruins M, Cathomas R. Compérat E, Efstathiou JA, Fietkau R, et al. EAU Guidelines on Muscle-invasive and metastatic Bladder Cancer 2020. European Association of Urology Guidelines 2022 Edition. presented at the EAU Annual Congress Amsterdam 2022. Arnhem, European Association of Urology Guidelines Office; 2022.
42. Kalble T, Anheuser P, Steffens J. Serosa-lined and tapered ileum as primary and secondary continence mechanism for various catheterizable pouches. BJU Int. 2012;110(5):756–70.

43. Kalble T, Roth S. Serosa lined and tapered ileum as primary and secondary continence mechanism for various catheterizable pouches. J Urol. 2008;180(5):2053–7.
44. Kalogirou C, Schwinger M, Kocot A, Riedmiller H. Troubleshooting of failed continence mechanisms in the ileocecal pouch: operative technique and long-term results of the intussuscepted ileal nipple valve. Int J Urol. 2021;28(11):1105–11.
45. Stenzl A, Jarolim L, Coloby P, Golia S, Bartsch G, Babjuk M, et al. Urethra-sparing cystectomy and orthotopic urinary diversion in women with malignant pelvic tumors. Cancer. 2001;92(7):1864–71.
46. Cheng KW, Yip W, Shah A, Medina LG, Ghoreifi A, Miranda G, et al. Stoma complications and quality of life in patients with Indiana pouch versus appendico/neo-appendico-umbilicostomy urinary diversions. World J Urol. 2021;39(5):1521–9.

Part X

Genitourinary and Pelvic Trauma: Iatrogenic and Violent Causes (War and Civil Causes)

Surgical Reconstruction of the Urinary Tract Following Obstetric and Pelvic Iatrogenic Trauma

60

Farzana Cassim, Jan Adlam, and Madina Ndoye

Contents

Introduction	1131
Anatomy	1131
Risk Factors	1131
Epidemiology of Ureteral Injuries	1132
Obstetric Injuries	1133
Gynecological Injuries	1133
Colorectal Surgery	1134
Vascular Surgery	1134
Spinal Surgery	1134
External Thermal Injuries	1134
Urological Injuries	1134
Epidemiology of Bladder Injuries	1135
Obstetric Injuries	1135
Gynecological Injuries	1136
Vascular Surgery Injuries	1136
Colorectal and General Surgery Injuries	1136
Urological Injuries	1137
Epidemiology of Urethral Injuries	1137
Urogynecological Surgery	1137
Urethral Diverticulum Repair	1137
Urethral Dilatation	1138
Prevention	1138

F. Cassim (✉)
Division of Urology, Stellenbosch University/Tygerberg Hospital, Cape Town, South Africa

J. Adlam
Department of Obstetrics and Gynaecoogy, Stellenbosch University/Tygerberg Hospital, Cape Town, South Africa

M. Ndoye
Department of Urology, Cheikh Anta Diop University/Hospital General Idrissa Poueye, Dakar, Senegal

© Springer Nature Switzerland AG 2023
F. E. Martins et al. (eds.), *Female Genitourinary and Pelvic Floor Reconstruction*,
https://doi.org/10.1007/978-3-031-19598-3_61

Investigations 1138
  Intraoperative 1138
  Postoperative 1139

Management 1139
  Stability of the Patient 1140

Timing, Position, and Level of the Injury 1146
  Injury of the Ureter 1146
  Injury of the Bladder 1147
  Obstetric Fistulae 1148
  Injuries at Multiple Levels 1149

Extent of Injury 1149
  Mucosal Ureteral Injuries 1149
  Partial Tears 1150
  Complete Tears/Transection 1151

Partial/Complete Occlusion of the Ureter with a Suture 1151

Damage or Excision of Tissue (Ureter/Bladder/Urethra) 1152
  Ureter 1152
  Bladder 1152
  Urethra 1152

Associated Injuries 1153
  Bowel 1153
  Vagina 1155
  Vascular 1155

Timing of Presentation 1155
  Delayed Presentation 1155
  Fistula Management 1156
  Urethral Stricture Formation 1157

Mechanism of Injury 1157

Comorbidities and Functional Status 1157
  History of Previous Radiotherapy 1157

Female Genital Mutilation (FGM) 1158

Conclusion 1159

References 1159

Abstract

The pelvic organs are always placed at risk when embarking on pelvic surgery. This is due to the compact nature of the human pelvis, with limited space for visualization and maneuverability. The increasing use of minimally invasive techniques such as laparoscopy, robotic-assisted laparoscopy, and increasing versatility of endoscopy has offered a solution to the challenges of visibility and the relatively limited operative field available. However, these solutions have presented their own challenges, and we have found that there is no substitute for in-depth anatomical knowledge and extensive operative experience when dealing with pelvic pathology surgically. The ureters, bladder, and urethra are all at risk during various transabdominal and transvaginal procedures. The various surgeries involved in the development of iatrogenic urinary tract injuries will be explored. Obstetric complications involving the urinary tract and female genital mutilation will also be explored. Management options for these complications will be described, but it is important to individualize care in order to improve long-term outcomes in terms of optimal renal function, continence, sexual function, and psychological well-being.

Keywords

Iatrogenic pelvic urinary tract injuries · Obstetric urinary tract injuries · Ureteral injury · Bladder injury · Urethral injury · Strictures · Fistulae · Urinary tract repair · Female genital mutilation

Introduction

Given the proximity of the ureters and urinary bladder to other pelvic organs and vasculature, it is easy to conceptualize how these organs are injured during various surgeries – urological and non-urological. It is therefore vital to have a clear understanding of the anatomy of the pelvis in order to prevent injuries from occurring. Ideally if an injury has occurred, the surgeon has a high index of suspicion, which will facilitate early diagnosis and repair – essential for optimal patient outcome and to prevent complications later. The majority of ureteral injuries occur during gynecological surgeries (64–82%), followed by general surgery (15–26%), and then urological interventions (11–30%) [1, 2]. The rate of ureteral injuries is approximately 3% of all genitourinary injuries [1].

This chapter will deal with obstetric and iatrogenic trauma to the female urogenital system, and how it may be managed. Any pelvic surgery places the ureters and bladder at risk of injury, including obstetric, gynecological, colorectal, vascular, and urological procedures. Some of these topics may have been covered in other chapters, allowing for this chapter to provide an overview of the various urological complications that may occur. The possible injuries to the urinary tract will be explored anatomically and each section will describe the potential surgeries that may put the urinary tract at risk.

Female genital mutilation (FGM) is a devastating entity that warrants discussion as well. While it is not a classical iatrogenic injury, it should be regarded as one and its practice should be stopped with immediate effect.

Anatomy

While familiarity with normal anatomy is vital, it is those cases with abnormal anatomy that pose the highest risk. The ureters are retroperitoneal structures running posterior to the renal vasculature from the renal pelvis to the trigone of the bladder. The ureters can be injured anywhere along its 22–30 cm path.

The right ureter descends over the duodenum, lateral to the inferior vena cava, and enters the pelvis as it crosses the external iliac artery. The left ureter descends lateral to the aorta, running closely to the sigmoid colon, and enters the pelvis as it crosses the common iliac artery. Both ureters are crossed anteriorly by the ovarian vessels and uterine arteries as they approach the pelvis and reach the mid-pelvis, respectively. Following the crossing of the uterine arteries the ureters tunnel into the cardinal ligaments, 1,5–2 cm lateral to the cervix, and enters the trigone of the bladder. This area is particularly prone to injury during hysterectomy.

The ureter's outer adventitial layer contains the blood and nerve supply. The renal, ovarian, common iliac arteries, and aorta contribute to the blood supply. In the abdomen the blood supply is received medially and within the pelvis it is received laterally.

Risk Factors

General risk factors for urinary tract injuries include:

- Pelvic irradiation: Irradiated tissue is at particular risk of delayed injury and breakdown due to obliterative endarteritis resulting in inherently weakened tissue.
- Atrophic vaginal epithelium due to hypo-estrogenic states, often seen in postmenopausal women not using topical or oral hormonal

replacement therapy, is less robust and more prone to damage and erosion.
- Inadequate preoperative imaging and planning: Ultrasound, voiding cystourethrogram, CT imaging, MRU, and examination under anesthesia all play a role in the workup and management of patients with urinary tract injuries.
- Inexperienced surgeon: There is no substitute for in-depth knowledge of anatomy and adequate surgical experience under guidance prior to embarking on independent surgical practice.
- Failure to fully empty the bladder and maintain this with a transurethral catheter throughout any pelvic procedure.
- Congenital abnormalities of the ureter, for example, an ectopic ureter or ureteral duplication
- Inflammatory or fibrotic conditions such as:
  - Endometriosis
  - Pelvic infections
  - Previous pelvic surgery
  - Resection of large bulky tumors [3]

Risk factors based on the level and mechanism of injury will be discussed more thoroughly throughout this chapter as certain risk factors are injury/organ-specific.

Epidemiology of Ureteral Injuries

The types of ureteral injuries that have been documented during surgical procedures (open and increasingly laparoscopic) include [4] (Table 1):

1. **Intra-ureteral damage** occurring with aggressive ureteroscopy or thermal injury. Laparoscopic diathermy of endometriotic lesions is increasingly the cause of thermal injuries to the ureter.
2. **Ligation** occurs when a suture is placed through the ureter; this may be partial or complete. This type of injury often occurs when the ureters are mistaken for bleeding vessels or when the uterine arteries are ligated.
3. **Kinking** of the ureter occurs when tension is placed on the ureteral wall or periureteral tissue by placement of a nearby suture.
4. **Transection** of the ureter may be partial or complete and occurs with sharp injury by a scalpel or scissors. Common sites of injury include: the pelvic brim (where the vascular pedicle to the ovary is in close proximity), the broad ligament (where the uterine artery crosses the ureter), and the ureteral canal in the cardinal ligament.
5. **Resection** may be inadvertent or planned – prior imaging confirming ureteral incorporation in a nearby mass or inflammatory process may make it necessary to resect a portion of the ureter. Inadvertent resection of part of the ureter is more likely to occur when a patient is not adequately imaged preoperatively, as well as with challenging surgery and distorted anatomy as a result of the underlying disease process.
6. **Devascularization** occurs when the periureteral tissue is aggressively stripped during dissection of the ureter, or when thermal injuries are caused by activation of energy-based surgical devices (ESD) in close proximity to the ureter. Devascularization leads to ischemic necrosis, and ultimately to the formation of a fistula or stricture.
7. **Avulsion** of the ureter can occur if the ureter is forcefully retracted, the ureters are

Table 1 Classification of ureteral injuries according to Moore et al. [5]

Injury grade	Findings
1	Hematoma (contusion or hematoma without devascularization)
2	Laceration (< 50% transection)
3	Laceration (> 50% transection)
4	Laceration (complete transection with <2 cm)
5	Laceration (avulsion with >2 cm of devascularization)

Advance one grade if multiple lesions exist

especially prone to such an injury if infection, or necrosis is present.
8. **Crushing** of the ureters may occur when clamps are used blindly, often to control hemorrhage; sites of these injuries are similar to transection injury. These injuries may also result in fistula and stricture formation.
9. **Fistula formation** can occur following transection, ischemic necrosis, or perforation if the distal ureter is not in continuity or is obstructed.
10. **Stricture formation** will ultimately lead to obstruction, hydronephrosis, and renal damage.
11. A combination of injuries.

There appears to be an increase in the prevalence of ureteral injuries in higher income countries, while the prevalence in middle to lower income countries appears to be stable [6]. There is no clear explanation for this increase. However, possible explanations include the increased rate of minimally invasive pelvic procedures, and the increased rate of elective Caesarean sections in certain countries. Surgeon experience with laparoscopic surgery plays a central role in the incidence of ureteral injuries, with the incidence of ureteral injury during laparoscopic gynecological surgery being 0.5–14%. Comparatively, the documented incidence of ureteral injury during open gynecological surgery is 0.5–1.5% [6, 7]. Laparoscopic-assisted vaginal hysterectomy resulted in the highest number of ureteral complications compared to other laparoscopic gynecological procedures [8].

Obstetric Injuries

Obstetric injuries to the ureter may occur in up to 24.5% of Caesarean sections [9]. However, the average incidence of ureteral injury during Caesarean section is 0.10–0.27% [10]. These are most commonly seen involving the left ureter during Caesarean section, or during Caesarean hysterectomy. It is unclear why the left ureter seems to be at higher risk of injury. Some theories include the variable path of the distal left ureter, making it more susceptible to injury and the handedness of the surgeon – a right-handed surgeon appears to place the left ureter at greater risk of injury due to positioning [6, 11].

Injuries to the ureters are generally a consequence of urgent control of massive hemorrhage. These often occur with placement of blind hemostatic sutures to the base of the bladder and the broad ligament. Delivery of the uterus out of the abdominal cavity during closure of the hysterotomy to avoid blind hemostatic sutures has been suggested to prevent inadvertent injury [12]. Pregnancies complicated by placenta percreta are particularly challenging due to the risks for both mother and baby, and the speed with which surgery needs to be performed.

Gynecological Injuries

Predisposing factors to ureteral injury appear to be surgeries involving extensive adhesiolysis (e.g., Endometriosis excision), oncological surgeries, and low surgeon case load [13, 14].

An in-depth knowledge of anatomy, adequate preoperative evaluation and imaging, as well as certain maneuvers such as mobilizing the ureter in the infundibulopelvic (IP) ligament, skeletonizing the distal ureter, and adequate upward traction on the uterus may prevent ureteral injuries [14, 15]. If the resection margin is in close proximity to the ureters, the ureters should be dissected. The ureter can be recognized by the glistening appearance of its sheath, visualization of stimulated peristalsis and the characteristic feel on palpation. The ureter is dissected using sharp dissection, with incorporation of a generous cuff of periureteral adventitia, in order to avoid ischemic injury. Should bleeding be encountered, bipolar electrocautery should be used in the vicinity of the ureter to avoid widespread devascularization.

Preoperative ureteral stenting has previously been advocated to identify the ureters easier to avoid injury. However, a randomized control trial by Chou et al. [16] in 2009 showed no statistical difference in the rate of ureteral injury when preoperative stenting is compared with no stenting for major gynecologic surgery.

In a review by Ostrzensky [17], only 8.6% of injuries during laparoscopic surgery were identified intraoperatively. In this review, documentation of the type of ureteral injury as well as location of the injury were both poorly documented.

Colorectal Surgery

Ureteral injuries during colorectal surgery occur in 0.25–1.1% cases [18]. The colorectal procedures posing the highest risk for ureteral injury include sigmoidectomy, and proctectomy (abdominoperineal resection and low anterior resection) [19].

Risk Factors [19]	
Patient Factors	
	Advanced malignancy
	Malnutrition
	Chronic steroid use
Disease factors	
	Rectal malignancy (highest risk)
	Diverticulosis
	Crohn's disease

According to Halabi et al. [18], open surgery appears to have a higher risk or ureteral injury; however selection bias may exist if more complex cases are treated by open procedures. Conversely, Palanniapa et al. [3] found an increased number of ureteral injuries in laparoscopic colorectal cases when compared to open cases (0.66% vs. 0.15%, respectively; p = 0.007).

Vascular Surgery

Injuries of the ureter during retroperitoneal vascular surgery are rare, with an incidence of 0.65–0.87% [20]. The risk increases during repeat surgery. The injury is often missed intraoperatively and presents a few weeks postoperatively. The vascular graft may need to be removed if the urine is infected. Vascular surgery may cause an exaggerated inflammatory process to occur peri-ureterally. This may result in stricture formation, or, rarely, in fistula formation between the ureter and vasculature [21]. The commonest defect is ureteral obstruction.

Uretero-arterial fistula formation may be a delayed, albeit a rare complication of long-term ureteral stenting, pelvic malignancy, surgery, or irradiation. Only 150 cases have been described in the literature, and a high index of suspicion is needed in order to diagnose this rare but potentially life-threatening entity. Presentation is classically nonspecific, and may range from hematuria in a stable patient, to a patient with hemorrhagic shock [22].

Spinal Surgery

The incidence of ureteral injuries during spinal surgery is uncommon, yet the complications are potentially devastating [23]. Recognition of these injuries are often missed or delayed as a result of their vague presentation with sepsis and a low index of suspicion by spinal surgeons. The ureters are at greater risk during anterior approach spinal surgeries; however injuries may also occur during posterior approach procedures. Distorted anatomy from the spinal disease process and the lack of visualization of the ureter during the posterior approach may increase the risk of a ureteral injury [23].

External Thermal Injuries

With an increase in the use of energy-based surgical devices, both in open and minimally invasive procedures, there has been an increase in thermal ureteral injuries [13]. The incidence during gynecological procedures is reported as being low (0.3–2%), but with poor reporting on the cause of ureteral injuries in general, it is difficult to ascertain the true incidence [14, 17, 24].

Urological Injuries

The majority of iatrogenic ureteral injuries occur during ureterorenoscopy (with or without the use of laser lithotripsy) for the management of renal or ureteral calculi. These injuries are preventable, yet relatively easy to sustain given the narrow caliber of a non-dilated ureter. Ureteral dilatation with dilators, an access sheath, or with a rigid ureterorenoscope may cause mucosal tears due to stretching of the ureteral lumen. The effect of these tears is to cause varying degrees of stricture formation due to scarring of the ureter.

Forcibly inserting a rigid ureterorenoscope or an access sheath may cause the proximal ureter to become semifixed to the ureter, and rapid removal of the scope or sheath may cause complete ureteral avulsion. This may also occur when trying to remove a large stone fragment in a basket using force.

Laser lithotripsy may also cause internal thermal injuries. The resultant burn may be mucosal, deeper, or completely through the ureter. Meticulous use of a laser by an experienced endoscopist is essential to prevent these injuries. Traxer and Thomas developed a grading system for ureteral injuries secondary to endoscopy in 2013 (Table 2) [25]. The injuries range from Grade 0 to Grade 4, with Grade 1 and 2 being regarded as low-grade injuries, and Grades 3–5 being high grade. Their study found that no patients in their center experienced a Grade 4 injury (ureteral avulsion). Karakan et al. had similar findings in their study, with no Grade 4 injuries [26]. The commonest injury is Grade 0 (69.4%), with grade 1, 2, and 3 occurring to a lesser extent (16.4%, 11.2%, and 2.7%, respectively) [26].

Percutaneous nephrolithotomy also places the proximal ureter at risk; large stone fragments can be pushed into the proximal ureter, and the ultrasonic lithotryptor or laser fiber being used on calculi in the renal pelvis may inadvertently damage the proximal ureter. Again, these injuries vary from small tears to through-and-through injuries with urine leaks and later stricture formation.

Table 2 Classification of ureteral wall injuries secondary to endoscopy [25]

Injury grade	Endoscopic findings
0	No lesion or only mucosal petechiae
1	Ureteral mucosal erosion without smooth muscle injury
2	Ureteral wall injury, including mucosa and smooth muscle, with adventitial preservation (periureteral fat not seen)
3	Ureteral wall injury, including mucosa and smooth muscle, with adventitial perforation (periureteral fat seen)
4	Total ureteral avulsion

Epidemiology of Bladder Injuries

Obstetric Injuries

Bladder injuries occur with increased frequency in patients who have undergone a previous Caesarean Section (C/S) or laparotomy for another pelvic procedure [27]. This is due to scarring and adherence of the dome of the bladder to the lower segment of the uterus. Surgical experience plays an important role in the prevention of bladder injuries during C/S. Failure to place a transurethral catheter preoperatively also places the bladder at significant risk during C/S. However, placement of a transurethral catheter alone is not adequate to prevent the occurrence of a bladder injury; meticulous surgical technique and careful dissection of the bladder off the uterus remains the most important measure to be taken.

If a bladder injury is sustained, it should ideally be identified and managed immediately during the Caesarean Section. A difficult dissection during the procedure with concomitant macroscopic hematuria should alert the surgeon to the possibility of a bladder injury. This suspicion should lead to an intraoperative cystogram under fluoroscopic guidance, instillation of dilute methylene blue intravesically, or a cystoscopy performed prior to closing the abdomen. It is important to note that Bonney's blue should not be used as a substitute for methylene blue due to the high ethanol content, causing it to be toxic to urothelium and placing the bladder at high risk of chemical cystitis [28].

In the case of a delayed presentation, the patient may present with either an intraperitoneal urine leak, or a vesicovaginal fistula. The upper tracts must be assessed due to the risk of concurrent ureteral injury.

Prolonged labor with poor access to health care services results in obstetric fistula formation [29]. While these injuries are rare in the developed world, they are more prevalent in developing countries where the health burden in general is already strained. Obstetric fistulae can be severe due to ischemia caused by the impacted fetal head against the pelvic outlet. The result may be circumferential fistulae with bladder neck and urethral tissue loss, extensive vaginal fibrosis, and also a rectovaginal fistula. The ureteral orifices may be visible on the edge of the damaged bladder wall. Education, family planning, and improved systemic infrastructure to offer better access to health care are needed to decrease the rate of obstetric fistulae.

Gynecological Injuries

Wong et al. [31] noted that bladder injuries were three times more likely to occur than ureteral injuries during gynecological procedures (0.24%, 95% CI 0.22–0.27 vs. 0.08%, 95% CI 0.07–0.10). As for ureteral injuries, laparoscopic hysterectomy (1.8%, 95% CI 1.2–2.6) and laparoscopically assisted vaginal hysterectomy (1.0%, 95% CI 0.9–1.2) had the highest rates of bladder injury. Adhesiolysis appeared to result in the highest rates of bladder injuries as opposed to electrosurgery; ureteral injuries are more commonly due to electrosurgery. If not identified and appropriately managed intraoperatively, bladder injuries during hysterectomy have a high risk of leading to vesicovaginal fistula formation (Fig. 1).

Other gynecological procedures that may result in a bladder injury include incontinence and pelvic organ prolapse (POP) procedures. Sacrocolpopexy (open or minimally invasive) involves the dissection of the bladder off the anterior vaginal wall to facilitate mesh placement. This plane may not always be clear, as in the case of patients with recurrent POP after a previous vaginal procedure. Over time, the mesh may also extrude into the bladder causing recurrent urinary tract infections (UTIs) and the formation of bladder calculi.

The placement of retropubic or pubovaginal slings may also result in bladder perforation with the trochar or Stamey needle that is used for these procedures. The reported rates of perforation during mid-urethral sling placement range from 4% to 9% [32]. Technical nuances of the procedure can decrease the likelihood of a bladder perforation, such as ensuring that the bladder is empty at the beginning of the procedure and asking the surgical assistant to place a cystoscope or a transurethral catheter on an introducer into the bladder and manually diverting the bladder away from the path of the trochar. These methods do not guarantee that the bladder will not be injured, but they do mitigate the risk of injury. It is important to perform a cystoscopy after sling insertion to assess the bladder and bladder neck area and thereby ensuring that the bladder has not been perforated. A 70° lens offers the best visualization of the area around the bladder neck.

Vascular Surgery Injuries

Bladder injuries are extremely rare during vascular procedures. Only a handful of cases have been reported, where the graft inadvertently traverses the bladder. This may present early or late after the surgery. Delayed presentation may be with recurrent UTIs, urinary incontinence, or most commonly with macroscopic hematuria [33].

Colorectal and General Surgery Injuries

Abdominal surgical procedures have a relatively low incidence of associated bladder injury. Colorectal procedures are clearly the most likely to have associated bladder complications due to the

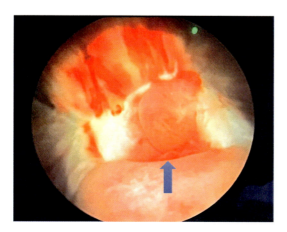

Fig. 1 Cystoscopic image showing a supratrigonal VVF

proximity of the involved organs. Malignancies infiltrating or abutting the bladder need to be thoroughly assessed preoperatively in order to plan a combined approach to management. Inadvertent bladder injury during colorectal surgery has an incidence of <1% [34]. It is important to assess for concomitant ureteral involvement in these cases.

Herniorrhaphy also has an associated risk to the bladder due to undiagnosed sliding hernias. These are more common in the pediatric male population where protrusion of the bladder through the internal inguinal ring has an incidence of 9% in infants under the age of 6 months [35].

Case reports of bladder injury during port insertion for laparoscopic appendicectomy can be found in the literature; however it is uncommon and easily avoidable.

Urological Injuries

The commonest urological bladder injury is due to perforation during bladder tumor resection. Tumors overlying the obturator area pose the greatest risk due to sudden hip adduction causing jerking of the resectoscope. This is prevented by competent surgical skill, anatomical understanding, and by use of electrical coagulation only when the patient is under deep general anesthesia with adequate neuromuscular blockade. The injury is usually extraperitoneal, although it is still necessary to exclude an intraperitoneal injury as the management for these injuries differ.

Patients with prolonged bladder outlet obstruction (prostatic pathology, strictures, or neurogenic bladder) causing bladder diverticula, as well as those with anatomically altered bladders as in the case of a bladder augmented with bowel are at risk of iatrogenic bladder rupture with aggressive transurethral catheterization [36]. Bladder instillations or manual bladder washouts with excessive pressure may also cause bladder rupture in a patient with an underlying bladder abnormality. In countries with a high prevalence of tuberculosis, spontaneous bladder rupture or rupture after minimal force (blunt trauma or during a gentle bladder washout) may indicate underlying urogenital tuberculosis. Biopsy of the rupture site during closure should be sent for histology to exclude malignancy, as well as TB culture. These incidents are rare.

Open and laparoscopic urological procedures rarely result in unplanned bladder injury.

Epidemiology of Urethral Injuries

Urogynecological Surgery

Given the proximity of the urethra and the vagina, it is understandable that urogynecological procedures carry a risk of urethral injuries. The rate of urethral injuries is <1% [37]. Patients who have undergone previous vaginal procedures are at greater risk due to local scarring and distortion of tissue planes.

Urethrovaginal fistulae are largely due to urogynecologic procedures in the developed world, with up to 70% of injuries being attributed to urethral diverticulectomy, anterior colporrhaphy, and anti-incontinence surgery [38]. The latter is associated with the greatest incidence of urethrovaginal fistula formation, which may occur due to a missed intraoperative urethral injury or para-urethral damage during the procedure, increasing the risk of mesh erosion and fistula formation. Conversely the leading cause of urethral tissue loss in developing countries is obstetric complications following obstructive and neglected labor.

Incontinence procedures such as synthetic or autologous sling placement may have associated urethral or bladder injuries with incorrect trochar positioning or due to periurethral scar tissue. The proximal urethra and bladder neck are at significantly greater risk than the bladder dome.

Urethral Diverticulum Repair

The urethra must be opened in order to excise the os of the diverticulum. However, extensive urethral damage may be caused by inexperienced surgeons performing diverticulectomy. The larger the diverticulum, the greater the risk. Saddle type diverticula pose the greatest risk not only to the urethra, but also to the dorsally placed external urethral sphincter. Recurrent sepsis in the area also results in scar tissue that may render the surgery more challenging.

Urethral Dilatation

Historically, urethral dilatation was used to manage most urinary complaints in women. With growing interest in female health, and increased publications on conditions such as primary bladder neck dysfunction, there is a greater understanding that there are very few acceptable indications for urethral dilatation in women. The dilatation may cause microtears in the urethral mucosa, resulting in long-term scarring requiring repeated dilatations. This ultimately increases the risk of iatrogenic urethral stricture formation and resultant bladder outlet obstruction (BOO). Approximately 2.7–8.0% of women experiencing lower urinary tract symptoms have BOO [39]. The BOO is caused by urethral strictures in 4–18% of these patients. Due to the rarity of urethral strictures in women, and the fact that the initial treatment for lower urinary tract symptoms is often urethral dilatation, it isn't always clear if the BOO is indeed iatrogenic, or due to an underlying pathology [36].

Prevention

While it is ideal to prevent injuries to the urogenital tract, it is not always possible. Several steps may be taken in order to facilitate prevention of iatrogenic injuries. A thorough history and preoperative examination is the first, and most essential step in managing any patient. Patients undergoing any form of surgery often also undergo radiological investigations. All of these findings must be assessed holistically, and as part of a multidisciplinary team if deemed complex and involving surrounding structures. Meticulously planned surgeries carry a lower risk of complications and iatrogenic injuries.

It is imperative to empty the urinary bladder prior to performing any pelvic or vaginal procedures to decrease the risk of bladder perforation. A transurethral catheter should be left in situ for the duration of the procedure, and it is important to confirm that it is draining optimally throughout the surgery.

Respecting tissue planes, and the use of sharp dissection (as opposed to blunt dissection and uncontrolled stripping of tissue), especially when mobilizing the bladder off the vagina and cervix (transabdominal or transvaginal), decrease the risk of inadvertent bladder injury.

For the prevention of ureteral injuries, preoperative placement of a ureteral stent may be useful, but this is not always the case. Several studies have shown no difference in the rate of ureteral injuries during gynecological surgery whether the patient was stented preoperatively or not. In a series of 145 complex laparoscopic surgeries published by Redan, in which illuminated or lighted ureteric stents were used, no ureteral injuries occurred [40]. The use of these stents should however be balanced against the risks or ureteral stenting and the additional costs incurred.

Intraoperatively, an experienced surgeon and sound knowledge of the anatomy are extremely important factors. Early identification of the urinary tract aides in its protection.

Investigations

Intraoperative

Cystoscopy and retrograde pyelography should be performed immediately if there is a suspicion of a bladder or ureteral injury that is not visible to the naked eye. An intraoperative voiding cystourethrogram (VCUG) may be useful to exclude a bladder injury. In the event that neither of these options is immediately available, instillation of dilute methylene blue via the transurethral catheter may exclude or confirm the presence of a bladder injury intraoperatively. Without cystoscopy, an injury may still be missed by using only the alternative investigations.

Importantly, cystoscopy, VCUG, and instillation of methylene blue into the bladder cannot be used to exclude a ureteral injury. Should there be any suspicion of a ureteral injury, retrograde pyelography should be performed. Indigo carmine or sodium fluorescein may be injected intravenously to identify any obvious ureteral defects as they discolor the urine and allow easier identification of ureteral injuries. Sodium fluorescein is somewhat more readily available, given its widespread use for ophthalmological assessment. Twenty-five milligrams of 10% intravenous sodium fluorescein (0.25 mL) is injected intravenously and the surgeon either watches the suspected injury site or the ureteral orifice via cystoscopy (or both simultaneously). The urinary jet is discolored green, facilitating visualization of any ureteral openings (normally positioned or in the location of the injury) [41]. Intravenous methylene blue and indocyanine green have also been used to visualize the ureters intraoperatively [42].

Postoperative

If there is any suspicion of an injury to the urinary tract, the patient should be investigated without delay. If the creatinine is normal, a CT intravenous pyelogram (IVP) with or without a high-pressure cystogram is the investigation of choice. A cystogram is unnecessary if there is no suspicion of a bladder injury. If CT facilities are unavailable, a traditional IVP may be performed. If the patient has abnormal renal function, or if neither CT IVP nor traditional IVP is possible, the minimum investigations would be an ultrasound to assess for hydronephrosis, followed by a retrograde pyelogram. These investigations allow for the identification of an injury, as well as delineating the extent and position of the injury. This step is essential for planning the approach to the management of the injury as the options include conservative management, minimally invasive options, or definitive repair.

Management

Despite the mechanism or complexity of injury, the basic underlying principles to manage iatrogenic injuries to the urinary tract remain universal. A tension-free water-tight repair is ideal, but, failing this, more complex reconstructive techniques may be used. Factors influencing the approach include:

- Stability of the patient.
- The position and level of the injury:
  – Ureter (proximal or distal)
  – Bladder
  – Urethra and bladder neck
  – Multiple levels of injury
- The extent of the injury:
  – Mucosal ureteral injuries
  – Partial or complete tears (transection)
  – Partial or complete occlusion of the ureter (tie or suture)
  – Damage or excision of a larger part of the organ involved
- Associated injuries:
  – Bowel
  – Vagina
  – Vascular
- Timing of presentation
  – Immediate (intraoperatively)
  – Early postoperatively
  – Late postoperatively, which is further influenced by the type of presenting complication:
    Hydronephrosis
    Pain
    Nonfunctioning kidney
    Ureteral stricture
    Urethral stricture with bladder outlet obstruction (partial or complete)
    Renal dysfunction
    Fistula (bladder/ureter/urethra to vagina/uterus/bowel)
- The mechanism of injury:
  – Sharp injury
  – Tear
  – Crush injury
  – Thermal injury (internal/external)
  – Ureteral stricture formation (delayed presentation)
- Comorbid disease and degree of functional impairment:
  – Indication for index surgery
  – Performance status (e.g., ECOG score)
  – Life expectancy
- History of previous radiotherapy

Depending on these factors, management options range from conservative to minimally invasive to genitourinary reconstruction, and in extreme cases, nephrectomy and/or urinary diversion.

Conservative management of a bladder injury with urethral catheter drainage alone may be attempted if the injury is extraperitoneal, small, and identified early postoperatively. Some suggest that in a patient with a vesicovaginal fistula diagnosed early, conservative management may be attempted if the patient is dry on a transurethral catheter. The catheter may then be kept in situ for several weeks. Cystography should be performed after 4 weeks and prior to catheter removal to assess for closure of the fistula. Persistent leakage beyond 4 weeks will need to be repaired surgically. Bladder neck and urethral injuries should not be managed conservatively due to the high rate of failure of this method, the risk of sepsis with ongoing urine leak, and poor long-term healing with scar tissue and stricture formation.

During the course of this chapter, we see that bowel, primarily ileum, is an important tool in the armamentarium of the Reconstructive Urologist. It is therefore important to understand the contraindications to the use of bowel in the urinary tract [43]. These include:

- Inflammatory bowel disease
  - Crohn's Disease
- Short or other bowel pathology
- Inability or unwillingness to perform self-catheterization
- Renal failure (GFR < 60 ml/min/1.73m^2)

Stability of the Patient

Injuries identified intraoperatively in a stable patient may potentially be repaired immediately. However, if the patient is unstable, it requires intraoperative inotropic support, or in patients with comorbidities associated with poor outcomes, it may be prudent to perform a temporizing procedure and return for definitive repair once the patient has been optimized. The aim of these temporizing procedures is to achieve maximal urinary drainage. This will not only prevent urinary leakage and subsequent renal dysfunction, but also improve the outcome of the definitive procedure.

Temporizing Procedures Include

- For ureteric injuries:
  - Ureteral stent insertion
  - Ligation of the injured ureter and subsequent nephrostomy tube insertion
  - Ureterostomy in situ with or without perinephric tube placement and formal repair at a later stage. This is usually done over a ureteral tube, which is tied to the distal ureter and brought out to the skin to allow drainage of the ureter
  - Cutaneous ureterostomy (less likely to be an option) – requires adequate ureteral length to be brought out directly to skin
- For bladder injuries:
  - Usually an attempt at repair is made in the initial setting
- For urethral injuries:
  - Suprapubic tube insertion
  - Should ideally be repaired without delay

If the patient's general status remains unchanged or if the injury is deemed to be irreparable, these temporizing procedures may evolve into the definitive procedure.

Types of and Principles of Definitive Ureteral Repairs

Ureteroureterostomy – Primary Ureteral Anastomosis (Fig. 2)

1. The ureter is mobilized without compromising its vascular supply, in order to obtain adequate length for a tension-free anastomosis
2. Both the proximal and distal edges of the injured ureteral segments are resected to ensure that viable tissue is anastomosed
3. Both ends are spatulated (if >50% transection)
4. The anastomosis is performed with interrupted, absorbable sutures over a ureteral stent
5. A drain should be placed at the anastomosis site

Fig. 2 Spatulated ureteroureterostomy

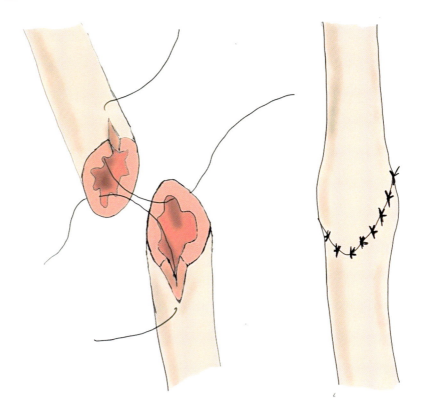

6. The anastomosis site is closed, ideally by closing the retroperitoneum, however if this is not feasible the anastomosis should be isolated by an omental flap

Ureteroneocystostomy – Ureteral Reimplantation
- Intravesical approach – Politano_Leadbetter (Fig. 3) [44]
  - The ureter enters the bladder superiorly, is tunneled under the mucosa and anastomosed directly to the bladder mucosa with interrupted absorbable sutures
  - The submucosal "flap valve" prevents reflux
- Extravesical approach – Lich-Gregoir (Fig. 4) [44]
  - The detrusor is incised and a trough is created for the ureter. The ureter is anastomosed to the mucosa and the trough is closed
  - This procedure also prevents reflux

Psoas Hitch and Ureteral Reimplantation
1. The bladder is mobilized on the ipsilateral and contralateral sides of the injury to facilitate a tension-free anastomosis
2. Cystostomy is performed on the anterior wall of the bladder
3. The bladder is anchored to the psoas tendon with nonabsorbable sutures
4. The ureter is reimplanted
5. The cystostomy is closed with absorbable suture
6. Ureteral and urethral catheters are left in place
7. The reimplantation site is drained

Boari Flap (with Psoas Hitch) (Fig. 5)
1. The bladder is mobilized on the ipsilateral and contralateral sides of the injury to facilitate a tension-free anastomosis
2. The bladder is distended with saline and the flap is marked with a sterile marker
   a. Rectangular flap is created on the anterior surface

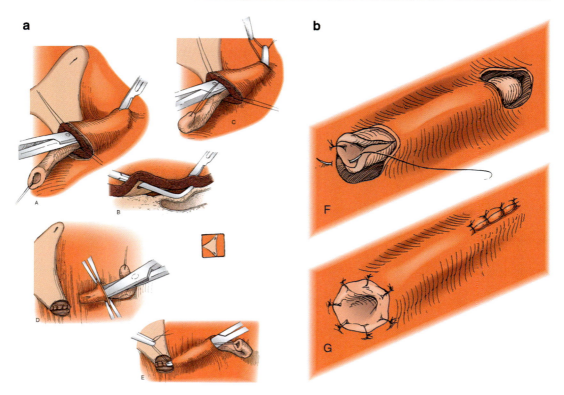

Fig. 3 Politano-Leadbetter Ureteroneocystostomy. (**a**) Mobilization of the ureter (intra- and extravesical) (**b**) Creation of submucosal tunnel and repositioning of the ureteral orifice

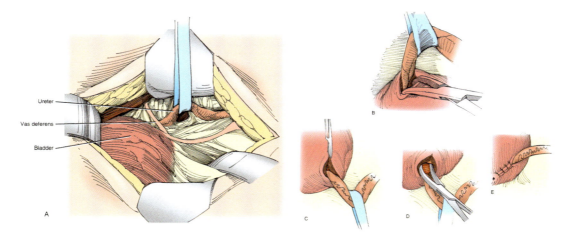

Fig. 4 Lich-Gregoir Ureteroneocystostomy. (**a**) Extravesical mobilization of the ureter. (**b**) Creation of tunnel

   b. The blood supply is preserved by ensuring a base of at least 4 cm and careful preservation of the superior vesical artery

3. The flap is sutured to the psoas tendon with nonabsorbable sutures
4. The ureter is tunneled through the proximal portion of the flap, creating a neo-orifice

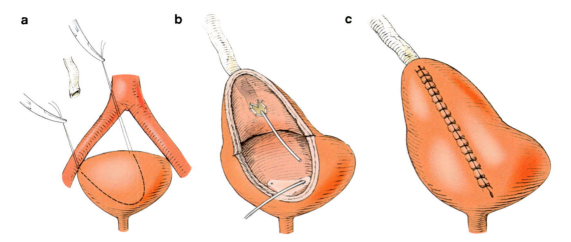

Fig. 5 Boari flap. (**a**) Marking of the flap after bladder mobilization. (**b**) Tunneling of the ureteral end into the bladder flap. (**c**) Bladder closure [45]

5. The bladder flap is tubularized with running absorbable sutures
6. The distal ureter is anastomosed to the flap using running absorbable suture – an end-to-side anastomosis with the creation of a submucosal tunnel in the bladder flap is done to decrease stricture rates and risk of vesicoureteral reflux
7. The anastomosis is stented and the site is drained
8. An indwelling transurethral catheter is placed

Transureteroureterostomy

An anastomosis between ureters is created, where the injured ureter crosses the midline to reach the contralateral ureter. This is only feasible if the patient does not have a history of renal stones and has a functioning contralateral kidney (Fig. 6).

1. Both ureters are mobilized, to ensure a tension-free anastomosis
2. The recipient ureter should not be angulated in order to reach the donor ureter
3. The donor ureter is spatulated
4. Stay sutures are placed in the recipient ureter
5. The anastomosis is preformed between the stay sutures with running absorbable suture with the knot on the outside of the posterior wall
6. The anastomotic site is drained

Autotransplantation

The injured ureter and ipsilateral kidney are moved to an ectopic site (e.g., Iliac fossa). This procedure should only be considered if no other options exist or if the contralateral kidney is poorly functioning or absent.

Ileal or Appendiceal Interposition Graft

As with autotransplantation this approach is only considered if no other options are feasible. The ileum is the preferred graft and the surgical technique is similar to the techniques used for the creation of an ileal conduit. The proximal and distal segments of the injured ureter are mobilized and an ureteral-ileal anastomosis is performed with absorbable sutures. The Yang-Monti technique (Fig. 7) is classically used in this setting. The required segment of bowel is measured, excised, detubularized, sutured together in a manner to cause narrowing of the caliber of the segment, and anastomosed primarily to the normal ureter over a ureteral stent. This procedure allows for longer strictures to be managed without replacing the entire ureter.

In the event that there is a pan-ureteral stricture with a functioning kidney, the entire disease portion must be excised. A segment of ileum is then placed from the renal pelvis to the bladder. This allows for drainage. A glomerular filtration rate of >60 ml/min/$1.73 m^2$ is required to make this a

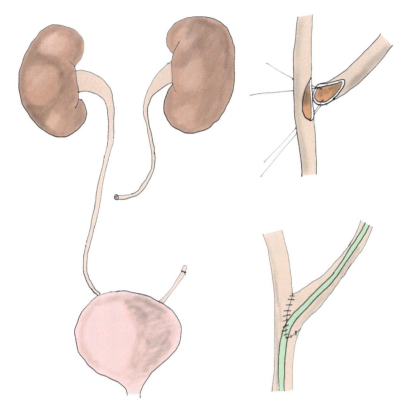

Fig. 6 Transureteroureterostomy

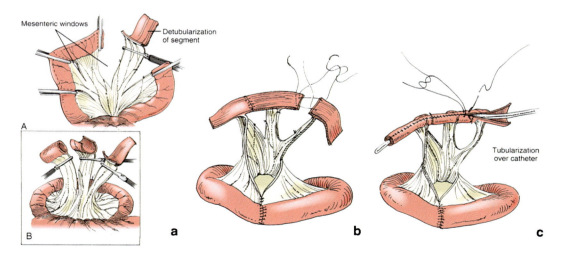

Fig. 7 Yang-Monti procedure. (**a**) Isolation of bowel (ileum) segments and detubularization. (**b**) Attachment of bowel segments to each other. (**c**) Tubularization over a catheter [46]

feasible option as there is an increased risk of a hyperchloremic hypokalemic metabolic acidosis and over the long term, renal failure.

Types of and Principles of Definitive Bladder Repairs

Primary bladder closure is a good option for simple incisions, tears, or partial excision of the bladder dome. Closure using one or two layers of absorbable sutures with adequate bladder drainage is generally enough to manage bladder injuries. A Transurethral catheter for 7–14 days may be sufficient to facilitate drainage and subsequent healing of the bladder repair. However, with extensive injuries or suspicion of tissue devascularization or a severe inflammatory response in close proximity to the bladder repair, one would also consider inserting a suprapubic cystostomy.

A covering wound drain (penrose, corrugated or closed-unit drain on free drainage) is useful to identify urinary leaks secondary to wound breakdown. Should the drain output increase dramatically, or not improve over 48–72 h, the effluent should be sent for assessment of fluid creatinine levels. Should the level be significantly higher than serum creatinine levels, then the effluent is most likely to be urine. A creatinine level that correlates with serum creatinine does not always exclude a urine leak due to the ability of the peritoneum to allow free passage of certain particles, thereby facilitating the equilibration of drain and serum creatinine levels over time.

More complex bladder injuries where surrounding structures may be involved are discussed elsewhere in this chapter. Trigonal involvement necessitates ureteral reimplantation and a thorough examination under anesthesia to exclude an associated rectal injury in a patient who has had a total hysterectomy.

Should a large portion of the bladder be excised, one needs to consider the value of attempting a primary repair compared to an ileocystoplasty or an ileal conduit. It is acceptable to attempt a primary repair in the acute setting, and reassessing the functional bladder capacity after 6 weeks once the inflammatory process is complete. Should the bladder capacity be suboptimal and causing a poorer quality of life for the patient, reconstructive or diversion options may be explored.

Augmentation Ileocystoplasty [43]

1. A standard lower midline incision is used (a Pfannenstiel incision may be used, but may limit vision in the operative field)
2. The terminal ileum is identified at the ileocecal junction
3. The terminal ileum is spared, with a 20–40 cm segment (starting 15–20 cm from the ileocecal junction) being harvested on a pedicle
4. Continuity of the remaining bowel is restored and mesenteric defects are closed
5. The bowel segment is detubularized using cautery or cold knife incision on the antimesenteric side
6. This segment is then sutured to the bladder with an absorbable suture, ensuring a spherical shape to optimize bladder function
7. A suprapubic tube is brought out through the native bladder tissue and externalized to allow maximal drainage
8. A catheterizable augmentation ileocystoplasty may also be performed using the cecum for the bladder augmentation and a small section of the terminal ileum (refashioned) to form a catheterizable stoma (Fig. 8)

Ileal Conduit (Wallace 2 Technique)

There are several techniques that may be used. Only one is described here, but the operating surgeon should perform the technique with which they have the most experience.

1. Steps 1–4 are as for augmentation ileocystoplasty, except that the bowel segment harvested should be as short as possible to avoid redundancy
2. The bowel is not detubularized
3. The distal ureters are identified, dissected out, clamped, cut, and ligated as close to the bladder as possible
4. A tunnel is made in the mesentery at the level of the sacral promontory
5. The left ureter is passed to the right via this tunnel (for a right-sided conduit)

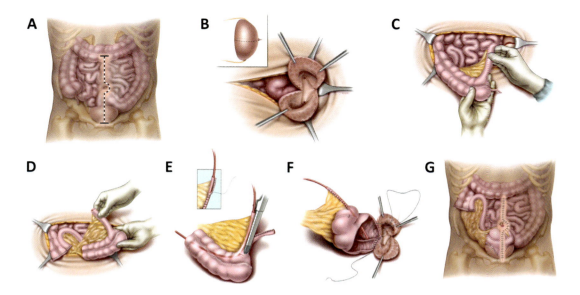

Fig. 8 Catheterizable augmentation ileocystoplasty. (**a**) Midline laparotomy. (**b**) Bivalved bladder. (**c**) Cecum, terminal ileum and appendix mobilized. (**d**) Cecum and terminal ileum stapled. (**e**) Refashioning of terminal ileum into catheterizable stoma with supporting second layer. (**f**) Cecum opened and sutured to bladder. (**g**) Closure of laparotomy with stoma brought out in an infra-umbilical position [47]

6. The ureters are spatulated, and one side wall of each ureter are sutured to each other
7. This is then sutured to the ileal segment
8. The distal opening of the ileal segment is brought through the anterior abdominal wall through an opening that can comfortably admit two fingers
9. The stoma is matured with absorbable sutures and the abdomen is closed

Timing, Position, and Level of the Injury

Injury of the Ureter

The timing of identification of the injury (intraoperatively vs. immediately postoperatively vs. delayed presentation) has a significant impact on the management options. The positioning of the injury (proximal vs. distal) also plays a role due to the blood supply to the ureter as described previously.

Injuries identified intraoperatively at the time the injury occurred allows for the option of immediate definitive repair over a ureteral stent. If the patient is stable, and the injury is reparable (a short defect with a well-perfused ureter), then positioning and extent of the injury are the next points to consider. The injury should be graded using Moore's system.

Proximal/Upper Ureter

Injuries involving the ureter from the uteropelvic junction to the upper border of the sacroiliac joint, as well as those in the mid-ureter (which extends from the upper border to the lower border of the sacroiliac joint), should ideally be repaired primarily over a ureteral stent. Grade 2 and 3 injuries may simply be approximated. Debridement of the edges may be necessary to optimize ureteral health and healing. Grade 4 injuries require spatulation (with or without debridement as necessary) and ureteroureterostomy if sufficient length can be mobilized for primary repair without tension. The ureter should not be mobilized in its entirety to avoid further devascularization and breakdown of the repair. Care must also be taken to ensure that the ureter is not stripped of all adventitial tissue in order to preserve its delicate blood supply. Fine, absorbable sutures such as 4.0 or 5.0 polyglycolic acid sutures are used. The risk of calculus formation on a nonabsorbable suture precludes its use in urothelial tissue.

Should the injury be more extensive whereby there is significant loss of part of the ureter (Grade 5 injury), or if a larger portion of the ureter is devascularized, then a primary tension-free anastomosis may not be possible. In this case, one has to consider if the injury is unilateral or bilateral, and if the bladder has been injured or is of normal capacity. Options would then include: use of an extensive Boari flap and psoas hitch, transureteroureterostomy, ileal, or appendiceal interposition graft, autotransplantation, or, as a last resort, a nephrectomy.

In the case of bilateral proximal ureteral injuries, options are more limited. A tension-free primary repair is ideal. If this is not possible, then one needs to consider more extensive reconstruction, such as a transureteroureterostomy and then a Boari flap and psoas hitch to the contralateral side. If the bladder is injured, or if the bladder has inadequate capacity for this procedure, then ligating the ureters and placing nephrostomy tubes is a reasonable option. One can then offer the patient delayed reconstruction of the ureters.

Distal/Lower Ureter

Injuries occurring between the inferior border of the sacroiliac joint to the ureterovesical junction are more amenable to primary repair due to the proximity to the bladder. Given the relatively poor blood supply of the distal ureters, primary ureteroureterostomy is not performed; there is a high risk of breakdown of the anastomosis. The ideal repair is a ureteral reimplantation. A modified Liche-Gregoire reimplantation has good outcomes in patients with obstetric or iatrogenic distal ureteral injuries. An anti-refluxing technique should be used in women of child-bearing age who wish to fall pregnant in the future. The risk of vesicoureteral reflux during a future pregnancy should be avoided due to the increased risk of pyelonephritis. The reimplantation may require a psoas hitch in order to achieve a tension-free repair.

Injury of the Bladder

Simple bladder dome injuries and extensive bladder resection has already been covered in this chapter.

Injuries Involving the Trigone

Injuries involving the trigone often involve surrounding structures and warrant careful assessment of the ureters, vagina, and uterine cervix or rectum in the event of a previous hysterectomy having been done. In the case of an associated:

- Ureteral injury: Ureteral reimplantation and primary bladder repair is required.
- Cervical injury: The patient's future fertility desires should be considered. These injuries can be complicated to repair, and a hysterectomy may be considered. When a primary bladder and cervical repair is attempted there is a significant risk of vesicocervical fistula formation. This can be avoided by interposing omentum or peritoneum between the bladder and cervix.
- Rectal injury: Colorectal surgeons should be involved in this repair. The development of a rectovesical fistula must be avoided. Depending on the extent, cause, and overall status of the patient, primary repair of the bladder and rectum with an interposition layer may be attempted. A covering loop colostomy may be considered if deemed necessary by the colorectal team. This is not always the case and primary repair may be enough.

Injuries of the Urethra and Bladder Neck

Iatrogenic urethral injuries are rare. However, once encountered, should be repaired by a surgeon comfortable with these repairs. The female urethra is short, and the external urethral sphincter needs to be considered when attempting repair.

The commonest cause for iatrogenic urethral injury in female patients occurs during urethral diverticulectomy. The more complex and the larger the diverticulum, the higher the risk of a large urethral injury. Once this occurs, a primary watertight closure over a silicone catheter should be performed while avoiding the risk of decreasing the caliber of the urethra. A Martius flap, also known as a pedicled labial fat pad (Fig. 9) may be used to support the repair, or as an interpositional layer between the vagina and the urethra.

Obstetric Fistulae

Complex obstetric fistula involving urethral tissue loss (Fig. 10) are difficult to manage [29]. High volume centers offer these patients the best outcomes. A multidisciplinary approach is often needed to optimally manage the patient and offer cure in one sitting. Sphincteric damage is almost always present due to ischemic damage from the impacted fetal head. Therefore, urethral repair alone is not enough to manage these patients. There is often associated bladder neck injury, with complete avulsion of the bladder from the urethra, as well as distal ureteral involvement in severe cases. Concomitant vaginal shortening from scarring, as well as a rectovaginal fistula often occur.

The principles of repair include complete excision of all scar tissue, primary apposition of urothelial tissue (with ureteral reimplantation if deemed necessary), improving vaginal length, and obtaining continence [29]. All of these may not be achievable in one procedure. The use of Gracilis or Singapore flaps (Fig. 11) may aid in achieving these aims. A labial flap may be necessary to reconstruct the urethra in the case of significant urethral tissue loss with the absence of healthy vaginal tissue for a vaginal advancement flap. A pubovaginal sling is often used to offer continence in these patients. The success rate for these patients is approximately 70–80% in high volume centers [29]. The first attempt at repair is

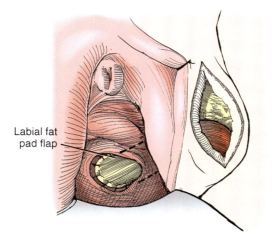

Fig. 9 Martius flap [48]

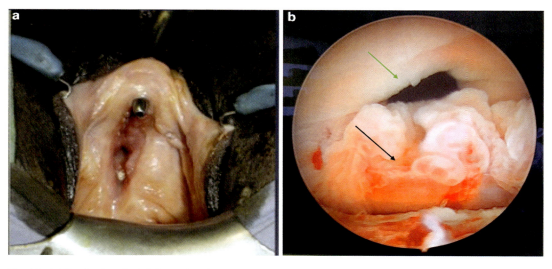

Fig. 10 (**a**) Proximal urethral defect and vaginal scarring. (**b**) Green arrow depicting bladder neck with extensive urethral tissue loss; Black arrow depicting fistula tract and inflammatory tissue

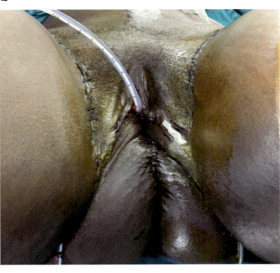

Fig. 11 (**a**) Development of bilateral Singapore flaps. (**b**) Flaps sutured to each other and onto the cervix – completed repair

the best chance to offer cure. The chances of cure decrease significantly if repeat surgery is needed. If it is not possible to reconstruct the injury, then urinary diversion is unfortunately the only option.

Bladder neck injuries, though uncommon, must be repaired as soon as they are identified. There is no role for conservative management of bladder neck injuries. These injuries are challenging to repair due to difficult accessibility. A combined transvaginal and transabdominal approach may be used. An episiotomy may help to improve with transvaginal access to the bladder neck.

Injuries at Multiple Levels

Injuries at multiple levels of the urinary tract must be carefully assessed and managed as a unit. The basic principles of tension-free, watertight closure and adequate drainage should be adhered to in order to ensure successful repair. Staged repairs may be considered to allow tissue healing in one area before repairing the next. Individualized management plans should be made for patients with complex multilevel injuries.

Extent of Injury

Mucosal Ureteral Injuries

Mucosal tears can be avoided by not manually dilating the ureter prior to ureteroscopy, along with gentle manipulation of the ureteroscope within the ureter. It is important not to proceed if there is any resistance to the passage of the ureteroscope. The same applies when passing an access sheath prior to flexible ureteroscopy. Stenting for 48–72 h prior to ureterorenoscopy allows for interruption of ureteral peristalsis and adequate vital dilatation of the ureter, which facilitates atraumatic ureteroscopy.

Stone extraction using a basket device may also result in ureteral mucosal damage and long-term stricture formation should any force be used during stone removal. Lithotripsy and ensuring that the fragments are small enough to be extracted without any tension are basic principles to be followed. This decreases the risk of mucosal injury. Mucosal injuries are graded according to the extent of injury as noted previously.

Mucosal injuries and perforation of the ureter may also be sustained during laser lithotripsy. It is key to ensure that an experienced endoscopist is performing the procedure in order to avoid these injuries. During training, an experienced surgeon should be present, guiding the trainee to avoid serious ureteral injuries. The operating surgeon should be comfortable performing basic ureteroscopy prior to embarking on using the laser within the ureter.

Smaller injuries may simply be observed, whereas more extensive mucosal damage should be managed by the passage of a ureteral stent to allow healing of this area. The damaged area may still heal with fibrosis and subsequent stricture formation. It is for this reason that patients with mucosal tears must always be followed up after stent removal with at least a renal ultrasound, and possibly a diuresis renogram to assess for obstruction to the ureter.

Partial Tears

Ureter

Partial injuries to the ureter are amenable to conservative management if they involve less than 50% of the ureteral diameter and are identified early. Delayed presentation makes conservative management less likely to succeed, but it may be attempted. Decisions regarding the management plan need to be individualized due to the various factors that impact on the decision to repair or not. A thermal injury often extends wider than is macroscopically visible. Conservative management may be attempted, but with caution and a low threshold to actively repair the ureter.

Conservative management entails passage of a ureteral stent under fluoroscopic guidance to ensure that a partial tear is not converted to a complete transection due to stent trauma.

The stent should be left in situ for 4–6 weeks and may then be removed. Following stent removal a retrograde pyelogram is performed. If the exam does not show an obvious ureteral stricture, a follow-up ultrasound to assess for hydronephrosis should be performed in 1–2 weeks as more subtle strictures may be missed. If hydronephrosis is present at this stage it is concerning for ureteral stricture formation and outflow obstruction. Further investigation is warranted in these cases.

One may choose to perform a diuresis renogram to assess for functional status and outflow obstruction in the affected kidney. If the overall renal function is normal, a CT abdomen with a delayed phase may be obtained to assess for anatomical and functional changes in the affected renal unit. Alternatively, one may repeat a retrograde pyelogram to assess for a ureteral stricture. If a stricture is noted, one may remove the ureteral catheter and repeat the fluoroscopy after 5–10 min to assess for adequate drainage of the affected kidney. If the kidney does not drain, a ureteral stent should be inserted and delayed definitive management should be planned. The chosen management option depends on various factors, which will be addressed later in this chapter.

Urethra

Partial injuries to the urethra occur most commonly during the insertion of slings for urinary incontinence. These should be identified intraoperatively during cystoscopy. Immediate primary repair using an absorbable suture (such as a 4.0 polyglactin suture) is warranted. A transurethral catheter is left in situ for 7–10 days to allow healing. The sling may be attempted again 6–12 weeks after healing of the injury.

Rarely a urethral injury is missed and presents at a later stage. Depending on the site of the injury, there may be total urinary incontinence (less common), or there may just be a spray of urine when voiding. Alternatively, the patient may also present with features of vaginal voiding. In this case the patient will void normally, but drips as soon as she stands up after voiding due to emptying of the vagina (paradoxical voiding). A VCUG in conjunction with cystoscopy and a careful examination under anesthesia should confirm the diagnosis. Repair should take place at 6 weeks post-injury to allow the inflammatory process to settle, thereby improving outcome.

Complete Tears/Transection

Ureter

Transection of the ureter must be repaired as soon as possible. Knowledge of anatomy and a high index of suspicion for ureteral injury will allow for early detection and repair. If the injury is above the pelvic brim, a spatulated repair over a ureteral stent using an absorbable suture should be done. The basic principles of a watertight tension-free closure should be followed in order to ensure a successful repair. If the injury is thermal, or if a portion of the ureter has been excised, then a simple end-to-end anastomosis may not be possible. The damaged area may need to be debrided, leaving a more extensive gap between the two ureteral ends. If this is the case, and an end-to-end repair is not possible, then alternative repair techniques will need to be used. These include:

- More extensive mobilization of the two ureteral ends (without devascularizing the ureter)
- Mobilizing the kidney and the proximal ureter
- Transposition of the renal vein to a lower position along with mobilization of the kidney and proximal ureter (not advised for inexperienced surgeons)
- A Boari flap and psoas hitch
- A transureteroureterostomy
- Ligation of the ureter with nephrostomy insertion and delayed definitive repair
- Yang-Monti bowel interposition
- Ileal ureter (ileal interposition)
- Renal autotransplantation
- Nephrectomy (last resort)

Bladder

The management of bladder injuries has been discussed previously in this chapter.

Urethra

Complete transection of the urethra is extremely rare. These injuries should be repaired immediately using the standard principles of a tension-free watertight repair over a transurethral catheter. The catheter may be removed 7–10 days after repair in the event of a normal peri-catheter urethrogram being performed.

Partial/Complete Occlusion of the Ureter with a Suture

The commonest scenario for this is when there is excessive bleeding in the pelvis and blind sutures are placed – seen largely during challenging Caesarean Sections. There may or may not be hematuria, and this sign can therefore not be used as a guide to exclude a ureteral injury.

If inadvertent suturing of the ureter is suspected, integrity of the ureter may be evaluated after the bleeding has been controlled by mobilizing the distal ureter, or with cystoscopy and retrograde pyelography (if the patient's hemodynamic state allows). The suture can then be removed immediately and is unlikely to cause long-lasting damage to the ureter. This option is unfortunately unsuccessful in the management of suture-related ureteral occlusion diagnosed postoperatively.

If the ureter is not evaluated intraoperatively and the surgeon suspects a possible ureteral injury, a CT IVP should be performed as soon as possible. Should there be a delay in obtaining CT imaging, then an ultrasound of the renal tract will be able to detect hydronephrosis of the affected side if the patient is well-hydrated.

Some patients may report flank pain postoperatively. This should be investigated even if there is no suspicion of a ureteral injury as they may occur without the surgeon realizing it intraoperatively. Initial investigations for these patients should include an ultrasound and serologic assessment of renal function.

If occlusion (partial or complete) of the ureter is confirmed, surgical repair should be expedited and should occur within 7–10 days of the initial surgery. The standard of care for patients with injuries that are only discovered later is to perform a temporizing percutaneous nephrostomy, followed by definitive repair in 6–12 weeks. Due to the intraperitoneal inflammatory process between 1 and 6 weeks following the injury, any definitive repair will be challenging and with a significantly higher risk of complications.

Definitive management involves ureteral reimplantation into the bladder if the occlusion occurs in the distal ureter. Should the distance from the bladder be too far for a tension-free repair, then a psoas hitch with or without a Boari flap may be required.

In the proximal ureter an end-to-end spatulated anastomosis may be performed if the blood supply seems adequate and a tension-free anastomosis is possible.

Repairs are done over a ureteral stent to allow vital dilatation of the ureter and aid in the healing process. A wound drain on free drainage is left in situ to allow drainage if there is urinary leak. A large, persistent leak warrants relook surgery as the repair has likely broken down. There is a higher risk of breakdown in the following circumstances:

- Tension on the repair
- Failure to connect mucosa to mucosa
- Stripping of the ureter resulting in compromised blood supply
- Sepsis
- Hemodynamic instability requiring inotropic support

A transurethral catheter is kept in situ for 7–10 days after a ureteral reimplantation and is removed only when a cystogram confirms that there is no anastomotic leak. After a ureteroureterostomy, the transurethral catheter may be removed after 3–5 days, but it is imperative to monitor the drain output. If the drain output remains <50 ml/24 h, the drain may be removed. If the drain output increases after removal of the transurethral catheter, this implies a leak due to secondary reflux in an incompletely healed ureter. Reinsertion of the transurethral catheter is usually adequate to allow drainage and subsequent healing of the ureter. A trial without catheter may be reattempted after another 5–7 days, or after a cystogram confirms reflux due to the stent, but no anastomotic leak.

Damage or Excision of Tissue (Ureter/Bladder/Urethra)

Ureter

Excision of a larger part of the ureter has already been covered.

Bladder

Excision of larger portions of bladder tissue may occur due to adherence to the surrounding structures as a result of previous surgery, malignancy, or an inflammatory process. The excision may be inadvertent or planned. The latter is clearly ideal, as it is possible to perform preoperative cystoscopy and examine the macroscopic extent of the disease process. This allows the surgeon to minimize tissue loss when dissecting in the region of the bladder. One may also assess the proximity of the disease process to the ureteral orifices, and can pass ureteral catheters preemptively if deemed necessary.

Once the bladder is opened, a primary repair is usually possible, as long as there is sufficient bladder volume after the closure. Primary repair may be in 1 or 2 layers using an absorbable suture such as polyglactin 2.0. A watertight closure is key to ensure healing. Adequate drainage by means of a transurethral catheter, a suprapubic cystostomy, and a wound drain is suggested.

Extensive resection of the bladder should be repaired by means of an augmentation ileocystoplasty as previously described. Prior to performing this procedure, it is necessary to check the patient's glomerular filtration rate (GFR). The GFR should be 60 ml/min/$1.73m^2$ or more, to allow any bowel being placed within the urinary system. If the GFR is below this level, or if it is unknown and suspected to be abnormal, an incontinent urinary diversion should be performed. It is possible to convert this to a bladder augmentation at a later stage and in a more controlled setting.

Urethra

Urethral injuries and/or excision are rare in female patients. The commonest cause for extensive urethral damage is a prolonged second stage of labor.

The basic principles of repair apply. If there is significant tissue loss, one must consider grafts. It is also important to measure the remaining vaginal length and assess for the position of the ureteral orifices. Due to tissue loss at the bladder neck and trigone, the ureteral orifices may be at the edge of the bladder wound (Fig. 12), necessitating ureteral

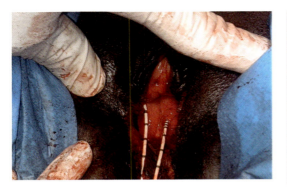

Fig. 12 Ureteral orifices at the edge of the defect

reimplantation. The ideal is to bring the ends of the urethra together primarily, without introducing other techniques. In the event of this not being possible, one may use one of the following options to repair the urethra:

- Bladder flap
- Vaginal advancement flap
- Tubularized labia minora flap
- Singapore flap
- Gracilis flap

Bladder flaps for complete urethral reconstruction are more prone to stenosis and are therefore not routinely used. Vaginal tissue may be used if healthy tissue is available. This may not always be the case, especially in patients with obstetric fistulae. Tubularized labia minora (Fig. 13) used as a pedicled flap for urethral reconstruction has a reasonable outcome in small studies. Fasciocutaneous and myofascial flaps such as the Singapore and Gracilis flaps, respectively, work exceptionally well for both urethral and simultaneous vaginal reconstruction. These pedicled flaps are relatively easy to create, and work well due to their predictable blood supply.

Should urethral reconstruction be deemed to not be feasible, or should the repair fail, the next step is a continent urinary diversion. The patient must be amenable to self-catheterize in order for this to be an option. The bladder neck is closed and a Mitrofanoff procedure may then be done. The commonest method is to perform an appendicovesicostomy (Fig. 14), with the opening either at the umbilicus, or to the right or left of the

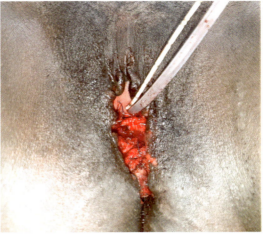

Fig. 13 Urethral reconstruction using bilateral labia minora flaps

lower abdomen (depending on the patient's handedness). If the appendix is unavailable, fallopian tube may be used. In the event that the use of the fallopian tube is also not an option, a small section of ileum may be detubularized and refashioned as with the Yang-Monti procedure to provide a catheterizable tube. Bladder tubularization has been done, but has higher rates of stenosis, and decreases the functional bladder capacity. An incontinent diversion (ileal conduit) is the last resort for these patients.

Associated Injuries

Concomitant injuries make repair of any organ more challenging. Due to the complexity of these injuries, and risk of fistula formation, adjacent viscous organs require repair simultaneously. Avoidance of overlapping suture lines and the use of omentum or peritoneum as an interpositional layer can improve the success rates of such a repair.

Bowel

Bowel injuries may be repaired primarily, with or without a covering stoma. The type of primary

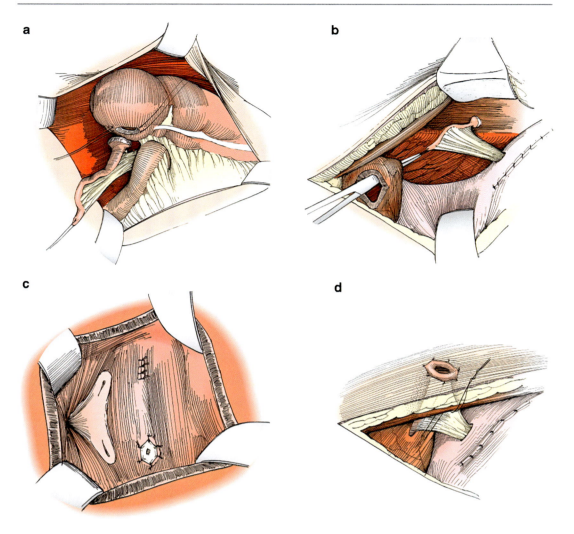

Fig. 14 Appendicovesicostomy. (**a**) Mobilization of appendix with appendiceal mesenteric pedicle. (**b**) Extraperitoneal transposition of the appendix and development of submucosal bladder tunnel. (**c**) Implantation of the appendiceal tip into the bladder mucosa, with closure of the bladder entry point. (**d**) Maturation of the appendiceal opening (proximal end) onto anterior abdominal wall [49]

repair may be simple suturing (in one or two layers), a wedge resection and primary repair, or an excision of a larger section of the bowel. Factors influencing the type of repair that is selected include:

- The portion of bowel that is injured
  - Small bowel
  - Sigmoid colon
  - Rectum
- Mechanism of injury
  - Sharp
  - Crush
  - Mesenteric devascularization
  - Thermal injury
- Extent of injury
  - Partial tear
  - Complete transection
  - Partial resection

Due to the risk of breakdown of the repair, and subsequent potentially life-threatening complications, enlisting the help of a colorectal surgeon intraoperatively is ideal. Complications include fistula formation, leakage of bowel content into the peritoneum, sepsis, necrotizing fasciitis, and death.

Vagina

Being a well-vascularized organ, the vagina heals well from the majority of injuries. Primary repair of the defect is usually performed while following the general principles mentioned previously. Healing by scarring is problematic if the scarring is severe enough to significantly decrease the vaginal caliber. Scar tissue must be excised and resultant denuded areas can be covered using Singapore or Gracilis pedicled flaps.

Vascular

The commonest site of vascular injury would be the iliac vessels – the veins being most susceptible to shearing forces during excision of pelvic masses and/or lymph nodes. Vascular injuries must be dealt with swiftly by the most experienced surgeon available due to the risk of hemorrhagic shock and death.

Timing of Presentation

Intraoperative and early postoperative presentation of obstetric and iatrogenic injuries to the urinary tract has already been discussed in this chapter.

Delayed Presentation

Ureter

Minor or partial injuries are more likely to present at a later stage. Less commonly, complete occlusion of the ureter with subsequent hydronephrosis and functional loss of the renal unit may also have a delayed presentation.

The management depends on the manner in which the patient presented. An incidental finding of a non-functioning kidney on follow-up imaging for another pathology does not warrant intervention should there be no associated complications. However, should the patient present with pain, infections, or hydronephrosis with any residual functionality (>15–20% on a MAG 3 renogram), then attempt to preserve the kidney should be made.

The first step would be to fully assess the patient clinically, with serologic markers, urine cultures, and imaging. A CT IVP (in the presence of normal renal function) is extremely useful in planning the further management of these patients. Alternatively, a retrograde pyelogram also delineates the position and extent of the injury, which has most likely resulted in stricture formation. A ureteral stent may be passed at the same time as the retrograde pyelogram, rendering it both diagnostic and therapeutic. Should stenting not be possible, or in the face of sepsis, then a retrograde pyelogram and stent placement should be avoided and a nephrostomy tube inserted to allow optimal drainage of the kidney.

Sepsis should be treated based on cultures. Furthermore, the overall functional status of the patient and life expectancy from the index pathology should be taken into account. In the event that the patient has a good functional status and life expectancy, then a temporizing procedure (ureteral stent or nephrostomy tube) should be done. Insertion of a nephrostomy tube allows the acquisition of a nephrostogram, which gives valuable anatomical information when planning the reconstruction. A repeat renogram may be considered if there is any doubt as to the functionality of the kidney.

Reconstruction may be done 6–12 weeks after the last intra-abdominal surgery that the patient underwent in order to avoid the early postoperative inflammatory effect and thereby improving the success rate of reconstruction. If the patient has a ureteral stricture, there are various options available for repair. These depend on the extent and position of the stricture. Some of the reconstructive techniques used with ureteral transection or excision apply, particularly if the stricture is short.

Simple excision of a short stricture may be carried out, with a spatulated ureteroureterostomy done over a ureteral stent with minimal ureteral mobilization or stripping. Should the stricture be longer, then other techniques for Grade 5 ureteral injuries may be employed. There are alternatives available for proximal ureteral stricture disease, namely, the Davis intubated ureterotomy with omental wrap, and buccal mucosal interposition grafting with omental wrap (Fig. 15). The former is performed endoscopically with a cold knife or laser, with an incision through the stricture laterally (proximal ureter), and subsequent ureteral stenting and wrapping with omentum. The latter procedure involves a similar approach, but with a buccal mucosal graft placed at the incision site (sutured to the ureteral incision), and wrapped in omentum.

Should the opposite be true in terms of ECOG score and life expectancy, and the patient has a poor functional status, or a very short life expectancy, then the risk of invasive surgery outweighs its benefit, and conservative management should be implemented to improve quality of life.

In countries with a high prevalence of TB, one should always exclude concomitant urinary TB prior to assuming that the stricture is purely due to an iatrogenic cause.

Fistula Management

Obstetric fistulae have been discussed earlier in this chapter, as have urethrovaginal fistulae. Vesicovaginal, rectovaginal, and ureterovaginal (as well as ureterouterine, ureterocervical, and vesicouterine) fistulae are covered in another chapter and will only be mentioned briefly. The basic principles of management include imaging (VCUG, ultrasound KUB, CT IVP, or MRU).

A three-swab test may also be carried out using intravenous indigocarmine and intravesical methylene blue with three swabs stacked in the vagina. The color and position of the wet swab directs the attending physician to the position of the fistula. A retrograde pyelogram may be considered if ureteral involvement is suspected. An examination under anesthesia and cystoscopy is also extremely

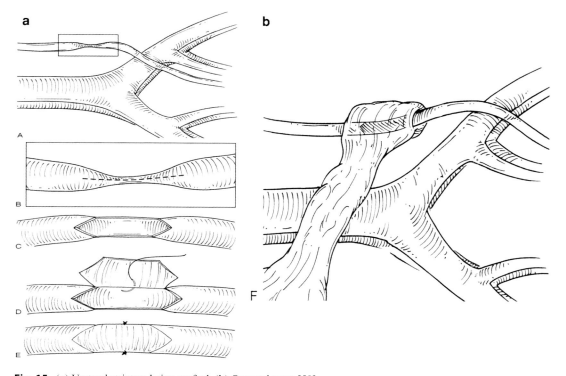

Fig. 15 (**a**) Ureteral stricture being grafted. (**b**) Omental wrap [50]

useful in order to fully assess the defect/s and plan the reconstruction.

Once the exact position is known, and concomitant injuries have been assessed, the repair may be undertaken, ideally 6–12 weeks after the index surgery. The patient should be counseled regarding the possibility of a hysterectomy, although this is not mandatory and should be avoided unless absolutely necessary. Again, the first repair has the highest chance of success. The repair may be transvaginal or transabdominal. If performed transabdominally, it may be laparoscopic, robotic-assisted, or open surgery.

The aim is to identify the fistulous tract (Fig. 16), consider excision of the tract if it will not enlarge the defect too much, repair both organs involved, and attempt to place an interpositional layer (omentum or peritoneum). Intraoperative testing and confirmation of the integrity of the bladder repair, by instilling water via the transurethral catheter, has been shown to correlate with successful repair. Adequate urinary drainage by means of a silicone transurethral catheter (and possibly a suprapubic cystostomy) should be ensured. The catheter may be removed after confirmation of complete healing by means of a VCUG after 7–14 days.

Urethral Stricture Formation

Urethral stricture formation is rare, as mentioned previously. The management may be minimally invasive with repeated urethral dilatation, and self-dilatation. This may, however, worsen the pathology and lead to long-term bladder outlet obstruction and a destroyed urethra. Urethroplasty using a buccal mucosal graft placed ventrally or dorsally has shown good outcomes for these patients. Care must be taken to not disrupt the external urethral sphincter when mobilizing for and placing a dorsal graft.

Should these options not be possible, as in the case with a pan-urethral stricture and damaged bladder neck, a continent diversion should be considered. In the event that the patient is unable or unwilling to perform self-catheterization, then an incontinent diversion such as an ileovesicostomy or ileal conduit may be considered.

Mechanism of Injury

This topic has been covered elsewhere in the chapter.

Comorbidities and Functional Status

These factors have been mentioned previously. When considering extensive reconstructive surgery, it is necessary to consider the patient's overall health and functional status. Should the patient have a poor Eastern Cooperative Oncology Group (ECOG) score or a short life expectancy, it is prudent to proceed with the least invasive procedure that will improve overall quality of life for the patient. If the patient is still of a reasonable ECOG status, then extensive reconstruction is an option. Discussion with the patient regarding possible complications and long-term outcomes of surgery must be addressed prior to proceeding.

History of Previous Radiotherapy

Radiotherapy causes damage and cell death to both normal and abnormal tissue. The resultant obliterative neovascularization that occurs leaves the residual tissue poorly vascularized. Repair of fistulae and strictures post-radiotherapy have

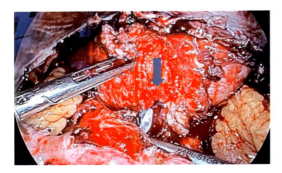

Fig. 16 Identification of the fistulous tract with a feeding tube traversing (blue arrow) between the bladder anteriorly and the vagina posteriorly

poorer success rates due to this reason. Hyperbaric oxygen therapy may be employed to improve tissue vascularity and overall health, allowing for better postoperative success rates. Meticulous patient assessment, planning, and counseling are vital in these patients due to the increased risk of complications.

Conservative management with ureteral stenting or nephrostomy tubes are fair options, depending on the underlying pathology and patient status. Urinary diversion with an ileal conduit may be done for patients with fistulae secondary to radiotherapy that are deemed irreparable. However, the tissue in these patients is often inflammatory and poorly vascularized, leaving an increased risk of complications. These include uretero-ileal stricture formation and subsequent hydronephrosis and renal dysfunction. They are also at higher risk of breakdown of the bowel anastomosis and subsequent enterocutaneous fistula formation. The ureters may be encased in fibrotic tissue, or inherently damaged and poorly vascularized, making mobilization and the formation of a diversion impossible.

Female Genital Mutilation (FGM)

A cultural practice in several regions of Africa and the Middle East, FGM involves the alteration and/or excision of parts of the female external genitalia (Table 3) [50, 51]. The most severe form of FGM is infibulation, where all the external genitalia including the labia are excised, and the vulva is sutured closed [50]. These procedures are carried out on young girls, from as young as the neonatal period. They are performed by religious leaders, midwives, or designated "circumcisers." There are no proven health benefits to FGM and it is a purely cultural ritual. Sterility and pain management are not considered during these procedures, and crying is seen to bring shame to the family [50]. In 2017, the World Health Organization (WHO) estimated that over 200 million women have been affected by FGM [52]. The practice of FGM has been nicknamed "three feminine sorrows" to symbolize the pain that the woman experiences at three main points during her lifetime: when the procedure is performed, during sexual intercourse, and during childbirth [52].

Table 3 Goh's classification of obstetric fistulae [30]

Classification	Criteria
Urethral length	
Type 1	Distal edge of fistula >3.5 cm from the external urethral meatus (EUM)
Type 2	Distal edge of fistula 2.5–3.5 cm from the EUM
Type 3	Distal edge of fistula 1.5–2.5 cm from the EUM
Type 4	Distal edge of fistula <1.5 cm from the EUM
Fistula size	
a	<1.5 cm
b	1.5–3 cm
c	>3 cm
Vaginal scarring	
I	No or mild fibrosis around the fistula/vagina and/or vaginal length > 6 cm or normal capacity
II	Moderate or severe fibrosis around the fistula and/or vagina and/or reduced vaginal length
III	Special considerations: circumferential fistula, involvement of ureteral orifices

There are both physiological and psychological complications of the procedure, and these may be short- and long-term in nature. Short-term physiological complications include sepsis, intractable pain, and hemorrhage. Type III FGM is associated with a higher rate of HIV infection, as well as Chlamydia trachomatis, Clostridium tetani, and Herpes simplex virus 2 [50].

Due to the issues surrounding reporting of complications and cultural taboo in doing so, it is difficult to accurately determine the incidence of complications secondary to FGM. The mortality rate is relatively high in the short term and is estimated to be approximately 1 in 500 circumcisions.

Scarring, keloid formation, and chronic neuralgia due to nerve entrapment occur in the intermediate to long term. Scarring may be severe and cause hematocolpos [50]. Fifteen percent of women interviewed in Sudan noted that it was necessary to undergo "cutting" in order to allow penetrative sex after a circumcision [50]. Childbirth after circumcision may be associated with significant tearing of the introitus. Perineal incision has been done for women who have undergone infibulation to facilitate safe delivery of the baby. Prolonged post-partum hospital stay and increased maternal complications have been noted. There is an increasing need for Caesarean Section in these patients. Urethral injuries may lead to long-term recurrent urinary tract infections, as well as urinary retention. These patients are also at risk of renal dysfunction.

Long-term psychosis, post-traumatic stress disorder, and anxiety disorders have been noted in these women. There is little support available to them as it is regarded to bring shame upon the family to speak about these issues [50–52].

Reconstruction is not really feasible as tissue is removed during the process of FGM. It is, however, possible to attempt to widen the residual os in order to allow drainage during menstrual cycles, improve the dyspareunia, and possibly improve on maternal outcomes during childbirth [50, 52] (Table 4).

Despite the practice of FGM being outlawed in many countries, and the declaration by the United Nations that FGM is a crime and a violation of one's basic rights, the practice continues. Advocates against the practice are rejected by their communities. It is necessary for these advocates to be supported in their endeavors to stop this destructive process.

Conclusion

Iatrogenic injury to the lower urinary tract Is a well-known complication of any surgical procedure involving the pelvic region. These injuries can be prevented with careful preoperative evaluation and preparation, meticulous attention to proper surgical technique, and knowledge of pelvic anatomy.

A high index of suspicion should allow intraoperative discovery with careful inspection, cystoscopy, or from concern of the proximity of suture, ligation, or thermal energy use. When an injury is identified intraoperative repair or a temporizing procedure should be done in order to avoid future morbidity, complications, and urogenital fistula formation.

References

1. Ledderose S, Beck V, Chaloupka M, Kretschmer A, Strittmatter F, Tritschler S. Management of ureteral injuries. Urologe. 2019;58(2):197–206.
2. Gild P, Kluth LA, Vetterlein MW, Engel O, Chun FKH, Fisch M. Adult iatrogenic ureteral injury and stricture–incidence and treatment strategies. Asian J Urol Editor. 2018;5:101–6.
3. Palaniappa NC, Telem DA, Ranasinghe NE, Divino CM. Incidence of iatrogenic ureteral injury after laparoscopic colectomy. Arch Surg. 2012;147:267.
4. Ade-Ojo IP, Tijani O. A review on the etiology, prevention, and management of ureteral injuries during obstetric and gynecologic surgeries. Int J Womens Health (Dove Medical Press Ltd). 2021;13:895–902.
5. Moore EE, Cogbill TH, Malangoni MA, et al. Organ Injury Scaling. Surg Clin North Am 1995;75(2):293–303
6. Lawal O, Bello O, Morhason-Bello I, Abdus-Salam R, Ojengbede O. Our experience with iatrogenic ureteric injuries among women presenting to University College Hospital, Ibadan: a call to action on trigger factors. Obstet Gynecol Int. 2019;2019:6456141.
7. Aarts JWM, Nieboer TE, Johnson N, Tavender E, Garry R, Mol BWJ, et al. Surgical approach to hysterectomy for benign gynaecological disease. Cochrane Database Syst Rev (John Wiley and Sons Ltd). 2015;2015:CD003677.

Table 4 World Health Organization Classification of FGM [53]

TYPE	
I – **CLITORIDECTOMY**	Excision of the prepuce, with or without excision of part or all of the clitoris
II – EXCISION	Involves clitoridectomy and partial or total excision of the labia minora and majora
III – INFIBULATION	Includes removing part or all of the external genitalia and reapproximation of the remnant labia majora, leaving a small neointroitus
IV	Any other injury to the female genital organs

8. Patil S, Guru N, Kundargi V, Patil B, Patil N, Ranka K. Posthysterectomy ureteric injuries: presentation and outcome of management. Urol Ann. 2017;9(1):4–8.
9. Browning A. Management of obstetric urogenital fistula. In: Cardozo L, Staskins D. (eds.) Texbook of Female Urology and Urogynecology, 4th Ed., CRC Press. Boca Raton, FL. USA. 109(2):1189–1200.
10. Ustunsoz B, Ugurel S, Duru NK, Ozgok Y, Ustunsoz A. Percutaneous management of ureteral injuries that are diagnosed late after cesarean section. Korean J Radiol. 2008;9(4):348–53.
11. Raassen TJIP, Ngongo CJ, Mahendeka MM. Iatrogenic genitourinary fistula: an 18-year retrospective review of 805 injuries. Int Urogynecol J. 2014;25(12):1699–706.
12. Rajasekar D, Hall M. Urinary tract injuries during obstetric intervention. Br J Obstet Gynaecol. 1997;104(6):731.
13. Selli C, Turri FM, Gabellieri C, Manassero F, de Maria M, Mogorovich A. Delayed-onset ureteral lesions due to thermal energy: An emerging condition. Arch Ital Urol Androl (Edizioni Scripta Manent s.n.c.). 2014;86:152.
14. Manoucheri E, Cohen SL, Sandberg EM, et al,. Ureteral injury in laparoscopic gynecologic surgery. Rev Obstet Gynecol. 2012;5(2):106-11
15. Janssen PF, Brölmann HAM, Huirne JAF. Recommendations to prevent urinary tract injuries during laparoscopic hysterectomy: a systematic Delphi procedure among experts. J Minim Invasive Gynecol. 2011;18(3):314–21.
16. Chou M-T, Wang C-J, Lien R-C. Prophylactic ureteral catheterization in gynecologic surgery: a 12-year randomized trial in a community hospital. Int Urogynecol J. 2009;20(6):689.
17. Ostrzenski A, Radolinski B, Ostrzenska KM. A review of laparoscopic ureteral injury in pelvic surgery. Obstet Gynecol Surv. 2003;58:794.
18. Halabi WJ, Jafari MD, Nguyen VQ, Carmichael JC, Mills S, Pigazzi A, et al. Ureteral injuries in colorectal surgery: an analysis of trends, outcomes, and risk factors over a 10-year period in the United States. Dis Colon Rectum. 2014;57(2):179–86.
19. Yellinek S, Krizzuk D, Nogueras JJ, Wexner SD. Ureteral injury during colorectal surgery: two case reports and a literature review. J Anus Rectum and Colon. 2018;2(3):71–6.
20. Dalsing MC, Bihrle R, Lalka SG, Cikrit DF, Sawchuk AP. Vascular surgery-associated ureteral injury: zebras do exist. Ann Vasc Surg. 1993;7:180.
21. Burks FN, Santucci RA. Management of iatrogenic ureteral injury. Ther Adv Urol. 2014;6:115–24.
22. Pillai AK, Anderson ME, Reddick MA, Sutphin PD, Kalva SP. Ureteroarterial fistula: diagnosis and management. Am J Roentgenol. 2015;204(5):W592–8.
23. Turgut M, Turgut AT, Dogra VS. Iatrogenic ureteral injury as a complication of posterior or lateral lumbar spine surgery: a systematic review of the literature, vol. 135. World Neurosurg (Elsevier Inc.); 2020. p. 280–96.
24. Shinohara S, Kasai T, Kasai M, Hirata S. Delayed detection of ureteral thermal injury in laparoscopic surgery. Gynecol Minim Invasive Ther (Elsevier B.V.). 2017;6:45.
25. Traxer O, Thomas A. Prospective evaluation and classification of ureteral wall injuries resulting from insertion of a ureteral access sheath during retrograde intrarenal surgery. J Urol. 2013;189(2):580–4.
26. Karakan T, Kilinc MF, Demirbas A, Hascicek AM, Doluoglu OG, Yucel MO, et al. Evaluating ureteral wall injuries with endoscopic grading system and analysis of the predisposing factors. J Endourol. 2016;30(4):375–8.
27. Raassen TJIP, Ngongo CJ, Mahendeka MM. Diagnosis and management of 365 ureteric injuries following obstetric and gynecologic surgery in resource-limited settings. Int Urogynecol J. 2018;29(9):1303–9.
28. Christmas TJ, Chapple CR, Payne SDW, Milroy EJG, Warwick RTT. Bonney's blue cystitis: a warning. Br J Urol. 1989;63(3):281.
29. Pope R, Beddow M. A review of surgical procedures to repair obstetric fistula. Int J Gynecol Obstet. 2020;148(S1):22–6.
30. Goh JTW, Browning A, Berhan B, Chang A. Predicting the risk of failure of closure of obstetric fistula and residual urinary incontinence using a classification system. Int Urogynecol J. 2008;19(12):1659–62.
31. Wong JMK, Bortoletto P, Tolentino J, Jung MJ, Milad MP. Urinary tract injury in gynecologic laparoscopy for benign indication: a systematic review. Obstet Gynecol (Lippincott Williams and Wilkins). 2018;131:100–8.
32. Schierlitz L, Dwyer PL, Rosamilia A, Murray C, Thomas E, de Souza A, et al. Effectiveness of tension-free vaginal tape compared with transobturator tape in women with stress urinary incontinence and intrinsic sphincter deficiency. Obstet Gynecol. 2008;112(6):1253.
33. Vincenzoni C, Sica S, Natola M, Sacco E, Totaro A, Bassi P, et al. Management of iatrogenic bladder injury due to vascular surgery: case report and literature review. Ann Vasc Surg. 2019;59:307.e13–6.
34. Rose J, Schneider C, Yildirim C, Geers P, Scheidbach H, Köckerling F. Complications in laparoscopic colorectal surgery: results of a multicentre trial. Tech Coloproctol. 2004;8(S1):s25–8.
35. Duess JW, Schaller MC, Lacher M, Sorge I, Puri P, Gosemann JH. Accidental bladder injury during elective inguinal hernia repair: a preventable complication with high morbidity. Pediatr Surg Int. 2020;36(2):235–9.
36. Teplitsky SL, Leong JY, Shenot PJ. Iatrogenic bladder rupture in individuals with disability related to spinal cord injury and chronic indwelling urethral catheters. Spinal Cord Ser Cases. 2020;6(1):47.
37. Morton H, Hilton P. Urethral injury associated with minimally invasive mid-urethral sling procedures for the treatment of stress urinary incontinence: a case

series and systematic literature search. BJOG. 2009;116(8):1120.
38. Enemchukwu EA, Brucker BM. Diagnosis of urogenital fistula. 2016.
39. Hoag N, Chee J. Surgical management of female urethral strictures. Translational Androl Urol (AME Publishing Company). 2017;6:S76–80.
40. Redan JA, Mccarus SD. Protect the ureters. JSLS. 2006;13(2):139–41.
41. Delbos L, Gareau-Labelle AK, Langlais EL, Lemyre M, Boutet M, Maheux-Lacroix S, et al. Sodium fluorescein for ureteral jet detection: a prospective observational study. J Soc Laparoendosc Surg. 2018;22(3):e2018.00019.
42. Slooter MD, Janssen A, Bemelman WA, Tanis PJ, Hompes R. Currently available and experimental dyes for intraoperative near-infrared fluorescence imaging of the ureters: a systematic review. Tech Coloproctol (Springer-Verlag Italia s.r.l.). 2019;23:305–13.
43. Nerli R, Ghagane S, Deole S, Dixit N, Hiremath M. Augmentation ileocystoplasty: operative steps. J Sci Soc. 2019;46(2):57.
44. Bacalbașa N, Bălescu I. Segmentary ureteral resection followed by ureteroneocystostomy associated with radical hysterectomy and partial cystectomy in a patient with bulky residual disease after chemoirradiation for invasive cervical cancer–a case report. J Med Life. 2014;7(4):558-62.
45. Padmanabhan P. (2019). Bladder Flap Repair (Boari). In: Smith JA, Howards SS, Preminger GM, Dmochowski RR, eds. Hinman's Atlas of Urologic Surgery. 4th Edition. Elsevier. 293.
46. Wolff B, Chartier-Kastler E, Mozer P, Haertig A, Bitker MO, Rouprêt M. Long-term functional outcomes after ileal ureter substitution: a single-center experience. Urology. 2011;78(3):692–5.
47. Cheng PJ, Myers JB. Augmentation cystoplasty in the patient with neurogenic bladder. World J Urol (Springer Science and Business Media Deutschland GmbH). 2020;38:3035–46.
48. Chapple C, Turner-Warwick R. Vesico-vaginal fistula. BJU Int. 2005;95(1):193–214.
49. Peterson AC, Webster GD. Management of urethral stricture disease: developing options for surgical intervention. BJU Int. 2004;94(7):971–6
50. Klein E, Helzner E, Shayowitz M, Kohlhoff S, Smith-Norowitz TA. Female genital mutilation: health consequences and complications – a short literature review. Obstet Gynecol Int (Hindawi Limited). 2018;2018: 7365715.
51. Lurie JM, Weidman A, Huynh S, Delgado D, Easthausen I, Kaur G. Painful gynecologic and obstetric complications of female genital mutilation/cutting: a systematic review and meta-analysis. PLoS Med. 2020;17(3):e1003088.
52. Almeer HH, Almulla AA, Almugahwi AA, Alzaher MZ, Alshammasi MM, Menezes RG. Female genital mutilation in Saudi Arabia: a systematic review. Cureus. 2021;13:e19300.
53. Zurynski Y, Phu A, Sureshkumar P, Cherian S, Deverell M, Elliott EJ. Female genital mutilation in children presenting to Australian paediatricians. Arch Dis Child. 2017;102(6):509–15.

Female Genital Mutilation/Cutting

Madina Ndoye, Serigne Gueye, Lamine Niang, Farzana Cassim, and Jan Adlam

Contents

Introduction	1164
Prevalence	1164
Epidemiology Trends	1165
Types of FGM/C	1165
Health Consequences	1167
Immediate Complications	1167
Short-Term Complications	1168
Long-Term Complications	1168
Dermatological Complications	1169
Urinary Tract Complications	1172
Sexual Health	1172
Neuropathic Clitoral Pain	1173
Gynecological Complications	1174
Obstetric and Perinatal Complications	1175
Psychological Disturbances	1175
Management of FGM/C	1176
Gynecological Care	1176
Obstetric Care	1177
Sexual Health	1177

M. Ndoye
Department of Urology, Cheikh Anta Diop University/ Hospital General Idrissa Poueye, Dakar, Senegal

S. Gueye · L. Niang
Cheikh Anta Diop University/Hospital General Idrissa Poueye, Dakar, Senegal

F. Cassim (✉)
Division of Urology, Stellenbosch University/Tygerberg Hospital, Cape Town, South Africa

J. Adlam
Department of Obstetrics and Gynaecoogy, Stellenbosch University/Tygerberg Hospital, Cape Town, South Africa

© Springer Nature Switzerland AG 2023
F. E. Martins et al. (eds.), *Female Genitourinary and Pelvic Floor Reconstruction*,
https://doi.org/10.1007/978-3-031-19598-3_63

Prevention Strategies 1178
Conclusion 1181
Cross-References 1181
References 1181

Abstract

Female genital mutilation/cutting (FGM/C) is the practice of removing or disfiguring the female external genitalia. This removal may be partial or complete. It is a practice predominantly occurring in some African, Middle Eastern, and Asian countries. However, with changing migratory patterns, FGM/C is a global health risk. The short-term and long-term health implications for girls and women undergoing FGM/C are potentially devastating, and it is for this reason that the United Nations (UN) has listed it under the Sustainable Development Goals (SDGs) as a practice to be eradicated by 2030. Although we are a long way from eradication of this practice, global advocacy for girls and women is gaining traction, and with a multisectoral approach, this goal may be achievable.

Keywords

Female genital mutilation/cutting · Gender-based violence · Infibulation · Defibulation · Women's health

Introduction

Female genital cutting (FGC) is the complete or partial removal of the external female genitalia or other injury to the genital organs for nonmedical reasons [1]. It is sometimes referred to as female genital mutilation (FGM), female circumcision, or female genital mutilation/cutting (FGM/C). The practice is highly concentrated in a swath of countries from the Atlantic coast to the Horn of Africa, in areas of the Middle East such as Iraq and Yemen, and in some countries in Asia like Indonesia, with wide variations in prevalence. Immigrant populations from countries where the practice still occurs and living in Europe, the United States, and other countries like Australia keep the practice alive [2]. While still having a significant prevalence, FGM/C is regarded as a form of gender-based violence (GBV) by the international community [3, 4]. Culturally however, FGM/C continues as it signifies the preservation of virginity and improves the child's marriage prospects, thereby improving the family's social standing [5].

Prevalence

The practice of FGM/C has impacted an estimated 200 million girls and women worldwide, and it continues to affect approximately 6000 girls every day in Africa [1]. Girls aged 0–14 make up a large proportion of the affected group, with approximately 70 million girls in this age group being subjected to FGM/C [6]. An estimated three million girls are subject to one of the four types of mutilations each year with more than 85% eventually having a medical complication sometime in their life as a result [7]. There are wide variations in prevalence across countries. In some countries such as Somalia, Guinea, and Djibouti, the practice is almost universal, while it affects no more than 1% of girls and women in other countries like Cameroon and Uganda [2, 8, 9]. Evidence suggests that FGM affects girls and women worldwide and exists in places including Colombia [8], India [10], Malaysia [10], Oman [11], Saudi Arabia [12], and the United Arab Emirates [13] with large variations in terms of the type performed, circumstances surrounding the practice, and size of the affected population groups. With extensive educational interventions, international pressure, and much lobbying for the discontinuation of FGM/C, the prevalence is slowly declining in certain countries [5]. However, it is still significant with many people ignoring the illegality of the practice.

Epidemiology Trends

Both ethnicity and location influence the likelihood of experiencing FGM/C, the way that it is performed within different cultures, and the age when it is performed. The regions in which FGM/C is most common are home primarily to ethnic groups among whom the practice is nearly universal, when in some others it's virtually nonexistent. In some countries, it is carried out very early in life in girls as young as five, while in others it is only performed in adolescence. The practice remains rare after the age of 15, with 30% of girls under the age of 15 having undergone FGM/C. In half of practicing countries, the average age at which FGM/C is performed is lower today than it was 30 years ago. This is illustrated in Gambia and Nigeria where the average age at which cutting is performed has dropped by 2 full years from the age of four to younger than the age of two and from the age of three to younger than a year old, respectfully. In Kenya, the average has dropped by over 3 years, from 12 to 9 years old.

More than just a harmful practice, FGM/C is a deeply rooted social norm enforced by community expectations around marriageability. By having a daughter cut, the family ensures that she will be a desirable marriage prospect. Compared to the health risks, the social consequences that uncut girls face are equally severe. A girl who is not cut is often ostracized by her community. In many countries where both child marriage and FGM/C are common, girls most at risk for each practice tend to share certain characteristics, such as low levels of education, rural residence, and living in poorer households. Opposition to FGM/C is highest among girls and women who are educated and tends to increase substantially as educational levels rise.

Migration to countries where FGM/C is not the norm also affects the prevalence of the practice. According to data from the United Nations High Commission for Refugees, nearly 300,000 women from areas practicing FGM/C applied for asylum in the European Union (EU) from 2013 to 2017 [6]. In 2017, 28% of all women seeking asylum in the EU were from FGM/C practicing countries, with Iraq, Nigeria, Eritrea, and Somalia being the top four countries represented [6].

Another changing trend is how the practice is done. In some countries like Egypt and Sudan, the practice is highly medicalized, about 8 in 10 girls are cut by medical personnel, whereas traditional practitioners are responsible for most cutting in Djibouti, Iraq, and Yemen. Communities may be increasingly turning to health-care providers to perform the procedure for a combination of reasons. An important contributing factor is the fact that FGM/C has been addressed for years as a health issue, using what is known as the "health risk approach." This approach has involved locally respected health experts expressing concern about the health risks of FGM/C, in the form of a didactic and factual delivery of messages. In several high-prevalence countries, this approach unfortunately did not result in individuals, families, or communities abandoning the practice but began to shift it from traditional circumcisers to modern healthcare practitioners in the hope that this would reduce the risk of various complications [14, 15].

Female genital mutilation/cutting is declining in many places, but progress is not fast enough in high- and low-prevalence countries alike. FGM/C for immigrant populations arriving in developed countries, particularly the United States of America (USA), presents a particular obstacle in the full-global abolition of female genital mutation practice as many seek to continue their cultural traditions [16, 17]. In some instances, parents fly their daughters back to their homeland to have the procedure done [18]. In the United States, for instance, girls and women at risk of having a FGM/C procedure live in cities or suburbs of large metropolitan areas. In particular, the tristate New York City area has an estimated 65,893 women who are at risk with more than 21,737 of them under the age of 18 (Fig. 1; Table 1).

Types of FGM/C

There is a wide range of variation in FGM/C with different degrees of severity, as well as clinical consequences and therapeutic needs. A slight trend toward less severe forms of FGM/C is noted in some countries. For example, in Guinea-Bissau, from those who experienced the practice, the share of women who underwent the

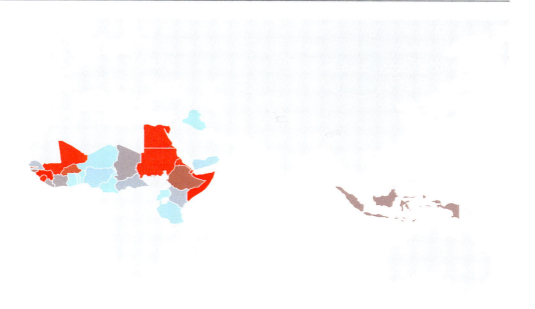

Fig. 1 Prevalence per country. (Source: UNICEF global databases, 2022, based on DHS, MICS and other national surveys, 2004–2021)

most severe form of FGM/C known as infibulation has nearly halved among younger girls compared to older women in the two regions where FGM/C is most common. The World Health Organization (WHO) classifies the mutilation of the female genitalia into four distinct categories [1, 19]. Three of the four categories are further broken down into subcategories that classify the specific type of mutilation that was performed.

Type I is known as clitoridectomy and includes any procedure that totally removes the clitoris and/or the prepuce.

- Type Ia is the removal of the clitoris hood or prepuce only.
- Type Ib includes the removal of both the clitoris and the prepuce.

Type II, or excision, is the partial or total removal of the labia minora unrelated to any mutilation performed on the labia majora.

- Type IIa includes the removal of the labia minora only.
- Type IIb is the removal of the labia minora and the partial or total removal of the clitoris.
- Type IIc involves the removal or the clitoris, labia minora, and labia majora.

Type III, or infibulation, is the third category of mutilation procedures defined as the narrowing of the vaginal orifice with the sealing of the perineum leaving a very small opening, about the size of a matchstick, to allow for the flow of urine and menstrual blood by cutting and repositioning the labia minora and labia majora with or without the excision of the clitoris.

- Type IIIa references specifically procedures done with the removal and apposition of the labia minora.
- Type IIIb includes procedures done with only the labia majora.

Type IV is a broad category that includes all other harmful procedures done without medical purpose to the female genitals. This includes any cutting, herbal treatments, or burns that alter or

Table 1 Prevalence per country (source below [18])

Prevalence	Countries
Prevalence ≥ 80%	Somalia
	Guinea
	Djibouti
	Egypt
	Eritrea
	Mali (89%)
	Sierra Leone (88%)
	Sudan (88%)
Prevalence 51–80%	Gambia (76%)
	Burkina Faso (76%)
	Ethiopia (74%)
	Mauritania (69%)
	Liberia (66%)
Prevalence 26–50%	Guinea-Bissau (50%)
	Chad (44%)
	Ivory Coast (38%)
	Kenya (27%)
	Nigeria (27%)
	Senegal (26%)
Prevalence 10–25%	Central African Republic (24%)
	Yemen (23%)
	United Republic of Tanzania (15%)
	Benin (13%)
Prevalence ≤ 10%	Iraq (8%),
	Ghana (4%)
	Togo (4%)
	Niger (2%)
	Cameroon (1%)
	Uganda (1%)

harm the patient's body and covers a variety of procedures including pricking, piercing, or incision of the clitoris and/or labia, stretching the clitoris and/or labia, burning of the clitoris and surrounding tissues, scraping of the vaginal orifice or cutting of the vagina, and insertion of substances into the vagina to cause bleeding or to tighten or narrow it (Figs. 2, 3, 4, and 5).

Health Consequences

FGM/C's negative health consequences are backed by strong evidence even though underreported. A number of well-designed studies have compared large samples of women and girls to identify these consequences which are both physical and psychological [21] and includes short- and long-term complications. The method in which the procedure is performed may determine the extent of the short-term complications [22]. If the process was completed using unsterile equipment, no antiseptics, and no antibiotics, the victim may have increased risk of complications. The ramifications of FGM/C affect the girl for the rest of her life and result in many health problems (problems with urination, cysts, infections, and complications during childbirth). Each of the most common complications occurred in more than one of every ten girls and women who undergo FGM/C. There were few differences in risk of immediate complications among different types of FGM/C, but there might be a greater risk of immediate complications for women with FGM/C type III (infibulation) compared to types I–II.

Immediate Complications

A systematic review that included 56 primary studies with over 133,000 girls and women who all had undergone the practice of FGM/C showed different results. The most common immediate complications of FGM/C are urinary retention, excessive bleeding, swelling, problems with healing, and pain. The results suggest that each of these five immediate harms occur in more than one of every ten girls and women who undergo FGM/C that include:

- Severe pain (11%) and genital tissue swelling (27%): pain and swelling arise from injury to nerves and lack of anesthesia.
- Urinary retention and pain (53%): problems urinating due to swelling, inflammation, injury to the urethra, and pain from urine on the wound.
- Shock and hemorrhage (43%): severe bleeding because arteries with high blood flow and pressure are cut. Shock resulting from blood loss, severe pain, and trauma, which can be fatal and lead to death. While data on the mortality of girls who underwent FGM/C are unknown and

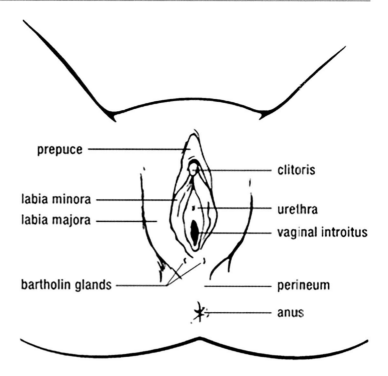

Fig. 2 The unaltered female genitalia [1, 20]

hard to procure, it is estimated that 1 in every 500 circumcisions results in death [8]. Death occurs from severe bleeding, trauma, infection, or a combination of these complications.

Short-Term Complications

- Problems with wound healing: it is estimated that just over 10% of girls have problems with healing such as failure of the wound to heal due to infection, irritation from urine, or chafing when walking.
- Infections: these develop from the use of unsterile equipment and conditions. Fever and infections are commonly experienced by 5% and 2% of the girls and women, respectively. The type and degree of infections vary and include potentially fatal septicemia and tetanus. If the process was completed using unsterile equipment, no antiseptics, and no antibiotics, the victim may have increased risk of complications. Primary infections include staphylococcus infections and urinary tract infections. Infections such as human immunodeficiency virus (HIV), *Chlamydia trachomatis*, *Clostridium tetani*, and herpes simplex virus (HSV) 2 are significantly more common among women who underwent type III mutilation compared with other categories [23]. After the area heals, victims suffer the long-term consequences of the abuse through both physiological and psychological complications and substantial complications during childbirth.

Long-Term Complications

Female genital mutilation/cutting can result in recurring, longer-term health problems for women and girls. Females who have undergone type II and III female genital cutting experience more long-term complications than those who have undergone type I and IV. These complications may have a domino effect leading to a multitude of complications related to pain, urinary symptoms, sexual dysfunction, and mental health problems. Figure 6 illustrates the consequences of some of these complications [24].

61 Female Genital Mutilation/Cutting

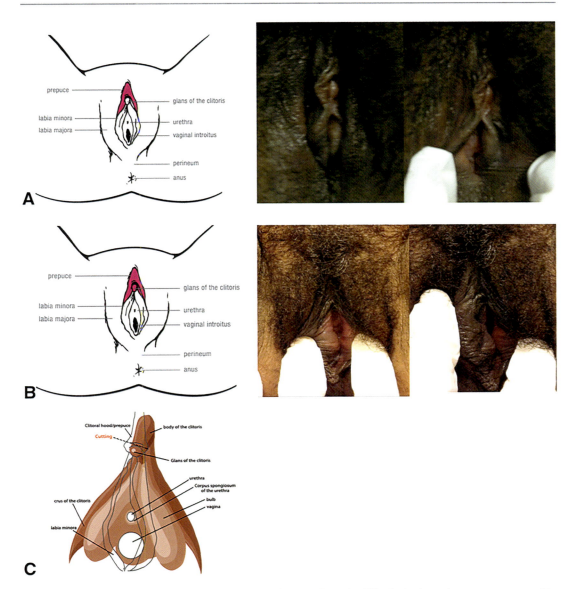

Fig. 3 Female genital mutilation type I: partial or total removal of the clitoris or the prepuce or both. (**a**) Female genital mutilation type Ia: removal of the prepuce of the clitoris or clitoral hood (female circumcision). (**b**) Female genital mutilation Ib: removal of the clitoris with the prepuce (clitoridectomy). In the World Health Organization (WHO) classification, when there is reference to removal of the clitoris, only the glans or the glans with part of the body of the clitoris is removed (**c**). 13 The recognition of type Ia can be difficult. As shown in **a**, an asymmetry of the prepuce can be noticed. (Illustrations in panels **a** and **b** reprinted from the World Health Organization. WHO guidelines on the management of health complications from female genital mutilation. Geneva, Switzerland: World Health Organization; 2016. Illustration in panel **c** modified from https://commons.wikimedia.org/wiki/File:Clitoris_anatomy_labeled-en.svg [1, 20])

Dermatological Complications

Dermatological complications due to tissue damage and abnormal healing often occur, especially in the setting of rudimentary cutting techniques. These complications include chronic pelvic pain from trapped or unprotected nerve endings, keloid scarring, epidermal inclusion cysts, neuroma formation, and damage to the vulvar lymphatic tissue [25].

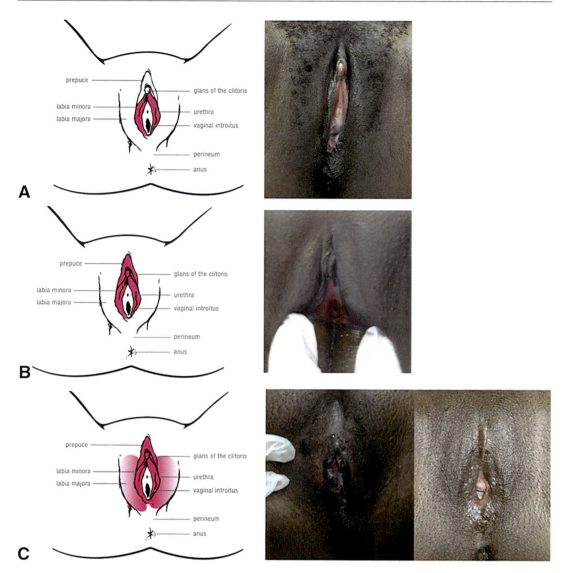

Fig. 4 Female genital mutilation type II: partial or total removal of the clitoris and the labia minora with or without excision of the labia majora (excision). (**a**) Female genital mutilation type IIa: removal of the labia minora only. (**b**) Female genital mutilation type IIb: partial or total removal of the clitoris and the labia minora. (**c**) Female genital mutilation type IIc: partial or total removal of the clitoris, the labia minora, and the labia majora. In the World Health Organization (WHO) classification, when there is reference to removal of the clitoris, only the glans or the glans with part of the body of the clitoris is removed.13 The examiner should be aware that the physiologic female anatomy of the labia minora can vary largely. The labia minora can physiologically overcome the labia majora or be asymmetric. (Illustrations in panels **a–c** reprinted from the World Health Organization. WHO guidelines on the management of health complications from female genital mutilation. Geneva, Switzerland: World Health Organization; 2016 [1, 20])

The most common dermatologic complication is the development of epidermal inclusion cysts (EICs) in the genital area. In a study of 118 women admitted to a hospital in Mogadishu, Somalia, with FGM/C complications, 55% of patients had EICs [26]. Epidermal inclusion cysts result from the invagination of squamous epithelium, which then desquamates into a closed

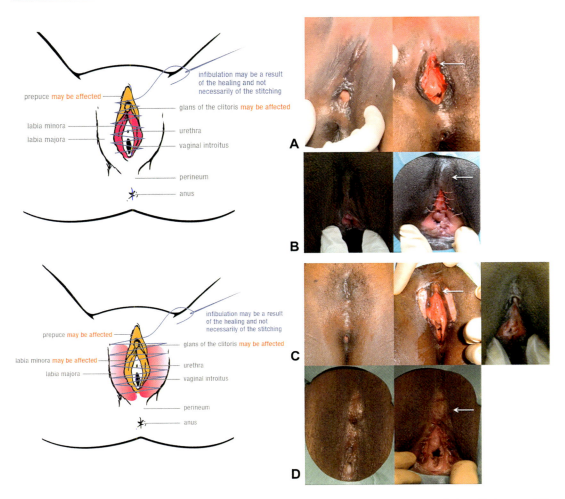

Fig. 5 Female genital mutilation type III: narrowing of the vaginal orifice with creation of a covering seal by cutting and appositioning the labia minora or the labia majora or both, with or without excision of the clitoris (infibulation). (**a**) Female genital mutilation type IIIa without cutting of the clitoris before and after defibulation, the surgery that opens infibulation. Arrow: intact clitoris uncovered after defibulation. (**b**) Female genital mutilation type IIIa with cutting of the clitoris before and after defibulation. Arrow: clitoral stump visible under the scar. (**c**) Female genital mutilation type IIIb without cutting of the clitoris before and after defibulation. Arrow: intact clitoris uncovered after defibulation. (**d**) Female genital mutilation type IIIb with cutting of the clitoris before and after defibulation. Arrow: clitoral stump visible under the scar. When the clitoris is excised, the clitoral stump is palpable and sometimes visible under the scar. When the clitoris is not excised, it lies under the scar and is re-exposed during defibulation. (Illustrations reprinted from the World Health Organization (WHO). WHO guidelines on the management of health complications from female genital mutilation. Geneva, Switzerland: World Health Organization; 2016 [1, 20])

space to form a cystic mass. These cysts are slow growing, beginning as a painless swelling at the wound site and gradually increasing in size over several years to form a large clitoral or vulvar mass [25]. If left untreated these cysts may cause pelvic pain, dyspareunia, pruritis, and discharge. Larger cysts may interfere with walking or sitting and pose complications to vaginal delivery. Treatment options include simple cyst excision with removal of the intact cyst or carbon dioxide laser surgery [27].

Keloid scarring results from progressive overgrowth of dense fibrous tissue after wound healing. In addition, inflammation secondary to

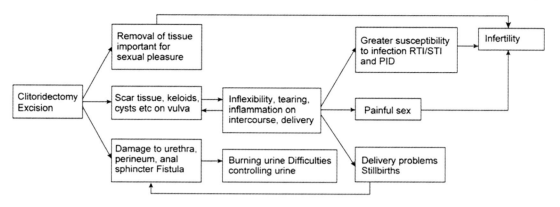

Fig. 6 Conceptual framework for long-term consequences of FGM/C [22]

both post-mutilation infections and poor urinary drainage may play a role in particularly severe keloid formation in these patients. Many women with genital keloid scarring delay treatment because of embarrassment and fear of surgical options [27].

Amputation neuromas of the clitoris may arise secondary to clitoral nerve entrapment in irregularly placed sutures or due to scar tissue that increases pressure on the nerve. These women may suffer from dyspareunia or pain at rest.

Vulvar lymphangiectasias result from damage to the lymphatic tissue and may occur as itchy, wart-like papules with or without lichenification due to chronic scarring [25].

Urinary Tract Complications

Urinary tract complications include urethral stricture formation, recurrent urinary tract infections, and urinary stones.

Due to the intimate relation of the urethra to the clitoris and labia, injury my occur at the time of FGM/C; the cephalad apex of the clitoral hood is only 12 mm from the urethral orifice at age 0–3 and only 17 mm at the age 4–8. Urethral injuries can result in scarring, stricture, or stenosis with subsequent lower urinary tract dysfunction [24].

Following FGM/C type III, a narrow neo-introitus is formed; this creates a moist and closed off space that surrounds the urethra. Urine can stagnate beneath the scar and promote abnormal bacterial growth. As a result, these women may experience recurrent urinary tract infections. Women who are infibulated may complain of a slow urinary stream and post-micturition dribbling. Some of these women may complain of straining and urinary retention, while others complain of overactive bladder symptoms. It is also possible for the obstructing scar to enable urinary crystals to deposit and, as a result, form urinary stones [28].

Sexual Health

Women with FGM/C are more likely to report dyspareunia and experience less sexual satisfaction than woman who had not been subjected to FGM/C [29]. FGM/C may cause injury to clitoral nerves and related receptors that may result in neuropathic pain. Additionally, vulva damage reduces the flexibility and sensitivity of critical genital tissue and may produce tearing during intercourse resulting in pain. This pain is further exaggerated in women with FGM/C type III, as the infibulation creates a narrow neo-introitus. For many of these women, the infibulation is opened either surgically or through penetrative sex, resulting in extremely painful coitus.

The clitoris contains specialized sensory tissue that is concentrated in a rich neurovascular area of a few centimeters. Due to direct damage of this tissue, surrounding scar tissue, and adhesions, the remaining tissue is less sensitive to tactile stimulation. Furthermore, critical vascular tissues may be absent impairing vasocongestion and subsequent lubrication to occur during the sexual response cycle. Dyspareunia is often described in women with decreased vaginal lubrication.

As the female sexual response cycle is not linear and multidimensional with interaction of neurophysiological and biochemical mechanisms, influenced by relationship dynamics and family and sociocultural issues, it is possible that women with FGM/C have an ability to compensate for anatomical damage to their genital tissue through enhancement of other sensory and erotic areas or emotions and fantasy. Psychological inputs from the partner and setting play a major role in sexual satisfaction. However, for the same reason, these women may experience even less sexual pleasure and satisfaction if lasting negative associations with intercourse were formed due to pain or a partner that is not sensitive toward the pain experienced.

Women with FGM/C have a greater likelihood of sexual desire than women without FGM/C [29]. This is possibly due to conditioning. As stated above women who have undergone FGM/C often experience pain with intercourse and impairment of sexual satisfaction. Repeated dissatisfaction may lead to reduced desire (learned inhibition). Although further research is warranted, it appears that women who had undergone FGM/C are likely to experience orgasm [29].

The extent that FGM/C impacts a woman's sexuality is probably related to the age when FGM/C was done, the healing process, and the extent of the excision of genital tissue (rather than suturing or closing off the vagina) (Figs. 7, 8, and 9).

Neuropathic Clitoral Pain

Pain after nerve injury is called neuropathic pain and is defined by the International Association for the Study of Pain as "pain directly resulting from a lesion or disease affecting the somatosensory system" [30]. Neuropathic pain can persist long after an injury has healed. It can include allodynia (pain induced by innocuous stimuli such as touch) and hyperalgesia (severe pain induced by painful stimuli), and it is often described as burning, needling, or electrical-type sensations [31]. Therefore, painful neuromas can severely impact quality of life and cause functional impairment and psychological distress [32]. Providers who care for women with FGM/C should consider a diagnosis

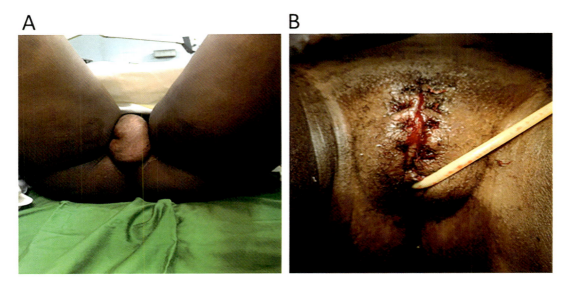

Fig. 7 (**a**) Cystic mass post-FGM. (**b**) After excision of the mass. (Images courtesy of Dr. M. Ndoye)

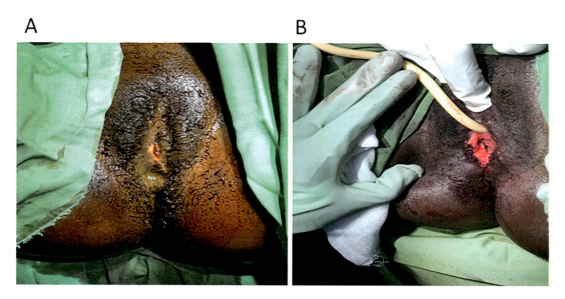

Fig. 8 (**a**) Infibulation with complete vaginal closure. (**b**) Vaginal opening post-corrective surgery. (Images courtesy of Dr. M. Ndoye)

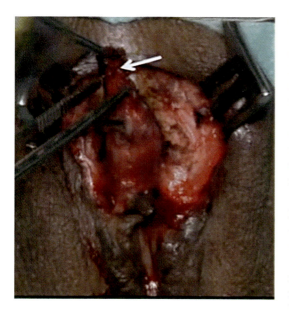

Fig. 9 Clitoral reconstruction of FGC type II. A post-traumatic neuroma was found within the peri-clitoral fibrotic tissue (arrow) removed around the clitoral stump

of clitoral neuroma in patients with neuropathic clitoral pain, even when a palpable or visible painful mass is not visible. Comprehensive multidisciplinary care should include counselling, psychosexual therapy, and surgical treatment.

Gynecological Complications

FGM/C is linked to a wide variety of gynecological health problems including menstrual difficulties, vaginal infections, increased cervical cancer rate, and infertility [25].

One of the most common long-term side effects of FGM/C is dysmenorrhea, occurring particularly in those who have undergone infibulation. Dysmenorrhea or severe pain associated with menses occurs in these patients due to congestion of obstructed menstrual flow which may lead to hematocolpos and hematometra. These women often do not understand the cause of their symptoms [25].

Recurrent and chronic vaginal infections occur more frequently in FGM/C patients. A study in rural Gambia showed that women with type II FGM/C had a 66% higher risk of bacterial vaginosis. The increased incidence has been speculated to be related to the removal of the protective labia minora. In the same study, all FCM/C patients had a 4.7-fold higher prevalence of herpes simplex 2 infection [22].

FGM/C appears to increase the risk of invasive cervical carcinoma due to recurrent infections, chronic inflammation, and scarring. A case control study conducted in Mali found 30% greater odds (95% CI 0.3–5.8) of developing cervical cancer in women who had undergone FGM/C. These findings are limited, however, by the study's small sample size (82 cases and 97 controls) and the fact that nearly all subjects had undergone FGM/C [33]. A more recent retrospective study of 2398 women, of which 26% had undergone FGM/C, found a substantially stronger association (OR = 2.50; CI 95%, 1.28–4.91) [34].

Anatomic and psychological barriers as well as possible recurrent pelvic infections contribute to potential infertility among women who have undergone FGM/C. Tubal factor infertility may arise in these women due to infections that arise after FGM/C in childhood that ascend to internal genitalia, causing inflammation and scarring. A case control study in Sudan investigating primary infertility not caused by hormonal, iatrogenic, or male-factor infertility showed a significantly higher risk than controls of having undergone the most extensive form of FGM/C, involving the labia majora (OR 4.69, 95% CI 1.49–19.7) [35].

Repeated attempts at penetration through the infibulated scar may be painful and difficult, and stretching of the infibulated introitus may take months. The learned association between sexuality and pain may have a significant negative effect on the woman's willingness to have intercourse, thereby, on fertility [28].

Obstetric and Perinatal Complications

Vaginal stenosis and obstruction around the introitus associated with more invasive forms of FGM/C may result in prolonged labor, and the inelasticity of vulvovaginal scarring predisposes the patient to perineal tears and hemorrhage. Obstetric fistulas develop due to necrosis of the urogenital structures caused by compression of the impacted fetal head during obstructed labor. Subsequent sloughing of the anterior vaginal wall and bladder leads to urinary incontinence, and sloughing of the posterior wall and rectum leads to fecal incontinence [25].

FGM/C has been proven to increase the rate of adverse obstetric and neonatal complications, including hemorrhage, obstructed labor, perineal injury, intrauterine fetal demise, and obstetric fistula formation [24]. The excess risk rises with the extent of cutting. This was illustrated in a large prospective collaborative study sponsored by the WHO in 2006 that examined 28,393 patients at 28 obstetric centers in Burkina Faso, Ghana, Kenya, Nigeria, Senegal, and Sudan (Table 2) [36].

It is important to note that maternal mortality rates are higher in countries that practice FGM/C compared with more developed regions, with hemorrhage being the leading cause of maternal mortality. However, countries in which the majority of women undergo extensive forms of FGM/C, such as Somalia and Djibouti, have a higher maternal death rate (>700 per 100,000 live births) than countries with a much lower prevalence of FGM/C but similar midwifery practices, such as Kenya and Tanzania (<500 per 100,000 live births) [37].

Psychological Disturbances

It appears that women who have undergone FGM/C may be more likely to have a psychiatric diagnosis and suffer from anxiety, somatization, phobia, and low self-esteem.

In a case control study, Behrendt and Moritz assessed the psychological effect of FGM/C. The examiners interviewed 42 Senegalese woman

Table 2 WHO study group on female genital mutilation and obstetric outcome [36]

Relative risk (95% CI)	FGM/C type I	FGM/C type II	FGM/C type III
Caesarean section	1.03 (0.88–1.21)	1.29 (1.09–1.52)	1.31 (1.01–1.70)
Postpartum hemorrhage	1.03 (0.87–1.21)	1.21 (1.01–1.43)	1.69 (1.34–2.12)
Extended maternal hospital stay	1.15 (0.97–1.35)	1.51 (1.29–1.76)	1.98 (1.54–2.54)
Infant resuscitation	1.11 (0.95–1.28)	1.28 (1.10–1.49)	1.66 (1.31–2.10)
Stillbirth and early neonatal death	1.15 (0.94–1.41)	1.32 (1.08–1.62)	1.55 (1.12–2.16)

(23 FGM/C; 24 controls). All the patients remembered the day of the cutting as appalling and traumatizing. Ninety percent of cases described feelings of intense fear, helplessness, horror, and severe pain, and over 80% were still suffering from intrusive reexperiences of their cutting. Of the cases just under 80% met criteria for a psychiatric diagnosis with post-traumatic stress disorder (PTSD), representing a particularly high proportion (30.8%) as compared with controls in which only one participant met criteria for a psychiatric disorder [38].

In developing countries, these conditions regularly go unrecognized. The physical harms arising from FGM/C may also affect women's and girls' social lives. For example, difficult penetration could affect women's sexual lives. Or women experiencing incontinence (loss of bladder control) as a side effect of being cut can face embarrassment and isolation. Chronic clitoral pain greatly impacts relationships, as well as daily social and psychosexual experiences.

Management of FGM/C

The management is based on guiding principles that females and girls with FGM/C are victims of a harmful practice and should be provided with quality healthcare. Few treatment options exist for victims of FGM/C, but psychological and emotional support from a therapist and support groups specializing in PTSD is mandatory.

Gynecological Care

It is important that when patients with FGM/C are seen the healthcare provider avoids verbal and nonverbal reactions that may make the patient feel stigmatized. Well-woman examinations and cervical screening need to be fully explained so the patient fully understands the need for these tests. A wide variety of small, narrow specula should be available to perform the exam with the least amount of discomfort. Women who experience apareunia/dyspareunia, dysmenorrhea, difficulty voiding, or those who are considering intercourse or pregnancy may be offered surgery, defibulation or excision.

Defibulation

Defibulation is a surgical process that attempts to reconstruct the labia by undoing the initial mutilation and is available at specialty hospitals throughout the world. If possible defibulation should ideally be performed prior to coitus, as this may prevent dyspareunia and lasting negative associations, or prior to pregnancy to prevent obstetric complications. Even though the procedure may be medically beneficial for the patient, she may prefer to decline surgery in order to prove that she has never had vaginal penetration when she marries.

Defibulation may be performed during pregnancy. However, many patients require several antenatal visits and counselling sessions before she would consent to the procedure. Counselling should include risks of delivery with an infibulated scar, bleeding, infection, scar formation, and preterm labor. The non-obstetric benefits of defibulation should also be discussed, and patients should be made aware that their urinary stream will feel increased. Surgery should ideally be done under regional anesthesia in the second trimester in order to minimize obstetric and fetal risks. Local anesthesia should be avoided as it may cause patients distressing flashbacks of the FGM/C procedure.

Technique

1. Provide regional or general anesthesia in addition to long-acting local anesthetic.
2. Delineate the length of the scar with the aid of a clamp inserted beneath the scar.
3. Assess if the clitoris is buried beneath the scar by gently palpating anteriorly.
4. Place two Allis clamps along the infibulated scar.
5. With a mayo scissor, divide the scar between the two clamps with special attention not to cut into the buried clitoris – the aim is to visualize the introitus and urethra easily.
6. Place subcuticular sutures (4–0) on each side to ensure hemostasis and approximation of the labial edges [39].

Other techniques using a carbon dioxide laser has also been described. Postoperatively patients should be given instruction to take sitz baths twice daily, after which a local anesthetic cream may be applied. Vaginal dilators may be appropriate for some woman to maintain vaginal caliber and avoid restenosis.

Contraceptive measures remain the same as for other women. Due to the increased infertility among women who have undergone FGM/C, artificial reproductive techniques may be considered; however these may be challenging because of the need of a vaginal approach for certain procedures (hysterosonogram, intrauterine insemination, transvaginal ovum retrieval).

Obstetric Care

It is important to treat pregnant and laboring patients with FGM/C with a professional and non-judgmental approach.

Antenatal Care

If defibulation will be necessary to allow vaginal birth, it is strongly recommended to be performed in the second semester; however some women prefer to wait until the time of birth and allow a trail of labor without defibulation. It is very important to discuss all possible scenarios and possible procedures antenatally to provide the patient an opportunity to ask questions and time to understand the reasoning.

Intrapartum Care

Monitoring the progress of labor may be challenging in the infibulated patient, as the neo-introitus can make a bimanual examination difficult, if not impossible. In these cases, the obstetrician may either defibulate the patient early in labor or monitor labor via rectal examination. Both options are suboptimal: early defibulation will require a very early epidural and irritation of the incision with every cervical assessment, while rectal examination of the cervix is uncomfortable and very few obstetricians have experience using this technique.

The infibulated scar can only prolong the second stage of labor, as it may obstruct the crowning and delivery of the fetal head. Defibulation may be performed with an episiotomy to facilitate the birth and minimize vaginal tearing. In some communities, it is customary to re-infibulate the genitals after each childbirth. The WHO and other international health organizations strongly oppose all medicalization of FGM/C, including re-infibulation [1]. FGM/C is not an indication for caesarean section. However, the risk for caesarean section may be reduced if defibulation is performed antenatally.

Sexual Health

In addition to currently accepted treatment for sexual dysfunction, women with FGM/C may be offered defibulation. As noted earlier it is possible for some women to have an ability to compensate for anatomical damage to their genital tissue through refocused development of other sensory and erotic areas or emotions and fantasy. Sexual therapy and education, individual and couple, could be offered to women with FGM/C who want that. Defibulation have been found to improve sexuality of women with FGM/C [39]. The use of lubricants, self-stimulation, and dilators may improve sexual function.

Clitoral Reconstruction

When FGM/C involves cutting or modification of the external clitoris, clitoral reconstruction can be considered. Clitoral reconstruction aims to restore and rebuild the clitoris. It is also known as "clitoral transposition" or "clitoral re-exposition." Claims have been made that it improves sexual function, restores genital appearance, and treats or decreases clitoral pain. However recent systematic reviews of studies reporting on safety and clinical outcomes associated with clitoral reconstruction illustrate that high-quality evidence to support these claims is largely lacking [40].

Technique

Clitoral reconstruction involves the removal and dissection of the scar tissue covering the clitoral body to form a neo-clitoris. The procedure is performed by urologists, gynecologists, and plastic surgeons. Table 3 describes varying techniques [40].

Table 3 Comparative techniques for clitoral reconstruction

Author	Technique
Thabet (Egypt), Foldès (France)	Dissection of scar tissue at the clitoral stump followed by mobilization of the remaining clitoris by transecting the suspensory ligament. The neo-clitoris is then anchored to bulbocavernosus muscles at a lower, more visible location
Ouedraogo (Burkina Faso)	Modified technique of above that does not involve anchoring sutures to the bulbocavernosus muscles
O'Dey	A more complex technique including an anterior obturator artery perforator flap (aOAP flap) for vulvar reconstruction, an omega domed flap (OD flap) for clitoral prepuce reconstruction, and a microsurgical procedure called neurotizing and molding of the clitoral stump (NMCS procedure) for the clitoral tip
Chang et al. (United States)	Wide circumferential release of the superficial scar between the labia followed by deep dissection to release the palpable clitoris to the pubic bone. The labia majora are then rolled and sutured to the periosteum. The clitoris is left to remucosalize and sutured nonstick dressing applied to prevent readherence of raw clitoris to surrounding tissue

In many countries it is mandatory for patients seeking clitoral reconstruction to first follow a multidisciplinary care pathway that involves education on sexual anatomy and function, care of other traumas (war, rape, forced marriage), or psychological or psychiatric comorbidities and sex therapy [40].

Potential risks:

- Anesthesia-related risks.
- Postoperative complications.
- Wound dehiscence, hematoma, infection.
- Hospital readmission.
- Revision surgery.
- Vaginal graft necrosis.
- De novo chronic pain.
- Hyperesthesia of the clitoris.
- Dysfunctional orgasm in women who were previously able to achieve orgasm.
- Recurrence of post-traumatic stress disorder.
- No change in sexual response, body image, and aesthetic appearance.

Potential benefits:

- More visible clitoris.
- Improved sexual function.
- Decreased pain.
- Improved gender identity.
- Improved body image.

As previously noted, there is not enough evidence to support the safety and efficacy of clitoral reconstruction. When examining all the available evidence, it appears that clitoral reconstruction cannot be medically indicated on physical or anatomical grounds, except in cases as a treatment for pain and potential improvement of associated sexual dysfunction when these have not responded to more conservative measures and following clear counselling regarding the risks introduced by clitoral reconstruction and the lack of strong evidence regarding its potential benefits (sexual, psychological, or symbolic).

For this reason, the Royal College of Obstetricians and Gynaecologists currently recommends against clitoral reconstruction. The WHO does not make recommendations in favor of clitoral reconstruction but suggests that before surgery is planned, less invasive treatments should be explored [40] (Table 4).

Prevention Strategies

There has been a global move toward aiming at prevention of the practice of FGM/C. As part of the Sustainable Development Goal 5, the United Nations aims to stop FGM/C by 2030 [41]. This falls under the category of stopping gender-based violence and inequality, as well as to empower women and girls. However, at this stage, an estimated 68 million girls will be at risk in 2030. Key

Table 4 WHO summary of the recommendations (R) and best practice statements (BP) [1]

Deinfibulation
R-1 Deinfibulation is recommended for preventing and treating obstetric complications in women living with type III FGM (strong recommendation; very low-quality evidence).
R-2 Either antepartm or intrapartum deinfibulation is recommended to facilitate childbirth in women living with type III FGM (conditional recommendation; very low-quality evidence).
R-3 Deinfibulation is recommended for preventing and treating urologic complications – specifically recurrent urinary tract infections and urinary retention – in girls and women living with type III FGM (strong recommendation; no direct evidence).
BP-1 Girls and women who are candidates for deinfibulation should receive adequate preoperative briefing (Best practice statement).
BP-2 Girls and women undergoing deinfibulation should be offered local anaesthesia (Best practice statement).
Mental health
R-4 Cognitive behavioural therapy (CBT) should be considered for girls and women living with FGM who are experiencing symptoms consistent with anxiety disorders, depression or post-traumatic stress disorder (PTSD) (conditional recommendation; no direct evidence).
BP-3 Psychological support should be available for girls and women who will receive or have received any surgical intervention to correct health complications of FGM (Best practice statement).
Female sexual health
R-5 Sexual counselling is recommended for preventing or treating female sexual dysfunction among women living with FGM (conditional recommendation; no direct evidence).
Information and education
BP-4 Information, education and communication (IEC)[a] interventions regarding FGM and women's health should be provided to girls and women living with any type of FGM (Best practice statement).
BP-5 Health education[b] information on deinfibulation should be provided to girls and women living with type III FGM (Best practice statement).
BP-6 Health-care providers have been responsibility to convey accurate and clear information, using language and methods that can be readily understood by clients (Best practice statement).
BP-7 Information regarding different types of FGM and the associated respective immediate and long-term health risks should be provided to health-care providers who care for girls and women living with FGM (Best practice statement).
BP-8 Information about FGM delivered to health workers should clearly convey the message that medicalization is unacceptable (Best practice statement).

[a]WHO defines information, education and communication (IEC) interventions as "a public health approach aiming at changing or reinforcing health-related behaviours in a target audience, concerning a specific problem and within a pre-defined period of time, through communication methods and principles." Source: Information, education and communication – lessons from the past, perspectives for the future. Geneva; World Health Organization; 2001
[b]Health education is the provision of accurate, truthful information so that a person can become knowledgeable about the subject and make an informed choice. Source: Training modules for the syndromic management of sexually transmitted infections: educating and counselling the patient. Geneva: World Health Organization; 2007

role players include community members; community leaders; local, national, and international governments; and healthcare providers.

Education is a fundamental element in the attempt to eradicate FGM/C as studies have shown that the practice decreases as the level of education, specifically the level of education of women, increases. Advocates for female health and body autonomy have the greatest impact when they are part of the community itself. However, this poses a security risk for these outspoken women who are sometimes seen as agitators.

Support of the local policing authorities is vital in aiding these women as FGM/C is illegal in most countries. Resistance from elders in the community, especially the elder women, appears to be a stumbling block in the plight to stop FGM/C.

Healthcare providers play an important role as well, a role which can be enhanced with training and knowledge around the subject. Reluctance to directly address the issue stems from concerns of causing offence due to cultural differences between the healthcare provider and the patient. This misunderstanding may lead to a breakdown in communication which will worsen the divide between patient and healthcare professional [4]. The only way in which to change this narrative is to educate healthcare professionals and to encourage them to open the dialogue with patients at risk or from countries where FGM/C is practiced. However, a survey conducted in France showed that only 24% of health professionals reported having received university training in FGM/C. Patients at risk are therefore not routinely asked or examined with a view to assess for FGM/C. Canada, the United States, Belgium, Switzerland, and the United Kingdom have published recommended procedures for screening protocols [4, 30].

Azadi et al. noted that women didn't always realize that they had been cut, as it was regarded as something that every girl goes through in their home country [4]. In this qualitative study, the women expressed distress at having been informed that they have been cut, but no further conversation or support was offered by the majority of healthcare professionals. Some did mention that there is the possibility of corrective surgery, but the benefit of it was poorly explained. These patients sought explanations from other healthcare providers. The consequences of having been cut were also not clearly discussed with the patients, leaving them feeling sad and confused rather than hopeful for assistance. That being said, studies have shown that medicalization of FGM/C alone does not decrease the rate at which it occurs [42]. The procedure is simply moved out of the hands of traditional leaders and into the hands of the healthcare provider.

As many people require an assessment at a travel clinic prior to traveling from Europe and the United States of America (USA) to FGM/C practicing countries, travel clinics are in the position to offer screening services for FGM/C. The legal implications of FGM/C should also be understood by all healthcare professionals but more so by those working in travel clinics as they are in the position to educate patients going to countries at risk. The impact that this may have in the prevention of FGM/C has yet to be determined, but it would be a step forward for young girls at risk.

Abidogun et al. reviewed the nature of preventative measures that have been put into place within the Arab League [43]. Eight of the 12 studies reviewed showed short-term improvement with education as the primary tool for prevention of FGM/C. However, no long-term changes resulted from these interventions. The different studies targeted different groups in terms of education: women and girls, religious leaders, and men in the general population. Social marketing and mixed media approaches were used in three studies where radio broadcasts and WhatsApp group messages were spread among the community. A multi-sectoral approach was only used in one study. The health belief model is most widely used as it focuses on attitude and knowledge around the subject [44]. However, there has been a shift away from this model as it does not offer guidance on how to effect change in health behavior, nor does it take into account societal and peer influences or motivation to stop the practice. Unfortunately, education alone, especially on an individual level, is unlikely to change FGM/C practices. A combination of enforcing legislation with community-level education largely targeting men and religious leaders, as well as girls at risk, may lead to a decrease in the practice of FGM/C. Non-government organizations may prove to be a valuable tool in the prevention strategy as they often have close ties and open channels of communication with the community [43].

Community involvement together with legal implications have led to a decline in FGM/C in Ethiopia [5]. There was a 24% decrease in the proportion of adolescents undergoing FGM/C between 2000 and 2016. However, there is still a significant number (28%) of girls aged 10–14 undergoing FGM/C. The overall attitude toward gender-based violence among both boys and girls in Ethiopia has decreased over the last decade [5]. With increasing education and a higher rate of primary school attendance, it is possible to change the narrative from early on. The rate-limiting factors include a high rate of discontinuing schooling before the end of primary school, as well as strong traditional and cultural beliefs that are being retained, especially in the rural parts of Ethiopia.

Conclusion

It is clear and widely acknowledged that FGM/C is a form of GBV and needs to be eradicated. Notwithstanding the immediate pain and suffering that the patient is experiencing, the long-term effects are significant on a physical and a psychological level. Education alone is not enough to stop this practice. Enlisting the aid of community leaders and separating cultural traditions from religious beliefs are vital for SDG 5 to be successful. It is only through a global multisectoral approach that we may be able to stop this procedure from being done.

Cross-References

▶ Female Sexual Dysfunction

References

1. WHO Geneva. WHO guidelines on the management of health complications from female genital mutilation. 2016 (May).
2. United Nations Children's Fund. Female genital mutilation/cutting: a statistical overview and exploration of the dynamics of change [Internet]. New York; 2013. Available from: https://www.unicef.org/reports/female-genital-mutilation-cutting
3. Lever H, Baranowski KA, Ottenheimer D, Atkinson HG, Singer EK. Histories of pervasive gender-based violence in asylum-seeking women who have undergone female genital mutilation or cutting. J Trauma Stress [Internet]. 2022;35(3):839–51. Available from: http://www.ncbi.nlm.nih.gov/pubmed/35170100
4. Azadi B, Tantet C, Sylla F, Andro A. Women who have undergone female genital mutilation/cutting's perceptions and experiences with healthcare providers in Paris. Cult Heal Sex [Internet]. 2022;24(4):583–96. https://doi.org/10.1080/13691058.2021.1982010.
5. Akwara E, Worknesh K, Oljiira L, Mengesha L, Asnake M, Sisay E, et al. ASRHR in Ethiopia: reviewing progress over the last 20 years and looking ahead to the next 10 years. Reprod Health [Internet]. 2022:1–10. https://doi.org/10.1186/s12978-022-01434-6.
6. Lurie JM, Weidman A, Huynh S, Delgado D, Easthausen I, Kaur G. Painful gynecologic and obstetric complications of female genital mutilation/cutting: a systematic review and meta-analysis. PLoS Med [Internet]. 2020;17(3):e1003088. Available from: http://www.ncbi.nlm.nih.gov/pubmed/32231359
7. Gele AA, Bø BP, Sundby J. Have we made progress in Somalia after 30 years of interventions? Attitudes toward female circumcision among people in the Hargeisa district. BMC Res Notes [Internet]. 2013;6:122. Available from: http://www.ncbi.nlm.nih.gov/pubmed/23537232
8. Reyners M. Health consequences of female genital mutilation. Rev Gynaecol Pract. 2004;4(4):242–51.
9. Ofor MO, Ofole NM. Female genital mutilation: the place of culture and the debilitating effects on the dignity of the female gender. 2015;11(14):112–21.
10. Ghadially R. All for "Izzat". Newsl Womens Glob Netw Reprod Rights [Internet]. 2018;(38):7–8. Available from: http://www.ncbi.nlm.nih.gov/pubmed/12285436
11. Al-Hinai H. Female genital mutilation in the Sultanate of Oman [Internet]. 2014. Available from: http://www.stopfgmmideast.org/wp-content/uploads/2014/01/habiba-al-hinai-female-genital-mutilation-in-the-sultanate-of-oman1.pdf
12. Alsibiani SA, Rouzi AA. Sexual function in women with female genital mutilation. Fertil Steril [Internet]. 2010;93(3):722–4. Available from: http://www.ncbi.nlm.nih.gov/pubmed/19028385.
13. Kvello A, Sayed L. Omskjering av kvinner i de forente arabiske emirater—er klitoridektomi i tradisjonell praksis et overgrep mot kvinner? (Concerning female circumcision in the United Arab Emirates: is clitoridectomy in a traditional context an assault against women? 2002.
14. Organization WH. Global strategy to stop health-care providers from performing female genital mutilation. World Health Organization (Geneva, Switzerland)/ iris. Insitutional Repository for Information SharingVernon, CA, USA).; 2010. p. 18.
15. Toubia NF, Sharief EH. Female genital mutilation: have we made progress? Int J Gynaecol Obstet [Internet]. 2003;82(3):251–61. Available from: http://www.ncbi.nlm.nih.gov/pubmed/14499972
16. New York governor signs ban on female genital mutilation. Reprod Free news [Internet]. 1997;6(16):6. Available from: http://www.ncbi.nlm.nih.gov/pubmed/12295180
17. Goldberg H, Stupp P, Okoroh E, Besera G, Goodman D, Danel I. Female genital mutilation/cutting in the United States: updated estimates of women and girls at risk. Public Health Rep [Internet]. 2012;131(2):340–7. Available from: http://www.ncbi.nlm.nih.gov/pubmed/26957669
18. Mather M, Feldman-Jacobs C. Women and girls at risk of female genital mutilation/cutting in the United States [Internet]. Population Reference Bureau. 2016. Available from: https://www.prb.org/resources/women-and-girls-at-risk-of-female-genital-mutilation-cutting-in-the-united-states/
19. Lee M, Strong N. Female genital mutilation: What Ob/Gyns need to know [Internet]. 2015. Available from:

20. Abdulcadir J, Catania L, Hindin MJ, Say L, Petignat P, Abdulcadir O. Female genital mutilation: a visual reference and learning tool for health care professionals. Obstet Gynecol [Internet]. 2016;128(5):958–63. Available from: http://www.ncbi.nlm.nih.gov/pubmed/27741194

21. Chibber R, El-Saleh E, El Harmi J. Female circumcision: obstetrical and psychological sequelae continues unabated in the 21st century. J Matern Fetal Neonatal Med [Internet]. 2011;24(6):833–6. Available from: http://www.ncbi.nlm.nih.gov/pubmed/21121711

22. Morison L, Scherf C, Ekpo G, Paine K, West B, Coleman R, et al. The long-term reproductive health consequences of female genital cutting in rural Gambia: a community-based survey. Trop Med Int Health [Internet]. 2001;6(8):643–53. Available from: http://www.ncbi.nlm.nih.gov/pubmed/11555430

23. Iavazzo C, Sardi TA, Gkegkes ID. Female genital mutilation and infections: a systematic review of the clinical evidence. Arch Gynecol Obstet [Internet]. 2013;287(6):1137–49. Available from: http://www.ncbi.nlm.nih.gov/pubmed/23315098

24. Payne CK, Abdulcadir J, Ouedraogo C, Madzou S, Kabore FA, De EJB. International continence society white paper regarding female genital mutilation/cutting. Neurourol Urodyn. 2019;38(2):857–67.

25. Farage MA, Miller KW, Tzeghai GE, Azuka CE, Sobel JD, Ledger WJ. Female genital cutting: confronting cultural challenges and health complications across the lifespan. Women's Heal [Internet]. 2015;11(1):79–94. https://doi.org/10.2217/WHE.14.63.

26. Dirie MA, Lindmark G. A hospital study of the complications of female circumcision. Trop Dr. 1991;21(4):146–8.

27. Dave AJ, Sethi A, Morrone A. Female genital mutilation: what every American dermatologist needs to know. Dermatol Clin [Internet]. 2011;29(1):103–9. https://doi.org/10.1016/j.det.2010.09.002.

28. Young J, Nour NM, Macauley RC, Narang SK, Johnson-Agbakwu C. Diagnosis, management, and treatment of female genital mutilation or cutting in girls. Pediatrics. 2020;146(2):e20201012.

29. Berg R, Denison EFA. Psychological, social and sexual consequences of female genital mutilation/cutting (FGM/C) [Internet]. A systematic REview of Quantitative Studies. 2010. Available from: www.kunnskapssenteret.no

30. Abdulcadir J, Rodriguez MI, Say L. A systematic review of the evidence on clitoral reconstruction after female genital mutilation/cutting. Int J Gynaecol Obstet [Internet]. 2015;129(2):93–7. Available from: http://www.ncbi.nlm.nih.gov/pubmed/25638712

31. Davis G, Curtin CM. Management of pain in complex nerve injuries. Hand Clin [Internet]. 2016;32(2):257–62. Available from: http://www.ncbi.nlm.nih.gov/pubmed/27094896

32. Foldes P. Reconstructive plastic surgery of the clitoris after sexual mutilation. Prog Urol [Internet]. 2004;14(1):47–50. Available from: http://www.ncbi.nlm.nih.gov/pubmed/15098751

33. Bayo S, Bosch FX, de Sanjosé S, Muñoz N, Combita AL, Coursaget P, et al. Risk factors of invasive cervical cancer in Mali. Int J Epidemiol [Internet]. 2002;31(1):202–9. Available from: http://www.ncbi.nlm.nih.gov/pubmed/11914322

34. Osterman AL, Winer RL, Gottlieb GS, Sy MP, Ba S, Dembele B, et al. Female genital mutilation and non-invasive cervical abnormalities and invasive cervical cancer in Senegal, West Africa: a retrospective study. Int J Cancer. 2019;144(6):1302–12.

35. Almroth L, Elmusharaf S, El Hadi N, Obeid A, El Sheikh MAA, Elfadil SM, et al. Primary infertility after genital mutilation in girlhood in Sudan: a case-control study. Lancet. 2005;366(9483):385–91.

36. Female Genital Mutilation and Obstetric Outcome: WHO collaborative prospective study in Six African countries. Obstet Gynecol. 2006;108(2):450.

37. Martinelli M, Ollé-Goig JE. Female genital mutilation in Djibouti. Afr Health Sci. 2012;12(4):412–5.

38. Behrendt A, Moritz S. Posttraumatic stress disorder and memory problems after female genital mutilation. Am J Psychiatry. 2005;162(5):1000–2.

39. Nour NM, Michels KB, Bryant AE. Defibulation to treat female genital cutting: effect on symptoms and sexual function. Obstet Gynecol. 2006;108(1):55–60.

40. Sharif Mohamed F, Wild V, Earp BD, Johnson-Agbakwu C, Abdulcadir J. Clitoral reconstruction after female genital mutilation/cutting: a review of surgical techniques and ethical debate. J Sex Med [Internet]. 2020;17(3):531–42. https://doi.org/10.1016/j.jsxm.2019.12.004.

41. Social Affairs UND of E and, Sustainable D. Goal 5: achieve gender equality and empower all women and girls, 2022.

42. Gruenbaum E. The female circumcision controversy: an anthropological perspective. Philadelphia University Pennsylvania Press, Philadelphia, Pensylvania, USA; 2001. p. 242.

43. Abidogun TM, Alyssa Ramnarine L, Fouladi N, Owens J, Abusalih HH, Bernstein J, et al. Female genital mutilation and cutting in the Arab League and diaspora: a systematic review of preventive interventions. Trop Med Int Health. 2022;27:468–78.

44. Jones CL, Jensen JD, Scherr CL, Brown NR, Christy K, Weaver J. The health belief model as an explanatory framework in communication research exploring parallel, serial, and moderated mediation. Health Commun [Internet]. 2015;30(6):566–76. Available from: http://www.ncbi.nlm.nih.gov/pubmed/25010519

Part XI

Vaginoplasty and Neovagina Construction in Congenital Defects, Trauma, and Gender Affirming Surgery

(Neo) Vaginoplasty in Female Pelvic Congenital Anomalies

Manuel Belmonte Chico Goerne, David Bouhadana, Mohamed El-Sherbiny, and Mélanie Aubé-Peterkin

Contents

Introduction	1186
Nonobstructive Anomalies	1187
Mayer-Rokitansky-Kuster-Hauser Syndrome	1187
Androgen Insensitivity Syndrome	1197
Longitudinal Vaginal Septum	1203
Obstructive Anomalies	1204
Imperforate Hymen	1204
Transverse Vaginal Septum	1204
Congenital Adrenal Hyperplasia	1205
Management	1206
Conclusion	1206
Cross-References	1206
References	1206

M. Belmonte Chico Goerne
Sexual Medicine and Genitourinary Reconstructive Surgery, McGill University Health Center, Montreal, QC, Canada

D. Bouhadana
McGill University, Montreal, QC, Canada
e-mail: david.bouhadana@mail.mcgill.ca

M. El-Sherbiny
Department of Surgery and Pediatric surgery, McGill University Health Center and Montreal Children's Hospital, Montreal, QC, Canada
e-mail: mohamed.el-sherbiny@mcgill.ca

M. Aubé-Peterkin (✉)
Department of Surgery/Urology, McGill University Health Center and Lachine Hospital, Montreal, QC, Canada
e-mail: melanie.aube-peterkin@mcgill.ca

Abstract

Congenital pelvic malformations are rare conditions characterized by specific common features resulting from an abnormal embryological development of the urogenital and anorectal apparatus. Anomalies in pelvic morphology caused by these malformations lead to complex management and surgical planning. Vaginal absence or hypoplasia is commonly found in females with these conditions. Vaginoplasty and neovaginoplasty are the surgical mainstays for functional, aesthetic, and reproductive restoration in these cases. These procedures aim to achieve an adequately sized and located vagina, as well as normal appearing external female genitalia.

A variety of vaginoplasty techniques exist with similar outcomes. Surgeon experience, complexity of vaginal defects and convergence between the vagina and the urethra are factors that impact surgical decision-making.

Management of congenital pelvic malformations in the context of disorders of sexual differentiation is often complex and sometimes controversial, and must be undertaken by trained specialists including a multidisciplinary team (e.g., endocrinologists, neonatologists, urogynecologists, etc.). These conditions may lead to long-term reproductive, psychological, and sexual health consequences.

This chapter covers the relatively common congenital pelvic malformations that require vaginoplasty. The individual pathophysiology, clinical presentation, diagnosis, and management options, both conservative and surgical, will be presented. The common surgical techniques of (neo)vaginoplasty will be discussed.

Keywords

Neovaginoplasty · Vaginoplasty · Female pelvic congenital anomalies · Female genital congenital anomalies · Disorders of sexual development

Introduction

Congenital pelvic malformations are uncommon, but when present may have a significant impact on psychological, sexual, and reproductive health. These conditions are characterized by specific features originating from abnormal embryological development of the urogenital apparatus. Depending on their severity, these anomalies can significantly modify pelvic morphology and impact surgical planning [1].

During the embryonic period, the Müllerian (paramesonephric) ducts appear from the mesoderm (7th week) as focal invaginations of the coelomic epithelium. These ducts are the precursors of the cervix, uterus, fallopian tubes, and upper two-thirds of the vagina. The lower third of the vagina develops as the sinovaginal bulb canalizes. The external genitalia differentiate between the 10th and 12th week of gestation [2].

There are three types of female reproductive tract congenital anomalies: (1) vaginal agenesis or hypoplasia, (2) lateral fusion defects, and (3) vertical fusion defects.

Vaginal hypoplasia and agenesis, commonly found in females with congenital pelvic malformations, can result from androgen insensitivity syndromes and inappropriate secretion of testosterone, which causes the fusion of vagina and urethra forming a common channel and external genitalia virilization. These can present concomitantly with Müllerian duct anomalies (MDAs). Mayer-Rokitansky-Kuster-Hauser syndrome (MRKH) and cloacal anomalies/bladder exstrophy may also cause vaginal hypoplasia or agenesis [3].

MDAs result from a faulty lateral or vertical merge, absent development, or a resorption failure of paramesonephric ducts. This leads to abnormal canalization, agenesis, fusion, and aberrant embryonic rests in the female reproductive tract [4]. When lateral merge anomalies happen, they can lead to longitudinal vaginal septum, and uterine defects such as bicornuate uterus, arcuate uterus, and uterus didelphys. If the merge between the Müllerian bulb and urogenital sinus (UGS) fails (vertical fusion), this can result in transverse vaginal septum, oblique vaginal septum, imperforate hymen, or cervical absence [5]. It is important to mention that MDAs have also a high correlation with urinary tract anomalies, notably renal (40%), spinal (15%), gastrointestinal (12%), and musculoskeletal anomalies (10–12%) [6, 7].

Clinical presentation can vary greatly between patients. Most of these anomalies are asymptomatic and are not diagnosed until early puberty or adolescence with symptoms such as cyclical pelvic pain, dysmenorrhea (94%), amenorrhea, and dyspareunia. Some cases may present with a palpable abdominal mass caused by hematometra (collected menstrual blood inside the uterus) [3].

The evaluation of a patient with suspected congenital pelvic malformations should include a full physical exam assessing for signs of female sexual secondary characteristics. Most of these patients will have normal height, breast development, pubic hair, and external genitalia, with the exception of patients with androgen insensitivity. Patients with the latter condition will present with decreased growth of pubic and axillary hair despite normal breast development. In sexually active patients, a vaginal examination is recommended and a short distal vagina and an absent cervix can be identified [8].

Psychological and social evaluation of the patient and their family is recommended due to the occasionally sensitive nature of these conditions, to prevent any long-term psychological impact [9].

These conditions are often accompanied with urinary, gastrointestinal, and musculoskeletal anomalies; therefore imaging is required to appropriately evaluate the extent of the condition [9]. Ultrasonography (US) – transabdominal, translabial, or transrectal using either 2D or 3D technology – is the initial diagnostic modality of choice. Magnetic resonance imaging (MRI) is considered the gold standard as it accurately assesses rudimentary Müllerian structures and pelvic organs to optimize clinical management and surgical planning. Computed tomography (CT) and genitography are also valid options but involve radiation exposure [9, 10].

Selection of laboratory tests is based on clinical findings, and can include karyotype, serum electrolytes, CYP17A1 gene, adrenal steroids (17-hydroxyprogesterone, deoxy-corticosterone, corticosterone, and cortisol), androgens (testosterone, dihydro-testosterone, and androstenedione), estrogens (estrone, estradiol, and estriol), Müllerian-inhibiting substance (MIS), and gonadotrophin levels (notably FSH) [9, 10].

Cystoscopy and vaginoscopy are useful for anatomic evaluation and surgical planning, and provide similar information than genitography. They are often performed at the time of surgical correction to assess the anatomic relation between the bladder neck and the confluence of the urinary tract with the vagina, to catheterize the urethra and vagina, and to facilitate the identification of these structures during surgery [11]. Laparoscopy is not necessary if the diagnosis has been obtained by clinical data supported by biochemical or genetics results and is only recommended to rule out ovotestis [12].

Once diagnosis is complete, treatment (medical or surgical) will depend on the type of malformation and involved organs. In the case of obstructive anomalies, initial medical treatment may be indicated if the patient is symptomatic (dysmenorrhea and/or abdominal pain) but wishes to delay surgical management. Medical suppressive therapy with hormonal contraception or progestin can be used. If suppression therapy is not available or ineffective, surgery may be performed by creating a vaginal space to allow for evacuation of the hematocolpos [3, 13, 14].

Vaginoplasty, or surgical creation of a neovagina, is reserved for patients with disorders of sexual differentiation (DSD) with absence or severe hypoplasia of the vagina. The objective of these procedures is to provide a normally positioned and sensate clitoris, a well-situated and adequately sized vagina, and to provide normal appearance of the external genitalia. Several surgical techniques have been described. Selection of the procedure depends on multiple factors, including type and severity of the defects, height of the confluence between the urethra and the vagina and surgeon experience [15].

Nonobstructive Anomalies

These anomalies in uterine and vaginal anatomy are frequently asymptomatic and present with normal appearing external genitalia. Patients who have symptoms will present during or after puberty with primary amenorrhea, infertility, dyspareunia, or recurrent miscarriages [16].

Mayer-Rokitansky-Kuster-Hauser Syndrome

Pathophysiology
Mayer-Rokitansky-Kuster-Hauser (MRKH) syndrome, also known as vaginal agenesis, refers to the congenital absence of the fallopian tubes,

uterus, cervix, and the upper two-thirds of the vagina, caused by a failure of the paramesonephric ducts in embryo. The incidence of this condition ranges from 4000 to 10,000 female births [17].

Clinical Presentation

Women with MRKH syndrome present with a normal female genotype (46, XX), normal appearing external genitalia and ovarian function, but with absent vagina and uterus. Mullerian aplasia is suspected if there is a history of amenorrhea with a normal appearing vulva and hymen, and the absence of a vaginal opening [18]. Endometrial activity is present in 6–10% of cases, which may cause cyclical abdominal pain. Dyspareunia, difficulties with sexual intercourse and/or primary infertility may be a concern [16] and may cause significant psychological distress [19, 20].

Diagnosis

On physical exam, these patients are phenotypical women with normal external genitalia, breast development, height, and body hair according to their age (Table 1). An absent or hypoplastic (small flush dimple-like) vagina and cervical absence are key features. Differential diagnosis includes androgen insensitivity syndrome (AIS) (Table 2) [8, 19]. Fifty percent of these patients have associated renal or musculoskeletal malformations [19].

MRI is the gold standard imaging study for MRKH, as MRI confirms the diagnosis and can provide information about endometrial presence and Müllerian remnants, which are often difficult to assess using US. MRI also helps to evaluate associated congenital anomalies like renal agenesis and scoliosis, has a 95% correlation with laparoscopic findings, and is the most useful tool for surgical planning [10, 19].

Laparoscopy is not mandatory for diagnosis, but findings include uterine absence and visualization of unilateral or bilateral Müllerian remnants. Laparoscopy can also aid in management of patients with cyclic pain who may have endometriosis or uterine horns, which can be removed in the same setting [21].

Classification

Two accepted forms of MRKH exist. The typical form, type 1, is characterized by the absence of the proximal two-thirds of the vagina, uterus agenesis and normal ovaries, fallopian tubes and urinary system. The atypical form, type 2, presents with other congenital defects including ovary and/or renal malformations including MURCS association (Mullerian, Renal, Cervicothoracic, and Somite abnormalities) [19].

Treatment

Psychological Counseling/Support

These women frequently suffer from anxiety, depression, self-esteem, and relationship issues and treatment should involve psychosocial, group, and parental counseling to help navigate treatments and surgical options [8, 22].

Vaginal Elongation/Dilation

Vaginal elongation via dilation is currently the first-line approach. Its goal is to increase vaginal size. It is a cost-effective, safe, and patient-driven approach [8]. Teaching of proper technique is essential to avoid injury and improve compliance [21]. Although not all patients perceive this option as acceptable [22], success rates in achieving a functional vagina can reach 90–96% [23].

Table 1 Tanner Staging Chart

Stage	Body hair characteristics	Breast characteristics
I	No hair	No breast development
II	Scarce and soft pubic hair on labia	Breast buds
III	Curly hair on mons pubis	Breast elevation and areolar enlargement
IV	Adult type but in small areas and absent on thigh	Areolae and papillate form secondary mound
V	Present on thighs, major quantity	Full development

Table 2 Comparative presentations of Mayer-Rokitansky-Kuster-Hauser syndrome, androgen insensitivity syndromes, and congenital adrenal hyperplasia

Abnormalities and findings	Mayer-Rokitansky-Kuster-Hauser (MRKH) syndrome	Complete Androgen Insensitivity syndrome (CAIS)	Partial Androgen Insensitivity syndrome (PAIS)	Congenital Adrenal Hyperplasia (CAH)
External Genitalia	Normal	Normal	Different degrees of virilization	Ambiguous, virilized
Vagina	Upper two-thirds absence	Short distal vagina	Labioscrotal folds, labial fusion	Labioscrotal folds, fused with urethra
Uterus	Absent	Absent	Absent	Present
Gonads	Ovary (some cases with abnormalities)	Testis (abdominal)	Testis	Ovaries
Breasts	Normal	Normal but pallid nipple	Normal	Subtle development[a]
Pubic Hair	Normal	Absent or scarce	Normal or scarce	Premature development
Testosterone	Unaltered	Elevated	Elevated	Decreased[b]
Karyotype	46, XX	46, XY	46, XY	46, XX[c]
Clinical presentation	Primary amenorrhea, infertility, impossible penetrative intercourse, and abdominal pain	Primary amenorrhea, facial acne	Hypospadias, micropenis, clitoromegaly, bifid scrotum, infertility, primary amenorrhea	Premature development of pubic hair, irregular cycles, oligomenorrhea androgenism signs (hirsutism, severe acne, etc.), clitoromegaly, hypertension
Imaging	Mullerian remnants and uterus absence (MRI)	Abdominal/Inguinal testicles, cervix, and uterus absence	Abdominal or scrotal testicles, uterus absence	Confirms presence of ovaries
Treatment	Vaginoplasty	Gonadectomy[d] with further estrogen replacement, neovaginoplasty and less frequent feminizing reconstruction surgery	Gonadectomy[d] with further estrogen replacement, feminizing reconstructive surgery and vaginoplasty	Glucocorticoid therapy, feminizing reconstructive surgery and vaginoplasty

[a]If patients are diagnosed and treated before puberty, the pubertal development is normal, even without hirsutism and amenorrhea
[b] Increased deoxycorticosterone and 11-deoxycortisol in plasma and their tetrahydrometabolites in urine
[c]46, XY is also possible, but we described only when it affects women (affected males have normal external genitalia)
[d]Important due to the risk of malignancy

Two methods of dilation/elongation are commonly used: Frank and Ingram methods [19]. Frank's method was described in 1938, using vaginal dilators (Pyrex tubes) to gradually increase vaginal length and width [18, 23]. This method can only be performed in patients with a short vaginal dimple and can take up to 6 months to achieve a 6–7 cm long vagina [18, 19]. Once achieved, dilation should be maintained 2–3 times per week or until the patient has regular penetrative intercourse [8, 18, 24].

Ingram described a variant of this technique with the creation of dilators attached to a bicycle seat. Using their own body weight, patients dilate the vaginal dimple progressively by sitting on the dilators for 2 h per day in 30 min intervals. The size of the dilator is changed progressively just as in Frank's method [19].

There is no official consensus regarding the minimum length to start penetrative intercourse, and vaginal coitus could successfully elongate the vagina in itself [8, 19, 24]. Dilation is successful regardless of the vaginal length achieved as long as the patient is satisfied with the outcomes [24–26]. Micro-fissures due to dilation may increase the risk of acquiring sexually transmitted infections (STIs) [24].

The most commonly reported adverse effects related to dilation are bleeding (0.5%), pain (0.5%), and urinary symptoms or infections (1%). Lubricating gels, vaginal estrogens creams, pelvic floor physiotherapy, and suspending dilations may prevent or treat complications [8, 18, 19, 24]. These patients may suffer from sexual dysfunction, dyspareunia, poor lubrication, and orgasmic dysfunction. Psychological counseling, peer support, and physical therapy may help in these cases [8, 19, 24].

(Neo) Vaginoplasty

Surgical management is indicated for patients who failed vaginal dilation or who prefer surgery as a first line approach. In the latter cases, patients must be informed that dilation is mandatory after surgery and that poor compliance could lead to complications including revision procedures [8, 15].

There is no consensus regarding the best surgical technique, and the elected method is based on the patient's needs and the experience of the surgeon. Surgery if avoided until after puberty and is most commonly performed during mid to late adolescence or in young adults. Patients must have enough mental maturity to take responsibility for their postoperative care and should be advised by a multidisciplinary team with expertise in DSD [22, 27].

The main objective of surgery is the creation of a functional ≥6 cm vaginal canal, with an appropriate vaginal pouch and introital transverse dimensions, with minimal wound contraction (≤25%) and resistant vaginal covering that permits painless penetrative intercourse [15, 26, 27] (Picture 1).

Since the second half of the nineteenth century, multiple neovagina techniques have been described, but none have yet to become a gold standard. Studies are often small, retrospective, and with variable outcomes. The main differences between these procedures are the type of tissue

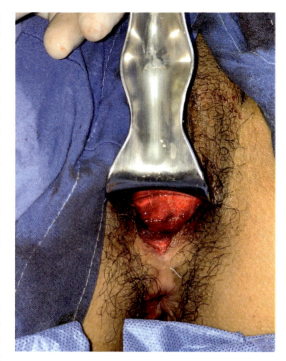

Picture 1 Neovaginal canal

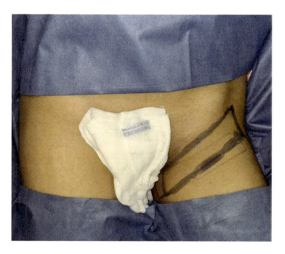

Picture 2 Donor site markings for inguinal split thickness skin graft

used, for example skin, bowel segments, pudendal-thigh flaps, labia minora flaps, fasciocutaneous, and gracilis myocutaneous flaps [27–29] (Picture 2).

Despite the wide number of options, the most frequently performed are the Abbé-McIndoe, Vecchietti (open and laparoscopic), and Williams procedures, with the common denominator that neither of them requires a bowel anastomosis nor laparotomy [26].

Abbé-McIndoe

This popular technique combines the retrovesical dissection described by McIndoe in 1938 and the use of a split thickness skin graft (STSG) developed by Abbé. Despite the procedure's relative simplicity and low complexity, complications like graft contraction, partial graft take, and fistula formation may occur [28, 29].

Advantages include minimal donor site morbidity, easy tissue harvesting, and avoidance of an abdominal approach. The most common drawbacks are vaginal dryness due to absence of lubricating properties of the skin, prolonged use of a vaginal support, and visible scars at the donor site [15, 27].

Functional success rates are around 80%. The surgery is successful when a ≥7 cm vagina with less than 25% of graft contracture and a normal looking functional neovagina are achieved [26].

Technique

Preoperative antibiotics and bowel preparation (to decrease inadvertent perforation) are recommended [12, 27]. The approach is done through a perineal transverse or "Y shaped" incision, then a space is created in the retrovesical space (between the urethra/bladder and rectum) with blunt dissection aiming to create a 12–13 cm length and 4.5–6 cm diameter cavity with the Douglas pouch as the upper and posterior limit. A <0.5 cm thick and 18 cm wide and long STSG is harvested from a non-hirsute area, usually the posterior aspect of the thigh, inguinal area, buttocks, or the suprapubic area (Picture 3). The graft is fenestrated and seated (with dermal surface facing toward the exterior) around a mold using mattress sutures with 4-0 polyglactin absorbable material. It is important to use a single suture line to secure the graft to the mold, since this reduces potential graft contraction) (Pictures 7, 8 and 4).

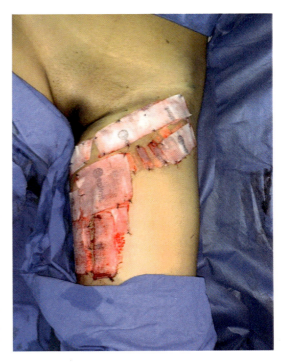

Picture 3 Donor site after harvesting inguinal skin graft

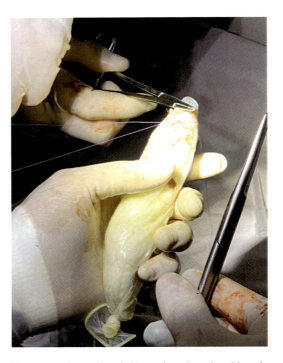

Picture 4 The mold and skin graft are introduced into the neovaginal canal

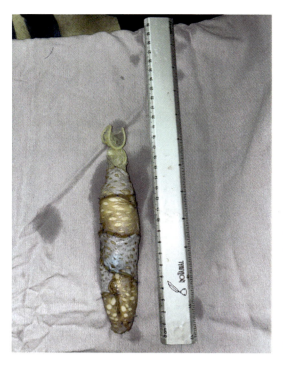

Picture 5 After introduction of the mold into the neovaginal canal, the margins of the skin graft are fixed

Picture 6 Neovaginal appearance after the mold is removed and the skin graft is in place

Once the STSG is secured to the mold, it is introduced into the created space and the free margins of the graft are fixed to the inner aspect of the labia and/or to the borders of the incision (Picture 5). This mold is kept in place for 7–10 days and if it has a channel, patients can irrigate daily the neovagina with saline or diluted povidone-iodine solution (1%). Once the mold is removed and the neovagina is well-healed, regular penetrative intercourse or dilation (at least three times per week) is indicated to prevent contraction [8, 15, 27–29] (Picture 6).

The mold is a key part of this procedure and can be created from different materials including a sponge, dental impression material, silicone or latex, which is wrapped with a soft sponge or a condom to ease insertion [29, 30] (Picture 8). Many graft tissue variants have emerged over the last 10 years, including artificial dermis, human amnion, or oral mucosa graft, all with promising outcomes and decreased donor site morbidity [28].

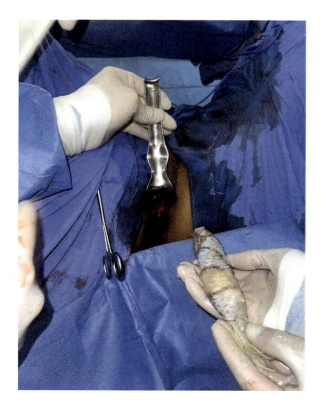

Picture 7 When placed around the mold, the dermal surface of the graft should face toward the exterior

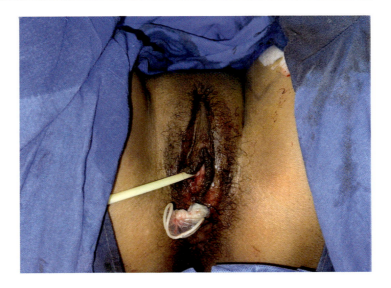

Picture 8 Final appearance of the molded skin graft. The mold is created using foam wrapped with a condom to ease insertion

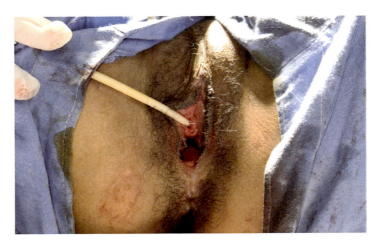

Complications and Troubleshooting

Complications occur in 14% of cases including inadvertent rectal, urethral, bladder, bowel perforation, partial graft take, complete graft failure/graft necrosis, bleeding, fistula (rectovaginal, vesicovaginal, and urethrovaginal), hair-growing vaginal skin, vaginal dryness, vaginal stenosis (pouch contracture), wound infection, keloid scar from donor site, and squamous adenocarcinoma [8, 27, 29].

The most common intraoperative complications with this technique are rare and include intraoperative hemorrhage (<1%) and rectal perforation (<1%). Meticulous hemostasis is usually sufficient, but in the case of uncontrollable bleeding, cavity packing and blood transfusion may be needed. Rectal perforation can be repaired, and the procedure finalized, but intestinal diversion should be concomitantly performed to avoid fistula formation [26]. Presence of fecal discharge and flatus through the neovagina are signs of fistula formation and a diverting colostomy should be performed as soon as possible with daily vaginal washing using saline, soap, or/and antiseptic. After confirming the cessation of the discharge (around 3 days after the colostomy is performed), the patient can replace a smaller mold to avoid putting pressure on the rectum [31]. After

12 weeks, a dye test can assess whether the fistula is still present and surgical repair can be planned. The use of a gracilis flap is recommended in these cases. After 4 weeks, the colostomy can be taken down and dilations resumed [31].

In case of urethral injury, a primary repair is often sufficient and should not affect outcomes. In case of bladder injury, the defect must be repaired and a catheter kept in place for 10–15 days to present postoperative fistula. These complications are rare [28, 32].

The most feared complications are those related to the graft because they can lead to loss of vaginal length or reoperation (<10% in experienced hands). Partial graft take usually occurs at sites of infection or bleeding, causing granulation or neovaginal discharge. Most cases are successfully treated conservatively with silver nitrate cauterization or excision [27, 32].

Complete graft failure is most often related to premature graft displacement or hematoma formation under the graft. Premature patient mobilization during the first postoperative week is the main cause of total graft failure, therefore bed rest is recommended. In these cases, reoperation with a new STSG is needed [27].

Donor site complications include bleeding, scarring, keloids, and hypertrophy, which may heal using topical treatments and corticosteroid injections [30, 32, 33]. Silver and the nanofibrillar cellulose dressings may promote donor site healing [29, 34].

Late complications include neovagina dryness, stricture, contracture, urinary incontinence, granulation tissue, and urinary tract infections (UTI) [32].

Dryness can lead to pain and dyspareunia and lubricants are useful to reduce these symptoms. Stricture and contracture of the neovagina can be corrected with relaxing incisions and progressive dilation. Granulation tissue may be cauterized with silver nitrate or excised [32].

Follow-Up

Regular speculum examination is suggested to rule out malignancy or ulceration [8]. Because MRKH patients who are sexually active are at higher risk of contracting STIs they should be screened annually and advised to use condoms. The Human papillomavirus vaccination is recommended to decrease the risk of neoplasia and genital warts [8].

Vecchietti Procedure

This graftless technique is a traction method because it creates a neovagina rapidly by an uninterrupted invagination, which results from a traction device. Originally described by Vecchietti in 1965 and then modified to a laparoscopic approach, this procedure is a trustable option for patients who failed primary auto dilation, or as a salvage surgery to lengthen a shortened vagina, or to reconstruct an obliterated neovagina. The advantages of this technique are its relative simplicity, low complication rates, the good long-term outcomes, and the fact that it preserves native vaginal tissue [26, 35].

A traction device, ligature carriers (straight and curved Vecchietti thread holders), and a 2.2 × 1.9 cm acrylic-shaped olive are necessary. Parenteral prophylactic antibiotics should be administered preoperatively and to reduce risk of perforation, a urethral catheter and a rectal probe during the procedure are recommended [35, 36].

Transabdominal Vecchietti Technique

After a Pfannenstiel incision is performed, the vesicorectal peritoneum is incised and dissected separating the bladder and rectum. Transabdominally and through the dissected vesicorectal space, the straight ligature carrier is passed perforating the perineum at the pseudohymen level preserving the pseudohymenal membrane. Then one end of a #2 polyglycolic acid suture is passed through the eye of the ligature carrier, which is pulled back into the peritoneal cavity as the ligature carrier is withdrawn. The olive is then threaded on to the external end of this suture. A second parallel pass with the ligature carrier brings the other perineal end of the traction suture into the peritoneal cavity. After that, the curved ligature carrier is introduced laterally to rectus muscle bilaterally in a subperitoneal fashion and is advanced along the pelvic side wall. The ipsilateral traction suture is threaded through the eye of the curved ligature carrier once the tip is visualized beneath the incised peritoneum. The ligature carrier is withdrawn, pulling the suture beyond the skin surface. The peritoneum at the vesicorectal junction and the abdominal incision are closed. The traction device is placed on the abdomen, and the ends of the extracorporeal suture are attached to the traction springs, finalizing the first phase of this technique, the position of the olive and traction sutures [35].

Laparoscopic Vecchietti Technique

The laparoscopic Vecchietti follows the same steps and uses the same instrumentation as the open approach. First, three port sites are created, including a 10 mm umbilical port (through which the laparoscope is introduced), and two lateral 5 mm trocar sites (chosen according to suture exit and surgical exposure). The straight ligature carrier with a number 2 polyglycolic acid suture is advanced from perineum to peritoneal cavity, passing through the vesicorectal space, safely guided by cystoscopy and laparoscopy. Once in the pelvis, the suture is unthreaded from the ligature carrier, and the latter is withdrawn. Then, the olive is threaded onto the external end of the same suture. The other suture end is brought into the peritoneal cavity using a second parallel pass. One of the lateral trocars is removed and the straight ligature carrier is passed and directed subperitoneally, aiming the opening in the peritoneum at the vesicorectal junction, once there, the carrier is passed through it. Same side traction suture is inserted through the eye of this ligature carrier. While removing the ligature carrier, the suture is pulled out of the cavity and beyond the skin surface. The previously removed trocar is reinserted, and the same procedure is done on the contralateral side. Finally, after the pneumoperitoneum is reduced, the traction device is connected to the traction sutures [35].

Postoperative Invagination Phase

For both approaches, during the invagination phase, the neovagina is created by applying constant traction to the olive. The traction device serves as the source of mechanical traction, which is transmitted constantly through the subperitoneal traction suture to the perineal olive. The invagination advances between 1 cm and 1.5 cm per day by steadily increasing traction, creating a neovagina of 10–12 cm length in only 7–9 days. During this phase early ambulation is advisable. Before patients are discharged, the traction device and olive are removed, and a vaginal mold is placed; patients need to be advised that nightly use of vaginal dilators until regular penetrative intercourse is started is necessary to maintain neovaginal length [15, 35].

The urethral catheter must be kept in place for 7–10 days and the patient is encouraged to start early mobilization. The mean postoperative stay is 8 days for post-laparotomy patients and 3 for post-laparoscopy patients [35, 36].

Complications and Troubleshooting

The main intraoperative complications are rectal or bladder injury (1.8%) and hemorrhage (<1%). Bladder perforation is more common in patients with previous failed surgery (9 vs. 1.6%) [26].

Borruto et al. reported a series of 522 patients with only five cases of surgical complications, including three cases of vaginal cavity bleeding and two cases of surrounding structure injury by the ligature carrier (one bladder and one rectum) [37]. Callens et al. conversely reported significant risk of intraoperative complications because of the limited retrovesical and rectal space into which the traction threads are placed [26].

Postoperative pain and need for strong analgesia due to daily tightening are reported. Complications include infections (2.1%), vaginal synechiae, hematuria, necrosis, dehiscence, fistulae, and stenosis (all <1%). Due to the fibrotic reaction in the pelvic connective tissue, there is an increased risk of vaginal prolapse, which can be avoided by preoperatively stretching the vaginal dimple with the Frank technique. The most common postoperative long-term complication is dyspareunia (up to 12%) usually secondary to neovaginal dryness [26, 36].

Outcomes

According to Langer et al., anatomical and functional results are excellent. Neovaginal length can reach 8–14 cm. Anatomical success is defined as a

≥6 cm of neovaginal length and to maintain a long-term success, patients must perform regular dilations or penetrative intercourse [26, 37].

The outcomes between laparoscopic and laparotomy Vecchietti technique are similar with regard to intraoperative complications, neovaginal length, vaginal dryness, and sexual satisfaction [36].

Williams' Neovaginoplasty

Vulvovaginoplasty was popularized by Williams as a method in which the rectovaginal space is not dissected, and the vaginal cavity is created using full-thickness skin grafts (FTSG) from the labia majora, resulting in a less invasive technique [27, 38].

The advantages of this technique are its relative technical simplicity, low complication rates, ease of postoperative care, minimal postoperative pain and rapid recovery, and high success rates of primary and even repeated procedures. In fact, the Williams technique was first used to treat patients with vaginal stenosis secondary to a previous failed repair [27, 38, 39].

The original characteristic horseshoe incision of this technique resulted in an increased risk of vaginal voiding and incorrect neovagina axis, resulting in the development of technical modifications and different materials substituting the FTSG to avoid the disadvantages of skin grafts (freeze-dried human amniotic membranes, buccal mucosa, artificial dermis, autologous in vitro-cultured vaginal tissue, and oxidized cellulose) [26, 27, 38]. FTSG can also be taken from mycocutaneous rectus abdominis or gracilis and pudendal thigh fasciocutaneous flaps [38].

The disadvantages of this technique are the use of hair bearing skin, the difficulty for intercourse due to angle of the external neovagina, insufficient neovaginal length, which can be expanded postoperatively with dilations or penetrative intercourse, lack of lubrication, stenosis, and hair regrowth [26].

Surgical Technique

The patient is positioned in lithotomy. The labia majora and posterior fourchette are infiltrated with 30 cc of 1 in 200,000 solution of adrenaline in normal saline. The labia are grasped with Allis forceps and are pulled laterally to visualize the inner aspects and their maximum extent. The posterior fourchette is incised horizontally and the incision is extended caudally on both sides of labia majora (U or Horse-shoe-shaped incision), following the hair line until the urethral level is reached but staying 4 cm away laterally in both sides. The incision is deepened until the bulbo-spongiosus and perineal muscles are seen and then, using chromic suture and marching from the perineum forward, the inner skin margins (left and right) are attached together; it is important to make sure the suture knots lie within the lumen of the neovagina. To gain the maximum thickness, the bulbo-spongiosus tissues are united and the adjacent connective tissue is brought in. Finally, the skin is closed with nylon and the two-finger test is performed, where the surgeon must be able to insert two fingers for their full length into the neovagina [40].

The key for surgical success relies on the use of sufficient skin to line the neovagina, that is why the mucosal incisions are as near as possible to the hair line and approximately 4 cm from midline, achieving a mucosa wide enough to line a 3 cm in diameter neovagina. A urethral urinary catheter is installed to avoid the contact with the neovagina suture line [40].

The patient is kept in the hospital for 1 week on bed rest. The wound must be scrubbed and irrigated daily with half-strength hydrogen peroxide and kept dry. The stitches are removed on day 7 and the smallest dilator can be used by then at least 2 times per day in progressively increasing diameter. After 3–4 weeks, the patient should be able to use the largest dilator [40].

Technical Modifications

Feroze et al. described a modified Williams' vulvovaginoplasty in which the initial adrenaline infiltration is not used as it may disguise bleeding that could cause a hematoma. They also suggest to preoperatively trim labia minora to the same level of the vulval skin if it is redundant. These authors describe long-term success in the absence of dilations and/or penetrative intercourse [39].

Creatsas' vaginoplasty is based on Williams' technique; the use of a skin flap from patient's perineum is necessary to create a perineal pouch. One advantage of this procedure is that postoperative dilation is not necessary [41].

Complications

Hair-bearing skin from the labia majora may cause further problems or undesirable esthetics, and can be treated using laser [38, 41]. Wound dehiscence, hematoma, and infection are rare and can be prevented with bed-rest, careful hemostasis, and prophylactic antibiotics [26, 41].

Vaginal voiding and micturition problems are rare but can be caused by elevation of the perineum creating a distorted urinary stream and postvoid dribbling. Due to the water-resistant properties of vulval skin, these are mild complications and patients can easily clean urine out of the neovagina. Creatsas modification avoids these complications because the perineum is not as high as in Williams' technique [39–41].

Regarding lubrication, Bartholin's glands will function normally but in case of neovaginal dryness, use of lubricating jelly is suggested [40].

Outcomes

Williams and colleagues reported satisfactory penetrative intercourse and orgasm for both patients and their partners [40].

Androgen Insensitivity Syndrome

Formerly called male pseudohermaphroditism, androgen insensitivity syndrome (AIS) is an X-linked recessive DSD caused by a large number and heterogeneity of Androgen Receptor (AR) mutations. It is one of the most common forms of XY DSD and is caused by cell incompetence to respond to the androgens (partially or completely). AIS presents in 46XY individuals as an absence of Müllerian structures and varying degrees of external genitalia virilization, resulting in a wide variety of syndromes. It is divided in two types, Complete Androgen Insensitivity Syndrome (CAIS) and Partial Androgen Insensitivity Syndrome (PAIS). The most frequent type is CAIS [15, 21].

Physiopathology

The mutation(s) of the gene in charge of AR production results in AIS. AR is what allows cells to respond to the androgens, testosterone, and dihydrotestosterone. The grade of androgen insensibility depends on the severity of these mutations. The inability of fetal cells to respond to androgens, even when serum testosterone levels are within normal range, result in suboptimal development of the reproductive system, making it common to find testes retained in the abdomen, the inguinal ring or in the labia majora [21, 42].

In CAIS, the presence of the SRY gene leads to the formation of testicles in the fetal abdomen, which will start producing testosterone by the 7th week. However, the testosterone activity is blocked because of AR malfunction. The testes, otherwise, produce MIS, and this hormone suppresses the formation of female genital organs, but the external genitalia will look normal since the lower vagina doesn't derive from the Müllerian duct. This is the reason why this entity is rarely diagnosed before puberty, as these patients have no signs of external virilization and are raised as females. Also, the testes produce testosterone in response to hypothalamic and pituitary gland stimulation. This testosterone is converted to estradiol, which when combined with androgen insensitivity leads to the development of a female phenotype [21, 42].

Diagnosis

History and physical exam allow to differentiate between CAIS and PAIS even before results of confirmatory laboratory tests and imaging [42]. The classic presentation for CAIS is a post-pubertal individual who identifies as a woman inquiring about primary amenorrhea. On physical exam, these patients have normal breast development (with a typically pallid nipple), absent or minor pubic and axillary hair growth, facial acne, normal-looking external genitalia, partially formed short distal vagina, and complete absence of uterus and cervix [15, 21] (Pictures 9 and 10).

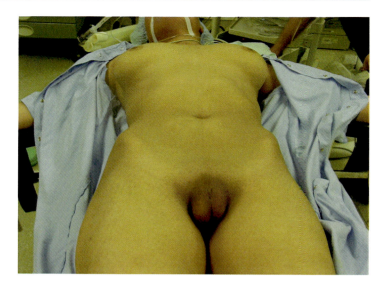

Picture 9 Patient with complete androgen insensitivity syndrome (CAIS). On physical exam, normal breast development and apparent normal female external genitalia are appreciated

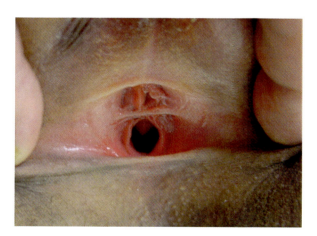

Picture 10 Once the labia are separated, vaginal hypoplasia is noted

In CAIS, blood tests will show serum testosterone levels at a normal male range with elevated antimüllerian hormone (MIS) the first year of child's life, then, normal values from there up to puberty and elevated again after the onset of pubertal development. Genetic testing shows a 46 XY karyotype and if gonads are found intraabdominally or in the inguinal canals, the vas deferens is blind [21].

PAIS is associated with variable presentations. Predominantly male phenotype may present with hypospadias, micropenis, bifid scrotum with or without intrascrotal testicles, and infertility. In some cases, the patient identifies as a phenotypical woman and may present with labial fusion, labioscrotal folds, normal breast development, normal to decreased pubic and axillary hair growth, and clitoromegaly [21, 42]. PAIS is sometimes difficult to diagnose during childhood and it is necessary to assess the type of mutation of the androgen gene. During puberty and adulthood, the diagnosis is done with the help of clinical and biochemical findings. A hormone profile will usually demonstrate an increase of luteinizing hormone (LH) and testosterone levels. To exclude androgen biosynthetic defect, testosterone precursors, DHT and testosterone before and after human chorionic gonadotropin (hCG) stimulation must be performed [42].

Treatment

Gonadectomy

These patients have increased risk of dysgerminoma formation due to the ectopic functional gonad. Gonadectomy is not offered until the patient's secondary sex characteristics are fully developed as it has been proved that breast development is better in patients who preserve their gonads during puberty. Delayed gonadectomy gives the opportunity to the patient to make a more conscious decision [21, 42]. Despite the low risk during of malignancy during childhood, it is mandatory to exclude a non-hormonally functional dysgenetic gonad with Y-chromosomal material, and ultrasound monitoring must be done early to rule out a pelvic mass. Once the gonadectomy is performed, the patients are started on estrogen replacement therapy [21, 42].

Genital Reconstruction/(Neo)vaginoplasty

CAIS patients usually present with normal external genitalia and a partially formed short vagina (vaginal hypoplasia), similarly to patients with MRKH syndrome (Picture 11). Therefore, these patients are managed similarly to patients with MRKH syndrome (see previous section) [42].

In PAIS, external genitalia virilization may result from the partially effective activity of testosterone [21].

Treatment

Gonadectomy

Unlike in CAIS, to avoid further virilization and germ cell neoplasia of the undescended testes, adolescents must undergo gonadectomy as soon as the diagnosis of PAIS is confirmed. If possible, this is performed before puberty to prevent further virilization and increased chances of malignant degeneration [21, 42].

After gonadectomy, estrogen treatment to induct puberty is required; psychological support and a close follow-up is necessary to make the patient aware of her condition and make acceptance process easier [42].

Feminizing Reconstructive Surgery

In PAIS, vaginoplasty combined with feminizing genital surgery may be required [42].

In cases where ambiguous genitalia are present and patient sexual identity is not defined, early gender assignment is suggested but controversial [15, 42]. To decide on gender assignation, the surgeon and patient's parents should consider the appearance of the external genitalia, the potential risk of virilization, complexity of reconstructive surgery, fertility feasibility, and eventual desired gender identity [15, 42]. Multidisciplinary approach and psychosocial evaluation is strongly

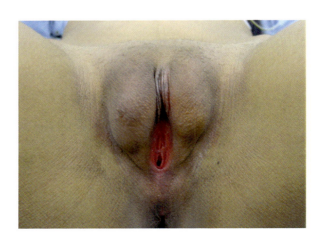

Picture 11 Normal external genitalia with vaginal hypoplasia in a patient with complete androgen insensitivity syndrome (CAIS)

recommended. This chapter will focus only on vaginoplasty and femininity surgery techniques.

The best timing to perform a feminizing genital reconstruction is not stipulated. While some maintain that is preferable between 6–12 months of age to facilitate gender acceptance, others state that adolescence is the best moment since the patient can provide informed consent, receive further advisement, the genitalia are fully developed, and vaginal skin is estrogenized, which facilitates the healing process and lowers complications rates (introital stenosis, need of revision or repeated procedures, etc.) [15].

Vaginoplasty and feminizing genital surgery are usually performed at the same time as a single stage procedure. As in vaginal agenesis/dysgenesia, the goal is to create a cavity by opening the lower malformed vagina. In general, there are three forms of vaginoplasty for urogenital sinus abnormalities: (1) the cutback vaginoplasty, which should be done only in those cases with mild anomalies and simple fusion of the vaginal posterior wall, (2) the flap vaginoplasty, which can be used for all low confluence UGS abnormalities, and (3) the vaginal pull-trough procedure, made for high confluence UGS. The type of vaginoplasty is chosen according to the severity of the vaginal defect (high or low confluence between vagina and urethra) and surgeon experience [15, 43].

Prior to surgery, it is important to assess the anatomy of the urogenital sinus, its length and the location of vaginal confluence in relation to the UGS orifice and the bladder neck. Recently, the length of the urethra from the bladder neck to the confluence has been shown to be a better predictor of surgical complexity. Genitography and endoscopy are the two important preoperative studies capable of revealing the UGS anatomy; however, endoscopy is more precise to demonstrate the confluence [15].

Low Confluence UGS

In Hendren's procedure, described in 1969 [44], a curved clamp is introduced into the UGS, lifting the perineal skin, then the fused perineal skin is incised posteriorly. The edges of the incised skin and mucosa are sutured together. The midline incision can be extended posteriorly, but ideally, a U-flap incision is preferred, which will join with the posterior vaginal wall, reducing the tension, especially in those cases where the vagina is not lying beneath the skin [45]. In this technique, clitorectomy can be performed at the same time after opening the vaginal introitus by incising the base of the clitoris in a circumferential fashion and then dissecting the corpora off the pubic rami. The corpora are removed to prevent pain during sexual stimulation and improve cosmetic outcomes. Nerve sparing techniques ensure adequate future sexual function [45].

Another common technique is the posterior skin flap vaginoplasty, also known as Fortunoff's procedure. In this surgery, an inverted U-flap is created from the perineum and then is placed inside the posterior distal vagina, increasing its caliber [15]. This procedure is used in the vast majority of feminizing genitoplasties since it is technically simple and has low complication rates [44]. However, this procedure does not achieve normal-appearing female anatomy. In fact, it shortens the perineum, resulting in abnormal genitalia. Other complications include hair bearing skin inside the vagina and vaginal stenosis since the posterior aspect of the vagina is entirely made of skin. This technique also impedes the posterior vaginal mucosa lining [44, 46].

High Confluence UGS and Cloaca

For these cases, the procedures are much complex than they are in low confluence UGS. These procedures include vaginoplasty, laboplasty, clitorectomy/clitoroplasty. The first procedure was described in 1969 by Hendren, using a Fogarty balloon, which was inserted into the UGS, to identify the vagina and then an incision was made over this balloon to separate the urethra from the vagina, and finally, using skin flaps, exteriorize the vagina [15].

Passerini and Glazel later described a single stage clitorovaginoplasty for virilized genitalia, where the UGS tissue is used for the anterior vaginal wall and skin flaps from the UGS are used to create a mucocutaneous bed for introitus and distal neovagina [15].

In 1997, Pena published an approach to correct the genitourinary and rectal anomalies caused by the persistent cloaca and named it total urogenital mobilization (TUM). The procedure consists in the UGS mobilization as a single unit in a circumferential fashion through a posterior sagittal approach and the use of a posterior skin flap, resulting in a superficial position vagina [15].

More recently, in 2001, Rink and Yerkes described a technique in which the Fortunoff skin graft is no longer needed by using the excess of UGS tissue as a mucosa-lined vestibule. Also, in 2006, they modified the TUM technique, which was reported to cause urinary incontinence and decreased clitoral sensation due to the proximal dissection above the pubo-urethral ligament, and created the partial urogenital mobilization (PUM), in which the proximal dissection is limited and still enough to achieve optimal mobilization [15].

Hendren Technique
In cases where the vagina and urethra communicate proximally to the external sphincter, a classic Hendren procedure may not be able to shift the vagina to the perineum or could even lead to stress urinary incontinence, and for that reason, a modification of the technique was described [45]. The patient requires bowel preparation with gauze packing to avoid contamination. First, endoscopically, a Fogarty catheter is placed into the vagina, inflated with 1 cc of air, and then is pulled to the lower vagina where the junction between the vagina and urethra is located. This will help to identify the lower vagina and prevent excessive dissection. Then, the urethra is incised posteriorly. The urethral mucosa is sutured to the skin up to 1 cm distal to the external sphincter. An inverted U incision is done at the perineum anteriorly to the anus, creating a flap. The flap is retracted posteriorly, and the dissection is performed along the anterior wall of the rectum behind the external sphincter. Insertion of a finger in the anus may help to dissect this plane. The next step is to encircle the lower vagina with a small catheter or penrose; the Fogarty balloon will help prevent injury to the urethra or bladder. Then, the vaginal posterior wall is transversally half transected, opening into the posterior wall of the urethra and the urethral opening is sutured with chromic sutures. A metal dilator is used to calibrate the urethra then an indwelling urethral catheter is inserted. The urethra and bladder neck are retracted forward using the catheter, and with blunt dissection in an upward fashion, the plane between bladder and vagina is dissected almost up to the cervix. The posterior perineal flap (flaps are essential to bring the vagina to the perineum) is sutured to the posterior margin of the vagina. In case the vagina is high, and the posterior perineal flap is not anterior enough, lateral flaps can be performed. A drain is placed to secure the evacuation of serum and prevent collections and the vagina is packed with Vaseline gauze [45].

A week after, the foley catheter and packing are removed and dilations are started. Parents can be taught to perform dilations if this surgery is done in an infant [45].

Clitorectomy can be performed at the same time for a single stage procedure treatment or at a separate operation before or after neovaginoplasty and is especially useful in cases with virilization features [45]. (See clitorectomy in Hendren technique for low confluence UGS.)

Issues with this technique include a difficult plane of dissection between the urethra and the vagina, and occasionally the vaginal opening is quite low and perineal, distant from the urethra [46].

Passerini-Gazel Technique (with Modifications)
This technique describes a single stage clitorovaginoplasty, used to address severe virilization [46]. The patient is placed in lithotomy, and the bladder, UGS, and vagina are inspected with a cystoscope. The vaginal cavity is canalized with a 6Fr Fogarty catheter [46]. The UGS is opened at 12 o'clock, and the mucosa inverted posteriorly to construct the distal anterior vaginal wall. This is the Passerini **perineal approach**, in which a U-shape incision is performed at the perineum above the anus, creating a U-shaped skin (and subcutaneous tissue) flap. The base of the flap will be located at the middle of the ischial tuberosities, meanwhile the apex posterior to the UGS opening. A second incision is made from the U-shape incision apex to the meatus and then it

is extended around the UGS opening bilaterally, completing a Y-shape incision. Once these are done, the incision is completed with a circumferential incision around the clitoris [46].

The dissection continues by deepening the incision (using the Fogarty catheter to traction and to identify the correct plane) until the flap can turn, then the lower part of the UGS is dissected and exposed. The lower part of the vaginal pouch is localized palpating the Fogarty catheter balloon and the anterior wall of the junction between the vagina and the urogenital sinus is incised over the balloon. The catheter is taken out through the UGS and the posterior wall of the junction between the vagina and the UGS is divided. The vagina is detached from the urethra and a short vaginal stump is conserved. A urethral catheter is installed. The posterior vaginal wall is dissected from inferior urethral wall until 1 cm length is reached, then the UGS is closed. It is preferable to remove as much as possible of the distal dysplastic vagina, until thick and highly vascularized vaginal walls are found [46] (Picture 12).

The **clitoroplasty** (Kogan technique with Passerini modification) is done using a circumferential incision around the clitoris (glans), then the prepuce and clitoral skin are dissected, degloving the clitoris meticulously to avoid vascular injury. A plane of cleavage between the corpora and neurovascular bundle is created dorsally through Buck's fascia, taking care to preserve the tunica. The tip of the corpora and the UGS are separated from the glans tissue. The glans is reduced by cutting two medial edges (instead of lateral edges as the original technique described) and removing tissue around the glandular hypospadiac groove or the urethral meatus. The corpora cavernosa is ligated proximally and resected 0.5 cm above. The UGS is preserved [46, 47].

The next step is to create the **mucocutaneous plate**. A vertical midline incision is done on the dorsal preputial and phallic skin surface until the pubis is reached. The proximal skin is sutured around the glans clitoris corona creating a preputial hood. The distal UGS part, which will be redundant, is taken and stretched to both sides and then is incised dorsally, maintaining an adequate urethral length, and creating a small dorsal inverted-V flap at the proximal end of the incision. The urethral V-flap is sutured to the clitoris' inferior part creating mucosa lining below it. Mucocutaneous plate is created by rotating downward and suturing side by side the cutaneous flaps to the urethra. The distal portion of the mucocutaneous plate is attached together with monocryl sutures creating a cylinder, which will be used to perform the vaginoplasty [46, 47].

Vaginoplasty is started bringing the cylinder posteriorly, and then its free end must be sutured to the native vagina forming the walls of the distal neovagina. The outer end of the cylinder is sutured to the inverted U-shaped cutaneous flap created with the first incision at the beginning of

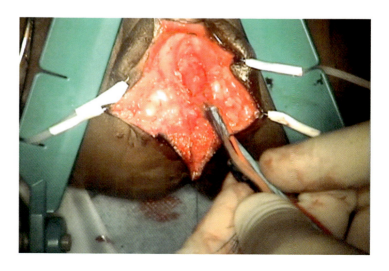

Picture 12 Removal of a distal dysplastic vagina during a cloacal repair

the surgery, completing the opening of the vagina at the perineum [47, 48].

Finally, a **labioplasty** is performed. The lateral labioscrotal folds are pulled down and sutured to the corners between the posterior U-flap and the labia majora lateral skin. The labia minora are created after the lateral edge of the proximal mucocutaneous plate and the medial edge of labia majora are sutured to a deep plane [48].

Posterior Sagittal Ano-Recto-Vagino-Urethroplasty (PSARVUP)

The PSARVUP was a technique created to treat high confluence UGS and cloaca to improve exposure to the complex visceral arrangements and the urinary and fecal sphincters. However, the technique is out of use due its complexity and the rectum splitting performed during the procedure, which requires the installation of a temporary diverting colostomy prior to surgery, therefore increasing its morbidity [46, 49].

TUM

Total urogenital mobilization (TUM) was described by Peña in 1997 as a modification of his PSARVUP technique for simple **cloaca repair** and **high confluence UGS** (<3 cm) since separation of vagina from urinary tract performed at PSARVUP showed an increased morbidity, with complications like urethrovaginal fistula, vaginal stricture, and vaginal atresia [50].

In TUM, the vagina and rectum are separated but vagina and UGS are mobilized together. The advantage of mobilizing UGS and vagina together is the avoidance of the vaginal-urinary tract dissection complications mentioned above [50].

In the original technique, TUM is performed through the same sagittal approach as in PSARVUP, and patients still need a diverting colostomy and occasionally urinary diversion prior to the procedure depending on the coexisting malformations. Cystoscopy is essential and bladder and vaginal catheter are installed [50, 51].

Surgery starts with the posterior sagittal approach. Once the rectum is separated from the vagina, the UGS is dissected and mobilized. Various series of 6-0 silk sutures are placed at the edge of the UGS and vagina, then, more silk sutures are placed across the common channel (UGS) between 5 mm and 10 mm dorsal to the clitoris. These sutures will facilitate to traction both structures at the same time avoiding tearing the tissue. The wall of the UGS is divided ventrally to the sutures [50]. A plane separates the UGS anteriorly from the pubis and the UGS must be dissected laterally and centrally to reach the retro public space. Then the vaginal edges are pulled, and the vagina and urethra are dissected. The fibrous ligaments holding the vagina and urethra to the pelvic rim must be divided. The dissection is extended circumferentially around the lateral and posterior vaginal walls and anterior wall of urethra and bladder until the vaginal edges are able to come together.

Urethra and vaginal openings are created, and the edges are sutured to the labia or perineal skin. The urethral opening and remaining UGS tissue is positioned between 5 mm and 8 mm from the clitoris [50].

The above-described technique can treat most cases of cloaca. However, there are complex anatomical variants for which additional maneuvers and approaches must be done.

Longitudinal Vaginal Septum

Longitudinal vaginal septum is a MDA caused by a deficient lateral merge of the paramesonephric ducts. It may be associated with uterine anomalies such as bicornuate uterus, arcuate uterus, and uterus didelphys. Renal malformations are found in up to 20% of patients. The septum may present as partial or complete [4, 38].

Many patients are asymptomatic since the septum is not obstructive, but some patients with obstructive septum may complain of dyspareunia, menometrorrhagia, dysmenorrhea, or abdominal pain [4, 38].

The diagnosis is done through physical exam as the septum can be visualized when the physician inspects the vaginal introitus using a speculum. A vaginoscopy can be performed under anesthesia the same day of the surgery. The treatment is surgical resection. The septum must be completely removed while avoiding cervix injury.

The cervix, or in some cases, cervices, are commonly inserted along the septum [38].

There are a variety of surgical techniques to resect a nonobstructive vaginal septum. The traditional approach is excision with scissors after clamping to avoid bleeding. Once the septum is excised, the edges are sutured [52]. Endoscopic resection is now more commonly used because it permits a better visualization of the defect and gives the possibility to use bipolar cutting forceps, Harmonic scalpel and Ligasure to cut and coagulate at the same time [52]. Potential complications include cervix injury, incidental bladder or rectal trauma and vascular injury, which can affect the cervix blood supply, cause scarring and cervical incompetence [38, 52].

Obstructive Anomalies

Imperforate Hymen

If the hymen is not perforated during the perinatal stage, various anomalies may occur, including imperforate hymen. These anomalies can be identified by the pediatrician during the routine newborn examination or later during gynecologic exam [38].

The clinical presentation in the neonatal period is hydrocolpos or mucocolpos, resulting from the stimulation of maternal estrogens, causing abdominal mass or perineal bulging of a translucent bluish or yellow-gray mass at the introitus. Some uncommon symptoms are urinary retention, and constipation. Large hydrocolpos can obstruct the ureters leading to hydronephrosis, and occasionally to respiratory distress. In some exceptions, this condition is asymptomatic and can resolve by reabsorption of the mucus when the estrogens decrease [38].

Even though the diagnostic is clinical, US or MRI can be ordered to confirm the obstruction and to decide on definitive treatment. Urgent hymen resection can be performed for symptomatic relief. Aspiration harbors the risk of infection and pyocolpos. Definitive surgery is usually delayed after onset of puberty but before menarche, and during that time the hymen is periodically monitored. The aim of the surgery (hymenotomy or hymenectomy) is to open the hymen allowing the evacuation of menstrual flow and sexual intercourse [38].

Technique

With patient in lithotomy and a urethral catheter in place, the hymen is incised with electrocautery performing an annular incision (hymenotomy), preserving circumferential tissue around 5 mm from the base. The hematocolpos is evacuated with help of suprapubic manual pressure. Patients can be discharged home on the same day. Complication rates are low and satisfaction rates are high. Minimal scarring is seen on follow-up since low-dose electrocautery is used [53].

Transverse Vaginal Septum

This condition is a rare type of MDA, it is thought to result from the incomplete vertical fusion between the Mullerian ducts and the urogenital sinus, leading to the formation of a transverse vaginal septum. The formation of a septum, which can be perforated or imperforated, can occur either in the lower, mid, or upper vagina. The septum can be found in different vaginal locations, but most of these usually occur in the upper vagina and are generally less than 1 cm long but vary in width (Table 3). The location of the septal defect is predictive of the degree of absence of the vagina with greater absence of the vagina being related to higher septal defects. Patients with imperforate septum will have amenorrhea, abdominopelvic pain, and, in some cases, a

Table 3 Classification of vaginal septa

Location (Distance from vaginal introitus to septum distal end)	Perforation	Thickness
Low (<3 cm)	No (Imperforate)	Thin (<1 cm)
Mid (3–6 cm)	Yes (Perforates, even microperforations)	Thick (>1 cm)
High (>6 cm)		

palpable abdominal mass. On the other hand, those cases with perforate septum will often have normal menstrual bleeding but have more chances of developing pyohematocolpos and will usually complain about dyspareunia and pain or difficulty with tampon insertion [9, 38, 54, 55].

On physical exam, a foreshortened vagina with a blind end vaginal pouch is seen. In some cases, a mass is palpated in the pelvic-abdominal area. Imaging studies are required (MRI or US) to evaluate the kidneys and for preoperative planning [38].

Surgical correction is the gold standard. The procedure consists of septum resection followed by a primary end-to-end anastomosis of lower and upper vagina. If the septum is thick, it may need undermining and mobilization of the upper and lower vaginal mucosa or even in rare cases, a section of intestine to bridge the gap. These can be done vaginally, laparoscopically, or via an abdominoperineal approach, depending on location and thickness of the septum [38, 55].

Resection of a thick septa may lead to scarring and further vaginal contracture and stenosis. Pyometra, wound infection, and recurrent menstrual obstruction are other potential postoperative complications. Postoperative cares include the use of vaginal molds and further need for temporary dilation to decrease risk of vaginal stenosis [38, 55].

Congenital Adrenal Hyperplasia

Congenital adrenal hyperplasia (CAH) accounts for most cases of female external genital virilization and about half of all patients with ambiguous external genitalia since it affects both sexes, but males with this condition do not develop genital abnormalities [56]. CAH is the result of various autosomal-recessive disorders of cortisol biosynthesis, determining aldosterone deficiency and androgen excess. This condition is also characterized by a 46 XX karyotype, the presence of ovaries, well-developed Müllerian duct structures, the absence of Wolffian duct structures, and different degrees of external

Table 4 Prader classification

Stage	Characteristic findings
I	Normal external genitalia except for clitoromegaly
II	Clitoromegaly, vaginal opening covered, UGS
III	Clitoromegaly, high UGS
IV	Small penis with small urogenital opening
V	Male external genitalia

genitalia virilization (see Table 4 "Prader classification"). Therefore, despite the appearance of their external genitalia, the sex assignment is usually female since these are considered to be genotypical females with ovaries and are potentially fertile [21]. Androgens given before the 14 weeks of gestation can cause complete fusion of the labial folds and clitoromegaly in the developing fetus mimicking CAH [57].

The endocrine imbalance in CAH influences in the location of the vagina and its relation to the urogenital system, causing a urogenital confluence. The urethra and vagina won't separate completely, and the junction of the urinary and reproductive tracts results in a common channel known as UGS. The place where the urethra and vagina joins is variable and can be from the bladder neck (high confluence UGS) to near the perineum (low confluence UGS). A very severe presentation, when the rectum joins the UGS, is called persistent cloaca [1].

There are three adrenal enzymes that may lead to CAH. In 95% of cases, CAH is due to a 21-hydroxylase deficiency, whereas the rest of the time it is due to a 11-hydroxylase deficiency or a 3-hydroxysteroid dehydrogenase deficiency [58]. Genetically, 21-hydroxylase deficiency is characterized by a recessive mutation in the *CYP21* gene, which encodes the P450c21 enzyme [59]. Seventy-five percent of patients with 21-hydroxylase deficiency also present with salt wasting. 11-hydroxylase deficiencies are characterized by mutations in the *CYP11B1* gene, which disrupt the activity of the P450C11B1 enzyme. In comparison to patients with 21-hydroxylase deficiency, these patients present with salt retention, volume expansion, and hypertension. Patients with a 3-hydroxysteroid dehydrogenase deficiency present with mild virilization, as the enzyme deficiency leads to the excess production of a weak androgen (DHEA) [59].

Management

Once laboratory studies are obtained, it is important to initiate glucocorticoid therapy as soon as possible to avoid salt wasting, which occurs after the 6th day of life, and the baby's weight, electrolytes, fluid status, and plasma renin activity should be closely monitored. Additionally, it is also possible to detect mutations in the *CYP21* gene, which can be useful for prenatal diagnoses in future pregnancies [59].

Despite the possible severe masculinization of the external genitalia, surgical therapy is also feasible. The feminizing reconstructive surgery includes genitoplasty (clitoroplasty and formation of labia) and vaginoplasty. The type and extent of surgery depends on the degree of masculinization and the location of the UGS and the techniques are the same as mentioned above for CAIS and PAIS. The higher the UGS, the more complex the reconstruction is. For example, low UGS can be fixed with a simple cutback procedure, meanwhile a high UGS will require TUM technique [1, 60, 61].

(The sub-sections "Low Confluence UGS" and "High Confluence UGS and Cloaca" are mentioned above.)

Conclusion

Female congenital pelvic malformations are a group of rare disorders characterized by specific features in which, depending on the severity, the pelvic morphology can change drastically making surgical treatment a real challenge. The pathologies causing these malformations include the MDAs, androgen insensitivity syndromes, CAH, hymenal, and uterine malformations.

A variety of vaginal abnormalities exist, ranging from common to rare resulting from the disorders mentioned above. It is important to keep all the differential diagnoses and possible associated anomalies in mind while evaluating and planning surgery in these patients.

Before any kind of treatment is attempted, the patient and their family require psychosocial counseling and multidisciplinary team management to determine ideal type and timing of management.

Vaginoplasty with or without clitoroplasty and feminizing surgery continues to be the mainstay treatments to restore the anatomical and functional normality of the female genitalia. Over the years, several techniques have been described and modified to reach safer, simpler, and more accurate results. Selection of surgical technique depends on type and severity of the malformation, patients factors, and surgeon experience.

Cross-References

▶ Clinical Evaluation of the Female Lower Urinary Tract and Pelvic Floor
▶ Embryology and Development of Congenital Anomalies of the Pelvis and Female Organs
▶ Endoscopic Evaluation
▶ Measurement of Urinary Symptoms, Health-Related Quality of Life, and Outcomes of Treatment of Genitourinary and Pelvic Floor Disorders

References

1. Laterza RM, et al. Female pelvic congenital malformations. Part I: Embryology, anatomy and surgical treatment. Eur J Obstet Gynecol Reprod Biol. 2011;159(1):26–34. https://doi.org/10.1016/j.ejogrb.2011.06.042.
2. Healey A. Embryology of the female reproductive tract. In G. Mann et al (Eds.), *Imaging of Gynecological Disorders in Infants and Children*, Medical Radiology. (Pp. 21–30). https://doi.org/10.1007/174_2010_128, Springer-Verlag Berlin Heidelberg 2012
3. Breech LL, Laufer MR. Müllerian anomalies. Obstet Gynecol Clin N Am. 2009;36(1):47–68. https://doi.org/10.1016/j.ogc.2009.02.002.
4. Junqueira BLP, et al. Müllerian duct anomalies and mimics in children and adolescents: correlative intraoperative assessment with clinical imaging. Radiographics. 2009;29(4):1085–103. https://doi.org/10.1148/rg.294085737.

5. Golan A, et al. Congenital anomalies of the Müllerian system. Fertil Steril. 1989;51(5):747–55. https://doi.org/10.1016/s0015-0282(16)60660-x.
6. Dietrich JE, et al. Obstructive reproductive tract anomalies. J Pediatr Adolesc Gynecol. 2014;27(6):396–402. https://doi.org/10.1016/j.jpag.2014.09.001.
7. Li S, et al. Association of renal agenesis and Müllerian duct anomalies. J Comput Assist Tomogr. 2000;24(6): 829–34. https://doi.org/10.1097/00004728-200011000-00001.
8. Committee on Adolescent Health Care. ACOG Committee Opinion No. 728: Müllerian agenesis: diagnosis, management, and treatment. Obstet Gynecol. 2018;131(1):e35–42. https://doi.org/10.1097/AOG.0000000000002458.
9. Edmonds DK. Congenital malformations of the genital tract and their management. Best Pract Res Clin Obstet Gynaecol. 2003;17(1):19–40. https://doi.org/10.1053/ybeog.2003.0356.
10. Preibsch H, et al. Clinical value of magnetic resonance imaging in patients with Mayer-Rokitansky-Küster-Hauser (MRKH) syndrome: diagnosis of associated malformations, uterine rudiments and intrauterine endometrium. Eur Radiol. 2014;24(7):1621–7. https://doi.org/10.1007/s00330-014-3156-3.
11. Vanderbrink BA, et al. Does preoperative genitography in congenital adrenal hyperplasia cases affect surgical approach to feminizing genitoplasty? J Urol. 2010;184 (4 Suppl):1793–8. https://doi.org/10.1016/j.juro.2010.05.082.
12. El-Sherbiny M. Disorders of sexual differentiation: II. Diagnosis and treatment. Arab J Urol. 2013;11(1): 27–32. https://doi.org/10.1016/j.aju.2012.11.008.
13. Ribeiro SC, et al. Müllerian duct anomalies: review of current management. Sao Paulo Med J Rev Paul Med. 2009;127(2):92–6. https://doi.org/10.1590/s1516-31802009000200007.
14. Rackow BW, Arici A. Reproductive performance of women with müllerian anomalies. Curr Opin Obstet Gynecol. 2007;19(3):229–37. https://doi.org/10.1097/GCO.0b013e32814b0649.
15. Guarino N, et al. Vaginoplasty for disorders of sex development. Front Endocrinol. 2013;4(29):11. https://doi.org/10.3389/fendo.2013.00029.
16. Counseller VS. Congenital absence and traumatic obliteration of the vagina and its treatment with inlaying thiersch grafts. Am J Obstet Gynecol. 1938;36: 632–8.
17. Templeman CL, Lam AM, Hertweck SP. Surgical management of vaginal agenesis. Obstet Gynecol Surv. 1999;54(9):583–91.
18. Frank RT. The formation of an artificial vagina without operation. Am J Obstet Gynecol. 1938;35(6): 1053–5.
19. Londra L, et al. Mayer-Rokitansky-Kuster-Hauser syndrome: a review. Int J Women's Health. 2015;7: 865–70. https://doi.org/10.2147/IJWH.S75637.
20. Patterson CJ, et al. Exploring the psychological impact of Mayer-Rokitansky-Küster-Hauser syndrome on young women: an interpretative phenomenological analysis. J Health Psychol. 2016;21(7):1228–40. https://doi.org/10.1177/1359105314551077.
21. Laufer MR. Structural abnormalities of the female reproductive tract. In: Emans SJ, Laufer MR, editors. Pediatric and adolescent gynecology. 6th ed. Philadelphia: Wolters Kluwer/Lippincott Williams & Wilkins; 2012. p. 177–237.
22. Adeyemi-Fowode OA, Dietrich JE. Assessing the experience of vaginal dilator use and potential barriers to ongoing use among a Focus Group of Women with Mayer-Rokitansky-Küster-Hauser syndrome. J Pediatr Adolesc Gynecol. 2017;30(4):491–4. https://doi.org/10.1016/j.jpag.2017.02.002.
23. Ismail-Pratt IS, et al. Normalization of the vagina by dilator treatment alone in Complete Androgen Insensitivity Syndrome and Mayer-Rokitansky-Kuster-Hauser syndrome. Hum Reprod. 2007;22(7):2020–4. https://doi.org/10.1093/humrep/dem074.
24. Oelschlager A-MA, et al. Primary vaginal dilation for vaginal agenesis: strategies to anticipate challenges and optimize outcomes. Curr Opin Obstet Gynecol. 2016;28(5):345–9. https://doi.org/10.1097/GCO.0000000000000302.
25. Willemsen WN, Kluivers KB. Long-term results of vaginal construction with the use of Frank dilation and a peritoneal graft (Davydov procedure) in patients with Mayer- Rokitansky-Kuster syndrome. Fertil Steril. 2015;103:220–7.e1.
26. Callens N, et al. An update on surgical and non-surgical treatments for vaginal hypoplasia. Hum Reprod Update. 2014;20(5):775–801. https://doi.org/10.1093/humupd/dmu024.
27. Eldor L, Friedman JD. Reconstruction of congenital defects of the vagina. Semin Plast Surg. 2011;25(2): 142–7. https://doi.org/10.1055/s-0031-1281483.
28. Allahbadia AG, et al. Vaginoplasty: a case series comparing three different operative techniques. Indian J Obstet Gynecol Res. 2018;5(1):148–53. https://doi.org/10.18231/2394-2754.2018.0033.
29. Jagadeb S, Bisoi S. Long term outcome of McIndoe's technique for vaginal agenesis & effect on quality of life, sexual function & body image. Int J Sci Res (IJSR). ISSN (Online): 2319-7064 Index Copernicus Value (2013): 6.14 | Impact Factor (2013): 4.438.
30. Avino A, et al. Vaginal reconstruction in patients with Mayer-Rokitansky-Küster-Hauser syndrome-one centre experience. Medicina (Kaunas, Lithuania). 2020;56(7): 327. https://doi.org/10.3390/medicina56070327.
31. Rao, et al. Recto-neovaginal fistula following vaginoplasty for vaginal agenesis: our experience and management guidelines. Sch J App Med Sci 2015;3 (3C):1187–1192.
32. Buss JG, Lee RA. McIndoe procedure for vaginal agenesis: results and complications. Mayo Clin Proc. 1989;64(7):758–61. https://doi.org/10.1016/s0025-6196(12)61747-9.
33. Herlin MK, et al. Mayer-Rokitansky-Küster-Hauser (MRKH) syndrome: a comprehensive update.

34. Serebrakian AT, et al. Meta-analysis and systematic review of skin graft donor-site dressings with future guidelines. Plast Reconstr Surg Glob Open. 2018;6(9): e1928. https://doi.org/10.1097/GOX.0000000000001928.
35. Veronikis DK, et al. The Vecchietti operation for constructing a neovagina: indications, instrumentation, and techniques. Obstet Gynecol. 1997;90(2):301–4. https://doi.org/10.1016/S0029-7844(97)00231-7.
36. Borruto F, et al. The Vecchietti procedure for surgical treatment of vaginal agenesis: comparison of laparoscopy and laparotomy. Int J Gynaecol Obstet. 1999;64(2): 153–8. https://doi.org/10.1016/s0020-7292(98)00244-6.
37. Langer M, et al. Vaginal agenesis and congenital adrenal hyperplasia. Psychosocial sequelae of diagnosis and neovagina formation. Acta Obstet Gynecol Scand. 1990;69(4):343–9. https://doi.org/10.3109/00016349009036159.
38. Miller RJ, Breech LL. Surgical correction of vaginal anomalies. Clin Obstet Gynecol. 2008;51(2):223–36. https://doi.org/10.1097/GRF.0b013e31816d2181.
39. Feroze RM, et al. Vaginoplasty at the Chelsea hospital for women: a comparison of two techniques. Br J Obstet Gynaecol. 1975;82(7):536–40. https://doi.org/10.1111/j.1471-0528.1975.tb00683.x.
40. Williams EA. Congenital absence of the vagina: a simple operation for its relief. Br J Obstet Gynecol. 1964;71:511–6.
41. Creatsas G, Deligeoroglou E. Creatsas modification of Williams vaginoplasty for reconstruction of the vaginal aplasia in Mayer-Rokitansky-Küster-Hauser syndrome cases. Women's Health (Lond Engl). 2010;6(3): 367–75. https://doi.org/10.2217/whe.10.13.
42. Gulía C, et al. Androgen insensitivity syndrome. Eur Rev Med Pharmacol Sci. 2018;22(12):3873–87. https://doi.org/10.26355/eurrev_201806_15272.
43. Rink RC, et al. Reconstruction of the high urogenital sinus: early perineal prone approach without division of the rectum. J Urol. 1997;158(3 Pt 2):1293–7.
44. Gosalbez R, et al. New concepts in feminizing genitoplasty – is the Fortunoff flap obsolete? J Urol. 2005;174(6): 2350–3; discussion 2353. https://doi.org/10.1097/01.ju.0000180419.62193.78.
45. Hendren WH, Crawford JD. Adrenogenital syndrome: the anatomy of the anomaly and its repair. Some new concepts. J Pediatr Surg. 1969;4(1):49–58. https://doi.org/10.1016/0022-3468(69)90183-3.
46. Rink RC, et al. Partial urogenital mobilization: a limited proximal dissection. J Pediatr Urol. 2006;2(4): 351–6. https://doi.org/10.1016/j.jpurol.2006.04.002.
47. Passerini-Glazel G. A new 1-stage procedure for clitorovaginoplasty in severely masculinized female pseudohermaphrodites. J Urol. 1989;142(2 Pt 2):565–8; discussion 572. https://doi.org/10.1016/s0022-5347(17)38817-1.
48. Lesma A, et al. Passerini-glazel feminizing genitoplasty: modifications in 17 years of experience with 82 cases. Eur Urol. 2007;52(6):1638–44. https://doi.org/10.1016/j.eururo.2007.02.068.
49. Peña A. The surgical management of persistent cloaca: results in 54 patients treated with a posterior sagittal approach. J Pediatr Surg. 1989;24(6):590–8. https://doi.org/10.1016/s0022-3468(89)80514-7.
50. Peña A. Total urogenital mobilization – an easier way to repair cloacas. J Pediatr Surg. 1997;32(2):263–7; discussion 267–8. https://doi.org/10.1016/s0022-3468(97)90191-3.
51. Rink RC, et al. Use of the mobilized sinus with total urogenital mobilization. J Urol. 2006;176(5):2205–11. https://doi.org/10.1016/j.juro.2006.07.078.
52. Chu K, et al. Resection of longitudinal vaginal septum using a surgical stapler. J Pediatr Adolesc Gynecol. 2020;33(4):435–7. https://doi.org/10.1016/j.jpag.2020.02.011.
53. Cetin C, et al. Annular hymenotomy for imperforate hymen. J Obstet Gynaecol Res. 2016;42(8):1013–5. https://doi.org/10.1111/jog.13010.
54. Rock JA, Reeves LA, Retto H, Baranki TA, Zacur HA, Jones HW Jr. Success following vaginal creation for Müllerian agenesis. Fertil Steril. 1983;39(6): 809–13.
55. Williams CE, et al. Transverse vaginal septae: management and long-term outcomes. BJOG. 2014;121(13): 1653–8. https://doi.org/10.1111/1471-0528.12899.
56. Krege S, Walz K, Hauffa B, Körner I, Rübben H. Long-term follow-up of female patients with congenital adrenal hyperplasia from 21-hydroxylase deficiency, with special emphasis on the results of vaginoplasty. BJU Int. 2000;86(3):253–8.
57. Shapiro E, Huang H, Wu X-R. New concepts on the development of the vagina. In: Hypospadias and genital development. Boston: Springer; 2004. p. 173–85.
58. Hendren WH. Urogenital sinus and cloacal malformations. Female Pelvic Med Reconstr Surg. 1995;1(3):149–60.
59. Speiser PW, White PC. Congenital adrenal hyperplasia. N Engl J Med. 2003;349(8):776–88.
60. Engert J. Surgical correction of virilised female external genitalia. In: Surgery in solitary kidney and corrections of urinary transport disturbances. Berlin: Springer; 1989. p. 151–64.
61. Bailez MM, Gearhart JP, Migeon C, Rock J. Vaginal reconstruction after initial construction of the external genitalia in girls with salt-wasting adrenal hyperplasia. J Urol. 1992;148(2):680–2.

ID# Genital Reconstruction in Male-to-Female Gender Affirmation Surgery

63

Marta R. Bizic, Marko T. Bencic, and Mirosav L. Djordjevic

Contents

History	1210
Introduction	1212
Preoperative Clinical Evaluation	1213
Overview of Surgical Techniques	1213
Orchiectomy	1213
Penectomy	1214
Clitoral Reconstruction	1214
Vulvoplasty	1214
Urethroplasty	1215
Creation of the Neovaginal Canal	1215
Vaginoplasty Techniques	1215
Penile Inversion Vaginoplasty	1215
Bowel Vaginoplasty	1216
Peritoneal Pull-Through Vaginoplasty	1218
Zero-Depth Vaginoplasty (Feminizing Vulvoplasty)	1219
Postoperative Care	1219
Complications	1220

M. R. Bizic (✉) · M. T. Bencic
Department of Urology, Faculty of Medicine, University of Belgrade, Belgrade, Serbia

Belgrade Center for Urogenital Reconstructive Surgery, Belgrade, Serbia
e-mail: martabizic@uromiros.com

M. L. Djordjevic
Belgrade Center for Urogenital Reconstructive Surgery, Belgrade, Serbia
e-mail: djordjevic@uromiros.com

© Springer Nature Switzerland AG 2023
F. E. Martins et al. (eds.), *Female Genitourinary and Pelvic Floor Reconstruction*,
https://doi.org/10.1007/978-3-031-19598-3_65

Early Postoperative Complications ... 1220
   Bleeding ... 1220
   Wound Dehiscence ... 1220
   Skin Necrosis ... 1220
   Clitoral Necrosis ... 1220
   Urethral Flap Necrosis ... 1220

Late Complications ... 1220
   Poor Cosmesis ... 1220
   Corpora Cavernosa Remnants ... 1221
   Formation of the Granulation Tissue ... 1221
   Hair Growth Inside the Neovagina ... 1221
   Neovaginal Prolapse ... 1221
   Excessive Mucus Production and Foul Smell ... 1221
   Diversion Colitis ... 1221
   Meatal Stenosis and Dysuric Problems ... 1221
   Corpus Spongiosum Bulging ... 1222
   Introital Stenosis ... 1222
   Vaginal Stenosis and Loss of Neovaginal Depth ... 1222
   Urinary and Enteric Neovaginal Fistulas ... 1222

Sexual Function ... 1222

Conclusions ... 1223

Cross-References ... 1223

References ... 1223

Abstract

Gender affirmation surgeries in male-to-female trans individuals (transwomen) present usually the last step in their transition. The genital gender affirmation surgery, commonly referred as vaginoplasty, includes the removal of masculine genitalia and creation of female genitals. There is a huge number of described vaginoplasty techniques but the gold standard is still the penile inversion technique. It is proved that gender affirmation surgeries have a positive impact to quality of life and overall satisfaction of transgender and gender-nonconforming individuals. Herein, we will review the options for vaginoplasty in transgender women and present in details the most commonly used surgical approaches and their outcomes and complications.

Keywords

Gender dysphoria · Transgender women · Transwomen · Male-to-female · Gender affirmation surgery · Genital gender affirmation surgery · Vaginoplasty · Penile inversion vaginoplasty · Peritoneal pull-through vaginoplasty · Bowel vaginoplasty

History

Gender refers to the socially constructed characteristics of women, men, girls, and boys. This covers the standards, behaviors, and roles that come with being a woman, man, girl, or boy, as well as interpersonal interactions. Gender as a social construct differs from society to society and can change through time. Gender is related to, but distinct from, sex, which refers to the biological and physiological differences between females, males, and intersex people, such as chromosomes, hormones, and reproductive organs. Gender and sex are intertwined, but different from gender identity. Gender identity refers to a personal conception of oneself, internal, and unique gender experience, which may or may not correlate to the person's physiology or sex assigned at birth [1]. Gender usually determines the gender roles that we have in society and how we are expected to dress, speak, behave, think, and interact within the society. Gender roles are culturally specific, and while the majority of cultures recognize two gender roles, there are some cultures that recognize more gender roles [2]. The desire to belong to the opposite gender and to have opposite gender role is strongly present in transgender individuals. During the history, we have witnessed that there were people throughout the ages and culture who challenged the cultural conventions and lived their lives as belonging to the opposite gender. In ancient Egypt in 1500 BC, Queen Hatshepsut became the pharaoh of Egypt and was portrayed as more masculine. In ancient Rome, Emperor Nero ordered the execution of his wife Poppaea Sabina and married his young male slave, Sporus, after he had him castrated. Another Roman emperor, Elagabalus, was known for cross-dressing and preferred to be called by female roles [3]. Throughout the history and around the world, there are individuals who do not categorize themselves into two genders – male or female – but as a third gender. In North America, the native Americans called such individuals "Nadleehi," which means two-spirited people. In India, there are Hijras who were respected in ancient India as they were participating in Hindu rituals and celebrating marriages and childbirth. However, after Great Britain's colonization of India, the Hijra community became socially marginalized which lead to their socioeconomic difficulties and stigmas [3].

Gender dysphoria presents the distress and inner conflict caused by discrepancy between an individual's gender identity and sex assigned at birth. Gender affirmation surgeries (GAS) are the last step in an individual's transition toward the desired gender. In the recent two decades, there have been an increased number of requests for GAS worldwide. Therefore, the awareness and acceptance of transgender minority lead to the formation of the multidisciplinary centers providing care and treatment for trans population globally [4].

The first known medical reference about transgender individuals dates from Jean Etienne Esquirol (1772–1840), the founder of psychiatric hospitals in France. Kraft-Ebbing (1842–1902) introduced the term "inversion sexuelle" in his book *Psychopathia Sexualis*. One of the most important milestones in acceptance of transgender individuals was when Magnus Hirschfeld (1868–1935) introduced the term "transsexual" and revolutionized gender theory by offering multiple axes to characterize gender development, gender identity, and sexual orientation [5]. He established the Institute for Sexual Science in Berlin, the world's first institute devoted to sexology, where the transgender individuals were offered psychiatric, endocrinologist, and even surgical treatment. The first documented GAS was performed on Dora Richter, born as Rudolph, who underwent bilateral orchiectomy in 1922 and later total penectomy and vaginoplasty performed by Erwin Gohrbandt (1890–1965). Even though Dora Richter was the first patient to undergo GAS, the most famous patient of the Hirschfeld's Institute was Lili Elbe, born as Einar Wegener, a Danish painter who was operated by the German gynecologist Kurt Warnekros. She underwent penectomy and bilateral orchiectomy and vaginoplasty and transplantation of the ovaries and uterus. She died after the rejection and sepsis due to uterus transplantation [3, 4, 6].

After the World War II, the modern era of genital reconstructive surgeries for transgender women started to develop widely. One of the first surgeons of the modern era was Danish plastic surgeon Paul Fogh-Andersen who performed full-thickness penile skin graft for vaginal reconstruction of the world famous Christine Jorgensen in Copenhagen [7]. Another significant surgeon who is credited for the innovation of GAS for transwomen is Dr. Georges Burou. Dr. Burou was a French gynecologist who practiced in Casablanca. He pioneered the anterior pedicled penile skin flap inversion vaginoplasty [8]. Father of modern plastic surgery, plastic surgeon, Sir Harold Gillies established surgical techniques that are still in use in plastic and reconstructive surgery. He applied his experience obtained during the World War I and II for genital reconstruction in wounded soldiers and was the first to perform the transmasculine GAS in 1946 with his colleague Dr. Ralph Millard. Gillies also performed vaginoplasty using the penile skin flap technique that became the standard for the next few decades [3, 4, 9].

Vaginal reconstruction for transgender women using the non-genital skin grafts was introduced by Abraham in the 1930s. The surgery was performed as a one-stage procedure with the creation of the hairless neovagina of an adequate depth and width for penetrative sexual intercourse. The disadvantages include scarring of the donor area, scarring of the neovagina with possible shrinkage, poor erogenous sensation, and absence of the natural lubrication and need for prolonged dilation [4].

As the transfeminine GAS was developing, the search for a new surgical approach that would provide better results for both patient and the surgeon lead to the use of non-genital skin flaps. There were different approaches from different centers such as Cairins and de Villiers with the medial thigh flap for vaginal lining and Huang with inguinopudendal flaps to create the neovagina [4, 10]. The advantages of these techniques are the creation of the neovagina of a sufficient depth and reduced period of postoperative dilatation. Disadvantages include scarring of the donor area and bulkiness of the flaps that impair the sexual intercourse [4].

Further development and search for the surgical approach that would provide natural looking vagina to the patient lead to the use of intestinal segments, like in cis-women with vaginal absence [11–14].

Additional improvement of the existing techniques brought other possibilities for vaginal reconstruction such as the use of the peritoneum that was initially pioneered for patient with vaginal agenesis, but later found acceptance among the patients and the surgeons performing GAS [15–18].

Also, there are few case reports on the use of biocompatible grafts for vaginal reconstruction, but the follow-up is insufficient and there are no large number of patients, so the conclusion of the success of the procedure cannot be made [19].

Nowadays, the most widespread techniques for neovaginal reconstruction for transgender women are penile inversion technique, with or without the combination of scrotal skin grafts or flaps, intestinal pedicled transplants, and peritoneal pull-through vaginoplasty in combination with penile skin flaps.

Introduction

Before undergoing GAS, transgender individuals must follow the guidelines from the World Professional Association for Transgender Health (WPATH), which include the evaluation from two independent mental health professionals with persistent and well-documented gender dysphoria and at least 12 months of hormonal substitution therapy under endocrinologist guidance, unless contraindicated. Also, the patients should be capable of informed consent and older than 18 years to undergo irreversible GAS [20]. Despite the fact that gender is not a binary phenomenon, GAS are often classed as either feminizing or masculinizing [21]. As this chapter is focusing on feminizing genital gender affirmation surgeries (GGAS), they will be described in details, while other feminizing GAS will be only mentioned.

According to the recent literature data, the prevalence of transgender women was found to be 6.8 per 100,000, which is higher than the transgender men [21]. Related to this fact, requests for feminizing GAS are more often and include facial feminization surgery, feminizing mammaplasty, body feminization surgery, and feminizing genital surgery [21] (Fig. 1).

The goal of GGAS in transgender women is to remove male genital organs – testes and penis – while creating a vagina and external genital organs that as feminine as possible in appearance and without excessive scars and neuromas. The urethra should be shortened so that the urinary stream is pointed downward in the sitting position, without fistulas or strictures. The neovagina should ideally be hairless, moist, and elastic. The dimensions of the neovagina should be at least 10 cm for depth and of about 3 cm for width, without introital stenosis. The sensation of the neovagina should be sufficient to enable acceptable erogeneity during the penetrative sexual intercourse. The neoclitoris should be small, concealed, and sensitive, providing complete

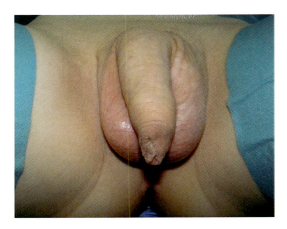

Fig. 1 Preoperative appearance of the external genitalia in a transgender woman

arousal to the patient. The labia minora and majora should not be bulky, but should look as much like a female vulva as possible anatomically [4, 14].

There are several different options for transgender women in order to create the female genital complex, but none of the described techniques is ideal. Each procedure for vaginoplasty requires shorter or longer or even lifelong dilation of the neovagina in order to maintain its functionality [22].

Preoperative Clinical Evaluation

Patients undergoing feminizing GGAS are advised to perform permanent hair removal using one of the available procedures. The critical points for hair removal are the penile shaft, the central portion of the scrotum, as well as the perineum toward the anal opening. The hair removal is very important to prevent hair growth inside the neovagina that can lead to malodor and infections [21].

Cessation of hormonal estrogen therapy is advised prior to the surgery since there is a risk for venous thromboembolism during the vaginoplasty procedure because of the patient position and length of surgery. The most common length for hormonal therapy temporary suspension is between 2 and 4 weeks depending on the center [20].

Patients undergoing any of the available vaginoplasty techniques are required to cease all nicotine use at least 6 weeks before and after the surgery because of present risk for flaps and graft necrosis in nicotine users [23]. Also, overweight (obese) patients are at increased risk for complications related to general anesthesia, potential positioning injuries, as well as postoperative complications such as infections and wound dehiscence that lead to prolonged and compromised healing. Technically, surgery in obese patients is more demanding for the surgeons, thus making the surgery lasts longer. The body mass index (BMI) should be up to maximum 35, preferably below so the rate of possible complications could be lower [23].

Furthermore, patients in whom previous surgeries or radiation included the space for neovaginal canal creation (prostate, rectum) can be at higher risk of bowel and bladder injury and subsequent formation of the fistulae that can compromise the healing and require additional surgical treatment. Also, in patients with a history of prostate surgery/radiation, urinary incontinence can be present and can increase after vaginal canal dissection, with no possibility for urinary incontinence treatment. Therefore, these candidates must be presented with possible additional risks for such surgeries and can be offered less invasive and safer procedure for them such as gender-affirming vulvoplasty (zero-depth vaginoplasty) [23].

Additionally, patients undergoing vaginal reconstruction must be willing and capable of neovaginal regular dilatation according to the instructions of the pelvic floor therapist, especially for the first postoperative year. Those who are unwilling or unable to perform self-dilations are not the best candidates for vaginal reconstruction and could be offered zero-depth vaginoplasty [23–25].

Overview of Surgical Techniques

Orchiectomy

Orchiectomy is the removal of both testicles, as a part of GAS. It can be done as a sole procedure, without the requirement for additional genital reconstruction, and it can be done prior to vaginoplasty or simultaneously with one of the available vaginoplasty techniques. The most common request for orchiectomy prior to vaginoplasty is the cessation of antiandrogens in therapy and potentially better effects of estrogen therapy. Orchiectomy is performed using the midline incision to minimize the scarring and vascularization of the future flap for vaginoplasty. Dissection is performed through the dartos fascia. Cremasteric layers are transected with caution to prevent bleeding and to reach the tunica vaginalis of one and then of the other testicle. The dissection continues to the external inguinal ring and two suture ligatures are placed to prevent slippage of a free ligature. The funiculus is transected and testicles are sent for histopathological verification. The wound is closed in layers using absorbable sutures. The disadvantage of prior orchiectomy can be additional surgical procedure, scarring of the scrotal skin due to scrotal incision to approach the testicles [20].

Penectomy

In situations where complete feminizing genital reconstruction is done, surgical treatment usually starts with penectomy, which is followed by bilateral orchiectomy (if not done before), vaginal reconstruction, and vulvoplasty. Penectomy refers to the removal of the corpora cavernosa of the penis with partial removal of the glans and urethra. The technique used for penectomy is called penile disassembly technique [26] (Fig. 2). A circumcision incision is made and penile degloving is performed. About 1cm of inner prepuce is left attached to the dorsal portion of the glans so clitoral hood could be fashioned later. Penile body is completely freed from the penile skin so the detachment of the urethra ventrally and neurovascular bundle dorsally could be performed. The dissection of the neurovascular bundle is performed together with Buck's fascia along the penile body with caution to avoid injury of the nerves that are positioned laterally. The dorsal part of the penile glans is marked to the size of the desired clitoris and dissected, so the complete liberation of the neurovascular bundle could be completed. Ventrally, the urethra is lifted from the corpora cavernosa with sharp dissection until the bulbar part so the crura of the penis could be detached from their attachment to the pubic bones, to completely remove corpora cavernosa and to prevent bulging during the arousal if left too long, as that can impair sexual functionality and quality of life of the patient [4, 20, 24].

Clitoral Reconstruction

In the literature, the first mention of creation of the clitoris dates back to 1976 with the reduction of the penile glans that remained fixed to the neurovascular bundle on the dorsal side [27]. Due to the relatively high percentage of complications in clitoral reconstruction, surgeons suggested various techniques: shortening of the neurovascular bundle with free transplantation of the glans penis, imitation of the clitoris with a part of the corpus cavernosum and covering with penile skin, and use of spongy tissue for vascularization. In one of the surgical techniques, the glans penis, on the neurovascular bundle, was placed entirely on the upper wall of the neovagina for the purpose of providing a vaginal orgasm during sexual intercourse [28, 29]. Most surgeons who perform feminizing GAS today reconstruct the clitoris using the dorsal part of the glans penis on the neurovascular bundle, without shortening the bundle, as described by Eldh, and then Perovic and Hage et al. [30–32] (Fig. 2).

Vulvoplasty

Creation of the labia minora and majora is usually done using the available genital skin. If the patient has not been previously circumcised, the labia minora are created from the penile prepuce, and in cases where they are, a skin fold is formed which then mimics the labia minora. The labia majora are created from the skin originating from the scrotum with the excision of excess skin and fatty tissue [33, 34].

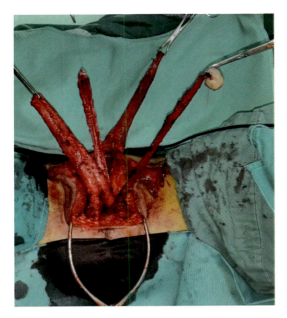

Fig. 2 Penile disassembly technique. Penile skin flap is dissected on the upper pedicle from the penis. The clitoris is created from the dorsal part of the penile glans. The urethra is completely dissected from the corpora cavernosa. Corpora cavernosa are completely freed and prepared for detachment

Urethroplasty

The creation of the urethral meatus in transgender women is done by shortening and spatulating the urethra and positioning the meatus above the neovaginal introitus, so that during the act of micturition in a sitting position, the urine stream goes down, in a physiological way. It is very important not to cause meatal stenosis when performing the urethroplasty, which makes it difficult for the patient to urinate and could need additional surgery.

Creation of the Neovaginal Canal

The canal for the neovagina is created between the rectum and urethra and bladder following Young's approach to perineal prostatectomy [23]. The creation of the neovaginal canal is one of the riskiest parts of feminizing genital gender affirmation surgery because of the possibility of injury to the rectum or the urethra and bladder.

The patient is positioned in lithotomy position. The 16Fr Foley catheter is placed into the urethra and bladder. Small triangular posteriorly based perineal flap is created to prevent introital stenosis. Then the midline incision is made superiorly across the scrotal raphe toward the penis. The bulbospongiosus muscle is dissected from the urethra on the posterior pedicle to allow it to be used as an interposition flap in case of bowel injury [20]. Then the urethra is completely dissected from the corpora cavernosa, and total penectomy is performed as described earlier. Further dissection continues through the perineal body using harmonic ultracision scalpel and blunt dissection toward the prostate capsule. Cautious dissection is necessary because of the close relationship between the prostate apex and rectum. Permanent palpation of the urethral catheter inside the urethra and palpation of the gauze inside the rectum can assure safe dissection in the Denonvilliers fascia. To widen the neovaginal canal, partial dissection of the levator muscles is performed and dissection is executed until the peritoneal reflection. Hemostasis is performed and gauze soaked in adrenalin solution is placed until the tissue for the vaginal canal is prepared.

Vaginoplasty Techniques

Vaginoplasty presents the main challenge for the surgeons treating transgender women. Historically, there are a vast number of described techniques with various success rates and follow-ups, but as mentioned before, few techniques are today used mostly for neovaginal creation in transgender women: penile inversion vaginoplasty, intestinal vaginoplasty, and peritoneal pull-through vaginoplasty.

Penile Inversion Vaginoplasty

Penile inversion vaginoplasty still presents the gold standard in genital reconstruction in transgender women, because of penile skin characteristics. Penile skin is thin, elastic, very sensitive, almost hairless, and well-vascularized.

Preoperative antibiotic prophylaxis is administered to the patient (ceftriaxone 2 g/day and metronidazole 500 mg/8 h) as well as anticoagulation prophylaxis. The patient is placed in dorsal lithotomy position. The urinary Foley catheter 16Ch is introduced into the bladder. Penile inversion technique includes the same subprocedures described above: bilateral orchiectomy (if not performed prior to GAS), penile disassembly, clitoroplasty, labiaplasty, urethroplasty, and vaginal canal dissection between the rectum and urethra and bladder. Penile skin flap of an adequate length is sutured at the distal end to form the neovagina and to line the neovaginal canal (Fig. 3). To prevent the neovaginal prolapse, neovagina can be fixed to the sacrospinous ligament or onto the prostate capsule [35, 36]. The neovagina is then packed with antibiotic gauze. In cases where the penile skin is limited for neovaginal creation (circumcision, puberty blockers, etc.), the augmentation of the neovagina can be performed either using the scrotal skin full-thickness graft or flap or urethral flap can be created after urethral dissection and its fixation on the upper neovaginal wall to increase the width of the penile skin flap as well as the length and to increase the neovaginal sensation and to provide lubrication [21, 23, 37] (Figs. 4 and 5).

Penile inversion vaginoplasty is found to have high percentage of satisfaction among the patients concerning neovaginal depth and esthetical appearance, ranging from 76% to 100% and from 90% to 100%, respectively [38, 39] (Fig. 6).

Bowel Vaginoplasty

Bowel vaginoplasty is usually performed as a secondary surgery for vaginal reconstruction in revision cases. However, in recent years, there is an increase in number of patients who are on puberty blockers and therefore have penoscrotal hypoplasia with lack of available penile skin for neovaginal reconstruction.

Bowel vaginoplasty was first performed in transgender women in 1974 by Markland and Hastings with cecum in five transgender women

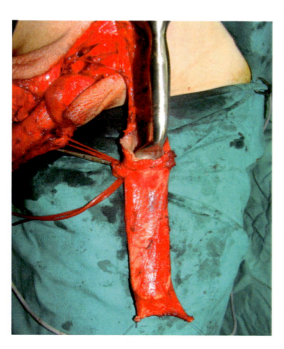

Fig. 3 Penile skin flap is inverted and sutured at the cranial end forming the apex of the neovagina

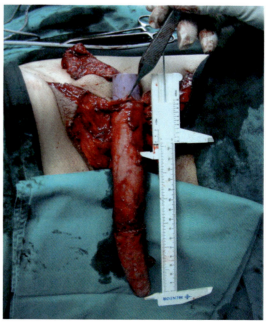

Fig. 4 Scrotal skin graft is harvested and defatted and anastomosed to the penile skin flap over the vaginal mold to increase the neovaginal depth

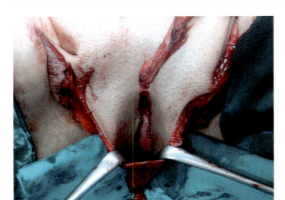

Fig. 5 The urethra is spatulated dorsally creating long vascularized urethral flap that is embedded onto the upper wall of the neovagina for neovaginal depth augmentation

with satisfying results in four patients [40–42]. The use of other intestinal segments with good postoperative results with satisfactory function has been announced by a number of centers worldwide [43, 44].

Proponents of the use of the sigmoid colon as an advantage of its use in the reconstruction of the neovagina emphasize its anatomical position, which greatly contributes to the easier surgical intervention. The position of the vascular pedicle and its mobility guarantee that the segment of the sigmoid colon can be transposed without tension to the perineum for further anastomosis and creation of the neovagina [41, 42, 45].

Preoperative antibiotic prophylaxis is administered to the patient (ceftriaxone 2 g/day and metronidazole 500 mg/8 h) as well as anticoagulation prophylaxis. The harvesting of the sigmoid colon is done after completion of the pelvic part of the surgery. The patient is placed in dorsal lithotomy-Trendelenburg position in stirrups. Three incisions are made: one of 12 mm in the right lower quadrant, one of 10 mm under the umbilicus, and one of 5mm to the left periumbilical area [46]. After pneumoperitoneum (12–14 mmHg) is created with carbon dioxide, the identification of the sigmoid colon is made. The dissection of the sigmoid colon is done from lateral to medial on vascular pedicle comprising the sigmoid artery and sigmoid vein. Vascular pedicle should be sufficient to allow the mobilization of the sigmoid

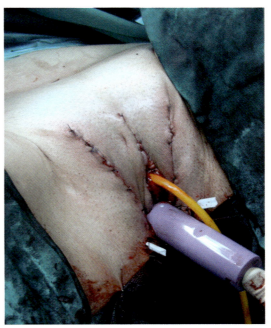

Fig. 6 Outcome at the end of surgery of penile inversion vaginoplasty

segment to the neovaginal canal for the anastomosis with the penile skin flap. Since the anatomy of the blood vessels varies widely among patients, intraoperative mapping should be done to avoid the damage to the sigmoid arteries and the common branch of Drummond, as the vascularization of the sigmoid colon is dependent on this branch [47]. A sigmoid segment of 10–15 cm is mobilized and both ends are closed with endo-GIA linear stapler of 65 mm. Minimal laparotomy of 4 cm is made on the left side for insertion of the circular stapler head. Bowel anastomosis is performed using the intraluminal 29 mm stapler. The peritoneal fold between the rectum and the bladder is carefully opened from the inside above the Denonvilliers fascia. The Ballinger forceps are introduced and the sigmoid colon is grasped and opened. The sigmoid colon is transposed in isoperistaltic way and anastomosed with interrupted monofilament sutures with the penile skin inverted flap. The proximal part of the neovagina is fixed to prevent neovaginal prolapse. The neovagina is then packed with antibiotic greasy gauze.

Also, the use of intestinal segments for vaginal reconstruction produces a self-lubricating vagina, which resembles a natural vagina, and the use of intestinal segments can create a vagina of satisfactory depth for penetrative sexual intercourse.

Peritoneal Pull-Through Vaginoplasty

Peritoneal pull-through vaginoplasty was first introduced by Davydov in 1969 and later by Rothman in 1972 [15, 16]. It was first used for patients with vaginal agenesis, but it found its use in patients with gender dysphoria.

Preoperative antibiotic prophylaxis is administered to the patient (ceftriaxone 2 g/day and metronidazole 500 mg/8 h) as well as anticoagulation prophylaxis. The harvesting of the peritoneal flaps is done after completion of the pelvic part of the surgery. The urinary Foley catheter 16Ch is introduced into the bladder. The patient is placed in dorsal lithotomy-Trendelenburg position. Three incisions are made: one of 10 mm under the umbilicus and two of 5 mm, one in the right lower quadrant, and the other in the left lower quadrant. After pneumoperitoneum (12–14 mmHg) is created with carbon dioxide, the inspection of the abdominal cavity is made. Sigmoid colon adhesiolysis is performed to fully expose the rectovesical space. The harvesting of two peritoneal flaps is then performed (Fig. 7). The horizontal peritoneal incision is made overlying seminal vesicles and widened laterally beneath the vas deferens to both sides [48]. One flap is harvested from the posterior aspect of the bladder in length of approximately 8–10 cm and width of about 7 cm using an ultracision harmonic scalpel. The posterior peritoneal flap is then raised adjacent to the rectum, having the ureters as lateral borders and promontory as the superior border. The mobilized flaps are then sutured laterally to form the tube. The incision is then made between the bladder and the rectum so the anastomosis between the inverted penile skin flap and peritoneal flaps could be made. The two Ballinger forceps are introduced into the neovaginal canal and peritoneal flaps are grasped and anastomosis with interrupted resorbable sutures was made with penile skin flap (Figs. 8 and 9). Intra-abdominally, both peritoneal flaps are sutured with the running suture creating the tube, and the apex of the neovagina was secured by its fixation to the sigmoid colon to prevent injury and perforation during the dilatations and sexual intercourse. Vaginal packing consisting of vaginal gauze soaked into the antibiotic ointment is placed.

Peritoneal pull-through vaginoplasty provides good esthetic and functional results and is considered a minimally invasive surgery. Also, pelvic peritoneum is in close proximity to the neovaginal canal, and therefore the neovagina created by peritoneal pull-through technique will have the axis suitable for penetrative sexual intercourse. On the other side, the peritoneum has very good

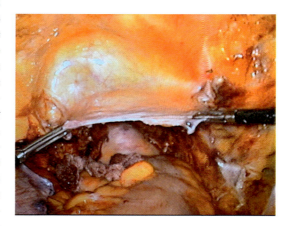

Fig. 7 Laparoscopic mobilization of the peritoneal flaps for neovaginal reconstruction

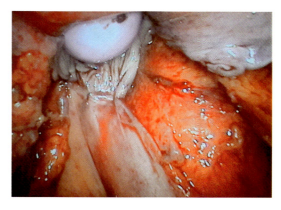

Fig. 8 Anastomosis of the peritoneal flaps with inverted penile skin

regenerative power and can go metaplasia and mimic vaginal epithelium which was proved by many literature data published so far [17, 18] (Fig. 10).

Zero-Depth Vaginoplasty (Feminizing Vulvoplasty)

Zero-depth vaginoplasty is a minimally invasive feminizing GAS that can be considered for those individuals in whom creation of the neovaginal canal is contraindicated or with high percentage of risk, for patients who are unable or incapable or unwilling to dilate and for patients who are not interested in penetrative vaginal sexual intercourse.

The patient is positioned in dorsal lithotomy position. Urinary Foley catheter is introduced into the bladder. Previously described subprocedures, e.g., bilateral orchiectomy, total penectomy, clitoroplasty and vulvoplasty, are performed completing the feminizing vulvoplasty (Fig. 11).

Feminizing vulvoplasty provides female external genitalia, with completely preserved clitoral sensation for orgasm to the patient. The surgery itself is much shorter as well as the hospital stay and postoperative recovery [25].

Postoperative Care

The patients undergoing any type of vaginoplasty is placed on prophylactic anticoagulant therapy until in bed rest. Antibiotic prophylaxis is also introduced until the Foley catheter is removed. The vaginal packing is removed after 6–7 days after the vaginoplasty surgery, and vaginal dilations and douching are started according to the instructions of the pelvic floor therapist. The regular vaginal dilations are advised to the patients for the period of at least 12 months postoperatively to maintain the patency of the neovaginal canal. Patients' cooperation and commitment is of utmost importance to preserve the full depth of the neovagina.

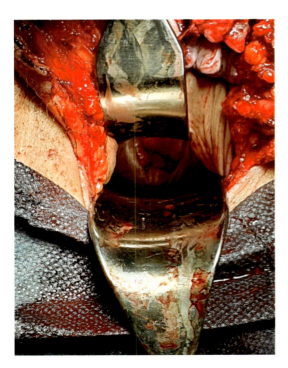

Fig. 9 Peritoneal pull-through vaginoplasty. Anastomosis of the peritoneal and penile skin flaps. Perineal view

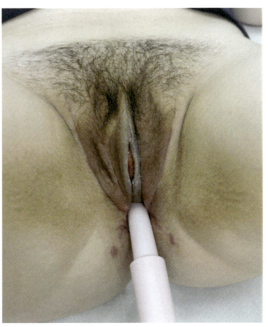

Fig. 10 Outcome 3 months after peritoneal pull-through vaginoplasty. A vaginal dilator is inserted into the neovagina. Labia majora and minora are symmetrical. The clitoris is anatomically positioned and hidden

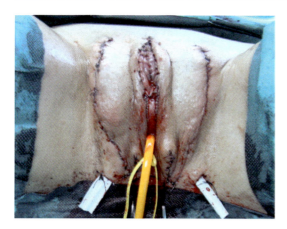

Fig. 11 Immediate outcome after zero-depth vaginoplasty with urinary catheter inserted into the bladder

Complications

Complications after vaginoplasty can be divided into early and late postoperative complications. Early postoperative complications include postoperative bleeding, hematoma formation, wound dehiscence, skin necrosis, clitoral necrosis, and urethral flap necrosis. Late postoperative complications related to vaginoplasty surgery involve poor cosmesis, corpora cavernosa remnants, formation of the granulation tissue, hair growth inside the neovagina, neovaginal prolapse, excessive mucus production, foul smell, dysuric problems, meatal stenosis, corpus spongiosum bulging, introital stenosis, loss of neovaginal depth, as well as urinary and enteric neovaginal fistulas [38, 49].

Early Postoperative Complications

Bleeding

Intraoperative bleeding occurs in 3–12% of patients undergoing vaginoplasty, and the majority of cases is from the corpus spongiosum during urethroplasty [49]. In less than 1% of patients, blood transfusion may be needed, while the formation of hematomas of the labia majora and suprapubic area may be present in up to 10% of the patients [49].

Bleeding can be prevented with the application of Satinsky clamp during urethroplasty and by application of compressive dressing over the spatulated urethra and application of the ice pack over the dressing.

Wound Dehiscence

Wound dehiscence is one of the most common early postoperative complications and varies between 5% and 33% [38, 49]. The treatment usually involves wound care with delayed healing. Sometimes the revision surgery consisting of wound suturing may be necessary.

Skin Necrosis

Neovaginal skin necrosis ranges from 1% to 4% according to the literature data [38, 49]. In case this happens, local wound care is needed. Sometimes the removal of necrotic tissue may be required. Also, in cases of partial neovaginal skin necrosis, the patients are advised to dilate to prevent complete vaginal shortening or stenosis.

Clitoral Necrosis

Necrosis of the neoclitoris is less frequent, but can happen in 1–3% of patients as described in the literature [38, 49]. In case of such occurrence, the sensation of the clitoris can be impaired and may be completely lost.

Urethral Flap Necrosis

Urethral flap necrosis is rare. It can happen in case the hemostatic clamp is applied very long or if during the urethral mobilization the bulbar arteries are injured. Wound care is advised to enable the flap to heal.

Late Complications

Poor Cosmesis

Unsatisfactory cosmetic results are among the most common reasons for the revision surgeries in transgender women with up to 50%

[38, 49]. The patients most commonly require excision of the scars, removal of the excessive skin, lipofilling, covering of the clitoris or reduction of the clitoris, and improvement of the look of their external genitalia

Corpora Cavernosa Remnants

Postoperative erection of the corpora cavernosa remnants presents one of the possible late complications in feminizing GAS [4, 38]. Depending on the length of the corpora cavernosa remnants, the patients may report inability to engage in sexual intercourse, pain and bulging during the arousal, and unclear sensations around the clitoris and deep inside the pelvis. To prevent corpora cavernosa remnants as a complication, we advise the approach of complete penile disassembly with the removal of the corporeal crura to their attachments on the pubic rami.

However, in cases with more extensive corpora cavernosa remnants that impair sexual activity of the patient, the revision surgery and removal of the remnants is required. The surgery is done using the pharmacological erection induced by prostaglandin E1 for the easier dissection [4].

Formation of the Granulation Tissue

Formation of the granulation tissue inside the neovagina with subsequent bleeding during neovaginal dilation or sexual intercourse is one of the described postoperative complications. The incidence is reported between 7% and 26% according to the available literature data. The treatment involves the application of the silver nitrate and antibiotic [49].

Hair Growth Inside the Neovagina

Hair growth inside the neovagina can happen in case when hair-bearing skin is used for the neovaginal lining. Hair growth within the neovagina can lead to infections, hairballs, malodor, and pain during the sexual intercourse and dilation. To prevent hair growth, the patients are advised to perform permanent hair removal prior to undergoing vaginoplasty.

Neovaginal Prolapse

The prevalence of the neovaginal prolapse is rare and varies between 1% and 2% [38]. As mentioned before, the prolapse can be prevented by fixation of the neovagina to the sacrospinous ligament or prostate capsule [22, 35, 36]. In sigmoid vaginoplasty to prevent the prolapse of the neovagina, its proximal part is fixed to the promontorium.

Excessive Mucus Production and Foul Smell

Excessive mucus production is one of the major complaints in patients after sigmoid vaginoplasty, but usually stops with first 6 months after the surgery. The patients are instructed to perform regular thorough douching of the neovagina to evacuate the mucus and to wear daily pads.

Diversion Colitis

Diversion colitis after sigmoid vaginoplasty presents colonic inflammation caused by the lack of luminal nutrients after surgical diversion from the fecal stream. Lack of luminal short-chain fatty acids, the nutrient of colonocytes, supposedly leads to apoptosis of colonocytes and subsequent to an inflammatory reaction of the colonic mucosa. It can present with tenesmus, sharp pain, and bleeding after sexual intercourse. The treatment is conservative with sodium butyrate enemas for at least 4 weeks. Even though diversion colitis is one of the main drawbacks of sigmoid vaginoplasty, only few cases are reported in the literature so far [50].

Meatal Stenosis and Dysuric Problems

Stenosis of the urethral meatus can occur in about 14% of the patients undergoing feminizing GAS and can lead to dysuric problems and urinary tract infection [49]. If stenosis of the urethral meatus is confirmed, the insertion of the urinary catheter is indicated if possible, or a suprapubic catheter if the patient is in urinary retention. The treatment includes the Y-V urethroplasty that can be repeated in about 15% of patients because of possible recurrence of the meatal stenosis [49].

Corpus Spongiosum Bulging

Bulging of the bulbar urethra during the arousal can impair the vaginal penetration or can make it painful. This can happen in case the bulbar muscle or corpus spongiosum is not removed during the dissection and urethroplasty. The treatment is surgical excision of the excessive spongiosal tissue of the urethra [24].

Introital Stenosis

Stenosis of the neovaginal introitus ranges between 4% and 15% [49]. The regular dilations of the neovagina with gradual increase of the vaginal dilator may prevent introital stenosis. In case of its occurrence, minor surgical intervention with perineal skin flap or Z-plasty may be performed.

Vaginal Stenosis and Loss of Neovaginal Depth

One of the most common reported complications after feminizing GAS is vaginal stenosis. It is more common in techniques where grafts are used, rather than flaps for vaginal reconstruction. The incidence of vaginal canal stenosis varies from 1% to 12% [49]. About 5% of patients will require revision surgery because of inadequate neovaginal depth.

To prevent the shortening of the neovagina, patients are advised and instructed on performing regular neovaginal dilations that in certain techniques must be performed lifelong. In case that the depth is lost and can't be gained by dilations, one of the revision surgeries can be proposed to the patient such as grafting and use of bowel or peritoneal flaps to augment the vaginal depth.

Urinary and Enteric Neovaginal Fistulas

One of the most difficult complications in feminizing genital gender affirmation surgery is formation of the rectovaginal or vesicovaginal fistula. Rectovaginal fistula can occur during the dissection for the neovaginal canal after overlooked rectal injury, infection, and dilation injury. The incidence of rectovaginal fistula varies from 0.8% to 17% across the centers and studies. Treatment is usually surgical and can include creation of diverting ileostomy or colostomy, especially in larger fistulas, or fistulectomy and primary closure in layers with interposition of pedicled flaps (exp. gracilis) [49]. Vesicovaginal or urethrovaginal fistula is rare and can develop secondary to a meatal stenosis. The repair of genitourinary fistula involves fistlectomy or fistulorraphy with interposition of pedicled flaps [49].

Sexual Function

Sexual function after vaginoplasty in transgender women is very important and requires a specific place in follow-up of these patients [51]. The majority of studies reported the sexual satisfaction of the patients by asking the patients to define the degree of their sexual satisfaction [52–54]. According to available studies, between 33% and 87% of patients reported having sexual intercourse after penile inversion vaginoplasty and between 63% and 79% after bowel vaginoplasty [38]. Hess et al. found more intense orgasm in their patients after performing vaginoplasty in 55.8% [54]. Also, patient satisfaction concerning neovaginal depth and esthetic appearance varied from 76% to 100% and from 90% to 100% according to the literature data [38] Buncamper et al. were the first to use Female Sexual Function Index (FSFI) to measure the sexual satisfaction in the cohort of 475 transgender women who underwent penile inversion vaginoplasty in their center [55]. According to the results from their study, 70% of the patients were pleased with the look of their external genitalia, while in 75%, the postoperative result met patient's expectations. Despite these high satisfaction rates, patients showed dysfunctional results on FSFI scale. One of the possible explanations could be that FSFI scale was not specifically created for transgender women. Concerning sigmoid vaginoplasty, some studies report 77.8% of their patients being satisfied with the sexual functioning of their neovaginas [42]. Only one study used standardized FSFI questionnaire created for operated transgender women, so further studies are needed so conclusions could be made [56].

Conclusions

Genital gender affirmation surgery for transgender women is challenging. Described techniques are safe procedures in the hands of experienced reconstructive surgeons and provide good results to majority of patients. Gender affirmation surgeries are proved to increase the quality of life and overall satisfaction of transgender and gender-nonconforming individuals.

In individuals undergoing transfeminine GAS, functional satisfaction is highly dependent on the depth of the neovagina as well as the sensation of the neoclitoris required to reach orgasm. Patients' overall happiness is also linked to the cosmesis of the neocreated vulva, scar visibility, and the necessity for revision surgeries.

Preoperative consultation with a surgeon is very important in terms of desired procedure, expectations, outcomes, and possible complications.

Cross-References

▶ Complications of Gender-Affirmation Surgery

Acknowledgments This chapter is supported by the Ministry of Science and Technological development, Republic of Serbia, project no. 175048.

References

1. https://www.who.int/health-topics/gender#tab=tab_1. Accessed on 2 Dec 2021
2. Richards C, Bouman WP, Barker MJ. Genderqueer and non-binary genders. London: Macmillan; 2017. p. 1–306.
3. Bhinder J, Upadhyaya P. Brief history of gender affirmation medicine and surgery. In: Nikolavsky D, Blakely SA, editors. Urological care for transgender patient. Switzerland: Springer Cham; 2021. p. 249–54.
4. Djordjevic ML, Bizic MR. Sexual reassignment surgery: male to female. In: Salgado CJ, Redett R, editors. Aesthetic and functional surgery of the genitalia. New York: Nova science Publishers, Inc.; 2014. p. 109–26.
5. Buncamper M. The Penile inversion vaginoplasty: From functional to the desired. Rotterdam: Optima Grafische Communicatie; 2016. p. 7–175.
6. Hoyer N, editor. Man into woman: the first sex change, a Portrait of Lili Elbe: the true and remarkable transformation of the Painter Einar Wegener. Chicago: Blue Boat Books Ltd.; 2004. p. 1–271.
7. Fogh-Andersen P. Transsexualism: an attempt at surgical management. Scand J Plast Reconstr surg. 1969;3:61–9.
8. Karim RB, Hage JJ. On the origin of pedicled skin inversion vaginoplasty: life and work of Dr Georges Burou of Casablanca. Ann Plast Surg. 2007;59:723–9.
9. Gillies H, Millard RD Jr. Genitalia. In: The principles and art of plastic surgery. London: Butterworth; 1957. p. 369–88.
10. Cairins TS, De Villiers W. Vaginoplasty. S Afr Med J. 1980;57:50–5.
11. Freundt I. Colocolpopoisis: the use of sigmoid colon in the treatment of conditions associated with absence of the vagina. The Netherlands: Erasmus University Rotterdam; 1994. pp. 11–128.
12. Baldwin J. The formation of an artificial vagina by intestinal transplantation. Ann Surg. 1904;40:398–403.
13. Karim RB, Hage JJ, Dekker JJ, Schoot CM. Evolution of the methods of neovaginoplasty for vaginal aplasia. Eur J Obstet Gynecol Reprod Biol. 1995;58(1):19–27.
14. Karim RB, Hage JJ, Mulder JW. Neovaginoplasty in male transsexuals: review of surgical techniques and recommendations regarding their eligibility. Ann Plast Surg. 1996;37:669–75.
15. Davydov SN, Zhvitiashvili OD. Formation of vagina (colpopoiesis) from peritoneum of Douglas pouch. Acta Chir Plast. 1974;16(1):35–41.
16. Rothman D. The use of peritoneum on construction of vagina. Obstel Gynecol. 1972;40:835–9.
17. Jacoby A, Maliha S, Granieri MA, Cohen O, Dy GW, Bluebond-Langner R, Zhao LC. Robotic Davydov peritoneal flap vaginoplasty for augmentation of vaginal depth in feminizing vaginoplasty. J Urol. 2019;201(6):1171–6.

18. Jun MS, Gonzalez E, Zhao LC, Bluebond-Langner R. Penile inversion vaginoplasty with robotically assisted peritoneal flaps. Plast Reconstr Surg. 2021;148(2):439–42.
19. Rodríguez ÁH, Lima Júnior EM, de Moraes Filho MO, Costa BA, Bruno ZV, Filho MPM, Amaral de Moraes ME, Rodrigues FAR, Paier CRK, Bezerra LRPS. Male-to-female gender-affirming surgery using Nile Tilapia Fish skin as a biocompatible graft. J Minim Invasive Gynecol. 2020;27(7):1474–5.
20. Pariser JJ, Kim N. Transgender vaginoplasty: techniques and outcomes. Transl Androl Urol. 2019;8(3):241–7.
21. Safa B, Lin WC, Salim AM, Deschamps-Braly JC, Poh MM. Current concepts in feminizing gender surgery. Plast Reconstr Surg. 2019;143(5):1081e–91e.
22. Bizic M, Kojovic V, Duisin D, Stanojevic D, Vujovic S, Milosevic A, Korac G, Djordjevic ML. An overview of neovaginal reconstruction options in male to female transsexuals. Scientific World Journal. 2014;638919 https://doi.org/10.1155/2014/638919.
23. Shoureshi P, Dugi D 3rd. Penile inversion vaginoplasty technique. Urol Clin North Am. 2019;46(4):511–25.
24. Djordjevic ML, Stanojevic D, Bizic M. Male-to-female gender affirmation skin-flap vaginoplasty. In: Salgado CJ, Monstrey SJ, Djordjevic ML, editors. Gender affirmation: medical and surgical perspectives. New York: Thieme Medical Publishers, Inc.; 2017. p. 83–93.
25. Jiang D, Witten J, Berli J, Dugi D 3rd. Does depth matter? Factors affecting choice of vulvoplasty over vaginoplasty as gender-affirming genital surgery for transgender women. J Sex Med. 2018;15(6):902–6.
26. Perovic S, Djordjevic M. Penile disassembly technique to surgical treatment of Peyronie's disease. Br J Urol. 2001;88:731–9.
27. Brown J. Creation of a functional clitoris and aesthetically pleasing introitus in sex conversion. In: Marchac D, Hueston JT, editors. Transactions of the sixth international Congress of plastic and reconstructive surgery. Paris: Masson; 1976. p. 654–5.
28. Hage JJ, Karim RB, Bloem JJ, Suliman HM, van Alphen M. Sculpturing the neoclitoris in vaginoplasty for male-to-female transsexuals. Plast Reconstr Surg. 1994;93(2):358–64.
29. Rubin SO. A method of preserving the glans penis as a clitoris in sex conversion operations in male transsexuals. Scand J Urol Nephrol. 1980;14:215–21.
30. Eldh J. Construction of a neovagina with preservation of the glans penis as a clitoris in male transsexuals. Plast Reconstr Surg. 1993;91(5):895–900.
31. Perovic S. Construction of a neoclitoris in male transsexuals. Plast Reconstr Surg. 1994;93:646–8.
32. Hage JJ, Karim RB. Sensate pedicled neoclitoroplasty for male transsexuals: Amsterdam experience in the first 60 patients. Ann Plast Surg. 1996;36(6):621–4.
33. Reed HM. Aesthetic and functional male to female genital and perineal surgery: feminizing vaginoplasty. Semin Plast Surg. 2011;25(2):163–74.
34. Goddard JC, Vickery RM, Qureshi A, Summerton DJ, Khoosal D, Terry TR. Feminizing genitoplasty in adult transsexuals: early and long-term surgical results. BJU Int. 2007;100(3):607–13.
35. Stanojevic DS, Djordjevic ML, Milosevic A, Sansalone S, Slavkovic Z, Ducic S, Vujovic S, Perovic SV, Belgrade Gender Dysphoria Team. Sacrospinous ligament fixation for neovaginal prolapse prevention in male-to-female surgery. Urology. 2007;70(4):767–71.
36. Sohn M, Bosinski HAG. Gender identity disorders: diagnostic and surgical aspects. J Sex Med. 2007;4:1193–208.
37. Perovic SV, Stanojevic DS. Djordjevic ML. Vaginoplasty in male transsexuals using penile skin and urethral flap. BJU Int. 2000;85:843–50.
38. Horbach SE, Bouman MB, Smit JM, Özer M, Buncamper ME, Mullender MG. Outcome of vaginoplasty in male-to-female transgenders: a systematic review of surgical techniques. J Sex Med. 2015;12(6):1499–512.
39. Krege S, Bex A, Lümmen G, Rübben H. Male-to-female transsexualism: a technique, results and long-term follow-up in 66 patients. BJU Int. 2001;88(4):396–402.
40. Markland C, Hastings D. Vaginal reconstruction using cecal and sigmoid bowel segments in transsexual patients. J Urol. 1974;111(2):217–9.
41. Bouman MB, van Zeijl MC, Buncamper ME, Meijerink WJ, van Bodegraven AA, Mullender MG. Intestinal vaginoplasty revisited: a review of surgical techniques, complications, and sexual function. J Sex Med. 2014;11(7):1835–47.
42. Djordjevic ML, Stanojevic DS, Bizic MR. Rectosigmoid vaginoplasty: clinical experience in 86 cases. J Sex Med. 2011;8(12):3487–94.
43. Perovic S, Stanojevic D, Djordjevic M, Djakovic N. Refinements in rectosigmoid vaginoplasty. Eur Urol. 1998;33:156–7.
44. Filipas D, Black P, Hohenfellner R. The use of isolated bowel segment in complicated vaginal reconstruction. BJU Int. 2000;85:715–9.
45. van der Sluis WB, Bouman MB. Al-Tamimi M, Meijerink WJ, Tuynman JB. Real-time indocyanine green fluorescent angiography in laparoscopic sigmoid vaginoplasty to assess perfusion of the pedicled sigmoid segment. Fertil Steril. 2019;112(5):967–9.
46. Bouman MB, Buncamper ME, van der Sluis WB, Meijerink WJ. Total laparoscopic sigmoid vaginoplasty. Fertil Steril. 2016;106(7):e22–3.
47. Bouman MB, van der Sluis WB, Buncamper ME, Meijerink WJ. Male-to-female gender affirmation colon vaginoplasty: total laparoscopic sigmoid vaginoplasty. In: Salgado CJ, Monstrey SJ, Dordjevic ML, editors. Gender affirmation: medical and surgical perspectives. New York: Thieme Medical Publishers, Inc; 2017. p. 95–108.
48. Dy GW, Jun MS, Blasdel G, Bluebond-Langner R, Zhao LC. Outcomes of gender affirming peritoneal

flap vaginoplasty using the Da Vinci single port versus Xi robotic systems. Eur Urol. 2021;79(5):676–83.
49. Schardein JN, Zhao LC, Nikolavsky D. Management of vaginoplasty and phalloplasty complications. Urol Clin North Am. 2019;46(4):605–18.
50. van der Sluis WB, Bouman MB, Meijerink WJHJ, Elfering L, Mullender MG, de Boer NKH, van Bodegraven AA. Diversion neovaginitis after sigmoid vaginoplasty: endoscopic and clinical characteristics. Fertil Steril. 2016;105(3):834–839.e1.
51. Weyers S, Elaut E, De Sutter P, Gerris J, T'Sjoen G, Heylens G, De Cuypere G, Verstraelen H. Long-term assessment of the physical, mental, and sexual health among transsexual women. J Sex Med. 2009;6(3):752–60.
52. De Cuypere G, T'Sjoen G, Beerten R, Selvaggi G, De Sutter P, Hoebeke P, Monstrey S, Vansteenwegen A, Rubens R. Sexual and physical health after sex reassignment surgery. Arch Sex Behav. 2005;34(6):679–90.
53. Selvaggi G, Monstrey S, Ceulemans P, T'Sjoen G, De Cuypere G, Hoebeke P. Genital sensitivity after sex reassignment surgery in transsexual patients. Ann Plast Surg. 2007;58(4):427–33.
54. Hess J, Rossi Neto R, Panic L, Rübben H, Senf W. Satisfaction with male-to-female gender reassignment surgery. Dtsch Arztebl Int. 2014;111(47):795–801.
55. Buncamper ME, Honselaar JS, Bouman MB, Özer M, Kreukels BP, Mullender MG. Aesthetic and functional outcomes of neovaginoplasty using penile skin in male-to-female transsexuals. J Sex Med. 2015;12(7):1626–34.
56. Vedovo F, Di Blas L, Perin C, Pavan N, Zatta M, Bucci S, Morelli G, Cocci A, Delle Rose A, Caroassai Grisanti S, Gentile G, Colombo F, Rolle L, Timpano M, Verze P, Spirito L, Schiralli F, Bettocchi C, Garaffa G, Palmieri A, Mirone V, Trombetta C. Operated male-to-female sexual function index: validity of the first questionnaire developed to assess sexual function after male-to-female gender affirming surgery. J Urol. 2020;204(1):115–20.

Complications of Gender-Affirmation Surgery

64

Silke Riechardt

Contents

Introduction	1228
General Perspective on Complications of Gender-Affirmation Surgery	1228
Localization by Organ of the Urinary Tract System	1228
Anatomical	1228
Urethral Fistulas:	1229
Functional: Incontinence	1230
Localization/Organ System: Genital	1230
Infection	1230
Localization/Organ System: Gastro/Bowel	1231
Localization: Gender-Specific: Prostate Hyperplasia/Cancer, Venous thromboembolism	1232
Conclusion	1232
Cross-References	1232
References	1232

Abstract

Gender affirming surgery means the complete reconstruction of the genital including interference on the pelvic floor resulting in a big wound area and complications in more than one organ system. Problems can occur in the urinary tract, the genital, or the bowel. Besides, problems like bleeding or infection can affect the whole surgery with all parts. So the overall complication rate is high compared to other surgeries. But fortunately most problems needing revision are minor complications with a good success rate in revisions.

Keywords

Gender affirming surgery · Gender dysphoria · Complications · Rectal injury · Rectal fistula · Meatal stenosis · Vaginal stenosis · Vaginal atrophy · Clitoris necrosis

S. Riechardt (✉)
Department of Urology, University Hospital Hamburg-Eppendorf, Hamburg, Germany
e-mail: s.riechardt@uke.de

Introduction

Talking about complications means to classify.

The possibilities to classify are various and depend on the point of view. If you are a surgeon, you need to know which event needs another operation. If you are a resident, you are interested to know which complication could occur on which organ. And as a patient, it is most important to know which complication has the highest impact on the quality of live (QoL).

This chapter tries to classify the complications of male-to-female gender reassigning surgery in a transparent way, so all different aspects could be found.

The complications are structured in:

Localization/Organ System: The gender reassignment affects more than one organ system, so the complications of different systems mean different limitations. They are split in: urinary tract, genital, bowel, and unspecific.

Time After Operation: Early/Late, Long Term. Some problems typically occur in the inpatient period, some only in the long term. If you only look at the 90 days period postoperatively long-term problems might be missed.

Severity/Consequences: Clavien Dindo, CCI

The Clavien Dindo classification (CDC) [1] is validated for any postoperative complication that means any deviation from the normal postoperative course. But it is useful only for the direct postoperative period, so it will be seldom used in this chapter

Grade I: With no need for pharmacological treatment
Grade II: Need for pharmacological treatment or blood transfusion
Grade III: Requires intervention, a/b: without/with general anesthesia
Grade IV: Life threatening a/b: single organ/multi-organ dysfunction
Grade V: Death

Comprehensive Complication Index (CCI): This is a tool to access the patients overall morbidity, sum of CDC single events, max 100 points. It is useful for such extensive surgery, because it adds the single event to a total score.

The two tools made for early surgical complications, only useful from the surgeon's point of view, can be used here for severity.

The Resultant Limitation: The limitation after a complication can have more than one aspect; it can be functional, a problem of cosmetics, or it can influence the sensibility/orgasm. The QoL is very important for the rating of success from the patients point of view, affecting the overall satisfaction.

Prevention: When surgery is done, complications do occur. But mostly there is a pitfall to avoid or a special technique to improve. Most tips and tricks are not validated, but results from long surgery experience.

General Perspective on Complications of Gender-Affirmation Surgery

Usually the complications in surgery procedures are counted by revisions and mortality and morbidity rates. Fortunately major complications classified by CDC as Grade IV or V are extremely rare in gender reassignment surgery. But there is a relevant complication rate of up to 50% that leads to surgical revision in 8–40% in the literature. It seems as if the longer (F/U) the more complications occur (Table 1).

Localization by Organ of the Urinary Tract System

The urinary tract is affected by the gender reassigning surgery only as a side effect. But complications concerning the urinary tract can be *anatomical* like bleeding, retention, strictures, and fistulas or *functional* like incontinence and might have a high impact on the QoL.

Anatomical

Early: Bleeding
One frightening early problem is serious bleeding from the urethral stump. This happens usually in the first days after operation or after the first change of dressing. Mainly it can be treated by compression; only seldom there is the need for revision or blood transfusion. Blood transfusion

Table 1 Reoperation rates

Author Year	n	(F/U)	Reoperation (%)	Main reason for Reoperation
Levy 2019 [2]	240	90 days	7.9	Cosmetic 3.8%
Dreher 2018 [3]	1684		21.7	Meatal stenosis 14.4%
Gaiter 2018 [4]	330	90 days	9	
Buncamper 2016 [5]	475	6 years	8.4	Vaginal scars 2.9%
Raigosa 2015 [6]	60	>12 months	28.2	Cosmetic 21.6%
Rossi Neto 2012 [7]	332	NR	51	Meatal stenosis 40%
Reed 2011 [8]	250	3 years	20	Cosmetic 12%
Kreege 2001 [9]	66	NR	15	Meatal stenosis 10.6%
Hage 2000 [10]	390	17.5 years	22	Introitus stenosis 10.2%

rates vary from 2–4.8% in the literature [5, 7, 8]. Buncamper [5] found 1.5% surgical revisions because of serious bleeding. Sometimes a serious bleeding with revision leads to a meatal stricture because of scar formations.

Severity/Consequences: CDC, CCI: Inside the CDC bleeding is classified as severe because of risk for transfusion or revision. For the patients' QoL, long-term outcome plays only a secondary role.

The Resultant Limitation: Bleeding postoperatively is frightening for the patients in the postoperative period. If it leads to blood transfusion, it means the risk for infection, which is quite low in a controlled hospital setting. Surgical revision is a small surgical procedure, which leads to stop the bleeding securely.

Prevention: The surrounding tissue of the urethra, the corpus spongiosum, is a sponge tissue with perfect blood supply. One possibility to prevent bleeding is an overcast suture to close the corpus spongiosum. Another possibility is any kind of comprehensive dressing staying for more than 2 days, to stop any bleeding in the area. But the compressing always means the risk of compromising the blood supply of other important structures like the clitoris. So the comprehensive dressing is a balance between no bleeding and enough blood supply.

Early: Urinary Retention

Urinary retention can happen after removal of the transurethral catheter. This effect is temporary due to swelling of the urethral stump and can be treated by watchful waiting, anti-inflammatory medication, or an indwelling catheter for another 1–2 weeks.

Some surgeons use a suprapubic tube to prevent postoperative urinary retention, but it is a minor complication, so it might not be needed for all patients and bears complications in itself like bleeding with bladder tamponade.

Late: Strictures of the Urethra

The common stricture after gender reassigning surgery affects the meatus. This is uncommon in the first weeks after surgery, but occurs within months. Most surgeons already plan the operation in a two staged manner, so that a meatotomy like y-v plasty or other techniques can be done planed in the second stage. In the literature the meatal stenosis has a rate up to 40%, which decreased the last years (Table 2).

Prevention: Spatulation of the urethral stump increases the outlet volume and prevents meatal stenosis.

Proximal Strictures: **Proximal strictures** or a complete breakdown of the lasting urethra are quite seldom (1.5% [9]). The treatment follows the guidelines for male strictures, because the anatomy is still male.

Urethral Fistulas:

Another problem are urethral fistulas, which are rarely reported in 1–4%, but occur [7, 11]. Usually they are a functional problem, because the fistula lies deep in the vagina and means a urine influx in the vagina resulting in postvoiding incontinence. If this is disturbing, they need a surgical closure.

Table 2 Rates of meatal stenosis

Author	Meatal stenosis (%)	Recurrence
Dreher [3]	14.4	
Levy [2]	0.5	
Rossi Neto [7]	40	12%
Reed [8]	6	
Kreege [9]	10.6	

The closure should be done in double layer technique, using the vaginal tissue as cover.

Limitation: All urinary tract problems are a disturbance for the patients, because they don't expect changes in voiding due to the operation. So, even a minor problem can be a serious decrease in QoL. A lot of transwomen are alarmed by urinary stream deviation, depending on bladder filling, pelvic floor tension, or sitting position, which are completely normal for *cis*-women. So it is important to explain the voiding changes before surgery.

Prevention: Complications of the urethra are triggered by a disturbance of the blood supply, due to an infection or extensive surgical preparation. The preparation should stay in the midline not to bother the arteriae bulbi coming from lateral, which support the urethral blood supply.

Functional: Incontinence

Urinary incontinence can look like stress or urge incontinence.

A real stress incontinence is uncommon because both male sphincter systems (sph. Ext. sph. Int.) are preserved. But the operation does disturb the anatomy by opening the pelvic floor muscles for the vaginal space. This disturbs the function of the pelvic floor, possibly resulting in an incontinence. Hoebeke [12] found in 2005 in 31 patients an incidence of 16% new incontinence resulting in discomfort without measurable LUTS.

A treatment possibility is pelvic floor exercises.

Urgency can be treated pharmacologically, but can be affected by exercises as well.

Limitations. Even mild functional incontinence is a major distress, especially for younger patients.

Prevention: The same principle is valid for the pelvic floor: the surgeons should avoid extensive preparation not to harm important structures like pelvis floor muscles and the nerves.

Localization/Organ System: Genital

Complications of the genital region are quite serious for the patients. They have high expectations regarding the benefits and new possibilities offered by their assigned gender.

Typical complications affect the neovagina like vaginal shortening, vaginal atrophy, or introitus stenosis: Besides, complications of the clitoris like necrosis or infection can decrease the sensibility and orgasm. Wound infection is related to the labia or the vulva affecting the cosmetical outcome.

Infection

Early: Infections of the genital region are a common postoperative problem. They mainly result in secondary healing with scars, which can be corrected in a second stage.

An early infection or reduced dilatation of the neovagina can lead to shortening or complete atrophy. To teach the patients the correct dilatation technique is utmost important for the long time success, because especially in the first months the neovagina tends to develop scars which narrow or shorten.

Vagina: If the infection affects the vagina, this can lead to introitus stenosis or complete atrophy because of necrosis of the neovaginal material or resulting reduced blood supply. Surgical revisions because of neovaginal problem are reported in 2–9% [2, 7] (Table 3).

Clitoris: If the infection affects the neoclitoris, it can lead to partial or complete necrosis. Rossi Neto [7] found a partial necrosis in 2%, a complete necrosis was seen in 0.8–4.5% [8, 9]. If it is only partial necrosis usually the sensibility is still present. A complete necrosis is final, but some patients report still sensibility under the skin, maybe because of the nerval stumps.

The Resultant **Limitation**: Every infection or reduced blood supply results in declined material:

Table 3 Rates of vaginal complications

Author	Introitus stenosis	Vaginal atrophy	Surgical revision
Levy [2]	2.1%		2.1%
Buncamper [5]	20%		2.9%
Raigosa [6]			3.3%
Rossi Neto [7]	15%	8%	9%
Reed [8]	1.2%	1.6%	
Kreege [9]			4.5%

A complete vaginal atrophy could be the result with the need of revision, for example, with using bowel or split skin.

Bowel is an often used material as neovagina, especially for revisions after PI and, for example, for young patient with a prepubertal genital after early hormone treatment, because the local skin might be not enough to form an adult vagina.

One can use sigma, cecum, or ileum; it depends on the length of the mesenterium, because it needs to reach the pelvic floor. Hadj. Moussa [13] found in a review in 2018 the use of bowel only in special cases.

Bouman [14] found in a review in 2014 of intestinal vaginoplasty in nearly 900, a revision rate of 5.3%, which is not worse than the classic PI. But it always means an abdominal surgery with all additional risks. Interestingly the revision rate was higher using sigma than ileum.

Reduced material of the neoclitoris can reduce the sensibility or the orgasmic options.

CDC: Even if the necrosis of the clitoris is rated a less severe complication because no revision is needed, it has a high impact on the QoL for the transwomen.

Prevention: To prevent an infection in the operation there are many proven aspects: sterile conditions, short operation time, single shot antibiotics, no bleeding, few people around.

Gender affirming surgery obtains particular characteristics: Because of the extensive wound and the risk for hematoma longer antibiotics might be useful.

In the penile inversion there is inverted skin closed for days with any kind of dilator and dressing. So trying to reduce the skin bacteria with washing the genital region preoperatively might reduce the risk of infections.

Localization/Organ System: Gastro/Bowel

The most frightening complication in gender reassigning surgery is rectal injury. Fortunately this happens seldom, in the literature up to 4.5% [9].

Early: The rectal injury is usually an early event happening intraoperatively while preparing the vaginal space. When noticed directly it can be repaired by just closing in multilayer technique, because most of the patients have healthy tissue without any surgery before. Only in special cases like obesity, deep injury, or bad visibility conditions there might be the need of an anus praeter (AP) to protect the closure.

Not all injuries leads to a rectal fistula, although it happens. This always leads to an AP for months, while the fistula has time to heal (Table 4).

Severity/Consequences: CDC, CCI: Consequences are often additional to the injury problems of the neovagina, because dilatation compromises fistula healing.

The Resultant **Limitation**: It can lead to a permanent AP if there is recurrence of the fistula and vaginal atrophy.

Prevention: Of utmost importance is careful and exact preparation of the vagina space. Some authors prepare the bowel preoperatively or put in disinfection sponges intraoperatively. Rectal guidance of the fingertip might help as well to

Table 4 Rates of rectal injury/rectal fistula

Author	Rectal injury	Rectal fistula	AP
Buncamper [5]	2.3%	0.6%	
Raigosa [6]		3.3%	
Rossi Neto [7]	3%	2.7%	
Perovic [15]		1.1%	
Van der Sluis [16]		1.2%	
Reed [8]	2.8%	0%	0%
Kreege [9]	4.5%		
Guevarra Martinez [17]		2–17%	

protect the rectum. But even with all efforts, the rectal preparation is a small region with sensitive structures, with the need of an experienced surgeon. And even with perfect preparation, the layers between rectum and neovagina are always thin.

Localization: Gender-Specific: Prostate Hyperplasia/Cancer, Venous thromboembolism

There are some complications resulting especially from the gender change: Results of the female hormone therapy are thromboembolic events, which are dangerous but rare. Reed [8] found in 2011 no thromboembolic complications in 250 surgeries, but they are reported.

Prevention lies in careful mounting of the patient in the lithotomy position, short operation time, early mobilization, and anticoagulation therapy.

Another long-term problem might be the remaining **prostate**. Usually because of the female hormone therapy the prostate stays small, but prostate hyperplasia can occur and even prostate cancer is possible. Patients need a long-term cancer surveillance.

Another rare event is cancer of the neovagina, especially squamous cell carcinoma of the neovagina. Transwomen need a lifelong cancer surveillance with a gynecologist and an endocrinologist.

Conclusion

Overall, the satisfaction besides all complications and revision is very high. In the literature there are less than 1% transperson regretting the surgeries [18]. Massie [19] found 94% of the patients would do the surgery again and 71% had no gender dysphoria anymore. Kreege [9] found >90% satisfaction with cosmesis and function and Horbach [20] identified in a review the most complications affecting the vagina, which can be solved.

Cross-References

▶ (Neo) Vaginoplasty in Female Pelvic Congenital Anomalies

References

1. Bolliger M, Kroehnert J-A, Molineus F, Kandioler D, Schindl M, Riss P. Experiences with the standardized classification of surgical complications (Clavien-Dindo) in general surgery patients. Eur Surg. 2018;50 (6):256–61. https://doi.org/10.1007/s10353-018-0551-z. Epub 2018 Jul 24.
2. Levy JA, Edwards DC, Cutruzzula-Dreher P, McGreen BH, Akanda S, Tarry S, Belkoff LH, Rumer KL. Affiliation male-to-female gender reassignment surgery: an institutional analysis of outcomes, short-term complications, and risk factors for 240 patients undergoing penile-inversion vaginoplasty. Urology. 2019;131:228–33. https://doi.org/10.1016/j.urology.2019.03.043. Epub 2019 Jun 14.
3. Dreher PC, Edwards D, Hager S, Dennis M, Belkoff A, Mora J, Tarry S, Rumer KL. Complications of the neovagina in male-to-female transgender surgery: a systematic review and meta-analysis with discussion of management. Clin Anat. 2018;31(2):191–9. https://doi.org/10.1002/ca.23001. Epub 2017 Nov 10.
4. Gaither TW, Awad MA, Charles Osterberg E, Murphy GP, Romero A, Bowers ML, Breyer BN. Postoperative complications following primary penile inversion vaginoplasty among 330 male-to-female transgender

patients. J Urol. 2018;199(3):760–5. https://doi.org/10.1016/j.juro.2017.10.013. Epub 2017 Oct 12.
5. Buncamper ME, van der Sluis WB, van der Pas RSD, Özer M, Smit JM, Witte BI, Bouman M-B, Mullender MG. Surgical outcome after penile inversion vaginoplasty: a retrospective study of 475 transgender women. Plast Reconstr Surg. 2016;138(5):999–1007. https://doi.org/10.1097/PRS.0000000000002684.
Heß J, Sohn M, Küntscher M, Bohr J. Gender reassignment surgery from male to female. Urologe A. 2020;59(11):1348–55. https://doi.org/10.1007/s00120-020-01337-z.
6. Raigosa M. Avvedimento S, Yoon TS, Cruz-Gimeno J, Rodriguez G, Fontdevila J. Male-to-female genital reassignment surgery: a retrospective review of surgical technique and complications in 60 patients. J Sex Med. 2015;12(8):1837–45. https://doi.org/10.1111/jsm.12936. Epub 2015 Jul 2.
7. Rossi Neto R, Hintz F, Krege S, Rubben H, Vom Dorp F. Gender reassignment surgery – a 13 year review of surgical outcomes. Int Braz J Urol. 2012;38(1):97–107. https://doi.org/10.1590/s1677-55382012000100014.
8. Harold Morgan Reed. Aesthetic and functional male to female genital and perineal surgery: feminizing vaginoplasty. Semin Plast Surg. 2011;25(2):163–74. https://doi.org/10.1055/s-0031-1281486.
9. Krege S, Bex A, Lümmen G, Rübben H. Male-to-female transsexualism: a technique, results and long-term follow-up in 66 patients. BJU Int. 2001;88(4):396–402. https://doi.org/10.1046/j.1464-410x.2001.02323.x.
10. Hage JJ, Goedkoop AY, Karim RB, Kanhai RC. Secondary corrections of the vulva in male-to-female transsexuals. Plast Reconstr Surg. 2000;106(2):350–9. https://doi.org/10.1097/00006534-200008000-00017.
11. van der Sluis WB, Steensma TD, Timmermans FW, Smit JM, de Haseth K, Özer M, Bouman M-B. Gender-confirming vulvoplasty in transgender women in The Netherlands: incidence, motivation analysis, and surgical outcomes. J Sex Med. 2020;17(8):1566–73. https://doi.org/10.1016/j.jsxm.2020.04.007. Epub 2020 May 17.
12. Hoebeke P, Selvaggi G, Ceulemans P, De Cuypere G, T'Sjoen G, Weyers S, Decaestecker K, Monstrey S. Impact of sex reassignment surgery on lower urinary tract function. Eur Urol. 2005;47(3):398–402. https://doi.org/10.1016/j.eururo.2004.10.008. Epub 2004 Dec 2.
13. Hadj-Moussa M, Ohl DA, Kuzon WM Jr. Feminizing genital gender-confirmation surgery. Sex Med Rev. 2018;6(3):457–468.e2. https://doi.org/10.1016/j.sxmr.2017.11.005.
14. Bouman M-B, van Zeijl MCT, Buncamper ME, Meijerink WJHJ, van Bodegraven AA, Mullender MG. Intestinal vaginoplasty revisited: a review of surgical techniques, complications, and sexual function. J Sex Med. 2014;11(7):1835–47. https://doi.org/10.1111/jsm.12538. Epub 2014 Apr 4.
15. Perovic SV, Stanojevic DS, Djordjevic ML. Vaginoplasty in male transsexuals using penile skin and a urethral flap. BJU Int. 2000;86(7):843–50. https://doi.org/10.1046/j.1464-410x.2000.00934.x.
16. van der Sluis WB, Bouman M-B, Buncamper ME, Pigot GLS, Mullender MG, Meijerink WJHJ. Clinical characteristics and management of neovaginal fistulas after vaginoplasty in transgender women. Obstet Gynecol. 2016;127(6):1118–26. https://doi.org/10.1097/AOG.0000000000001421.
17. Guevara-Martínez J, Barragán C, Bonastre J, Zarbakhsh S, Cantero R. Rectoneovaginal fistula after sex reassignment surgery. Description of our experience and literature review. Actas Urol Esp (Engl Ed). 2021;45(3):239–44. https://doi.org/10.1016/j.acuro.2020.08.012.
18. Wiepjes CM, Nota NM, de Blok CJM, Klaver M, de Vries ALC, Annelijn Wensing-Kruger S, de Jongh RT, Bouman M-B, Steensma TD, Cohen-Kettenis P, Gooren LJG, Kreukels BPC, den Heijer M. The Amsterdam Cohort of Gender Dysphoria Study (1972–2015): trends in prevalence, treatment, and regrets. J Sex Med. 2018;15(4):582–90. https://doi.org/10.1016/j.jsxm.2018.01.016. Epub 2018 Feb 17.
19. Massie JP, Morrison SD, Van Maasdam J, Satterwhite T. Predictors of patient satisfaction and postoperative complications in penile inversion vaginoplasty. Plast Reconstr Surg. 2018;141(6):911e–21e. https://doi.org/10.1097/PRS.0000000000004427.
20. Horbach SER, Bouman M-B, Smit JM, Özer M, Buncamper ME, Mullender MG. Outcome of vaginoplasty in male-to-female transgenders: a systematic review of surgical techniques. J Sex Med. 2015;12(6):1499–512. https://doi.org/10.1111/jsm.12868. Epub 2015 Mar 26.

Functional and Aesthetic Surgery of Female Genitalia

65

S. Pusica, B. Stojanovic, and Mirosav L. Djordjevic

Contents

Introduction	1236
Anatomy of Female Genitalia and Changes with Aging	1237
Etiopathogenesis	1238
Genital Surgery for Congenital Adrenal Hyperplasia	1239
Genital Surgery for Vaginal Agenesis	1241
Creatsas Vaginoplasty	1242
Vecchietti Procedure	1242
Davydov Procedure	1242
Mcindoe Procedure	1243
Sigmoid Vaginoplasty	1243
Genital Surgery for Female Mutilation	1243
Genital Surgery for Lichen Sclerosus	1244
Aesthetical Genital Surgery	1245
Labiaplasty	1245
Techniques	1246

S. Pusica · M. L. Djordjevic (✉)
Belgrade Center for Urogenital Reconstructive Surgery,
Belgrade, Serbia
e-mail: djordjevic@uromiros.com

B. Stojanovic
Belgrade Center for Urogenital Reconstructive Surgery,
Belgrade, Serbia

School of Medicine, University of Belgrade,
Belgrade, Serbia

© Springer Nature Switzerland AG 2023
F. E. Martins et al. (eds.), *Female Genitourinary and Pelvic Floor Reconstruction*,
https://doi.org/10.1007/978-3-031-19598-3_67

Labia Majora Augmentation 1247

Vaginal Rejuvenation 1248
Surgical Vaginal Rejuvenation 1248
Nonsurgical Vaginal Rejuvenation Procedures 1248

Hymenoplasty 1250

Conclusions 1250

References 1250

Abstract

Acceptable appearance of female genitalia have significant impact in functional, as well as in aesthetical sense, since there are many anomalies, either congenital or acquired, which require proper correction. Certainly, attention should be paid to the growing demands and needs for aesthetics in the field of genital surgery, and these women should be helped to prevent the development of genital dysmorphophobia. Various specialties are involved in the work in this specific field, from plastic surgeons, through gynecologists and urologists. The genital surgeon must have sufficient training in sexual medicine to withhold these procedures from women with sexual dysfunction, mental impairment, or body dysmorphic disorder. There is a variety of surgical procedures for better functioning of genitalia such as reduction of enlarged clitoris or creation of new vagina. Many new and redefined techniques are emerging, but very few long-term results and follow up studies are published. Also, reconstruction of missing organs due to trauma or mutilation injuries represents new challenges. Finally, new trends in cosmetic surgery offer better aesthetic appearance and recruit more and more new non-surgical procedures. Patients should always be made aware that the results of surgery or procedures to alter sexual appearance or function are always prone to subjectivism, and must be presented with realistic expectations.

In our chapter we will evaluate all the modalities of treatment for this pathology, and we will also pay special attention to a new trend in cosmetic surgery, aesthetic correction of female genitalia. It will be an overview of the possible surgical procedures for women with congenital and functional disorders as well as general principles of aesthetic surgery of the female genitalia. Some details are already fully described in other chapters and will be poorly contributed in our chapter as a reminder of this very important issue.

Keywords

Female genitalia · Genital reconstruction · Vaginoplasty · Vulvoplasty · Clitoroplasty · Labioplasty

Introduction

Female genitalia have a various roles relating to genital identity as well as urinary, sexual and reproductive functions. In last decade, aesthetical surgery of female genitalia presents a great challenge. It includes a wide spectrum of different elective cosmetic procedures that change the structure and appearance of the healthy external female genitalia, or internal in the case of vaginal tightening. Since these procedures have become widely performed, surgical approach should continue to be optimized, resulting in satisfactory outcomes. Despite the fact that there is no medical reason for this surgery in this population, female genital cosmetic surgery presents a new field with increasing number of new candidates. It is important to state that these women do not have clinical indication for this type of surgery, such as female sexual dysfunction, dyspareunia, problems with athletic performance, history of genital injuries, vaginal prolapse, or gender affirming surgery. This definition expands to diverse procedures, such as labiaplasty, labia majora augmentation, clitoral hood reduction, hymenoplasty, vaginal rejuvenation, vaginoplasty, or G spot amplification.

Unlike the centuries-old obsession with the size of a male sex organ, female genitals and their appearance has always been a taboo subject. With increased availability of pornography, as well as changing trends concerning the removal of pubic hair, women's external genitals have become more exposed and with that, general assumption is that these factors have led to dissatisfaction and the cause of increased demand for these types of interventions. According to national data base, aesthetic surgery of female genitalia is increasingly sought by women in the United States, and there was more than 40% increase in labioplasty between 2012 and 2013 and more than 50% increase between 2014 and 2018 [1, 2]. Another study from Australia reported the highest incidence in women aged between 25 and 34 (32.6%) and 35 and 44 years (25.8%), respectively [3]. They found similar interest for cosmetic surgery in younger population between 15 and 24 years (25.3%).

Operative techniques for aesthetic surgery of female genitalia have evolved from vulvoplasty, which refers to external female genitalia and involves either augmentation or reduction of clitoral and labial tissue (labiaplasty, hymenoplasty, perineoplasty, clitoroplasty, monsplasty) to vaginoplasty that includes reconstruction of internal part of female genitalia (surgical vaginal tightening, laser vaginal rejuvenation, G-spot augmentation or amplification). Preoperative evaluation and operative approaches should be tailored to enable ideal contours of the external genitalia, to resize and place all structures in good anatomical relationship and prevent functional complications.

Anatomy of Female Genitalia and Changes with Aging

There are large variations in the appearance of the female external genitalia, which depend on the influence of estrogen during intrauterine development. More estrogen means more prominent genitals and vice versa. However, in general, the appearance and shape of the female genitalia do not affect their function. Understanding of female anatomy helps medical practitioners with the coming of solution that female genitals can be aesthetically pleasing and also functional. Vulvar complex is a term that encompasses the externally visible structures, including the mons pubis and the labia majora. Underneath the vulva is the vestibule protected by the hymenal ring, comprising of an outer tunnel and a deeper tunnel. The outer tunnel consists of the clitoris, the clitoral prepuce, the labia minora, hymen, and the urethral meatus – all structures, which are nonhairy and mucosal, lined by secretory glands, and having nerve endings. The vestibule is whatever part of genitals that is visible in lithotomy position, except the labia majora and mons pubis. Mons pubis is a mass of fatty tissue located directly anterior to the pubic bones. Its functions are buffing during sexual intercourse and also secretion of pheromones for sexual attraction.

Labia majora are Latin words for the larger lips. The labia majora are prominent pair of cutaneous skin folds that form the lateral longitudinal borders of the vulval clefts. The labia majora form the folds that cover the labia minora, clitoris, vulva vestibule, vestibular bulbs, Bartholin's glands, Skene's glands, urethra, and the vaginal opening. The anterior part of the labia majora folds comes together to form the anterior labial commissure directly beneath the mons pubis, while the posterior part of the labia majora comes together to form the posterior labial commissure. The length varies from 7 cm to 12 cm from the crura of the clitoris to the posterior fourchette. Hystologically, the labia majora has several layers, the skin, a finger-like subcutaneous layer with investing colles fascia, and the deep scarpa fascia. Labia minora are a pair of small cutaneous folds that begin at the clitoris and extend downward. The anterior folds of the labia minora encircle the clitoris forming the clitoral hood and the frenulum of the clitoris. The labia minora then descend obliquely and downward, forming the borders of the vulva vestibule. Eventually, posterior ends of the labia minora terminate as they become linked together by a skin fold called the frenulum of the labia minora. The labia minora will encircle the vulva vestibule and terminate between the labia majora and the vulva vestibule. The length varies from 20 mm to 100 mm, and width from 7 mm to 15 mm. On the medial surface of the labia minora is a Hart line, a landmark junction between the mucosal and squamous epithelial surfaces, i.e., the junction between endodermal and ectodermal-derived tissues [4]. Clitoris consists of the erectile bodies (paired bulbs and paired corpora, which are continuous with the crura), the glans clitoris, the neurovascular bundle dorsally, and the wide urethral plate ventrally. The glans is a midline, densely neural, nonerectile structure that is the only external manifestation of the clitoris. Vestibular bulbs are structures formed from corpus spongiosum tissue. This is a type of erectile tissue closely related to the clitoris. The vestibule bulbs are two bulbs of erectile tissue that start close to the inferior side of the body of the clitoris. Vagina is an elastic, muscular tube connected to the cervix proximally and extends to the external surface through the vulva vestibule. The distal opening of the vagina is usually partially covered by a membrane called the hymen. The vaginal opening is located posterior to the urethra opening. Blood supply is through the external and internal pudendal artery systems, besides an arborization from the inferior abdominal wall system. The internal, external, and transverse superficial perineal arteries, all branches of the internal pudendal artery, anastomose with the branches of the deep external pudendal artery. Nerve supply is from the pudendal nerve, which is derived from the second to the fourth sacral nerve roots. It enters the pelvis from the lesser sciatic foramen, then through the pudendal canal onward to the ischial spine. The pudendal nerve has three branches: the dorsal nerve of clitoris, the perineal nerve for external genitalia, and the inferior rectal nerve. These, as well as branches of the ilioinguinal, iliofemoral, and posterior genitofemoral cutaneous nerves, supply the sensory nerves to the perineum and external genitalia. Erogenous nerve supply also comes from the pudendal nerve to supply the glans clitoris [5–7].

Anatomy of female external genitalia undergoes transformations at several stages in life. Labia minora grow and become pigmented during puberty, while clitoral prepuce becomes wrinkled to cover the clitoris. Increased fat accumulation and relaxation of the superficial fascial system happen with age. Also, the vaginal canal relaxes and the pelvic outlet becomes weaker. Pregnancy initiates more growth of the labia minora and it starts hanging down externally even more. With gravity, the labia minora have increased hypertrophy, pigmentation, wrinkling, nerves, and sebaceous glands. Excessive weight loss causes fat reduction from the labia majora and the mons, and subsequent wrinkling and ptosis of the labia. With advancing age, the perineal ptosis becomes prominent, and the atrophy of external genitalia starts. There is a significant loss of subcutaneous fat and reduced secretions from the vaginal mucosal tissues, leading to dryness of the lining of vulva and vestibule, and consequently further mucosal atrophy. However, these changes do not strictly follow the above stages in life, but genetic and individual factors also play a role.

Etiopathogenesis

There is a great variety of indications for female genital surgery, which dictate the type of procedure. Surgical and nonsurgical treatments are available, with the main purpose being to correct functional and aesthetical problems of female genitalia. Both functional and aesthetical indications are recommended for congenital or acquired anomalies of female genitalia, such as congenital adrenal hyperplasia, genital trauma, morphological changes of skin or mucosal parts, and genital mutilation. In the last decades, aesthetical reasons present a great challenge for new surgical and nonsurgical procedures. Changes with age, deformities, asymmetry, or size of parts of female genitalia are the main reasons for aesthetic procedures. Treatment modalities vary, and despite traditional surgical methods, there are nonsurgical procedures, such as energy-based interventions and injections. All of them are based on indications, and suitable procedure should be chosen in each case. According to etiopathogenesis, indications for female genital surgery could be divided in three groups:

1. **Congenital Anomalies of Female Genitalia.** The most difficult congenital anomalies of female genitalia are vaginal agenesis and congenital adrenal hyperplasia. Mayer–Rokitanky–Kuster–Hauser (MRKH) syndrome is a rare disorder that affects one in 4500 women as a form of primary amenorrhea and abnormalities of internal genitalia, mainly the absence of the uterus and upper two-thirds of the vagina. Surgical treatment is advised after careful therapeutical counseling and noninvasive vaginal dilatation, ensuring that the patient is mature enough for advised surgical option. Female patients with congenital adrenal hyperplasia can present with hyperpigmented or fused labioscrotal tissue, enlarged labia majora, urogenital sinus, and clitoromegaly. Clitoromegaly can express itself in different forms, in most severe cases showing greatly enlarged clitoris with similar anatomy to penis. Many intermediate forms can also be seen. The main goals of surgical treatment are adequate clitoral appearance, satisfactory sexual function, and proper development of gender identity.
2. **Genital Mutilation.** Between 130 and 140 million women worldwide have undergone female genital mutilation in the past 10 years, including 92 million girls in Africa. Three million girls every year are estimated to be at risk of undergoing the procedure [8].

    The World Health Organization (WHO) classifies female mutilation in four types:

    Type 1: This is the partial or total removal of the clitoral glans (the external and visible part of the clitoris, which is a sensitive part of the female genitalia), and/or the prepuce/clitoral hood.

    Type 2: This is the partial or total removal of the clitoral glans and the labia minora (the inner folds of the vulva), with or without removal of the labia majora (the outer folds of skin of the vulva).

    Type 3: Also known as infibulation, this is the narrowing of the vaginal opening through the creation of a covering seal. The seal is formed by cutting and repositioning the labia minora, or labia majora, sometimes through stitching, with or without removal of the clitoral prepuce/clitoral hood and glans.

    Type 4: This includes all other harmful procedures to the female genitalia for non-medical purposes, e.g., pricking, piercing, incising, scraping, and cauterizing the genital area.

    The main goals of genital reconstruction in this type of surgery are improvement of sexual life, general genital appearance, and pain relief.
3. **Aesthetic Female Genital Surgery.** Indication for this type is based on a patient's desire, mainly related to patient's displeasure by the appearance of genitalia. It can be sorted in the same category with breast augmentation or any other cosmetic surgery. Although motives and reasons for this type of surgery can be strictly aesthetic, sometimes patients can feel pain and discomfort, and at the same time have functional and aesthetic discomfort. It is designed to improve the appearance subjectively, and potentially provide psychological and functional improvement in sexual stimulation and satisfaction [9].

Genital Surgery for Congenital Adrenal Hyperplasia

Patients suffering from congenital adrenal hyperplasia (CAH) have varying degrees of genital virilization, which results in a number of anatomical issues. There is usually clitoral hypertrophy, which occurs within a spectrum of normal size and configuration (Prader 0) to severe hypertrophy with a phallic urethra exiting the glans (Prader 5) [10]. In CAH the urethra and vagina usually share a distal common channel or urogenital sinus that exits to the perineum. This confluence may occur anywhere in a spectrum from near the perineum (low confluence) to near the bladder neck (high confluence). Labia disorders mirrored itself in some degree of fusion. The most extreme form of this fusion is certainly complete masculinization, where labia majora form scrotal like appearance. The labia minora are usually absent.

Considering these anatomical variations, the most surgical reconstructions include: clitoroplasty, labioplasty, and vaginoplasty. In the past surgery was done in several stages that could lead to more scaring, fibrosis, and poor cosmetic results. Single stage procedure gives hope for a better outcome than multistage genital surgery, with an expected 88% incidence of good cosmetic results [11, 12]. Another important decision for medical practitioners, as well as patient's parents, is right timing for the surgery. Most practitioners suggest that surgery should take place early from the newborn to 3-year-old period. Reasons for this early intervention include better compliance with dilatation, lessening of parents concerns regarding their child, and the assumption that the child later in life does not remember early intervention [13]. Many additional advantages have been contemplated for early surgery, including genitourinary tract infection prevention and relative ease of surgery in childhood compared with adolescence.

Preoperative Evaluation. Prior to surgery, the urogenital sinus should be examined radiographically by genitography and endoscopy. This usually allows identification of the level of urethrovaginal confluence and assessment of the size of the vagina. Endoscopy is very important procedure that requires metabolically stable child. Most children require only an enema preoperatively but, in the very high vaginal confluence, a gentle bowel preparation may be necessary.

Procedures. Genital reconstruction is performed under general anesthesia. The patient is placed in a gynecological position on the operative table. The operative field is prepped and draped in a standard fashion. Intravenous broad-spectrum antibiotics are administered before the incision. Injection of 0.5% lidocaine with 1–200,000 epinephrine subcutaneously can help with the hemostasis.

Clitoroplasty has passed through many changes ranging from amputation of the organ to its complete preservation (clitoral recession). The main goals of surgical treatment should be adequate sexual function, promote consistent female gender identity development, and ensure anatomically correct clitoris appearance. Reduction clitoroplasty is the most widely accepted and practiced surgical approach for clitoromegaly as it provides clitoral aesthetic while preserving sexual function through neurovascular preservation. Operative procedure includes complete disassembly of the clitoris into glans with neurovascular bundle and cavernosal bodies. Urethral plate is mobilized with Buck's fascia. Dissection is continued toward the glans cap, and neurovascular bundle is dissected under Buck's fascia in order to preserve its structures. This is how vascularization and sensitivity of glans are preserved. Glans cap is separated from the tips of the corporeal bodies, avoiding the injury of the arteries. Reduction of corporeal bodies and glans are performed, followed by glans reconstruction and reassembly of all entities, in order to attain normal clitoral morphology (Figs. 1a-d).

Labioplasty. After clitoroplasty, remaining of clitoral skin is used for creation of labia minora. This skin is divided in the midline for the creation of equal flaps that can be mobilized in anatomically correct position, thus providing normal appearance to the external genitalia The division of skin should be done carefully, minding the appearance of clitoral hood. The labia majora are virtually always anteriorly displaced and therefore must be moved inferiorly if the vagina is to exit between them. Therefore, to complete the labioplasty, a Y–V plasty with movement of the labia majora inferiorly is required. Complications include poor cosmetic results and labia minora atrophy.

Vaginoplasty and Urethroplasty. Urogenital mobilization techniques are necessary in almost every patient with CAH. Pena initially described total urogenital mobilization (TUM) in 1997 [14]. In this procedure the entire urogenital complex (urogenital sinus, urethra, vagina, and bladder) is mobilized circumferentially and moved toward the perineum. This allows the vagina to reach the perineum and usually avoids having to separate the vagina from the urinary tract, which historically has been the most difficult part of vaginoplasty and also renders the most blood

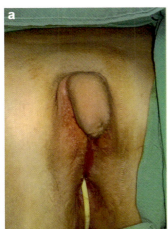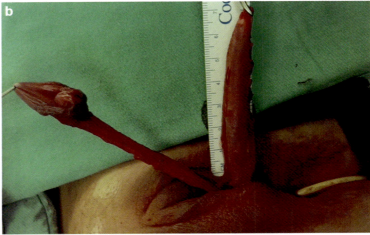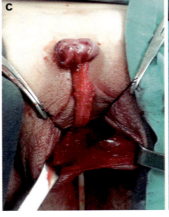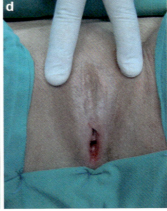

Fig. 1 Clitoral disassembly for congenital adrenal hyperplasia (CAH). (**a**) Preoperative appearance. Virilized genitalia with clitoromegaly; (**b**) Clitoral disassembly is performed. Enlarged, 7 cm-long corpora cavernosa are completely separated from glans cap with neurovascular bundle; (**c**) Corpora cavernosa are totally removed; (**d**) Result 2 years after surgery

loss. However, urethral meatus should be placed and fixed in a proper position, in order to avoid hypospadiac position and voiding difficulties. Rink et al. showed that this mobilized urogenital tissue is very beneficial and can be used to create three structures: (1) a mucosal lined vestibule; (2) an anterior vaginal wall; or (3) a posterior vaginal wall [15]. This urogenital tissue is not only cosmetically superior to the use of skin flaps, but it is also non-hairbearing and less likely to result in vaginal stenosis. There have been concerns regarding the risks of incontinence with TUM, but this appears to be a rare occurrence [16]. The most common complication is vaginal stenosis or stenosis of the introitus (Figs. 2a, b).

Genital Surgery for Vaginal Agenesis

The etiology of Mayer–Rokitanky–Kuster–Hauser (MRKH) syndrome is still inconclusive. However, newer studies suggest genetic causes and novel genomic techniques are moving research toward recurrent genetic anomalies in some patients. The burden of diagnosed MRKH syndrome should not be underestimated, and all patients should have counseling sessions and psychological support from medical professionals. Several different methods of neovaginoplasty were described during the years. These include the Creatsas vaginoplasty, the Vecchietti procedure, Davydov procedure, and Sigmoid colon

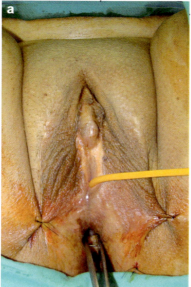 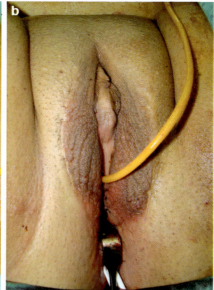

Fig. 2 Introitoplasty after CAH repair. (**a**) Introital stenosis after genital reconstruction for CAH; (**b**) Result after introitoplasty. Normal appearance of vaginal introitus is achieved

vaginoplasty. Thus yet, the gold standard for surgical treatment is not determined. Suiting surgical method should be chosen and based on the surgeon's expertise and experience.

Absolute uterine factor infertility is direct consequence of MRKH syndrome, leaving patients who wanted to become mothers with surrogacy as only option. Recently, Swedish team in Gothenburg, performed first successful uterus transplantation, allowing other women suffering from MRKH syndrome fertility treatment, and chance for biological motherhood [17].

Creatsas Vaginoplasty

Creatsas modification of Williams vaginoplasty is a surgical technique used frequently in patients with MRKH for the creation of neovagina [18]. Patient is placed in lithotomy position. The labia majora and minora are put under tension. The hymen, which is almost always present in these cases, should be removed using cautery. Incision is made in U-shape, starting in the vulva, across the perineum, and up to the medial side of the labia up to the urethral meatus. The tissues are mobilized and a first layer of interrupted sutures is put between the inner skin margins using absorbable material, with the knots lying inside the neovagina. A second layer of the same material is used to approximate the subcutaneous fat and the perineal muscles and finally, the external skin is sutured with absorbable interrupted stitches.

Vecchietti Procedure

The Vecchietti procedure is considered as a surgical version of Frank's Method [19]. An olive-shaped bead is wedded to the vaginal stump, using laparoscopy-assisted or robot-assisted approach, an olive-shaped bead is Through the assistance of laparoscopy, an olive-shaped bead is wedded to the vaginal stump. The bead is then attached to a thread that runs from the female's peritoneum, into the pelvis, and cut through the abdomen where it is attached to a tension device placed on top of the abdomen. The goal is to lengthen the vagina about 1.5 cm per day, as tension is increased daily. Expected depth of the neovagina is about 7 cm and then the procedure is stopped. For maintenance and prevention of vaginal stenosis, daily vaginal dilatation is advised.

Davydov Procedure

In this procedure, peritoneal flaps are designed to serve as lining for the neovagina. Neovaginal space is created using perineal skin flap made by

U-fashioned incision. The vaginal stump is located and opened using H-shaped incision. Using laparoscopic approach, peritoneal flaps are created, pulled down into newly created vagina, and anastomosed with the vaginal opening. The top portion of the neovagina is created by sealing the peritoneum. Usually adequate length of neovagina is achieved and patients are ready for sexual intercourse 3–6 months after the procedure. Intermittent vaginal dilatation is necessary for satisfying long-term results.

Mcindoe Procedure

Skin grafts are the material of choice in this procedure, where they serve as lining for the neovagina. Donor sites are usually thigh or gluteal area. Grafts are wrapped around an acrylic mold and placed into neovaginal space, created between urethra, bladder, and rectum. However, this method is associated with scars at the donor area, which can be disturbing for already burdened patients. Graft failure can also occur, as neovaginal stenosis and contractures.

Sigmoid Vaginoplasty

Sigmoid vaginoplasty is surgical procedure where a segment of the sigmoid colon is isolated on a vascular pedicle and used to create the inner lining of a neovagina. The most comfortable approach for the patient is laparoscopic or robot assisted, where the chosen segment, in an adequate length, is inspected for proper color and vascularization. Neovaginal space is created between urethra, bladder, and rectum using sharp and blunt dissection. The segment is then pulled into neovagina and anastomosed with vaginal introitus. The caliber of the sigmoid colon is nearly comparable with the width of the normal vagina. Strong muscle tissue of the bowel and mucosal secretion enable lubrication and adequate sexual intercourse. Sigmoid vaginoplasty, with its advantages, represents one of the widely accepted options for MRKH syndrome (Figs. 3a-d).

Complications. Despite their association with variety of complications, patients are leaning to surgical procedures, as they ultimately result in desirable vaginal caliber. In the literature, postoperative complications have been recorded, such as rectovaginal fistula, vaginal stricture, bleeding, recurrent infections of the urinary system, urinary incontinence, or rectocele [20]. Laparosopic approach carries its own risks, such as ureter and bladder injuries.

Genital Surgery for Female Mutilation

In the past, surgical treatment for patients who suffered female genital mutilation (FGM) was reserved for complications of infubilation in cases of pregnancy and genitourinary syndromes. Extreme cases of FGM can lead to complete stenosis of vaginal introitus or significant vaginal scaring, which by itself is risk in pregnancy as well as in delivery. During this time, women were subjected to defibulation or cesarean section, in order to avoid vulvar complications during delivery. Reopening of narrowed and scared vaginal introitus is called defibulation, and this procedure was also frequently used by gynecologist for treatment of dysmenorrhea, apareunia and dyspareunia [21, 22].

Literature on defibulation showed that this is rather a simple procedure, with no significant risk and good satisfaction rates for non-complicated delivery and other long-term complication from infibulated introital stenosis. Urology specialists also have important role, as this excessive scaring can lead to recurrent urinary tract infections and obstructive voiding disorders, facilitating reconstructive treatment, together with gynecologists and plastic surgeons. Patients with Type III FGM carry greater risk of recurrent urinary tract infections, urinary retention and incontinence [23, 24].

Reconstruction of vulvar anatomy is an important factor for alleviation and elimination of obstructive micturition disorders and lower urinary tract symptoms. Foldes et al. reported results of 2938 women with FGM Type II and III, who have been treated with reconstructive genital surgery. Their results showed reduced pain, improved pleasure and sexual health [8]. Clitoral reconstruction is also very important part of

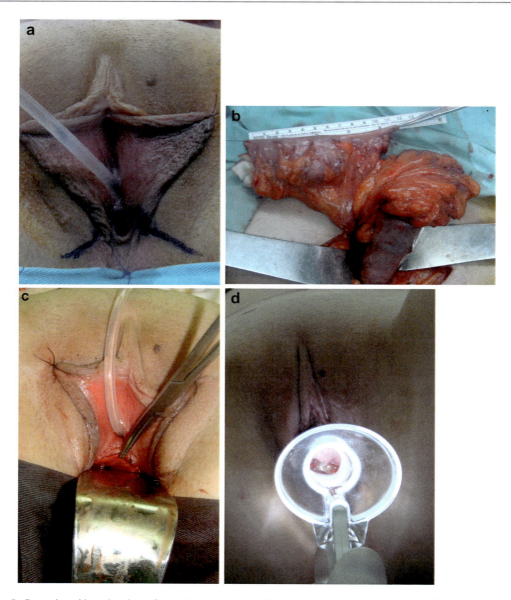

Fig. 3 Rectosigmoid vaginoplasty for vaginal agenesis. (**a**) Preoperative appearance. Introital skin flaps are designed; (**b**) A 10 cm-long rectosigmoid segment is harvested for neovaginal reconstruction; (**c**) Rectosigmoid flap is anastomosed with introital flaps using perineal approach; (**d**) Outcome 3 months after surgery. Good depth of the neovagina is achieved

reconstructive surgery in this case. Clitoroplasty, together with psychosexual therapy benefited reduced pain during intercourse, improved sexual function and self-confidence. Unfortunately, till this day, there is no consensus for reconstructive treatment and psychosexual therapy. Readers can find more details on this topic in another chapter.

Genital Surgery for Lichen Sclerosus

Lichen sclerosus (LS) is a chronic inflammatory disease, and involves hypopigmentation and atrophy of genital skin. The affected area varies from a small area to large surface, which includes entire vulva and perineum. It may cause entrapment of

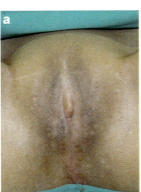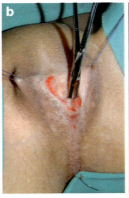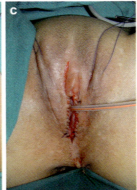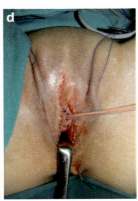

Fig. 4 Genital reconstruction in case of lichen sclerosus. (**a**) Preoperative appearance. Complete fusion of labia minora and clitoral prepuce due to lichen sclerosus; (**b**) Sharp opening of introital stenosis; (**c**) Outcome after introitoplasty, labioplasty, and urethroplasty; (**d**) Normal appearance of the vulva and wide introital opening are achieved

the clitoris, urethral meatus and scarring and stenosis of the vaginal introitus, fusion of labia minora, resulting in voiding issues, disabled sexual intercourse, and sexual dysfunction. In these cases of functional impairment, surgical reconstruction is necessary in order to remove affected sclerotic skin, achieve normal appearance of the vulva and vaginal introitus, as well as normal voiding pattern and sexual functioning [25] (Figs. 4a-d).

Aesthetical Genital Surgery

Labiaplasty

Labiaplasty involves aesthetical improvement, in most cases surgical reduction in the size of hypertrophied labia minora. This type of surgery was first described in medical literature by Hodgkinson and Hait in 1984 [26]. Although this was the first description of labiaplasty in plastic surgery literature, trimming of the labia minora, a social custom in some cultures, had been described in other literature, and external genital surgery had previously been performed by medical professionals for a variety of indications. The main reason for this procedure is condition where labia minora are protruding out of the vulva in a standing position. Beside aesthetic motivation, sometimes functional problems can be reason for women to decide for this procedure. Hypertrophy of the labia minora can result in dyspareunia, interference with sports, difficulties with cleanliness, chronic urinary tract infections, and irritation. Psychological symptoms related to the appearance of the genitalia should not be underestimated; the appearance of the labia minora can cause significant emotional distress (Figs. 5a-c).

Motakef classification describes the length of labia minora protrusion over the labia majora: [27]

Class I: 0–2 cm protrusion beyond the edge of the labia majora
Class II: 2–4 cm beyond the edge of the labia majora
Class III: More than 4 cm, beyond the edge of labia majora

There are several surgical techniques described, including deepithelialization, W-shaped resection, edge resection, wedge resection, composite reduction, and laser excision [28].

Preoperative Care. Broad-spectrum antibiotics should be administered, such as cefazolin or cefotaxime intravenously. These procedures can be performed in local or general anesthesia. General anesthesia is mostly used for patients undergoing concurrent procedures.

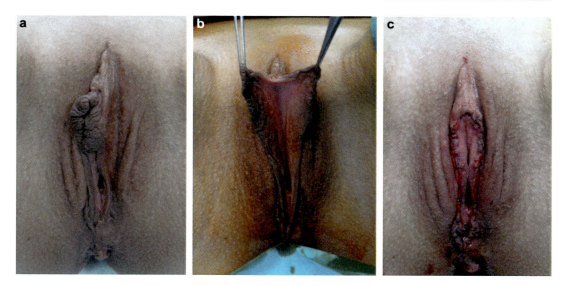

Fig. 5 Hypertrophy of labia minora. (**a**) Labial hypertrophy causing aesthetical disturbance and dyspareunia; (**b**) Excessive labia minora skin is present; (**c**) Final result after labiaplasty

Techniques

Deepithelialization. Choi and Kim introduced the deepithelialization technique in 2000 [29] The central part of the inner aspects of each labia is incised superficially in an oval manner, and the epithelial layer is removed, leaving the subcutaneous tissue largely intact. This is followed by re-approximation of the two edges. They performed labia minora reduction in six patients by deepithelialization of the central portion and re-approximation. Cao et al., in 2012, described a modified version of this technique in which the deepithelialization is widened to the posterior aspect of the labia minora [30].

W-Shaped Resection. Also in 2000, Maas and Hage first performed W-shaped resection with interdigitated suturing of the protuberant labia minora [31]. The closure of the opposing W-shaped incisions results in a tensionless zigzag suture line running obliquely across the edge of the labium. This technique leaves intact the anterior and posterior commissure and the tissue around the base of the labia minora. It does not affect the branches of the superficial perineal nerve entry, thus preserving sexual function and sensation.

Wedge Resection. In 1998, Alter introduced the wedge resection technique [32]. Its main indication is protrusion of the labia minora extending at least 2 cm beyond the fourchette. The excess of labia is estimated by pinching between thumb and finger. As the tissue is held in a pinch, the excess labia minora fold looks like a dog ear, and this dog ear is excised. Continuous overrunning suturing produces hemostasis at the edges, and also does away with cut ends of the suture that are usually hurtful to the patient in the postoperative period. In 2006, Munhoz et al. published a reconstruction technique that involved creation of a superior flap. The grade of resection in their technique depends on the quantity of tissue excess and the degree of cutaneous/mucosal laxity. The superior wedge-shaped flap is designed on the remaining upper part of the labia minora [33]. Kelishadi et al. described in 2013 posterior wedge resection [34]. Posterior wedge boundaries resection is initially outlined with intraoperative marking, first along the lateral border of the labia minora to preserve the natural pigment and tissue. The marking continues inferosuperiorly and proceeds medially down to the base of the labia minora, approximately 1 cm up to the frenulum. The marking then continues posteriorly, to the posterior fourchette and is stopped prior to reaching the midline. Parallel markings are made on the mucosal side.

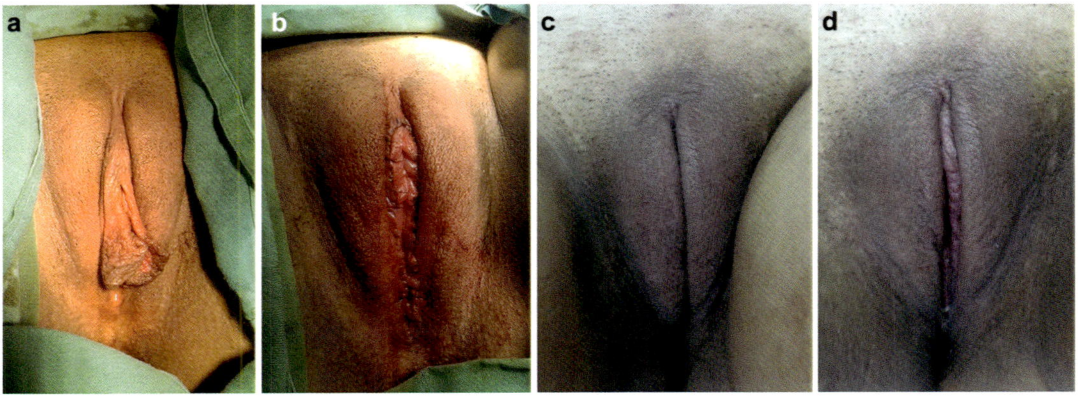

Fig. 6 Reduction labiaplasty. (**a**) Preoperative appearance. Excessive labia minora; (**b**) Result after reduction of hypertrophied labia; (**c**) Outcome 3 months after surgery; (**d**) Good shape and appearance of labia minora are achieved

Composite Reduction. Gress described this technique in 2013 [35]. All other procedures until this were focused on labia minora portion bellow the clitoris. Composite reduction beside labial reduction removes tissue that is anatomically closer to clitoris. This way labia minora are reduced across their entire length, thus clitoral glans is more exposed and available for stimulation, if needed.

Edge Resection. This is the original and first described labiaplasty technique [36]. It consists of simple resection of tissues at the free edge. One resection-technique variation features a clamp placed across the area of the labial tissue to be resected in order to decrease bleeding. The edges are then sutured together (Figs. 6a-d).

Laser Excision. A retrospective series of 55 patients treated with laser labiaplasty was presented in 2006 by Pardo et al. [37]. The authors concluded that laser labiaplasty may be simpler to perform than conventional cautery or knife excision.

Postoperative Care. In general, to avoid postoperative infection, oral and topical antibiotics should be administered. Bathtubs and sexual intercourse should be avoided for at least 4 weeks. Pain management by analgesics and ice pads should be taken into consideration.

Complications. The most common complications described in literature are wound dehiscence, hematoma, postoperative bleeding, and urinary retention. Besides purely surgical complications, patients who underwent labiaplasty can suffer from over-repair, disfigurement, scarring and "scalloping" of the labial edge, hypersensitivity or hyposensitivity, dyspareunia, partial or complete separation of the repair, infection, cosmetic results not up to the patient's expectations [9].

Labia Majora Augmentation

Labia majora augmentation is considered to be a solely aesthetical procedure, used to improve look of this external genitalia that with age can get atrophied, hypoplastic, or loose. This aged look can be improved using fillers, autologous fat-grafting, or hyaluronic acid fillers. Fat can be harvested from any body region with sufficient fatty tissue. The fat graft is prepared through techniques such as a washing centrifuge; the Coleman technique is the most frequently used [38]. As with every other fat filler, reabsorption is expected, so enough fat must be harvested and injected. With the increased use of hyaluronic acid fillers, this filler also gained popularity in aesthetic domain of female genitalia. It is easily accessible, ready to use, and relatively simple for application. In the USA, filling of the labia majora is not as popular as in Europe. The preference for American women is a sleeker and more petite appearance, which labia majora plasty or radio-frequency shrinkage can help achieve. In Europe, there is more use of filling techniques, specifically hyaluronic acid. However, this is not a procedure without postoperative complications, such as inflammation or granuloma formation.

Vaginal Rejuvenation

Vaginal rejuvenation, or vaginoplasty, involves surgical procedures of the vaginal entrance, deeper canal, and epithelium. These procedures are usually mostly requested by women who went through one or more vaginal childbirths. Childbirth alone or combined with episiotomy can lead to poor quality of sex life for both partners. The most important part of this procedure is dialogue with the patient, as limits of the planned vaginal diameter must be presented and sometimes patients can have unrealistic expectations. There are several options for vaginal rejuvenation and all of them can be separated in two groups, surgical and nonsurgical procedures.

Surgical Vaginal Rejuvenation

Vaginal rejuvenation refers to more than one procedure, often combining excision of redundant vaginal tissues, muscular tightening by imbrication of the median levator muscles, remodeling of the perineal body, and excision of the surplus skin for bigger patient satisfaction. Since there is no golden standard for vaginal tightening, surgeons often combine anterior with high posterior colporrhaphy and possible excision of lateral vaginal mucosa.

Preparation. Antibiotics of choice should be administered preoperatively. Patient is positioned in lithotomy position. With patient's permission, preoperative photographs should be taken for documentation. Operative field is prepared with 10% povidone-iodine solution and draped sterilely.

Anterior Colporrhaphy. A trapezoid-shaped incision is made at introitus site, and later the same incision will be used in perineoplasty stage of the intervention. Then, the posterior wall of the vagina is incised in a vertical fashion, vaginal epithelium is freed from rectovaginal fascia laterally until the levator muscles. Dissection should take place up to the apex of the vagina, thus not excluding posterior wall, since it is needed for the maintenance of vaginal width. Perioneoplasty includes lateral incisions, preserving the deep and superficial transverse perineal muscles, which leads to consistency on the same level as the posterior wall. The lower part of the labia major will now serve as posterior fourchette of vaginal opening. Finally, remaining introital and perineal skin should be excised giving the maximal cosmetical result.

Posterior Colporrhaphy. Two triangular shaped incisions are made, first on the posterior vaginal wall and another at the perineum, creating a diamond-shaped appearance. Their meeting point should be at the level of the hymenal ring, which represents the widest point of the planned excision. Hymenal remnants should be identified and serve as a point for best reachable neowidth. Increased tension of the margins should be avoided and checked before the procedure. Undermining presents optimal option for dissection preserving vaginal stenosis postoperatively. External perineal incisions will be made in posterior fourchette fashion. This portion includes repair of the superficial transverse perineal muscles, lengthening of the perineal body, reparation of the the posterior fourchette, and correction of the gap at the posterior vaginal vestibule.

Postoperative Care. At the end of the procedure, vaginal canal should be packed. All patients are instructed to wear a protective pad due to possible vaginal discharge. Package should be removed the next day. All wounds should be cleaned daily minimizing the risk of infection and scab formation. Vaginal dilatation is not advised. Painkillers and postoperative antibiotic regimen are recommended.

Complications. Possible complications include hematomas; iatrogenic injuries of bladder, urethra, or rectum; infection; abscessus; excessive blood loss; incomplete wound healing with postoperative scars; dyspareunia, and incontinence [39].

Nonsurgical Vaginal Rejuvenation Procedures

As vaginal rejuvenation became more common in practices worldwide, the question becomes how to improve outcomes by using minimally invasive procedures. Laser technology (i.e., fractional CO2 laser, erbium YAG laser) is publicized as noninvasive and conservative technique for vaginal tightening. It is suggested as a technique of choice for women suffering from dyspareunia or vaginal fibrosis as complications from episiotomy or vaginal deliveries. As increased collagen production was demonstrated, laser therapy is used for women in menopause, who suffered vaginal atrophy due to hormonal changes. Besides higher collagen production, other effects as neovascularization, higher elasticity, better vaginal lubrication, and hydration were noticed. Another popular method is the use of the radiofrequency devices that create an electrical field in the tissue that causes molecular motion of charged particles and thereby generate heat. Radiofrequency has been found to reduce skin laxity, improve the mechanical strength of skin, and induce neocollagenesis and elastogenesis. As platelet-rich plasma (PRP) gained its popularity in aesthetic medicine, its usage in vaginal rejuvenation was explored. Some studies showed that that PRP promotes the wound healing process by releasing growth factors. In this case, PRP is combined with fillers, such as hyaluronic acid or fat for better results. However, the clinician must understand the benefits that each minimally invasive procedure can provide, thereby matching the desired goals of a given procedure to the correct results.

Carbon Dioxide Lasers. Fractional CO2 lasers (10,600 nm) allow for focused energy delivery and targeted ablative islands surrounded by adjacent healthy tissue with water as the chromophore. The energy leads to heating of underlying tissues at 45–50 °C and induces shrinkage of collagen and stimulates fibroblasts to produce new collagen in the treated tissue. The physiological response to CO2 laser is based on inflammatory and wound healing mechanisms that stimulate elastin and collagen production. Some reports showed good outcomes of vaginal mucosa reaction to CO2 laser and confirmed by small vaginal biopsies. Histological studies in ex vivo experiments confirmed the effects of CO2 laser and impact on increased fibroblast and collagen production. However, there is no precise protocol for CO2 laser use in vaginal rejuvenation procedures. Protocol can differ depending from the type of laser, its power, and dwelling time. Each treatment will ultimately depend on the type of the device and it should be conducted with great caution [40–42].

Er:YAG Laser. This is a nonablative laser with a coefficient of absorption that is 16 times lower than CO2. In turn, it has a lower depth of penetration of 1–3 μm leading to minimal thermal injury to surrounding tissue and less pain, discomfort, swelling, and erythema. Histological effects of this laser included increased production of collagen and elastin but more reports and long-term follow-up are needed for better estimation of the procedure [40–42].

Radiofrequency Therapy (RF). It has been found to reduce skin laxity, improve the mechanical strength of skin, and induce neocollagenesis and elastogenesis. RF activity is based on reducing tissue compliance without inducing true scar formation. Despite the fact that some of the devices have FDA clearance for use in electrocoagulation and hemostasis in dermatologic and general surgical procedures, there is no FDA-approved device for the treatment of vaginal laxity and rejuvenation procedures. These devices have been classically used for firming up both the face and neck skin without anesthesia [40].

Platelet-Rich Plasma (PRP) and Fillers. There is limited data regarding the use of PRP in vaginal rejuvenation. PRP contains growth factors as PDGF, TGF-B, IGF, EGF, VEGF released by platelets that have an important role in inflammation reduction, angiogenesis stimulation, and collagen III synthesis. PRP injections can be used for increased lubrication in cases of vaginal dryness. Hyaluronic acid is a dermal filler widely used in cosmetic medicine, but its use in the vaginal sphere is very recent and poorly documented. One study showed a case report of lipofilling of the posterior vaginal wall, in combination with hyaluronic acid and PRP in the subcutaneous tissue of the surrounding perineum, but effectiveness and safety need further studies [43]. Generally, more experience and studies are needed to confirm safety and efficiency of these minimally invasive procedures.

Hymenoplasty

Reconstruction of the hymen or revirgination can be requested from various reasons, usually for cultural or social reasons, or sometimes after penetrative sexual assault. The technique used must be adjusted based on the state of the original hymen. If the hymenal remnants are present, they are sutured and joined to create hymenal ring. It is also possible to suture together skin tags far from one another across the introitus. In case hymenal remnants are absent, two trap door flaps are raised from opposing sides of the vaginal wall. The raw surfaces of flaps are opposed and sutured together. Care must be taken to leave enough space for menstruation. Postcoital bleeding cannot be guaranteed.

Conclusions

Female genital cosmetic surgery includes various aesthetical procedures that enable quality of life improvement and well-being for majority of women who desire better appearance and functioning of their genitalia. These procedures are increasingly being requested by women who expect excellent aesthetical outcomes with minimal complication rates. Otherwise, there is a group of women with deformities of external genitalia, either due to congenital anomalies or genital mutilation. In both groups, the main principle should include choice of appropriate operative technique based on each woman's unique genital anatomy and aesthetical desires.

References

1. Cosmetic Surgery National Data Bank Statistics. Aesthet Surg J. 2015;35(Suppl 2):1–24.
2. Lista F, Mistry BD, Singh Y, Ahmad J. The safety of aesthetic labioplasty: a plastic surgery experience. Aesthet Surg J. 2015;35(6):689–95.
3. Ampt AJ, Roach V, Roberts CL. Vulvoplasty in New South Wales, 2001–2013: a population-based record linkage study. Med J Aust. 2016;205:365–9.
4. Georgiou CA, Benatar M, Dumas P, et al. A cadaveric study of the arterial blood supply of the labia minora. Plast Reconstr Surg. 2015;136(1):167–78.
5. Corton MM, Cunningham FG. Anatomy. In: Hoffman BL, Schorge JO, Schaffer JI, et al., editors. Williams gynecology. 2nd ed. New York: McGraw-Hill Education LLC; 2012. p. 918–46.
6. Puppo V. Anatomy and physiology of the clitoris, vestibular bulbs, and labia minora with a review of the female orgasm and the prevention of female sexual dysfunction. Clin Anat. 2013;26(1):134–52.
7. O'Connell HE, Sanjeevan KV, Hutson JM. Anatomy of the clitoris. J Urol. 2005;174:1189–95.
8. Foldès P, Cuzin B, Andro A. Reconstructive surgery after female genital mutilation: a prospective cohort study. Lancet. 2012;380:134–41.
9. Goodman MP. Female genital cosmetic and plastic surgery: a review. J Sex Med. 2011;8(6):1813–25.
10. White PC, Speiser PW. Congenital adrenal hyperplasia due to 21-hydroxylase deficiency. Endocr Rev. 2000;21:245–91.
11. Lean WL, Deshpande A, Hutson J, et al. Cosmetic and anatomic outcomes after feminizing surgery for ambiguous genitalia. J Pediatr Surg. 2005;40:1856–60.
12. Stoianovic B, Bizic M, Bencic M, Vukadinovic V, Korac G, Djordjevic M. Reduction clitoroplasty by clitoral disassembly as an approach for the treatment of congenital adrenal hyperplasia. Eur Urol Suppl. 2019;18(2):e2360.
13. Graziano K, Teitelbaum DH, Hirschl RB, et al. Vaginal reconstruction for ambiguous genitalia and congenital absence of the vagina: a 27-year experience. J Pediatr Surg. 2002;37:955–60.
14. Pena A. Total urogenital mobilization – an easier way to repair cloacas. J Pediatr Surg. 1997;32:263–7.
15. Rink RC, Metcalfe PD, Cain MP, Meldrum KK, Kaefer MA, Casale AJ. Use of the mobilized sinus with total urogenital mobilization. J Urol. 2006;176:2205–11.
16. Palmer BW, Trojan B, Griffin K, et al. Total and partial urogenital mobilization: focus on urinary continence. J Urol. 2012;187:1422–6.
17. Brännström M, Brännström M. Uterus transplantation in a Nordic perspective: a proposition for clinical introduction with centralization. Acta Obstet Gynecol Scand. 2021;100(8):1361–3.
18. Creatsas G, Deligeoroglou E, Makrakis E, Kontoravdis A, Papadimitriou L. Creation of a neovagina following Williams vaginoplasty and the Creatsas modification in 111 patients with Mayer–Rokitansky–Kuster–Hauser syndrome. Fertil Steril. 2001;76:1036–40.
19. Borruto F, Camoglio FS, Zampieri N, Fedele L. The laparoscopic Vecchietti technique for vaginal agenesis. Int J Gynaecol Obstet. 2007;98:15–9.
20. Hojsgaard A, Villadsen I. McIndoe procedure for congenital vaginal agenesis: complications and results. Br J Plast Surg. 1995;48:97–102.
21. Carcopino X, Shojai R, Boubli L. Female genital mutilation: generalities, complications and management during obstetrical period. J Gynecol Obstet Biol Reprod. 2004;33:378–83.

22. Nour NM, Michels KB, Bryant AE. Defibulation to treat female genital cutting: effect on symptoms and sexual function. Obstet Gynecol. 2006;108:55–60.
23. Iavazzo C, Sardi TA, Gkegkes ID. Female genital mutilation and infections: a systematic review of the clinical evidence. Arch Gynecol Obstet. 2013;87:1137–49.
24. Obermeyer CM. The consequences of female circumcision for health and sexuality: an update on the evidence. Cult Health Sex. 2005;7:443–61.
25. Perez-Lopez FR, Vieira-Baptista P. Lichen sclerosus in women: a review. Climacteric. 2017;20(4):339–47.
26. Hodgkinson DJ, Hait G. Aesthetic vaginal labioplasty. Plast Reconstr Surg. 1984;74:414–6.
27. Motakef S. Rodriguez-Feliz J, Chung MT, Ingargiola MJ, Wong VW, Patel A. Vaginal labiaplasty: current practices and a simplified classification system for labial protrusion. Plast Reconstr Surg. 2015;135(3):774–88.
28. Oranges CM, Sisti A, Sisti G. Labia minora reduction techniques: a comprehensive literature review. Aesthet Surg J. 2015;35(4):419–43.
29. Choi HY, Kim KT. A new method for aesthetic reduction of labia minora (the deepithelialized reduction of labioplasty). Plast Reconstr Surg. 2000;105:419–22.
30. Cao YJ, Li FY, Li SK, et al. A modified method of labia minora reduction: the de-epithelialised reduction of the central and posterior labia minora. J Plast Reconstr Aesthet Surg. 2012;65:1096–102.
31. Maas SM, Hage JJ. Functional and aesthetic labia minora reduction. Plast Reconstr Surg. 2000;105:1453–6.
32. Alter GJ. A new technique for aesthetic labia minora reduction. Ann Plast Surg. 1998;40:287–90.
33. Munhoz AM, Filassi JR, Ricci MD, et al. Aesthetic labia minora reduction with inferior wedge resection and superior pedicle flap reconstruction. Plast Reconstr Surg. 2006;118:1237–47.
34. Kelishadi SS, Elston JB, Rao AJ, Tutela JP, Mizuguchi NN. Posterior wedge resection: a more aesthetic labiaplasty. Aesthet Surg J. 2013;33:847–53.
35. Gress S. Composite reduction labiaplasty. Aesthet Plast Surg. 2013;37:674–83.
36. Capraro VJ. Congenital anomalies. Clin Obstet Gynecol. 1971;14:988–1012.
37. Pardo J, Sola V, Ricci P, Guilloff E. Laser labioplasty of labia minora. Int J Gynaecol Obstet. 2006;93:38–43.
38. Coleman SR. Structural fat grafts; the ideal filler? Clin Plast Surg. 2001;28:111–9.
39. Wilkie G, Bartz D. Vaginal rejuvenation: a review of female genital cosmetic surgery. Obstet Gynecol Surv. 2018;73(5):287–92.
40. Juhasz MLW, Korta DZ, Mesinkovska NA. Vaginal rejuvenation: a retrospective review of lasers and radiofrequency devices. Dermatol Surg. 2021;47(4):489–94.
41. Eppley BL, Dadvand B. Injectable soft-tissue fillers: clinical overview. Plast Reconstr Surg. 2006;118(4):98e–106e.
42. Hashim PW, Nia JK, Zade J, Farberg AS, Goldenberg G. Noninvasive vaginal rejuvenation. Cutis. 2018;102(4):243–6.
43. Aguilar P, Hersant B, SidAhmed-Mezi M, Bosc R, Vidal L, Meningaud JP. Novel technique of vulvovaginal rejuvenation by lipofilling and injection of combined platelet-rich-plasma and hyaluronic acid: a case-report. Springerplus. 2016;5(1):1184.

Index

A
Abdominal approach, 817
Abdominal-perineal resection (APR), 873
Abdominal sacrocolpopexy (ASC), 88, 597, 632, 646
    complications, 637, 639
    historical background, 633–634
    outcomes for, 638
    patient evaluation, 633
    postoperative care, 637
    preoperative preparation, 634–635
    surgical technique, 635–637
    use of mesh, 637
Abdominal wall reconstruction, 1080–1082
Abdominoperineal resection (APR), 295
Abdominoplasty, 1088
Ablative surgery, 1102
Abol-Enein pouch, 1107, 1111
Accidental bowel leakage, see Anorectal dysfunction
Acetaminophen, 927
Acontractile detrusor, 208
Acucise, 876
Acupuncture, 231
Acute spinal cord injury, 459
Acute/transient urinary retention (AUR), 198
Acute urinary retention (AUR), 401, 442
Adenocarcinomas, 193
Adenomyosis, 916
Adhesiolysis, 1133, 1136
Adipose-derived stem cells, 497–499
Adjustable continence devices (ProACT™ and ACT™), 477
Adnexa, 118
Adrenergic stimulation, 56–57
Afferent communication
    anatomy, 60
    Aδ and C fibers, 60–61
Aggravating factors, 328
Air cystoscopy, 182
AirSeal® trocar, 423
Alcock's canal, 266, 338, 353
Alcohol-based solutions, 184
Alkalinized lidocaine, 948
Allogenic grafts, 381
Alpha 1 adrenergic receptor, 56

Alpha 2 adrenergic receptor, 57
Alpha-blockers, 478
Altemeier operation, 1026
Alvimopan, 481
Ambulatory urodynamics, 170–171
American College of Obstetricians and Gynecologists (ACOG), 910
American Urogynecological Association (AUGA), 576
American Urological Association (AUA), 198, 576
    guidelines, 466
Amitriptyline, 947
Amniotic fluid stem cells, 500
Amniotic membrane
    See also Interposing graft
AMS-800™ model, 410
Anal fissure, 345
Anal manography, 812
Anastomotic leakage, 1057
Anastomotic urethroplasty, 844–845
Anchor based approach, 108
Androgen insensitivity syndrome (AIS), 588, 1197
    clitoroplasty, 1202
    diagnosis, 1197
    feminizing genital reconstruction, 1200
    genital reconstruction/(neo)vaginoplasty, 1199
    gonadectomy, 1199
    Hendren technique, 1201
    high confluence UGS, 1200
    labioplasty, 1203
    low confluence UGS, 1200
    mucocutaneous plate, 1202
    Passerini perineal approach, 1201
    physiopathology, 1197
    PSARVUP technique, 1203
    in TUM, 1203
    vaginoplasty, 1202
Anorectal dysfunction, 998
Anorectal malformations (ARM), 36
Anorectal manometry, 1004, 1019
Anorgasmia, 962
Antegrade nephrostogram, 736
Anterior cingulate cortex (ACC), 65
Anterior colporrhaphy, 523, 535, 537, 540, 546–548

Anterior compartment prolapse
  anterior colporrhaphy with/without graft reinforcement, 546–548
  apical suspension procedure, 546
  definition, 534
  incidence of, 534
  paravaginal repair for (see Laparoscopic paravaginal repair)
  pathogenesis of, 536
  surgical approach for, 535
  vaginal procedure, 537
Anterior prolapse, 290
Anterior proximal vaginal flap urethroplasty, 713–714
Anterior vaginal compartment prolapse, 82
Anterior vaginal repair, 979
Anterior vaginal support defects, 535–537, 548
Anterior vaginal wall prolapse, 557–560
Antibiotic prophylaxis, 741, 815
Antibiotics, 741
Anticholinergics, 215–216
Anti-incontinence procedures, 82, 401
Anti-lincontinence surgery, 1073–1074
Antimicrobial prophylaxis, 184
Anti-Müllerian hormone (AMH), 31, 32
Antimuscarinic medications, 470
Antispasmodics, 865
Anti-stress urinary incontinence surgery, 979
Anxiety, 975
Apical prolapse, 292, 594
Apical suspension procedures, 546, 632
Appendiceal tunneling, 1048
Appendicovesicostomy, 1153, 1154
Arcus tendineus fascia pelvis (ATFP), 72, 73, 644
Arcus tendinous fasciae rectovaginalis (ATFR), 644
Armamentarium Chirurgicum, 10
Artificial urinary sphincters (AUS), 477, 847, 1074
  AMS-800™ AUS model, 416–418
  contraindications, 415
  early post-operative complications, 401, 429
  evaluation and diagnosis, female patient, 411–414
  future research, 433
  history and development, 409
  indications, 415
  laparoscopic implantation, 421
  late post-operative complications, 401, 402
  long-term complications, 429–430
  mechanism of action, 410–411
  neurogenic patient groups, 401
  open trans-abdominal impantation, 418–420
  open trans-vaginal implantation, 420–421
  patient preparation, 416
  perioperative complications, 425–429
  placement, 401
  postoperative care, 425
  robotic-assisted implantation, 421–425
  second-line treatment for female SUI, 415
  technique of implantation, 416–425
Augmentation cystoplasty
  description, 1053
  neurogenic lower urinary tract dysfunction, 1054–1055
  non-neurogenic bladder, 1053–1054

Augmentation ileocystoplasty, 1036
Autoaugmentation, 307
Autologous ear chondrocytes, 500–501
Autologous fascial slings, 399, 400, 663
Autologous pubovaginal rectus sling, 280
Autologous pubovaginal sling, 286–288
Autologous slings, 374–380
Autonomic dysreflexia (AD), 464
Autonomic nerve fibers, 1103
Autotransplantation, 1077

B

Baclofen, 478
Baden-Walker system, 539
β3-adrenoreceptors (β3-ARs), 77
B3 agonists, 216
Balloon dilation, 875
Balloon expulsion test, 1004
Barrington's nucleus, 77
Barry technique, 901–902
Bartholin glands, 807, 968
Behavioral therapy, OAB
  bladder training, frequency volume charts, 228–229
  habit training, scheduled voiding regimens, 229–230
Behcet's syndrome, 807
Bevacizumab, 733
Bilateral gracilis total vaginectomy, 1087
Bilateral ileococcygeal fixation, 613
Bilateral innominate bones, 72
Bile acids, 1119
Bilharzia, 1044
Bimanual exam, 118
Biofeedback therapy, 234–239
BioGlue©, 813
BK polyomavirus, 934
Bladder
  augmentation, 1074–1075
  exstrophy, 904
  flaps, 851–853
  neck closure, 1074
  neck reconstruction, 1073
  transection, 845
  wall flap, 851
Bladder architecture
  detrusor, 53–54
  extracellular matrix, 54–56
  lamina propria, 52–53
  urothelium, 51–52
Bladder augmentation, 302
  indications and patient selection, 303–304
  postoperative care, outcome and complications, 307–309
  preoperative investigation, 305
  reconstructive options, 304–305
  surgical technique, 306–307
Bladder biomechanics
  bladder architecture, 51–56
  bladder storage and emptying, 56–59
Bladder cancers, 188, 192, 1042–1043

Bladder compliance, 164
Bladder contractility index (BCI), 214
Bladder diverticulum, 189
Bladder drainage, 203
Bladder dysfunction, 399
    drugs and radiation-induced cystitis, 1045
    schistosomiasis, 1044–1045
    urogenital tuberculosis, 1044
Bladder emptying, 279–281, 287, 302
Bladder endometriosis, 189
Bladder exstrophy (BE), 44, 320, 1045
Bladder injuries, 661, 666
    colorectal procedures, 1136, 1137
    conservative management, 1140
    gynaecological injuries, 1136
    obstetric injuries, 1135–1136
    urological injuries, 1137
    vascular surgery injuries, 1136
Bladder neck closure, 477
    abdominal approach, 722–723
    outcomes of, 723–725
    transvaginal approach, 722
Bladder neurophysiology, 209–210
Bladder outlet, 474
Bladder outlet obstruction (BOO), 81, 82, 199, 202, 203, 208, 211, 276, 278–281, 286, 288, 291, 295, 296
Bladder pain syndrome (BPS), 191, 917–918
    animal studies, 950
    biomarkers, 942–944
    classification, 942
    conservative measures, 945
    conventional pharmacotherapy, 945–946
    cystoscopy and bladder biopsy, 941–942
    diagnosis, 936–944
    epidemiology, 933–934
    etiology, 934–935
    history, 936–940
    interventional pharmacotherapy, 945–946
    intramural treatments, 948–949
    intravesical pharmacotherapy, 948
    laboratory tests, 940
    management, 944–950
    oral pharmacotherapy, 946–948
    pathology, 935
    phenotyping patients, 944
    physical examination, 940
    surgical treatments, 949–950
    terminology, 932–933
    urodynamics, 940
Bladder schistosomiasis, 188
Bladder spasms, 750
Bladder stones, 187
Bladder storage and emptying, 302, 479
Bladder tubularisation, 1152, 1153
Blue-light cystoscopy (BLC), 192, 193
Boari flap, 878, 888, 890–893, 895, 1141, 1143

Boari-Ockerblad flap, 888
Body mass index (BMI), 224
Body part discomfort (BPD) scale, 753
Bone marrow-derived stem cells (BMSCs), 499–500
Botulinum neurotoxin A (BoNT-A), 218
Botulinum toxin, 216
    type A, 948
Botulism syndrome, 472
Bowel anastomosis, 1041
Bowel dysfunction, 1025
Bowel function assessment, 305
Bowel injuries, 399, 667, 1152, 1153, 1155
Brachytherapy (BT), 1064
Breisky–Navratil retractors, 598
Bremelanotide, 986
Bricker method, 318
Bricker technique, 1042
Bricker/Wallace technique, 1046
Bridges, 182
Bristol stool chart, 1003
Bristol stool scale, 1015
Buccal mucosa, 882
Buccal mucosa graft, 834–836
Buck's fascia, 1214
Bulbospongious muscle, 1215
Bulkamid®, 397, 441
Bupropion, 986
Burch colposuspension, 286, 287, 296, 364, 400
    complications, 454
    history, 450, 451
    laparoscopic, 367
    midurethral sling, 365–366
    outcomes and complications of MMK repair, 364–365, 452–454
    pubovaginal sling, 366–367
    surgical technique, 451
Buttock pain, 599

C

Cadaveric fascia lata (CFL), 380
Cadaveric slings, 380–381
Caffeine, 226–227
Cajal function, 53
Calcified synthetic mesh, 284
Calcitonin-gene-related peptide (CGRP), 60
Caliectasis, 823
Cancers, rectovaginal fistula (RVF), 808
Cannabinoids, 471
Capio® device, 600
Carbon-coated zirconium, 397
Carcinoma in situ (CIS), 192
Cardinal ligaments (CL), 74, 595
Caregivers, 480
Carnett test, 913
Catheter drainage, 659
Catheterisable augmentation ileocystoplasty, 1145, 1146

Catheterization, 471
Cauda equina syndrome (CES), 464, 923
Central nervous system
    ACC, 65
    locus coeruleus, 65
    PAG, 64–65
    PMC, 65
    prefrontal cortex, 65
    storage, 64–65
    voiding, 65
Cerebral palsy, 461
Cerebrovascular accidents (CVA), 461
Cervical cancer, 981, 1100
Cervix, 118
Chemodenervation, 471
Chemoprophylaxis, 741
Childbirth complications, 1158, 1159
Cholestyramine, 1059
Cholinergic stimulation, 57–58
Chronic intestinal pseudo-obstruction, 201
Chronic metabolic acidosis, 1059
Chronic pelvic/bladder pain syndrome, 190, 664
Chronic pelvic pain (CPP), 265
    causes of, 910–912
    definition, 910, 932
    diagnosis, 911
    differential diagnosis, 915–926
    etiologies, 912
    gastrointestinal system, 920
    gynecological system, 915–916
    initial assessment of, 912–914
    laboratory and imaging studies, 915
    male genitalia, 916–917
    medical history, 912–913
    multifocal pain, 926
    musculoskeletal system, 918–920
    neurological structures, 922–926
    physical examination, 913–914
    special populations, 914–915
    treatment, 926–927
    urological system, 917–918
    validation, 912
    vascular disorders, 921–922
Chronic/persistent urinary retention (CUR), 198
Chronic prostatitis, 916
Cimetidine, 947
Clavien-Dindo complications grade, 429
Clean intermittent catheterization (CIC), 248, 662
Clitoral reconstruction, 1177
    aims, 1177
    benefits, 1178
    multidisciplinary care pathway, 1178
    potential benefits, 1178
    potential risks, 1178
    risks, 1178
    techniques, 1177, 1178
    WHO recommendations, 1179
Clitorectomy, 1201
Clitoridectomy, 1166

Clitoris
    components, 968
    external, 969
    internal, 969
Clostridium tetani, 1157, 1158
Coaptite™, 397, 442, 443
Coccygeus-sacrospinous ligament (C-SSL), 595
Coccygodynia, 350
Coccyx, 72
Cognition, 480
Cognitive behavioral therapy (CBT), 927, 985
Cognitive function, 466
Cognitive sexual arousal, 972
Cold knife endopyelotomy, 876
Colon, 1039
Colon conduit, 1047
Colonic inertia, 1001
Colon transit studies, 1006–1007
Colopopexy and urinary reduction efforts (CARE) trial, 575
Colorectal, 76
Colorectal surgery, 295
Common cloaca (CC), 36
Common Era (CE), 6
Complementary alternative medicine (CAM), 230–232
Complete blood count (CBC), 575
Complications of vaginal surgery
    diverticulectomy, 660
    slings, 661–663
    urethral prolapse, 661
    urethrovaginal/vesicovaginal fistula repair, 659
    vaginal hysterectomy, 665–669
    vaginal mesh surgery, 663–669
    vaginal prolapse repair, 669–672
    vaginoplasty, 658–659
Computerized tomography (CT), 42
Computer tomography, 736
Concomitant bilateral oophorectomy, 612
Concomitant hysterectomy, 636
Concomitant urethrovaginal fistula, 843, 845, 851, 853
Congenital adrenal hyperplasia (CAH), 1205, 1239
    adrenal enzymes, 1205
    anatomical variations, 1240
    clitoroplasty, 1240
    endocrine imbalance, 1205
    labioplasty, 1240
    preoperative evaluation, 1240
    urogenital tissue, 1241
    vaginoplasty, 1240
Congenital pelvic malformations, 1186
Congenital renal anomalies, 37
Congenital urogenital anomalies, 1045
Conservative management, 738
Constipation, 1014
    treatment, 1025
Construct validity, 107
Content validity, 107
Content validity ratio (CVR), 107
Contigen®, 441

Continent catheterizable channel, 309
  continent cutaneous/catheterizable ileocecocystoplasty, 312–314
  hemi-Kock system, 314
  Mitrofanoff, 309
  Yang-Mont, 310–312
Continent catheterizable ileal cecocystoplasty (CCIC), 1076–1077
Continent cutaneous reservoir, 1108
  outcome, 1121–1122
  risks, 1119–1120
Continent cutaneous urinary diversions, 315–317
Continent urinary channels
  continent catheterizable ileal cecocystoplasty (CCIC), 1076–1077
  Kock nipple valve, 1076
  Mitrofanoff appendicovesicostomy, 1075–1076
  Yang-Monti channel, 1076
Continent urinary diversion, 1046
  early risks of, 1118
  long term risks, 1118–1122
  patient selection, 1105–1106
Continuous bladder drainage, 749
Contrast-enhanced CT, 790
Conventional laparoscopy, 752
Convergent validity, 107
Cook Biotech© Biodesign Fistula Plug sets, 813
Cooper's ligament, 450–452
Cough stress test (CST), 413
C-reactive protein, 575
Creutzfeldt-Jakob disease (CJD), 380
Criterion validity, 107
Crohn's disease, 807, 809, 812–815, 817, 818
Cross-trigonal (Cohen) ureteral reimplantation technique, 897–898
CT intravenous pyelogram (IVP), 1139, 1140
Cumulative distribution function (CDF), 107, 108
Cutaneous catheterizing pouch
  components and types of, 1047, 1048
  continence mechanisms, 1048–1049
  Mitrofanoff procedure, 1049
  Yang-Monti procedure, 1049
Cutaneous ureterostomy, 317
Cyanoacrylate, see Tissue sealants
Cyclosporine, 946
Cystectomy
  anatomical borders, 1102
  forms, 1101–1102
  indications, 1101–1102
Cystocele, 508, 534, 546, 547
Cystocele repair
  anterior colporrhaphy, 523
  complications, 525
  outcomes, 524–526
  paravaginal repair, 524
  transverse defect repair, 524
Cystogram, 737
Cystography, 823

Cystoplasty, 306
  and Hemi-Kock CCC, 314
  pregnancy, 319
Cystoscopy, 180, 181, 284, 331, 413, 468, 523, 736, 742, 769, 789, 790, 823
Cystotomy, 744
Cysto-urethroscopy, 180, 193, 284, 699, 711, 765, 859
Cytokines, 943

D

da Vinci Surgical System, 554
da Vinci Xi system, 893
Deep infiltrating endometriosis (DIE), 294
Dees-Leadbetter procedure, 851
Defecatory dysfunction, 998
  acupuncture and neuromodulation, 1010
  anatomical structures, 1000
  approach to care, 1000
  behavior modification and biofeedback, 1007–1008
  causes, 1001
  colonoscopy, 1004
  colon transit studies, 1006–1007
  correlation between anatomy and function, 1003–1004
  defecography, 1005–1006
  definition, 998–999
  differential diagnosis, 1000–1002
  epidemiology, 999
  evaluation, 1002–1007
  management, 1007–1010
  medications, 1008
  motility studies, 1004–1005
  physiology, 999
  surgical management, 1008–1010
  testing, 1004–1007
Defecography, 1017
Defibulation, 1176
Deflux™, 397
Delayed injury, 669
Delorme method, 1026
Dementia, 461
Denovilliers fascia, 1215
Depression, 975
Desmopressin, 471
Detrusor, 53–54
Detrusor contraction strength, 214–215
Detrusor external-sphincter dyssynergia (DESD), 81–82, 475
Detrusor leak point pressure, 62
Detrusor overactivity (DO), 79–80, 160, 164, 208, 222, 283, 1054–1055
Detrusorrhaphy (Hodgson-Firlit-Zaontz) technique, 902
Detrusor-sphincter dyssynergia (DSD), 64, 169, 460
Detrusor underactivity (DUA), 81, 199, 200, 203, 208, 210, 213, 246
Detubularization of bowel, 1036
Devastated bladder outlet, 303
Dextranomer hyaluronic acid (Deflux™), 397, 887

Diabetic cystopathy, 464
Diethylentriamine penta-acetic acid (DTPA), 38
Diethylstilbestrol (DES), 32, 34
DIGNITY trials, 472
3D image-guided adaptive brachytherapy (IGABT), 1064
Dimethyl sulfoxide (DMSO), 948
Direct vision internal urethrotomy, 833
Disorders of sexual differentiation (DSD), 1187
Disseminated central disease, 465
Distal defects, 521
Distal diverticulum, 861
Distribution-based approach, 108
Diuretic renography, 876, 895
Diurnal urinary continence, 847
Divergent/discriminant validity, 107
Diverticulectomy, 660
Dnamic MRI defecography, 1006
Doppler ultrasonography, 349
Dorsal lithotomy, 742
Double balloon positive pressure urethrography (PPU), 860
Double hydrodistention-implantation technique (Double HIT), 887
Double-stapled trans-anal rectal resection (STARR) procedure, 1009
Drains, 1090
Dribbling, 858
Drug metabolism abnormalities, 1059
Drugs and radiation-induced cystitis, 1045
Durasphere™, 397, 442
Dye testing, 122
Dynamic graciloplasty, 1024
Dynamic imaging, 129
Dysfunctional voiding, 200
Dysmenorrhea, 1174
Dyspareunia, 344, 661, 671, 858, 861, 962
Dysuria, 858

E
Eastern Cooperative Oncology Group (ECOG) score, 1156, 1157
Ectopic kidneys, 37
Electrical stimulation (ES), 217–218, 248
  at home without caregivers, 241
  in hospitals/continence clinics, 239–241
Electrical stimulation of peripheral nerves, 473
Electroacupuncture, 231
Electrofulguration, 739
Electrolyte abnormalities, 1058–1059
Electromyography (EMG), 173, 349
  autonomic fibers, 153
  clitoro-cavernosus, 154
  concentric needle, 147, 152
  concentric needle electrode, 144
  diagnostics of, 142
  interference pattern of MUPs, 145
  kinesiologic, 142
  motor control, 143
  motor evoked potentials (MEPs), 149
  motor unit, 143
  muscle denervation, 145
  muscle reinnervation, 145
  needle electrode insertions, 144
  in neurophysiological laboratory, 147
  overview, 141
  pelvic floor muscle, 142
  primary muscle disease, 149
  somatic sensory and somatic motor systems, 150
  urethral sphincter, 144
  vaginal delivery, 148
  women in urinary retention, 148
Electrophysiological evaluation, 140
EMBRACE-I trial, 1069
Endoanal and transperineal ultrasounds, 811
Endometriosis, 188, 915
Endometriosis surgery, 293, 295
Endopelvic fascia, 73, 595
Endorectal advancement flap (ERAF), 815, 816
Endoscopic evaluation, 735
  complications, 185
  contraindications, 185
  equipment types, 181–185
  history, 180, 181
  indications, 185
  normal findings, 185, 186
  pathologic bladder findings, 186–193
  pathologic urethral findings, 186
  personnel and preparation, 184
  technique, 184
Endoureterotomy, 887
Enhanced recovery after surgery (ERAS) protocols, 559
Enterocele, 508, 514
Enterocystoplasty, 307
Epidermal inclusion cysts (EICs), 1170
Epirubicin, 1045
Epithelized fistula tract, 744
Erythrocyte sedimentation rate (ESR), 575
Estradiol, 976
Ethylene Vinyl Alcohol copolymer, 439
European Association of Urology (EAU), 211, 738, 1074, 1115
European Association of Urology Robotic Urology Section (ERUS), 792
European Organization for Research and Treatment of Cancer (EORTC), 1066, 1067
External anal sphincter (EAS), 1000
External beam radiation therapy (EBRT), 1064
External clitoris, 969
External genitalia, 116
External tunnel (Barry) technique, 901–902
External urethral meatus, 860, 863
External urinary sphincter (EUS), 76, 459
Extracellular matrix, 54–56
Extra-peritoneal conduit (EPIC) procedure, 318
Extravesical approach, 745–747
Exuberant exophitic bladder neoplasm, 192

F

Face validity, 107
Fasciae, 72
Fascial sparing VRAM for vagina, 1084
Fasciocutaneous, 1152
Fasciocutaneous flaps, 1153
Feasibility, 105–106
Fecal incontinence, 998, 1014
    clinical examination, 1016–1017
    imaging, 1017–1019
    investigations, 1019–1021
    multidisciplinary approach, 1014–1015
    pathophysiological considerations, 1015–1016
    patient history, 1016
    primary treatment, 1021–1022
Female circumcision, *see* Female genital mutilation/cutting (FGM/C)
Female continence, 459
Female genital cutting (FGC), 1164
    clitoral reconstruction, 1177
    clitoris and the labia minora, 1170
    community involvement, 1180
    cystic mass post, 1173
    defibulation, 1176
    dermatological complications, 1169
    education, 1179
    epidemiology trends, 1165
    gynaecological care, 1176
    gynaecological complications, 1174
    health consequences, 1167
    immediate complications, 1167
    immigrant populations, 1165
    infibulation, 1174
    intrapartum care, 1177
    longer-term complications, 1168
    migration, 1165
    neuropathic clitoral pain, 1173
    obstetric and perinatal complications, 1175
    prevalence per country, 1164–1167
    prevention strategies, 1178, 1180
    psychiatric diagnosis, 1175
    sexual dysfunction women, 1177
    sexual health, 1172
    short term complications, 1168
    types of, 1165
    urinary tract complications, 1172
    vaginal orifice, 1171
Female genitalia
    aging changes, 1237
    anatomy, 1238
    congenital adrenal hyperplasia (CAH), 1239–1241
    congenital anomalies, 1239
    esthetic surgery, 1237, 1239
    genital mutilation, 1239
    hymenoplasty, 1250
    labia majora, 1237
    labia majora augmentation, 1247
    labiaplasty, 1245–1247
    lichen sclerosus (LS), 1244
    overview, 1236
    surgical treatment, 1243
    vaginal agenesis, 1241–1243
    vaginal rejuvenation, 1248, 1249
Female genital mutilation (FGM), 1131, 1157, 1243
    urogenital fistula, 681
    WHO classification, 1159
Female genital mutilation/cutting (FGM/C), 1131, 1158, 1159, 1164
    antenatal care, 1177
    defibulation, 1176
    dermatological complications, 1169–1172
    epidemiology trends, 1165
    gynecological care, 1176–1177
    gynecological complications, 1174–1175
    immediate complications, 1167–1168
    intrapartum care, 1177
    long-term complications, 1168
    management, 1176–1178
    neuropathic clitoral pain, 1173–1174
    obstetric and perinatal complications, 1175
    prevalence, 1164
    prevention, 1178–1180
    psychological disturbances, 1175–1176
    sexual health, 1172–1173, 1177
    short-term complications, 1168
    types, 1165–1167
    urinary tract complications, 1172
Female genitourinary
    Aldrich's technique, 21
    Andreas Vesalius, 8, 9
    antiquity, 4, 6
    antiseptic surgery and preventative medicine, 15, 16
    bladder and pelvic cavity, 8
    bladder and ureteric injury, 23
    cervical cancer, 18, 24
    Charrière vaginal speculum, 13
    Cusco vaginal speculum, 13, 14
    early hysterectomies, 23
    eighteenth century, 11
    enormous progress, 4
    evolution, 25
    factors, 4
    Fallopian tube, 9
    female reproductive system and ovarian follicles, 10, 11
    Foley Y-V pyeloplasty, 19
    Gabriele Fallopio, 9
    Goebell-Fragenheim-Stoeckel sling technique, 20
    gynecologic diseases, 18, 19
    gynecology and urology, 18
    innovative procedure, 19
    intra-abdominal pressure, 4
    James Marion Sims, 13, 14
    laparoscopic hysterectomy, 24
    ligaments of Douglas, 11
    Mackenrodt ligaments, 16, 17
    Marshall-Marchetti-Krantz operation, 22
    Maximilian Carl-Fredrich Nitze, 19

Female genitourinary (cont.)
  medieval era, 6, 7
  modern breast surgery, 15
  nineteenth century, 11, 13–18
  Nitze endoscope, 19
  operations, 20
  pasteurization, 15, 16
  Pawlik's procedure, 20
  peritoneum, 11, 12
  pioneer of antisepsis, 14, 15
  placement, 9, 10
  post-menopausal population, 4
  pouch of Douglas, 11
  radical abdominal hysterectomy, 24
  refinements, 25
  renaissance period, 7–9
  seventeenth century, 10, 11
  sims' double bladed vaginal speculum, 15
  subfundic radical hysterectomy, 24
  succussion, 5
  surgical technique, 23
  symphysis pubis, 21
  treatments, 20
  urethrovesical junction, 21
  uterine fibroids, 23
  uterine prolapse, 9, 10, 19
  vaginal hysterectomy, 7, 11, 12, 22, 23
  vaginal radical trachelectomy, 24
  vesicourethral junction, 21
  vesicovaginal fistula repair, 20
Female genitourinary reconstruction
  augmentation cystoplasty, 1053–1055
  bowel anastomosis, 1041
  bowel in, 1035
  colon, 1039
  complications of bowel use in, 1056–1060
  conduit, 1046–1047
  cutaneous catheterizing pouch, 1047–1049
  history, 1036
  ileocolonic segment, 1038–1039
  ileum, 1037–1038
  jejunum, 1037
  neovaginal reconstruction, 1055–1056
  orthotopic neobladder, 1049–1052
  patient evaluation, 1040
  physics of bowel, 1036–1037
  preoperative preparation, 1040–1041
  stomach, 1037
  surgical anatomy, 1037–1039
  surgical techniques, 1041–1042
  ureterointestinal anastomosis, 1041–1042
  ureterosigmoidostomy, 1052–1053
  ureter substitution, 1055
  urinary diversion, 1042–1046
  urinary stoma, 1042
Female lower urinary tract and pelvic floor
  dye testing, 122
  history, 114–116
  pad test, 118
  physical exam, 116–118
  post void residual, 121–122
  self-reported questionnaires, 119–121
  urinalysis, 121
  void diary, 118–120
Female neurologic patient
  history, 465
  low risk patients, 466
  physical examination, 466
  questionnaires, 465
  surveillance, 468
  unknown risk patients, 467
  urinalysis, 466
Female pelvic cancer
  anterior compartment, 1100
  middle compartment, 1100
  posterior compartment, 1100
Female pelvic medicine and reconstructive surgery (FPMRS), 576
Female pelvis
  anatomy, 965–974
  clitoris, 968–969
  female sexual response, 970–974
  G-spot, 966–967
  innervation, 969–970
  vagina, 965–966
  vascular supply, 970
  vulva, 967–968
Female reproductive system
  arcuate uterus, 34
  bicornuate uterus, 34
  categories, 33
  cervix and vagina, 35
  clinical anomalies, 30
  cloacal division, 30
  congenital cervical and vaginal atresia, 35
  congenital cervical atresia, 33
  early zygote and embryogenesis, 30
  external genitalia, 32
  gartner's duct cyst (GDC), 41
  genital ducts, 31
  gonads, 32
  malignancy, 40
  McIndoe vaginoplasty, 35
  McKusick-Kaufman syndrome (MKKS), 43, 44
  MRKH syndrome, 42, 43
  Mullerian anomalies, 33
  multiple anomalies, 35
  pelvic anomalies, 44
  posterior sagittal approach, 36
  primitive Mullerian duct development, 30, 31
  radiological imaging, 34
  rectovaginal fistula, 36
  rectovestibular fistula, 36
  renal calculi, 40
  reproductive ducts, 32
  sacral deformity, 36
  septate uterus, 34
  septate vaginal abnormalities, 36

Index   1261

sexual differentiation, 32
3D sonar, 35
transverse vaginal septum, 34
T-shaped uterus, 34
unicornuate uterus, 33
ureteric bud anomalies, 37–40
uterus, 31, 32
uterus didelphys, 33
vagina, 31, 32
vesicoureteric reflux, 40
Female sexual arousal (FSA)
   mechanisms, 974–975
Female sexual dysfunction (FSD), 1177
   after pelvic surgeries, 979–984
   after treatment of pelvic malignancies, 981–984
   with aging, 984
   awareness and management, 960
   classification, 962–963
   definition, 961–962
   etiology and pathophysiology, 975–977
   evaluation of, 984–985
   organic/physical causes, 976–977
   and pelvic organ prolapse/urinary incontinence, 978
   in post-partum period, 977–978
   prevalence, 963
   psychological causes, 975
   risk factors, 963–965
   treatment, 985–987
Female sexual function index (FSFI), 754, 1222
Female sexual response cycle, 970
   arousal, 971–972
   desire, 971
   orgasm, 972–974
   physiology and biochemistry, 974–975
Female stress urinary incontinence, 488
   amniotic fluid stem cells, 500
   animal studies, 491–493
   autologous ear chondrocytes, 500–501
   bone marrow-derived stem cells, 499–500
   human clinical trials on AMDC injections, 493–496
   umbilical cord blood stem cells, 500
Female urethra, anatomy and function, 695, 708–709
Female urethral diverticula (UD)
   aetiology, 858
   algorithm, 861
   classification systems, 860
   clinical presentation, 858
   conservative management, 860
   cysto-urethroscopy, 859
   different variations, 859
   double balloon positive pressure urethrography (PPU), 860
   magnetic resonance imaging (MRI), 859
   marsupialisation technique, 862
   outcomes, 865
   pathogenesis, 858
   periurethral fascia, 864
   pre-operative preparation, 862
   surgical techniques, 861

   transvaginal urethral diverticulectomy, 862
   ultrasonography, 860
   urine studies, 859
   voiding cystourethrogram (VCUG), 860
Female urethral diverticulum
   definition, 830
   diagnosis of, 831
   management, 833
   outcomes, 837
   procedural approach, 835
Female urethral injuries, 708
   complete-or transverse-type injuries, 842
   concomitant urethrovaginal fistula, 843, 845, 851, 853
   diagnosis, 711–712
   iatrogenic postsurgical urethral injury, 709–710
   meatal stenosis, 843, 845, 848
   mechanisms of severe, 709–711
   preoperative evaluation, 711–713
   surgical management, 713–726
   surgical reconstruction, 842
   trauma, 710–711
   types, 844
Female urethral stricture
   diagnosis, 831
   outcomes, 837
   procedural approach, 836
   treatment, 833
Female urinary retention, 198, 199, 204
Fiberoptic lens system, 181
Fiberoptic telescope, 181
Fibrin glue, *see* Tissue sealants
Fibrofatty martius flap, 289, 290
Fibrosis, 1068–1069
Filling cystometry, 163–165
Fistula, 1057
Fistula post abdominal hysterectomy, 790
Fistula-tract laser closure (FiLaC) procedure, 817
Fistulotomy, 815
Flatal incontinence, 998
Flexible cystourethroscopy, 183, 184
Flexible endoscopes, 181
Flexion, abduction, external rotation (FABER) test, 913, 919, 920
Flibanserin, 985
Fluoroquinolone, 184
Flush stoma, 1042
Focused urologic history
   general voiding patterns, 114
   incontinence, 114
   overactive bladder, 115
   pelvic pain, 115
   prolapse, 115
Foley catheter, 864
Food and Drug Administration (FDA), 650
Fowler's syndrome (FS), 199–200
French Association of Urology (AFU), 1074
16Fr Foley catheter, 1215
Fr measurement system, 183
Frykman-Goldberg operation, 1027

Functional anorectal pain disorders, 920
Functional tests, 141
Functional urethral length (FUL), 98
Fuoroscopic defecography, 1005–1006

G
GABA-B receptor agonist, 478
Gartner's duct cyst (GDC), 41
Gastrocystoplasty, 307
Gastrointestinal system, 1034
Gender affirmation surgeries (GAS), 1211, 1231
    clitoral reconstruction, 1214
    neovagina canal, 1215
    orchiectomy, 1213
    penectomy, 1214
    preoperative clinical evaluation, 1213
    transfeminine, 1212
    urethroplasty, 1215
    vaginoplasty techniques, 1213 (*see also* Vaginoplasty)
    vulvoplasty, 1214
Gender dysphoria, 1211
Gender identity, 1210
Gender reassigning surgery, 1228
    complications, 1228
    gastro/bowel, 1231
    genital region, 1230
    prostate hyperplasia/cancer, VTE, 1232
    ReOperation rates, 1229
    reoperation rates, 1229
    urinary tract, 1228, 1229
General anesthesia, 180
General medical history, 115–116
Genital gender affirmation surgeries (GGAS), 1212
Genital hiatus (GH), 603
Genital prolapse, 611
Genitourinary injury, 733
Genitourinary Pain Index (GUPI) questionnaire, 937–938
Genitourinary syndrome of menopause (GSM), 985
Genitourinary tuberculosis, 1044
German method, 20
Ghoneim pouch, 1107, 1111
Gil-Vernet technique (Gil-Vernet Trigonoplasty), 898–899
Glenn-Anderson Technique, 898–899
Glenn-Anderson technique, 898
Glucocorticoid therapy, 1206
Glutaraldehyde cross-linked bovine collagen, 438
Gluteal fold flap, 1089
Glycosaminoglycan layer, 51
Goal attainment scale (GAS), 104
Goh classification, 763, 764, 1158
Goh genitourinary fistula classification, 679
Goh's classification, 1158
Gore BIO-A© tissue reinforcement or fistula plug, 813
Gracilis flaps, 775, 1150, 1152, 1153, 1155
Gracilis muscle flap, 702, 703
Gracilis vagninal fistula, 1086
Grading system, 108
Graft-augmented posterior colporrhaphy, 645–646

Graft stenosis, 658
Griffith's point, 1039
Gynecare TVT®, 386
Gynecologic, 76
Gynecologic injuries, 873

H
Haematuria, 858, 859
Hammock hypothesis, 78
Hautmann neobladder, 1110, 1111
Healthcare system, 1176, 1180
Health-related quality of life (HRQL), 103–104, 1068
Hematocolpos, 43
Hematometra, 43
Hematuria, 187
Hematuria-dysuria syndrome, 1037
Hemi-Kock CCC, 314
Hemorrhagic cystitis, 187, 1068
Hemorrhoids, 1017
Hemostasis, 665
Herlyn-Werner-Wunderlich (HWW) syndrome, 33
Herniated disc, 923
Herniorrhaphy, 1137
Herpes simplex virus, 1157, 1158
Herpes zoster infection, 146
Heterotopic continent cutaneous reservoirs, 1108
Heterotopic continent urinary diversions, 1111–1112
    ileal heterotopic cutaneous pouch, 1113–1115
    Mainz I pouch, 1112–1114
Heterotopic ileocecal pouches, 1108
Hodgson-Firlit-Zaontz technique, 902
Holmium laser, 876
Home care therapy, 241
Hopkins rod-lens system, 181
Hormonal estrogen therapy, 1213
Horseshoe kidney, 39
Hunner's lesion, 191, 934, 935
Hydrodistension, 191
Hydronephrosis, 902, 903, 1044
Hydroxyzine, 947
Hymenoplasty, 1250
Hyperammonemia, 1059
Hypertonicity, 344
Hypoactive sexual desire disorder, 962, 985
Hypogastric nerves, 276
Hyponatremia, 1059
Hypoxia-inducible factor-1 (HIF-1), 1066
Hysterectomy, 515, 680, 681, 686, 980
Hysteropexy, 515, 603, 610
Hysteropexy suspension technique, 600
Hysterosalpingo-contrast-sonography, 35
Hysteroscopy, 35

I
Iatrogenic bladder outlet obstruction, 402
Iatrogenic postsurgical urethral injury, 709–710
Iatrogenic ureteral injuries, 872–874

Iatrogenic urinary tract injuries
  anatomy, 1131
  bladder injury, 1147, 1148
  bowel injuries, 1153, 1155
  comorbidities and functional status, 1157
  complete tears/transection, 1151
  damage excision of tissue, 1152, 1153
  definitive bladder repairs, 1145, 1146
  definitive ureteral repairs, 1140, 1145
  delayed presentation, 1155, 1156
  female genital mutilation (FGM), 1158, 1159
  fistula management, 1156, 1157
  intraoperative investigations, 1138, 1139
  management, 1139, 1140
  mucosal ureteral injuries, 1149
  multiple levels injury, 1149
  obstetric fistulae, 1148, 1149
  partial/complete occlusion of the ureter with a suture, 1151, 1152
  partial injuries, 1150
  postoperative investigations, 1139
  prevention, 1138
  previous radiotherapy, 1157, 1158
  risk factors, 1131, 1132
  stability of patient, 1140
  timing, position, and level of injury, 1146, 1147
  ureteral injuries, 1149
  urethral stricture formation, 1157
  vascular injuries, 1155
Idiopathic detrusor overactivity (IDO), 222
Idiopathic detrusor underactivity, 200
Idiopathic urinary retention
  chronic intestinal pseudo-obstruction, 201
  dysfunctional voiding, 200
  Fowler's syndrome, 199
  idiopathic detrusor underactivity, 200
  primary bladder neck obstruction, 200
Ileal conduit, 1046
Ileal heterotopic cutaneous pouch, 1113–1115
Ileal segment, 852
Ileal ureter, 880–881
Ileocolonic segment, 1038–1039
Ileocystostomy, 880
Ileopectineal line, 451
Ileum, 1037–1038
Iliococcygeus, 75
Iliococcygeus suspension, 603
Iliopsoas pain, 919
Ilium, 72
Impaired (low) compliance, 80
Implacer™-guided device implantation, 440
Inadvertent ureteral ligation, 900, 901
Incontinence, 72, 78–82, 114, 126, 127, 129, 130
  treatment, 1022–1025
Incontinence impact questionnaire, 283
Incontinence questionnaire-urge incontinence-short form (ICIQ-UI SF), 101
Incontinence symptom severity (ISS), 101
Incontinent ileovesicostomy, 1075

Incontinent urinary channels, 1075
Indiana pouch, 316, 1047
Indwelling catheters, 471
Infibulation, 1166
Inflammatory bowel disease, 807, 920
Informed consent, 184
InhibiZone™ coating, 410, 429
Inner (paraurethral) layer, 76
INSITE trial, 264
Integral theory, 78, 278
Intensity-modulated radiation therapy (IMRT), 1064
Interleukins, 943
Intermittent catheterization, 471
Intermittent flow, 160
Intermittent self-catheterization (ISC), 203, 248
Internal anal sphincter (EAS), 1000
Internal clitoris, 969
Internal consistency, 106
Internal iliac arteries and veins, 76
Internal iliac lymph nodes, 76
Internal pudendal artery, 970
Internal urethral sphincter (IUS), 76
International Consultation on Incontinence (ICI), 98, 108
International Consultation on Incontinence Questionnaire Overactive Bladder (ICIQ-OAB), 101
International Continence Society (ICS), 754, 1074
International Society for the Study of BPS criteria (ESSIC), 191
Inter-observer/inter-rater reliability, 106
Interposing graft, 749
Interposition tissue flap, 796
Interrupted nonabsorbable suture, 637
Interstitial cells (ITC), 52
Interstitial cystitis, 188, 190, 265, 917
  animal studies, 950
  biomarkers, 942–944
  classification, 942
  conservative measures, 945
  conventional pharmacotherapy, 945–946
  cystoscopy and bladder biopsy, 941–942
  diagnosis, 936–944
  epidemiology, 933–934
  etiology, 934–935
  history, 936–940
  interventional pharmacotherapy, 945–946
  intramural treatments, 948–949
  intravesical pharmacotherapy, 948
  laboratory tests, 940
  management, 944–950
  oral pharmacotherapy, 946–948
  pathology, 935
  phenotyping patients, 944
  physical examination, 940
  surgical treatments, 949–950
  terminology, 932–933
  urodynamics, 940
Intestinal anastomosis, 1118
Intestinal dysfunction, 308
Intra-abdominal pressure, 78

Intracorporal neobladder, 1121
Intraepithelial lymphocytes, 935
Intraextravesical technique (Paquin), 902
Intraoperative electron beam radiotherapy (IOERT), 1069
Intraperitoneal entry, 742
Intrasphincteric botulinum toxin, 218
Intrasphincteric onabotulinumtoxinA injection therapy, 478
Intravaginal pessaries, 594
Intravesical electrostimulation (IVES), 248
Intravesical electrotherapy (IVE), 217
Intrinsic/intramural, 76
Intrinsic properties of the urethra, 79
Intrinsic sphincter deficiency (ISD), 80–81, 327, 411
    imaging, 414
    urodynamic studies, 413–414
Intussuscepted ileal nipple valve, 314
Intussusception method, 1048
Inversion sexuelle, 1211
I-Pouch, 1109–1110
Irritable bowel syndrome, 920, 1001
Ischium, 72
Isotonic irrigating fluids, 184

J
Jejunal conduit, 1046
Jejunum, 1037
"Jumping man" z-plasty, 1091

K
Kaplan's hypothesis, 961
Ketamine cystitis, 1045
Kock ileal neobladder, 1110
Kock neobladder, 1107
Kock nipple valve, 1076
Kock pouch, 1048

L
Labial pedicle grafts, 718–719
Labia majora, 967
Labia minora, 967–968, 1214
Labiaplasty, 1245
    complications, 1247
    composite reduction, 1247
    deepithelialization technique, 1246
    edge resection, 1247
    laser labiaplasty, 1247
    Motakef classification, 1245
    postoperative care, 1247
    wedge resection technique, 1246
    W-shaped resection, 1246
lacZ reporter gene, 492
Lamina propria, 52–53
Laparoendoscopic single-site surgery (LESS), 750, 751
Laparoscopic and transvaginal uterosacral colpopexy, 609
Laparoscopic AUS implantation, 421, 427
Laparoscopic Burch, 450, 453

Laparoscopic or robotic approach for extravesical reimplantation, 900–901
Laparoscopic paravaginal repair
    clinical examination, 538–539
    cystoscopic insertion of ureteric catheters, 541
    cystoscopy and abdominal closure, 544
    diagnostic tests, 539–540
    efficacy and safety of, 545–546
    evaluation of abdominal cavity and abdominopelvic organs, 542
    patient counselling, 540–541
    patient history, 538
    peritoneal cavity, 542
    postoperative care, 544
    pre-operative steps, 541
    technique of, 543–544
Laparoscopic pectopexy, 561–563
Laparoscopic sacrocolpopexy, 553, 620, 622
    prevalence, POP, 553–554
    procedure for POP, 555
    single-port, 565
Laparoscopy, 35
Laparotomy, 1056
Late-plate cells, 491
Lateral pelvic lymph node dissection (LFLD), 295
Latzko procedure, 754
Latzko technique, 771–772
Left labial incision, 864
Leukoplakia, 189
Levator ani, 75
Levator ani muscles, 977
Levator plication or levatorrhaphy, 1009
Lichen sclerosus (LS), 1244
Lich-Gregoir technique, 899–900
Lich-Gregoir ureteroneocystostomy, 1141, 1142
Lidocaine, 940
Lifting and strenuous activity, 1090
LIFT procedure, 815, 816
Light walking, 1090
Liposuction, 1071
Locus coeruleus (LC), 65
Longitudinal vaginal septum, 1203
Long-term bladder function after hysterectomy, 285
Long-term urethral catheterization, 710
Loperamide, 1021
Low anterior resection (LAR), 295, 873
Lower urinary tract, 180, 184, 1040
Lower urinary tract dysfunction (LUTD), 458
    pattern, 460
    sacral lesions, 461
    suprapontine lesions, 459
    suprasacral cord lesions, 459
Lower urinary tract symptoms (LUTS), 72, 79, 82, 115, 185, 208, 224, 465, 858, 859, 861, 865, 1067–1068
Low-resource countries, 687, 1165
Lumbar disc herniation, 464
Lundiana technique, 317
Lymphatic drainage of the vagina, 966

M

Mackenrodt's ligaments, 15
Macroplastique™, 397, 443
Magnetic resonance imaging (MRI), 202, 859
MAINZ I pouch, 1108
Mainz I pouch, 1112–1114
Male urogenital distress inventory (MUDI), 109
Malignancy, 40
Malignant bladder lesions, 191
Manchester operation, 608
Manual dexterity, 480
Markov model, 626
Marshal/Bonney test, 413
Marshall-Marchetti-Krantz (MMK)
    operation, 450
    procedure, 286, 296, 373
Marshall-Marchetti-Krantz repair, 364
Marshall-Marchetti-Krantz retropubic urethrovesical
    suspension procedure, 400
Marshall-Marchetti-Kranz bladder neck suspension
    technique, 538
Marsupialisation technique, 862
Martius fat pad for grafting, 864
Martius flaps, 685, 701, 721, 772–774, 864, 1148
Mast cells, 934
Matrix metalloprotein 2 (MMP-2), 56
Maximum urethral closure pressure (MUCP), 98, 277
Mayer–Rokitanky–Kuster–Hauser (MRKH) syndrome,
    42, 43, 588, 1187, 1241
    antibiotics and bowel preparation, 1191
    classification, 1188
    clinical presentation, 1188
    comparative presentations, 1189
    complications, 1193
    diagnosis, 1188
    neo vaginoplasty, 1190
    pathophysiology, 1187
    psychosocial, group and parental counseling, 1188
    STSG, 1192
    vaginal elongation, 1188
Mayo-McCall culdoplasty, 626
May-Thurner syndrome, 921
McCall's culdoplasty, 603, 611
McKusick-Kaufman syndrome (MKKS), 43, 44
Meatal stenosis, 843, 845, 848, 1229, 1230
Medical, Epidemiological, and Social Aspects of Aging
    (MESA), 101
Medications, 115
Mental sexual arousal, 972
Mercaptoacetyltriglycine-3 (MAG-3), 38
Mesenchymal proliferation, 30
Mesh augmentation, 597
Mesh complications
    abdominal removal, 584
    asymptomatic, 580
    bladder/urethra, 581, 582
    cystoscopy, 578
    dyspareunia and pain, 580
    history, 578
    imaging studies, 578
    infection, 581
    midurethral sling exposure, 582, 583
    physical examination, 578
    rectum, 585, 586
    symptomatic, 580, 581
    ureter, 584
    vaginal approaches, 583, 584
    vaginal mesh exposure, 580
    visceral injury, 581
Mesh erosions, 284, 399, 664
Mesh removal, 402, 403
Mesoappendix, 1113
Metabolic acidosis, 308
Metabolic imbalances, 1107
Meyer-Rokitansky-Küster-Hauser syndrome, 658
Miami pouch, 1048
Micturition, 72, 77–80, 458, 459, 464, 479, 481
Micturition dysfunction
    urinary emptying, abnormalities of, 81–82
    urinary storage, disorders of, 79–81
Micturition patterns, 400
Middle compartment prolapse, 608, 613
Mid-urethral sling (MUS), 129, 279, 281, 283, 286, 287,
    398, 438, 441, 488
    intraoperative complications, 398
    overactive bladder symptoms, 398
    postoperative complications, 399
    retreatment rates, 399
    types, 398
    visceral injury, 398
Mindfulness therapy, 927
Minimal clinically important difference (MCID), 107, 108
Minimal important difference (MID), 108
Minimally invasive prolapse surgery, 553
    cost-effectiveness, 556
    ERAS protocols, 559
    in older women, 555
    vs. open abdominal sacrocolpopexy, 553
    patient selection, 555
    trends in usage of, 554–555
Minimally invasive sacrocolpopexy
    anterior vaginal dissection, 621–622
    complications, 625–626
    cost, 626–627
    dissection of the sacral promontory, 620–621
    future research, 627
    outcomes, 623–625
    patient selection and pre-operative evaluation,
        618–620
    port placement, 620–621
    posterior vaginal dissection, 622
    retroperitonealization of graft, 623
    sacral fixation of graft, 622–623
    sub-peritoneal tunnel creation, 621
    surgical technique, 620
    vaginal fixation of graft, 622
Minimally invasive surgical repair of ureterovaginal
    fistula, 827

Minimally invasive ureteral reimplant, 893–894
Minitape®, 387
Mitrofanoff appendicovesicostomy, 1075–1076
Mitrofanoff CCC, 309
Mitrofanoff/Mainz-type procedure, 849
Mitrofanoff procedure, 724, 1049
Mitrofanoff stoma/procedure, 1108
Mixed augmentation ileum and c(z)ecum, 1112–1114
Mixed urinary incontinence (MUI), 92–93, 324, 522
Monarc™, 386
Mons pubis, 967
Monti/double-Monti channel, 1077
Mood disorders, 975
Motor unit potentials (MUPs), 147
MRI defecography, 1018
Müllerian duct anomalies (MDAs), 1186
Müllerian duct (MD) growth, 32
Müllerian inhibiting substance (MIS), 31
Multicenter analysis, 87
Multichannel UDS assess bladder storage, 468
Multiple sclerosis (MS), 465
Münchausen syndrome, 304
Muscular dystrophies, 491
Musculofascial control, 327
Musculogenic FSD, 977
Mycobacterium tuberculosis, 1044
Mycoplasma genitalium, 917
Myofascial flaps, 701–702, 1152, 1153
Myofascial pain, 356
Myofascial syndrome, 340
    pelviperineal muscle contraction, 340
    postural disorder and global, 340
Myogenic, 210

N
Nantes criteria, 922
National Aeronautics and Space Administration Task Load Index (NASA-TLX), 753
National Cancer Institute Common Terminology Criteria for Adverse Events (CTCAE) tool, 1065
National Center for Complementary and Integrative Health, 231
National Institute for Health and Clinical Excellence (NICE), 98
National Institute of Diabetes and Digestive and Kidney Diseases (NIDDK), 191, 932
National Overactive Bladder Evaluation (NOBLE), 91
National Surgical Quality Improvement Program (NSQIP), 875
National Trauma Data Bank, 842
Necrosis, 1118
Negative predictive value (NPV), 115
Neoadjuvant radiation, 1071
Neourethral reconstructions, 849
Neovaginal reconstruction, 1055–1056
Nephrectomy, 1077
Nephrolithiasis, 872
Nerve conduction latency studies, 174

Nerve growth factor (NGF), 943
Nerve injury, 667, 669
Nerves and nervous pathways, 149
Nerve sparing radical hysterectomy, 285
Neural control, 326
Neuralgia, 266
Neuroanatomy and neurophysiology
    bladder biomechanics, 51–59
    central nervous system, 64–66
    peripheral nervous system, 59–64
Neurogenic, 210
Neurogenic bladder (NGB), 458, 465, 473, 481
Neurogenic detrusor overactivity (NDO), 222, 470
Neurogenic FSD, 976
Neurogenic lower urinary tract dysfunction (NLUTD), 303, 458, 463, 466, 476, 478
    bladder capacity, 1054
    bladder compliance, 1054
    detrusor overactivity, 1054–1055
Neurological control of micturition, 459
Neuromodulation, 216–217, 257, 473, 1022
Neuropathic clitoral pain, 1173–1174
Neuropathic injury, 277
Neurophysiology, 173
Neurotransmitters, 934
Nitric oxide, 943, 974–975
Nitric oxide/cyclic guanosine monophosphate (NO/cGMP), 58
Nocturia-quality of life (N-QOL), 107
Nocturnal incontinence, 847
Noninvasive assisted bladder emptying, 469
Nonionic irrigants, 184
Non-organ-sparing reconstruction
    pelvic exenteration, 1078
    urinary diversion, 1078–1080
Nonsteroidal antiinflammatory drugs (NSAIDs), 927
Nonthrombotic iliac vein lesion, 922
Non-tunneling technique, 636
Non-urological pelvic tumor, 1043–1044
Norepinephrine, 943
Normal detrusor, 164
Nuclear factor kappa B (NF-kB), 1066
Nutcracker syndrome, 921
Nutriments, 227–228
Nutritional abnormalities, 1059

O
Obesity, 224–225, 326, 363, 480
Obstetric fistulas, 679, 681, 686–688, 765, 1147, 1153, 1156, 1158
Obstetric trauma, 710
Obstructed defecation, 1002
Obstructed labor, 696
Obstructive anomalies
    imperforate hymen, 1204
    transverse vaginal septum, 1204
Obstructive sling, 132
Obturator fascia, 73

Obturator internus, 75
Occlusion tests, 215
Occult SUI, 672
O'Conor technique, 744
Office therapy, 239–241
O'Leary-Sant IC Symptom Index and Problem Index score, 937, 938
Omental flap, 774, 1082
Omental pedicle flap, 798
Omentum, *see* Interposing graft
OnabotulinumtoxinA, 471, 472
Onuf's nucleus, 326
Open abdominal sacrocolpopexy, 553
Open abdominal technique, 556
Open Burch colposuspension
    midurethral sling, 365–366
    pubovaginal sling, 366–367
    steps, 367–368
Open surgery neobladders and, 1117
Open trans-abdominal implantation, 418–420
Open trans-vaginal implantation, 420–421
Open ureteral reimplant, 888–890
Operations and pelvic muscle training in the management of apical support loss trial (OPTIMAL), 602
Oral pharmacotherapy, 203
Orchalgia, 917
Organ-sparing reconstruction, 1073
Orgasmic disorder, 962
Orthotopic ileal neobladder, 1103
Orthotopic neobladder, 1049–1050, 1107–1108
    Abol-Enein and Ghoneim pouch, 1111
    components and types, 1050–1051
    continence, 1052
    contraindications, 1050
    Hautmann neobladder, 1110, 1111
    I-Pouch, 1109–1110
    Kock ileal neobladder, 1110
    long term risk, 1119
    outcome, 1120–1121
    Padua ileal neobladder, 1111
    quality of life, 1052
    Studer neobladder, 1109
    T-Pouch, 1110–1111
    urinary retention, 1052
Osmotic laxatives, 1008
Ospemifene, 985
Osteitis pubis, 400
Osteomalacia, 1059
Osteomyelitis/spondylodiscitis, 575, 576, 625
Osteopenia, 1060
Outer (periurethral/extramural) layer, 76
Outlet obstruction, 1025
Ovarian cancer, 1100
Overactive bladder (OAB), 936
Overactive bladder innovative therapy trial (OrBIT), 269
Overactive bladder (OAB) syndrome, 80, 86, 115, 159, 167, 218, 221, 264, 401, 469
    aetio-pathogenesis, 210
    anticholinergics, 215–216
    B3 agonists, 216
    behavioral therapy, 228–230
    biofeedback therapy, 234–239
    bladder irritants, 227
    botulinum toxin, 216
    caffeine, 226–227
    CAM, 231–232
    conservative management, 215
    definition, 91, 208
    electrical stimulation, 239–245
    epidemiology, 91–92
    examination, 211
    fluid intake, 225–226
    food and dietary habits, impact of, 225
    history, 211
    investigations, 213–215
    lifestyle interventions, 223–228
    nutriments, 227–228
    obesity, 224–225
    pelvic floor muscle training, 232–233
    pharmacological management, 215–217
    prevalence, 209
    PTNS, 217
    risk factors, 92
    sacral neuromodulation, 216–217
    self-rehabilitation at home, 245–246
    smoking, 224
    socioeconomic impact, 92
    symptoms of, 222
    urgency inhibition and suppression techniques, 233–234

P

Pad testing, 118, 159
Padua ileal neobladder, 1111
Pad weight test, 412
Painful bladder syndrome, 191
Palliative procedures, 801
Pancake kidneys, 37, 38
Parastomal hernia, 1047
Parasympathetic innervation, 77
Parasympathetic nerves, 276, 277, 295
Paravaginal autonomic nerves, 3D reconstruction, 1104
Paravaginal defect repair, 364, 524, 538, 557
Parkes retractor, 863
Parkinson's disease (PD), 461
Partial urethral injury, 853
Past physical trauma, 975
Pathophysiology
Pathophysiology, of micturition dysfunction, 79–82
Patient global impression of improvement (PGI-I), 104
Patient reported outcome (PRO) data, validated questionnaire
    HRQL, 103–104
    satisfaction, 104
    screening, 100–101
    symptom severity, 101
Pedicled tubularized labia minora flap, 851

Pelvic anatomy and clinical correlations, 72–76
Pelvic area test
   autonomic reflexes, 153
   bulbocavernosus reflex, 152
   motor conduction, 150
   sensory conduction, 151
Pelvic bones, 72
Pelvic congestion syndrome, 921
Pelvic dead space, 1082–1084
Pelvic exenteration, 1078
Pelvic floor disorders (PFD), 86, 92
Pelvic floor dysfunction, 82, 509, 510, 512, 611
Pelvic floor impact questionnaire (PFIQ), 521
Pelvic floor muscle training, 232–233, 594
Pelvic floor musculature, 117
Pelvic floor myofascial pain syndrome, 918
Pelvic floor nerve injury, 277
Pelvic floor physiotherapy, 469
Pelvic floor reconstruction, *see* Female genitourinary
Pelvic floor surgical anatomy, 277
Pelvic floor tension myalgia, 916, 918
Pelvic floor ultrasound
   imaging modalities, 126–127
   pelvic organ prolapse, assessment of, 135–136
   sling and mesh complications, evaluation of, 129–135
Pelvic fracture urethral injury
   algorithm for management of, 848
   anastomotic urethroplasty, 844–845
   artificial urinary sphincter, 847
   bladder flap tube, 850
   bladder neck transection, 845
   bladder wall flap, 851
   clinical presentation, 844
   evaluation, 842–843
   meatus transection, 846
   mid-urethral level transection, 845–846
   Mitrofanoff/Mainz-type procedure, 849
   neourethral reconstructions, 849
   nocturnal incontinence, 847
   outcomes after surgical repair, 849
   proximal urethra level transection, 845–847
   pubectomy, 845–847
   reverse Boari flap, 851
   surgical approach, 845
   surgical reconstruction, 849
   total urethral loss
   urethral loss, 848–853
   vaginal wall flap, 852
Pelvic kidney, 37
Pelvic musculature, 74
Pelvic nervous system, 276
Pelvic organ prolapse (POP), 87, 135, 136, 168, 283, 286, 288–290, 293, 326, 402, 534, 553, 571, 611, 618, 619, 632, 859, 1119
   abdominal sacrocolpopexy (*see* Abdominal sacrocolpopexy)
   abdominal *vs.* vaginal approach, 513
   anatomy, 520
   classification, 508
   clinical presentation, 521
   colpocleisis, 516
   cystoscopy, 523
   definition, 508
   diagnosis, 521
   dynamic imaging, 522
   epidemiology, 87
   etiology, 520
   grafts, 513, 515
   hysterectomy/hysteropexy, 515, 562–564
   incidence and prevalence, 510
   laparoscopic pectopexy, 561–563
   laproscopic *vs.* robotic surgery, 553
   observation, 512
   pelvic floor muscle exercises, 512
   pessaries, 512
   prevalence of a cystocele, 520
   race/ethnicity, 88
   risk factors, 87–88, 510
   socieconomic burden, 88–89
   staging, 508–510
   surgery, 512, 513
   symptoms/presentation, 510, 511
   types, 514
   urodynamics (UDS), 522
   workup, 511, 512
Pelvic organ prolapse distress inventory (POPDI), 603
Pelvic organ prolapse quantification (POPQ) system, 119, 288, 520, 633, 634
Pelvic organ prolapse symptom score (POP-SS), 649
Pelvic organ prolapse/urinary incontinence sexual questionnaire (PISQ-12), 755
Pelvic organs, 76
Pelvic organ support defects, 1002
Pelvic pain, 115
Pelvic physiotherapy, 1021
Pelvic reconstructive surgery, 98
Pelvic surgery, 276, 278–280, 283, 286, 293, 295, 296
Penile skin flap, 1215, 1216
Pentosan polysulfate sodium, 946
Percutaneous nephrostomy tube, 874, 875
Percutaneous nerve evaluation, 260
Percutaneous tibial nerve stimulation (PTNS), 92, 204, 217, 242–245, 473
Periaqueductal gray (PAG), 64, 65, 77
Perineal repair, 1086–1087
Peripheral nervous system
   afferent communication, 60–61
   bladder outlet coordination, 61–62
   parasympathetic, 61
   pudendal, 61
   sympathetic, 61
Peristalsis, 1049
Peritoneal flap
Periurethral and transurethral routes, 449
Periurethral fascia, 862, 864
Periurethral glands, 858
Perivesical fascia, 771
Persistent/recurrent vesicoureteral reflux, 903

Pfannenstiel/transverse incision, 795
Phosphodiesterase 5 inhibitors (PDE5-I), 58, 986
Photosensitizing drugs, 192
Physical exam, 116–118
Physiology
    of stress urinary continence, 78–79
    of urinary storage and emptying, 77–78
Piriformis, 74
Pituitary adenylate cyclase activating polypeptide (PACAP), 60
Plastic reconstructive surgery
    abdominal wall reconstruction, 1080–1082
    abdominoplasty, 1088
    APR sacrectomy vaginectomy, 1083
    APR sacrectomy VRAM, 1083
    APR with vaginectomy, 1085
    bilateral component release, 1081
    bilateral gracilis total vaginectomy, 1087
    component with stoma and mesh, 1082
    drains, 1090
    fascial sparing VRAM for vagina, 1084
    gluteal fold flap, 1089
    gracilis after VRAM resected, 1087
    gracilis vaginal fistula, 1086
    lifting and strenuous activity, 1090
    pelvic dead space, 1082–1084
    perineal repair, 1086–1087
    postoperative revisions, 1091
    primary fascial reapproximation after VRAM with stoma, 1084
    sexual activity, 1090–1091
    sitting protocols, 1089–1090
    vaginal dilation, 1090–1091
    vaginal reconstruction, 1084–1086
    vulvar and perineal defect, 1089
    vulvar repair, 1087–1089
Plastic surgery, 1070–1071
Plateau flow, 161–162
Pneumodissection, 451
Pneumoperitoneum, 564, 620, 799
Poiseuille law, 158
Politano-Leadbetter technique, 898
Politano-Leadbetter ureteroneocystostomy, 1142, 1143
Polytetrafluoroethylene (PTFE), 385, 438
Pontine micturition center (PMC), 64, 65, 77, 256
POP-quantification system, 283
PORTEC-2 trial, 1069
Positive predictive value (PPV), 115
Posterior colporrhaphy, 644, 645, 647
Posterior prolapse, 293
Posterior vaginal repair, 979–980
Post-hysterectomy, 737
Post mid urethral sling surgery, 284
Postoperative dyspareunia, 613
Postoperative Radiation Therapy for Endometrial Cancer (PORTEC-2) trial, 1068
Postoperative urinary retention, 283, 287, 293
Post void residual (PVR), 121–122, 126, 279, 280, 331, 466

Potassium channel blockers, 59
Potassium chloride test, 940, 941
Potts scissors, 890
Practica Copiosa, 9
Prader classification, 1205
Prefrontal cortex, 65
Premature ejaculation, 343
Pre-operative urodynamics, 737
Pressure-flow studies, 165–169
Primary bladder neck obstruction, 82, 200
Proctalgia fugax, 920
Profunda artery perforator (PAP) flap, 1085
Projected isovolumetric pressure (PIP), 214
Prolapse, 115
Prolapse repair, 595, 619, 621
Prolonged flow, 160
Protophallus anterior, 30
Protruding stoma, 1042
Prune belly syndrome, 1045
Psoas hitch technique, 877–878, 888, 890–891, 894
Psychometric analysis
    feasibility, 105–106
    linguistic and cultural validation, 108
    reliability, 106
    responsiveness, 108
    validity, 106–107
Psychosomatic mechanism, 961
Pubectomy, 845–847
Pubis, 72
Pubocervical fascia (PCF), 72
Pubococcygeus, 75
Pubococcygeus muscles, 277, 278
Puborectalis, 75
Pubourethral ligaments (PUL), 73, 708
Pubovaginal slings (PVS), 372, 374–376, 379–381, 384, 386, 388, 399, 400, 663
Pubovesical fascia, 772
Pubovesical ligaments, 277
Pudendal entrapment, 334
    anatomy, 334
    arterial aspects, 345
    associated pathology, 346
    clinical aspects, 342
    compression, 338
    conservative treatment, 350
        drugs, 352
        postural control, 351
        postural physiotherapy, 351
        psychiatric support, 352
        pudendal nerve infiltratio, 352
    contralateral decompensation, 356
    diagnosis
        clinical exam, 346, 347
        complementary exams, 348
        digital examination, 347
        infiltration test, 349
        nantes criteria, 350
        patient history, 346
    differential diagnosis, 336

Pudendal entrapment (cont.)
    epidemiology, 337
    erectile dysfunction, 352
    external factors, 338
    hypersensitivity of neurons, 356
    laparoscopic pudendal decompression, 353
        decompression, 354
        hernia, 353
        postoperative recovery, 354
        second-line treatment after failure, 356
        umbilical artery, 353
    myofascial pain, 356
    myofascial syndrome, 340
    neurological aspects, 343
        motor fibers, 344
        sensory fibers, 343
        sympathetic fibers, 343
    nocturnal symptoms, 342
    pyriformis muscle, 339
    sport activity, 343
    stretching, 338
    stretching problem, 356
    trigger event, 341
    uterosacral ligament, 339
    venous aspects, 345
Pudendal nerve, 265
    branches, 266
    complications of pudendal neuromodulation, 267
    damage to, 266
    pudendal neuromodulation, 266–267
Pudendal nerve terminal motor latency (PNTML), 1020, 1021
Pudendal neuralgia, 922
Pudendal neuropathy, 151
PureWick™ female external catheter, 475

Q
Q-tip test, 116, 412
Quality-adjusted life year (QALY), 87, 103
Quality of life (QoL), 101, 211, 649
Quantitative sensory tests, 141
Questionnaire
    scale development, 104
    scale evaluation with psychometric analysis, 105
    theorization and item development, 104

R
Radiation
    cystitis, 188
    rectovaginal fistula (RVF), 808
Radiation induced fistulae, 800–801
Radiation therapy (RT) in pelvic cancer, 1064
    anti-Iincontinence surgery, 1073–1074
    bladder augmentation, 1074–1075
    bladder neck closure, 1074
    bladder neck reconstruction, 1073
    clinical presentation, 1065
    conservative/non-reconstructive, 1072
    continent urinary diversion (see Continent urinary channels)
    epidemiology, 1065
    fibrosis, 1068–1069
    genitourinary complications, 1067
    hemorrhagic cystitis, 1068
    incontinent ileovesicostomy, 1075
    lower urinary tract symptoms (LUTS), 1067–1068
    non-organ-sparing reconstruction
        (see Non-organ-sparing reconstruction)
    organ-sparing reconstruction, 1073
    plastic surgery, 1070–1071
    radiation stigmata, 1071
    secondary malignancy, 1069–1070
    sexual dysfunction, 1069
    supravesical diversion, 1077–1078
    urethroplasty, 1073
    urethrovaginal fistula, 697
    urinary fistulae, 1068
    urinary strictures, 1068–1069
    urinary tract reconstruction, 1073
    urology, 1070
Radiation Therapy Oncology Group (RTOG), 1066, 1067
Radical cystectomy, 983, 1101, 1120
Radical hysterectomy, 285, 295
Raised U-shaped vaginal flap, 864
Randomized controlled trials (RCTs), 98
Reconstructive plastic surgery, 1065
Reconstructive surgery, 218
Rectal barostat test, 1007
Rectal cancers, 983
Rectal exam, 118
Rectal intussusception, 1018
Rectal prolapse, 1026, 1027
    diagnoses, 1026
    ventral mesh rectopexy, 1027
Rectoanal manovolumetry, 1020
Rectoceles, 508, 670
    graft-augmented posterior colporrhaphy, 645–646
    site-specific posterior colporrhaphy, 645
    traditional posterior colporrhaphy, with midline plication, 645
    ventral rectopexy, abdominal sacrocolpopexy, 646–647
Rectopexy, 1010
Rectovaginal fascia, 644
Rectovaginal fistula (RVF), 671, 682, 683
    abdominal approach, 817
    cancers, 808
    chronic inflammation, 807
    clinical presentation, 809
    endoanal and transperineal ultrasounds, 811
    endorectal advancement flap (ERAF), 815, 816
    etiology, 809
    expectant management, 812
    fistula-tract laser closure (FiLaC) procedure, 817
    fistulotomy, 815
    incidence, 806

inflammatory bowel disease, 807
LIFT procedure, 815, 816
location, 808
medical management, 812–813
obstetric causes, 806–807
optimization prior to surgical repair, 814–815
physical exam, 809–810
postoperative complications, 817–818
postsurgical care and expectations, 817
prosthetic insertions, 813–814
radiation, 808
seton placement, 812–813
"simple" vs. "complex," 809
size, 808
surgeries, 807–808
tissue flaps, 816–817
transanal or transrectal repair, 815
transperineal ultrasound, 811–812
vaginal repairs, 815
vaginography/anal manography, 811, 812
video-assisted fistula repair, 817
Rectus abdominis muscle flaps, 702, 721
Rectus fascia, 72
Rectus fascial sling, 380, 382
Recurrent UTI (rUTI), 284, 285, 469, 577, 862
Refluxing system, 37
Regenerative technologies, 489
Reliability, 106
Renal and bladder ultrasound, 468
Renal deterioration, 1058
Renal fusion anomalies, 37
Renal insufficiency, 305
Renal sonogram, 736
Reoperative ureteral reimplantation, 903
Reproducibility, 106
Resiniferatoxin, 948
Responsiveness, 108
Retrograde pyelogram, 736
Retroperitonealization of graft, 623
Retropubic approach, 419
Retropubic colposuspension, 450, 451, 453
Retropubic suspension operations
    age, 363
    comorbidities, 363
    concomitant detrusor overactivity, 363
    concomitant prolapse, 364
    contraindications, 363
    indications, 363
    Marshall-Marchetti-Krantz repair, 364
    obesity, 363
    paravaginal repair and vagino-obturator shelf repair, 364
    patient selection, 363–364
    previous SUI surgeries, 363
Retropubic tension-free vaginal tape (TVT), 398
Retropubic urethrovesical suspension procedures, 400
Reverse Boari flap, 851
Reversible causes of incontinence, 469
Revised female sexual distress scale (FSDS-R), 755

Rhabdosphincter, 326
Rheumatological disorders, 926
Rigid cystourethroscopy, 181, 183
Rigid endoscopes, 181
Ripstein procedure, 1027
Robot-assisted radical cystectomy, 1115
Robot-assisted sacrocolpopexy, 553
    da Vinci surgical system, 554
    ergonomics of surgery, 556
    prevalence, POP, 554
    procedure for POP, 555
    single-port, 565
Robotic-assisted Burch colposuspension, 451
Robotic-assisted implantation, 421–425, 428
Robotic-assisted laparoscopy, 744
Robotic Burch procedure, 451
Robotic surgery, 618, 624, 626
Robotic ureteroureterostomy, 881–882
RVF, see Rectovaginal fistula (RVF)

S
Sacral and peripheral nervous system lesions
    cauda equina syndrome (CES), 464
    diabetes, 464
    lumbar disc herniation, 464
    multiple sclerosis (MS), 465
Sacral fixation, 622
Sacral lesions, 461
Sacral nerve entrapment, 602
Sacral nerve modulation, 1022
Sacral nerve stimulation (SNS), 92
Sacral neuromodulation (SNM), 203, 216–217, 473, 474, 1022
Sacral plexus, 257
    chronic pelvic pain, 265
    complications for SNM, 261
    indications, 264
    nerve branches of, 258
    overactive bladder, 264
    percutaneous nerve evaluation, 260
    programming, 261–264
    staged sacral neuromodulation, 258–260
    urinary retention, 265
Sacral tumor, 925
Sacrospinous ligament (SSL), 73, 595, 596
Sacrospinous ligament fixation (SSLF)
    complications, 599, 600
    surgical technique, 598, 599
Sacrotuberous ligament, 73
Sacrum, 72
Salpingo-oophorectomy, 636
Satellite cells, 491
Schistosoma haematobium, 1045
    infection, 192
Schistosomiasis, 1044–1045
Sciatic nerve injury, 600
Scientific Committee on Emerging and Newly Identified Health Risks (SCENIHR) report, 572

Scottish Intercollegiate Guidelines Network (SIGN), 98
Secondary malignancy, 1069–1070
Seldinger technique, 260
Self-Assessment Goal Attainment (SAGA), 104
Self-rehabilitation, 245–246
Self-reported questionnaires, 119–121
Sensory-type C fibers, 948
Seton, 812–813
Sexual abuse, 975
Sexual activity, 1090–1091
Sexual arousal disorder, 961, 962
Sexual aversion disorder, 962
Sexual counselling, 945
Sexual differentiation, 32
Sexual dysfunction, 960, 1069
Sexual function, 1078
Sexual pain disorder, 962
Sheath approximation (Gil-Vernet) technique, 898–899
Sigmoidoplasty, 658
Sildenafil, 947, 975
Silicone catheters, 471
Silk fibroin microspheres, 498
Single incision sling (SIS), 398
Single-port robotic, 752
SISTEr trial, 453
Site-specific posterior colporrhaphy, 645
Site-specific posterior vaginal repair, 1009
Sitting protocols, 1089–1090
Sjogren syndrome, 935
Skeletal muscle, 491
Skene's glands, 858
Sling erosion, 132–134
Sling failure, 130
Slings, 661–663
Small fiber polyneuropathy, 912, 926
Smoking, 224
Smooth sphincter dyssynergia, 82
Social support, 480
Society of Urodynamics, Female Pelvic Medicine and Urogenital Reconstruction (SUFU), 576
Somatic efferent pathways, 277
Somatic innervation, 76
Somatosensory evoked potentials (SEPs), 150
Spatulated nipple technique, 899
Spatulated ureteroureterostomy, 1141, 1156
Spence-Duckett marsupialization procedure, 661
Sphincteroplasty, 1022, 1023
Sphincters, 76
Spina bifida/myelomeningocele (SB/MM), 464
Spina bifida occulta, 923
Spinal cord injury (SCI), 463, 976
Spinal dysraphism, 904
Spinelli technique, 266
Spinobulbospinal reflex pathways, 78
Spiral Monti, 311
Split thickness skin graft (STSG), 1191
Squamous cell carcinomas, 193
Stamey endoscopic needle suspension, 286
STAR method, 266

Stimulant laxatives, 1008
Stomach, 1037
Stoma incontinence, 1120
Stress incontinence, 453, 454
Stress urinary continence, physiology of, 78–79
Stress urinary incontinence (SUI), 98, 279, 286, 288, 290–292, 324, 372, 438, 439, 441, 444, 445, 450, 521, 659–661, 672, 699, 709, 1119
  abnormal physiology, 327
  adipose-derived stem cells, 497–499
  age, 325
  animal models for, 489–490
  anti-incontinence procedures, 401
  AUS, 401, 402
  autologous slings, 374–380
  Burch colposuspension, 400
  cadaveric slings, 380–381
  cystoscopy, 331, 413
  definition, 89, 362, 408
  epidemiology, 89
  evaluation of recurrent or persistent after AUS implantation, 432–433
  history of present illness, 328
  history of stress incontinence management, 372–374
  intra-abdominal pressure, 396
  management for women with, 488
  medications, family history, social history and review of systems, 328–329
  mesh removal, 402, 403
  MUS, 398–399
  musculofascial control, 327
  neural control, 326
  normal physiology and continence, 326–327
  obesity, 326
  pad weight, 330
  paraclinical testing, 413
  past medical history, 328
  past surgical history, 328
  pathophysiology, 326–327
  patient medical history, 411–412
  patient-reported measures, 412
  physical exam, 329–330
  physical examination, 412–413
  POP, 326
  post-void residual, 331
  pregnancy, 325
  prevalence and risk factors, 324–326, 408
  on prolapse reduction, 327
  PVS, 399, 400
  race/ethnicity, 90, 326
  rates of complications, 576
  risk factors, 89–90
  smoking status, 326
  socioeconomic impact, 90–91
  surgery, 396, 403
  synthetic slings, 382–387
  treatments for women with, 409
  UBAs, 396–398
  UDS, 331

Index 1273

urethrolysis, 402
urinalysis, 330
urinary tract infection, 577
use of AUS in women (see Artificial urinary sphincter (AUS))
voiding diary, 330
voiding dysfunction, 577
xenografts, 381–382
Strictures, 661, 664, 670, 1137, 1138, 1143, 1150, 1157
Studer neobladder, 1107
Subjective arousal, 972
Sub-peritoneal tunnel, 621
Substance P (SP), 60
Subtotal hysterectomy, 285
Suburethral hammock, 277
Sudeck's point, 1039
Suprameatal urethrolysis with Martius flap (SMUM), 288
Suprapontine lesions, 459
    cerebral palsy, 461
    cerebrovascular accidents (CVA), 461
    dementia, 461
    Parkinson's disease (PD), 461
Suprasacral cord lesions, 459
Suprasacral lesions
    spina bifida/myelomeningocele (SB/MM), 464
    spinal cord injury (SCI), 463
Supravesical diversion, 1077–1078
Surfactants, 1008
Surgeon ergonomics, 753
Swedish cost-analysis study, 91
Sympathetic fibers, 1103
Sympathetic innervation, 76
Sympathetic preganglionic pathways, 276
Sympathetic skin response (SSR), 153
Synthetic mesh materials
    abdominal sacrocolpopexy, 574
    anterior compartment mesh, 574
    Australia, 572
    Canada, 571, 572
    characteristics, 572
    European Union, 572
    loss of vaginal length/canal stenosis, 588
    mesh excision, 578, 580, 581, 586
    mesh wight, 573
    New Zealand, 572
    osteomyelitis/spondylodiscitis, 575, 576
    pelvic organ prolapse (POP), 571
    persistent/worsening pain, 587
    polypropylene mesh, 573
    pore size, 572, 573
    posterior compartment mesh, 574
    recurrent prolapse, 587, 588
    recurrent vaginal mesh exposure, 588
    regenerative medicine, 589
    risk factors, 573, 574
    sacrocolpopexy, 589
    sacrocolpopexy surgery, 574
    short-and-long-term complications, 570
    surgical management options, 588, 589
    surgical repair of POP, 570
    synthetic midurethral sling removal, 586, 587
    terminology, 570
    transvaginal mesh, 589
    United Kingdom, 572
    United States, 571, 572
    vaginal dilation, 588
    vaginal mesh trends, 574
Synthetic midurethral slings, 476
Synthetic sling surgery, 382–387, 725
Synthetic suburethral sling, 281

T
Tabulae Anatomicae, 9
Tamm-Horsfall protein, 934
Tanagho bladder flap urethroplasty, 720
Tanagho flap, 850, 851
Tandem cystoscopy, 736
Tanezumab, 947
Tanner staging chart, 1188
Tapered tunneled ureteral reimplant, 894
Tarlov cysts, 923
Teflon™, 438
Tension-free vaginal tapes (TVT), 376, 382, 384–386, 453, 1119
Testis-determining factor (TDF), 31
Testosterone, 31, 976
Tethered spinal cord, 923
Therapeutics, 62–63
3D-conformal radiation therapy (3D-CRT), 1064
3D ultrasound, 129, 132, 134–136
Tibial nerve, 268
    complications of PTNS, 269
    percutaneous tibial nerve stimulation, 269
    stimulation, 473
Tissue flaps, 816–817
Tissue inhibitor metalloproteiniase 2 (TIMP-2), 56
Tissue sealants, 739
Total abdominal hysterectomy (TAH), 738
Total urogenital mobilization (TUM), 1203, 1240
T-Pouch, 1107, 1110–1111
Tramadol, 352
Transabdominal repair, VVF, 793
    abdominal incision, 795
    bladder closure, 798
    cystoscopy, 794–795
    drains, 798
    excision of the fistula tract, 795
    interposition tissue flap, 796
    leak testing, 798
    omental pedicle flap, 798
    patient positioning, 794
    reconstructive principles, 794
    steps of VVF repair, 794
    vaginal closure, 798
Transabdominal surgery, 597
Transabdominal ultrasound, 126
Transabdominal ureteroneocystostomy, 825

Transanal/transrectal repair, 815
Transcutaneous electrical nerve stimulation (TENS), 204, 241–242, 244, 473
Transcutaneous tibial nerve stimulation (TTNS), 473
Transforming growth factor beta-1 (TGF-ß1), 1066
Transgender woman
  genital reconstructive surgeries, 1211
  preoperative appearance, 1213
  vaginal reconstruction, 1212
Transgluteal approach, 268
Transient receptor potential (TRP) channels, 52
Transitional cell carcinoma, 188
Translabial, 135
Translabial ultrasound (TLUS), 579, 582
Transobturator (TOT), 398
Transobturator midurethral sling, 287, 291
Transobturator sling, 853
Transperineal imaging, 126, 129
Transperineal ultrasound, 811–812
Transplant kidney ureteroneocystostomy, 904
Transureteroureterostomy, 879, 880, 890
Transurethral incision of the bladder neck (TUIBN), 479
Transvaginal approaches, 768–771, 860–862
Transvaginal mesh (TVM) repair, 283
Transvaginal needle suspension procedures, 373
Transvaginal sacrospinous fixation procedure, 980
Transvaginal slings (TVT), 91
Transvaginal surgical repair
  anatomic considerations, 594, 595, 597
  apical defects, 594
  surgical options, 603–604
  techniques, 597–603
  vaginal approach, 597
Transvaginal ultrasound, 790
Transvaginal urethral diverticulectomy, 862
Transverse defect repair, 524
Transversely tubularized bowel segments (TTBS), 310–312
Transverse vaginal septum, 843
Transvesical approach, 744
Trattner catheter, 860
Traumatic urethral injury, 710–711, 851
Trial of Mid-Urethral Slings (TOMUS), 98
Trimethroprim-sulfamethoxazole, 184
Tubularised labia minora, 1152, 1153
Tubularized vaginal flap urethroplasty, 714–715
Tunneling technique, 635
2D dynamic ultrasound, 134

U

Ueteroureterostomy, 1140, 1146, 1151, 1152, 1156
Ulcers, 191
Ultrasonography, 860, 915
Ultrasound
  assessment of pain, 134–135
  dynamic imaging, 129
  multiple slings, patient with, 134
  obstructive sling, 132

  pelvic organ prolapse, assessment of, 135–136
  sling erosion, 132–134
  sling failure, 130
  transabdominal ultrasound, 126
  video urodynamics, 129
Umbilical cord blood stem cells, 500
Underactive bladder (UAB), 218, 474
  causes of, 246
  conservative management, 217, 247–248
  definition, 209
  electrical stimulation, 217–218
  examination, 211
  history, 211
  intrasphincteric botulinum toxin, 218
  investigations, 213–215
  long-term effects of, 246
  pharmacotherapies, 217
  prevalence of, 209, 246
  reconstructive surgery, 218
Underactive outlets, 475
Unilateral renal agenesis, 39
UPOINT system, 938, 939
Upper tract imaging, 736
Upper urinary tract, 1040
Ureaplasma, 917
Ureteral defects, 872
  Boari flap, 878
  buccal mucosa, 882
  diagnosis, 874
  endoscopic management, 875–876
  iatrogenic ureteral injuries, 873–874
  ileal ureter, 880–881
  malignancy, 873
  preoperative stenting, 874–875
  psoas hitch, 877–878
  radiation, 872–873
  robotic and laparoscopic approaches, 881
  robotic ureteroureterostomy, 881–882
  timing of repair, 874
  transureteroureterostomy, 880
  trauma, 873
  ureteroneocystostomy, 877, 882
  ureteroureterostomy, 876–877
Ureteral dilation, 823, 875
Ureteral injuries, 666, 822–824, 826, 827, 886, 887
  anatomy, 1131
  anti-refluxing technique, 1146
  augmentation ileocystoplasty, 1144
  boari flap, 1143
  bowel injuries, 1152
  classification, 1132
  colorectal injuries, 1134
  colorectal surgery, 1134
  ECOG score, 1155
  ECOG status, 1156
  endoscopy findings, 1135
  epidemiology, 1132, 1133
  excision of tissue, 1151
  external thermal injuries, 1134

Index   1275

  fistula management, 1155
  gynaecological Injuries, 1133
  gynecological injuries, 1133, 1134
  injuries involving the trigone, 1146
  intra-operative, 1138
  laser lithotripsy, 1135
  mucosal tears, 1148
  at multiple levels, 1148
  obstetric fistula, 1147
  obstetric injuries, 1133
  partial/complete occlusion, 1150
  partial tears, 1149
  post-operative, 1139
  prevention. 1138
  radiotherapy, 1156
  risk factors, 1131
  spinal surgery, 1134
  stable patient, 1140
  stricture formation, 1156
  surgical procedures, 1132
  tension-free water-tight repair, 1139
  timing, position, level of injury, 1145
  transection tears, 1150
  transureteroureterostomy, 1144
  ureter, 1154
  ureteral dilatation, 1135
  ureteroureterostomy, 1141
  urethra, 1150
  urethral dilatation, 1138
  urethral diverticulum repair, 1137, 1138
  urogenital fistula, 1137, 1138
  urogynecological surgery, 1137
  urological injuries, 1134, 1135
  uteropelvic junction, 1145
  vagina, 1154
  vascular injury, 1154
  vascular surgery, 1134
Ureteral injury, 886–888
Ureteral kinking/injury, 600
Ureteral obstruction, 669, 874
Ureteral orifices, 743
Ureteral reconstruction, 825, 886–888
Ureteral reimplantation, 886
  anti-refluxing techniques, 895
  Barry technique, 901
  bladder closing, 900
  Boari flap, 890–893
  Boari-Ockerblad flap, 888
  into bowel segment, 904–905
  closing the bladder, 899
  complications, 895, 902
  cross-trigonal (Cohen) ureteral reimplantation technique, 897–898
  da Vinci Xi system, 893
  detrusorrhaphy (Hodgson-Firlit-Zaontz) technique, 902
  dissecting down to bladder, 900
  duplication anomalies, 903–904
  endoscopic management, 887

  external tunnel (Barry) technique, 901–902
  extravesical reimplantation, 899
  extravesical ureteral reimplantation, 899
  Glenn-Anderson technique, 898
  indications, 887–888, 895, 896
  initial dissection, 896
  intraextravesical (Politano-Leadbetter) technique, 898
  intraextravesical technique (Paquin), 902
  intravesical techniques, 896
  laparoscopic or robotic approach, 900–901
  laparoscopic or robotic approach for extravesical reimplantation, 901, 902
  Lich-Gregoir technique, 899, 900
  minimally invasive ureteral reimplant, 893–894
  obstruction, 903
  open Lich-Gregoir technique, 899–900
  open ureteral reimplant, 888–890
  patient positioning, 896, 897, 900
  patient positioning and dissecting down to the bladder, 899
  persistent or recurrent vesicoureteral reflux, 903
  persistent/recurrent vesicoureteral reflux, 903
  Politano-Leadbetter technique, 899
  postoperative management, 895, 902
  postoperative obstruction, 902–903
  preoperative considerations, 887–888, 895, 896
  psoas hitch, 890–891
  psoas hitch technique, 890
  reimplant into bowel segment, 904
  reoperation, 903
  sheath approximation (Gil-Vernet) technique, 898–900
  spatulated nipple technique, 899
  transplant kidney, 904
  transplant kidney ureteroneocystostomy, 904
  ureteral advancement (Glenn-Anderson) technique, 898
  ureter mobilization, 896–897
  ureteroneocystostomy with tapering, 894–895
Ureteral stents, 875, 887–891, 893–895, 902–904, 1108, 1112
Ureteral stricture, 887, 888, 904
Ureteral trauma, 887
Ureteric and urethral catheters, 864
Ureteric bud anomalies, 37–40
Ureteric stricture, 1119
Uretero-ileal conduit, 317–318
Ureterointestinal anastomosis, 1041–1042
Ureteroneocystostomy, 826, 877, 882
  See also Ureteral reimplantation
Ureterorenoscopy, 1134, 1149
Ureteroscopy, 874
Ureterosigmoidostomy, 315, 1052–1053
Ureteroureterostomy, 876–877
Ureterovaginal fistula
  cystoscopy, 823
  definition, 822
  endoscopic management, 824
  etiology, 822
  imaging, 823

Ureterovaginal fistula (*cont.*)
   surgical management, 825–827
   symptoms, 822
   vaginoscopy, 822
Ureters, 188
Ureter substitution, 1055
Urethra, 116–117, 1217
Urethral and vaginal closure, 864
Urethral atrophy, 402
Urethral avulsion injury, 712, 843–845, 847, 853
Urethral bulking agents (UBAs)
   Bulkamid, 441
   coaptite, 442, 443
   complications, 396
   durasphere, 442
   history, 438
   individual analyses, 396, 398
   injection techniques, 440, 441
   intrinsic sphincter deficiency, 396
   macroplastique, 443
   mechanism of action, 439, 440
   periurethral technique, 396
   transurethral technique, 396
   urolastic (Urogyn BV), 443
Urethral caruncle, 116
Urethral crest, 185
Urethral diverticulectomy, 830, 833
Urethral diverticulum, 186
Urethral erosion, 279, 284, 296, 399, 401
Urethral fistulas, 1229
Urethral hypermobility, 80
Urethral injections, 439
Urethral injuries, 398
   bladder, 1151
   bladder flaps, 1152
   dilatation, 1138
   diverticulum repair, 1137
   gracilis flaps, 1152
   tubularised labia minora, 1152
   urogynaecological surgery, 1137
   vaginal tissue, 1152
Urethral meatus, 116
Urethral mobility, 116
Urethral pressure profile, 171–173
Urethral prolapse/caruncle repair, 661
Urethral reconstruction
   anterior proximal vaginal flap urethroplasty, 713–714
   autologous fascial pubovaginal sling, 725–726
   bladder flaps, 719–721
   bladder neck closure, 722–725
   labial pedicle grafts, 718–719
   outcomes of vaginal flap reconstruction, 715–718
   primary closure or anastomotic repair, 713
   repair after eroded synthetic sling, 725
   timing of extensive, 712
   tubularized vaginal flap urethroplasty, 714–715
   urinary diversion, 725
Urethral slings, 476
Urethral stricture, 849, 853

Urethral stricture formation, 1157
Urethra open post-diverticulectomy, 864
Urethra-sparing cystectomy, 1104
Urethra-sparing radical cystectomy, 1102
Urethritis, 917
Urethrocele, 508
Urethro-cystoscopy, 202
Urethrolysis, 402
Urethropelvic ligaments, 708, 858
Urethroplasty, 833, 837, 838, 1073
Urethrovaginal fistula, 682, 844–847, 849 851, 853, 861
   in adults, 694
   clinical presentation, 698
   diagnosis, 694, 698–700
   epidemiology, 694–695
   etiology and pathogenesis, 696–697
   inflammation, 697
   postsurgical (iatrogenic), 697
   prevention, 697–698
   radiation therapy, 697
   risk factors, 695–696
   traumatic injury, 697
   treatment and outcomes, 700–703
Urethrovaginal/vesicovaginal fistula repair, 659
Urethrovesical junction (UVJ), 185
Uretic stents, 1118
Urgency, 208
Urgency urinary incontinence (UUI), 208, 324, 522, 699
Urinalysis, 121, 279, 330, 413, 466
Urinary bladder, 256
Urinary distress inventory (UDI) questionnaire, 624
Urinary diversion, 302, 725, 801, 1078–1080
   bladder dysfunction, 1044–1045
   classification, 1101
   congenital urogenital anomalies, 1045
   continent cutaneous, 315–317
   follow-up, 1122–1123
   immediate postoperative patient care, 1116–1117
   incontinent, 317–318
   malignancy, 1042–1044
   orthotopic neobladder, 1107–1108
   orthotopic or heterotopic, 1102–1105
   outcomes, 1120
   patient selection, 1105–1106
   preoperative patient preparation, 1106
   reservoir, 1106–1107
   robot-assisted surgery, 1115–1116
Urinary emptying, 77
   abnormalities of, 81–82
Urinary fistulae, 1068
Urinary incontinence (UI), 208, 324, 466, 1230
   definition, 89
   prevalence, 89
Urinary incontinence in female neurologic patient
   adjustable continence devices, 477
   antimuscarinic medications, 470
   artificial urinary sphincters (AUS), 477
   beta-3-adrenergic receptor agonists, 470
   bladder neck closure, 477

Index 1277

bladder outlet, 474
cannabinoids, 471
caring for patients, 479
catheterization, 471
chemodenervation, 471
cognition, 480
combined storage and emptying disorders, 479
conservative measures, 469
desmopressin, 471
end stage bladder dysfunction, 474
intrasphincteric botox, 478
manual dexterity, 480
neuromodulation, 473
obesity, 480
overactive bladder, 469
overactive outlet, 478
perioperative considerations, 481
pharmacologic therapies, 475, 478
reversible causes of incontinence, 469
sacral neuromodulation, 473
social support and caregivers, 480
surgical management, 475
transcutaneous/percutaneous options, 473
transurethral incision of bladder Neck (TUIBN), 479
underactive bladder, 474
underactive outlet, 475
urethral bulking, 476
urethral slings, 476
Urinary infection, 859
Urinary leakage, 822, 823
Urinary microbiome, 944
Urinary obstruction, 1057
Urinary reservoir, 304, 305, 309
Urinary retention, 198, 662, 1229
  bladder drainage, 203
  etiology of, 199
  history and physical exam, 201–202
  investigations, 202
  oral pharmacotherapy, 203
  pathophysiology of, 201
  surgical therapy, 203–204
Urinary stoma, 1042
Urinary storage, 72, 77–79, 82
Urinary strictures, 1068–1069
Urinary symptoms/signs, 58–59
Urinary tract, 1228–1229
  bleeding, 1228–1229
  neuroanatomy of, 76–77
  prevention, 1229
Urinary tract fistulae, 189
Urinary tract infections (UTIs), 208, 279, 285, 440, 442, 660, 917, 1058, 1118, 1119
Urinary tract injuries, 454
Urinary tract reconstruction, 1073
Urinary tract repair, 1139, 1140
Urinary urgency, 283, 286, 344
Urinoma or abscess, 823
Urodynamic assessment, 82, 200

Urodynamics, 127–129, 379, 940
Urodynamic studies (UDS), 158, 202, 280, 281, 283, 331, 522, 712, 1040
  ambulatory urodynamics, 170–171
  cystometry and pressure-flow studies, 162–169
  in female settings, 158
  neurophysiology, 173
  pad testing, 159
  urethral pressure profile, 171–173
  uroflowmetry (*see* Uroflowmetry)
  videourodynamics, 169–170
  voiding diaries, 159
Uroflowmetry, 159, 467, 1040
  detrusor overactivity, 160
  intermittent flow, 160
  normal flow, 160
  plateau flow, 161–162
  prolonged flow, 160
  PVR determination, 162
Urogenital distress inventory (UDI-6), 101, 283
Urogenital fistulae, 678, 788, 1137, 1138, 1175
  aetiology of, 680
  classification system, 678
  diagnosis of, 682
  female genital mutilation (FGM), 681
  HES data, 681
  maternal mortality ratio, 679, 680
  outcomes, 688–690
  resource-limited countries, 679, 682
  schematic representation of, 678
  symptoms, 682
  treatment, 684, 685, 687
  urethral catheterisation, 687
Urogenital trauma, 1168
Urogenital tuberculosis, 1044
Urogynaecology, 548
Urolastic (Urogyn BV), 443
Urolithiasis, 1057–1058
Urologic, 76
Urological cystourethroscopes, 181
Urologic laparoscopic procedures, 451
Uroneurophysiological tests, 153
Urothelial cancer, 1100
Urothelium, 51–52
U-shaped vaginal flap, 863, 864
USLS *vs.* SSLF, 602, 603
Uterine preservation procedure, 609
Uterine-preserving techniques, 554
Uterine prolapse, 5, 608, 612
Uterosacral ligaments (USL), 74, 595, 596
Uterosacral ligament suspension (USLS), 559–562, 609
  complications, 601, 602
  surgical technique, 600, 601
Uterovaginal prolapse, 608
  hysterectomy (*see* Vaginal hysterectomy)
Utero-vesical fistulae (UtVF), 682, 687
Uterus, 118, 603

V

Vagina, 965–966
Vaginal agenesis
   complications, 1243
   creatsas modification, 1242
   Davydov procedure, 1242
   Mcindoe procedure, 1243
   MRKH syndrome, 1241
   sigmoid vaginoplasty, 1243
   Vecchietti procedure, 1242
Vaginal anatomy, 825
Vaginal apex, 595
Vaginal approach, 597
Vaginal canal dissection, 1213
Vaginal complications, 1230, 1231
Vaginal cuff cellulitis, 668
Vaginal dilatation, 1090–1091, 1248
Vaginal estrogen therapy, 403
Vaginal flap, 700–701, 836
   advancement, 815
Vaginal hypoplasia, 1186
Vaginal hysterectomy, 286, 292, 665–669, 873
   concomitant bilateral oophorectomy, 612
   genital prolapse prevention, 611
   ileococcygeal fixation, 613
   and pelvic organ prolapse, 610–611
   postoperative dyspareunia, 613
   role of, 610–611
   on sexual function, 612
   vault dehiscence, 612
Vaginal laceration, 844, 847
Vaginal mesh exposure, 584
Vaginal mesh kits, 604
Vaginal mesh surgery, 663–669
Vaginal packing, 671
Vaginal posterior compartment prolapse
   biologic graft, 647–648
   concomitant intussusception/rectal prolapse, 650
   recurrent prolapse, 650
   surgical outcomes, 647–650
   surgical repair for rectoceles, 645–647
   synthetic delayed-absorbable mesh, 648
   synthetic permanent mesh and biologic graft, 648–649
   synthetic permanent polypropylene mesh *vs.* biologic graft, 649
Vaginal prolapse, 632
Vaginal prolapse repair, 669–672
Vaginal reconstruction, 1084–1086
Vaginal rejuvenation
   anterior colporrhaphy, 1248
   carbon dioxide lasers, 1249
   Er:YAG laser, 1249
   posterior colporrhaphy, 1248
   PRP and fillers, 1249
   radiofrequency therapy (RF), 1249
Vaginal repairs, 815
Vaginal salt packing, 696
Vaginal septa, 1204
Vaginal stenosis, 843, 845, 848–850, 852, 1069

Vaginal vault, 117–119
Vaginal wall flap, 770, 852
Vaginismus, 962, 963
Vaginography, 812
Vagino-obturator shelf repair, 364
Vaginoplasty, 658–659, 1055–1056, 1215
   bowel vaginoplasty, 1216
   clitoral neoclitoris, 1220
   corpora cavernosa remnants, 1221
   corpus spongiosum, 1222
   diversion colitis, 1221
   dysuric problems, 1221
   excessive mucus production, 1221
   granulation tissue, 1221
   hair growth inside the neovagina, 1221
   intraoperative bleeding, 1220
   introitus stenosis, 1222
   laparoscopic mobilization, 1218
   meatal stenosis, 1222
   neovaginal prolapse, 1221
   penile inversion, 1215, 1217
   perineal view, 1219
   peritoneal pull-through vaginoplasty, 1218
   poor cosmesis, 1220
   rectovaginal fistula, 1222
   scrotal skin graft, 1216
   sexual function, 1222
   skin necrosis, 1220
   urethral flap necrosis, 1220
   vaginal dilator, 1219
   vaginal stenosis, 1222
   wound dehiscence, 1220
   zero-depth vaginoplasty, 1219
Vaginoscopy, 285, 736, 765, 822, 843–846, 848
Validated questionnaire
   ideal properties of, 105
   PRO data, 100–104
Validity, 106–107
Valsalva leak point pressure (VLPP), 98, 327
Value of uterus (VALUS) instrument, 610
Vascular disorders, 921–922
Vascular injuries, 625, 873
Vascular surgery injuries, 1136
Vascular thromboembolic events (VTEs), 668
Vasculogenic FSD, 975, 976
Vault dehiscence, 612
Vecchietti procedure, 1194
   complications, 1195
   invagination phase, 1195
   laparoscopic, 1195
   outcomes, 1196
   transabdominal, 1194
Venous drainage of the vagina, 966
Ventral HerniaWorking Group (VHWG), 1080
Ventral mesh rectopexy, 1027
Vertical rectus abdominis myocutaneous (VRAM) flap, 1071, 1072, 1083–1085, 1087 1088
Vertical ureterotomy, 879
Vesical neck, 709

Index 1279

Vesicoenteric fistula, 190
Vesicoperineal dyssynergia, 348
Vesicoureteral reflux (VUR), 40, 170, 895–897, 903
Vesicovaginal fistula (VVF), 190, 678, 679, 681–687, 786, 787, 801, 830, 832, 1135, 1136, 1140
  aetiology, 787–788
  amniotic membrane, 776
  bladder layer closure, 747
  classification, 788
  classification systems, 762–764
  clinical evaluation, 788–792
  clinical presentation and evaluation, 763–766
  conservative management, 792
  conservative management options, 738–739
  cost for robotic sacrocolpopexy, 753
  diagnostic investigations, 735–737
  etiology and epidemiology, 733–734
  etiology and incidence, 762
  extravesical approach, 745–747
  gracilis flap, 774–775
  history, 734
  interposing tissue layer, 748–749
  laparoscopic and robotic approaches, 740
  Latzko technique, 771–772
  long-term sexual function, 754–755
  management, 791, 834
  Martius flap, 772–774
  minimally invasive approach, 800
  modified laparoscopic approaches, 750–751
  omental flap, 774
  outcomes, 793, 838
  palliative procedures, 801
  perineal loss, 682
  peritoneal flap, 774
  physical examination, 735, 765–766
  positioning and entry, 741–743
  post operative care, 800
  post-operative catheterization, 749–750
  post-operative management, 776–782
  pre-operative management, 766–767
  preoperative work up, 790–791
  primary closure, 688
  procedural approach, 836
  radiation-associated and complex VVF repair, 772–776
  radiation induced fistulae, 800–801
  recto-vaginal fistula, 683
  retrograde filling of the bladder, 748
  risk factors, 765
  robotic approach, 751–753
  spontaneous closure, 684
  surgical approach, 768
  surgical outcomes, 782
  surgical repair options, 739–740
  timing of repair, 737–738, 767–768
  transabdominal repair, 793–799
  transabdominal vs. transvaginal approach, 793
  transvaginal approaches, 768–771
  transvesical approach, 744
  urethra and bladder neck, 683
  urethrovesicovaginal fistula, 683
  urinary symptoms, 754
  vaginal closure, 748–749
  vaginal flap/flap-splitting technique, 768–771
  vaginal repair, 686
Vestibule, 968
VICTO®, 433
VICTO PLUS®, 433
Video-assisted fistula repair, 817
Videourodynamic studies (VUDS), 129, 281, 414, 464, 712
Visceral organs, 256
Visual analogue scale (VAS), 937
Visualization, 181
Vitamin B12 deficiency, 1119
Voiding, 170, 326, 329, 331
Voiding cystography, 304
Voiding cystourethrogram (VCUG), 38, 40, 765, 860, 896, 1138, 1150, 1157
Voiding diaries, 118, 120, 159
Voiding dysfunction after pelvic surgery
  after colorectal surgery, 295
  after radical hysterectomy, 285–288
  cystoscopy, 284
  endometriosis surgery, 293, 295
  history, 278
  pathophysiology of, 278
  pelvic organ prolapse (POP), 288–293
  physical examination, 279
  post void residual (PVR), 279, 280
  for stress urinary incontinence, 286–288
  urinalysis, 279
  urodynamics, 280–283
Voiding phase, 78
Vulva
  labia majora, 967
  labia minora, 967–968
  mons pubis, 967
  vestibule, 968
Vulvar and perineal defect, 1089
Vulvar atrophy, 917
Vulvar repair, 1087–1089

W
Waaldijk genitourinary fistula classification, 679
Waaldijk system, 763, 764
Williams' neovaginoplasty, 1196
  adrenaline infiltration, 1196
  complications, 1197
  horseshoe incision, 1196
  outcomes, 1197
  surgical technique, 1196
Wireless motility capsule, 1007
Women's quality of life, 396
Women's sexuality, 1177
World Professional Association for Transgender Health (WPATH), 1212
W-shaped ileal plate, 1110

X
Xenografts, 381–382
X-ray hysterosalpingography, 35

Y
Yang-Monti channel, 1076
Yang-Monti procedure, 1049
Yang-Monti technique, 852
Yoga, 231

Young-Dees-Leadbetter procedure, 720, 721
Youssef's syndrome, 682

Z
Zero-depth vaginoplasty, 1219, 1220
z-plasties, 1091
Zuidex™, 397